LANGUAGES AND LINGUISTICS

COMPREHENSIVE PERSPECTIVES ON SPEECH SOUND DEVELOPMENT AND DISORDERS

PATHWAYS FROM LINGUISTIC THEORY TO CLINICAL PRACTICE

LANGUAGES AND LINGUISTICS

Additional books in this series can be found on Nova's website under the Series tab.

Additional e-books in this series can be found on Nova's website under the e-book tab.

LANGUAGES AND LINGUISTICS

COMPREHENSIVE PERSPECTIVES ON SPEECH SOUND DEVELOPMENT AND DISORDERS

PATHWAYS FROM LINGUISTIC THEORY TO CLINICAL PRACTICE

BEATE PETER
AND
ANDREA A. N. MACLEOD
EDITORS

nova
publishers
New York

For permission to use material from this book please contact us:
Telephone 631-231-7269; Fax 631-231-8175
Web Site: http://www.novapublishers.com

LIBRARY OF CONGRESS CATALOGING-IN-PUBLICATION DATA

Comprehensive perspectives on speech sound development and disorders : pathways from linguistic theory to clinical practice / [edited by] Beate Peter (University of Washington, Seattle, WA), Andrea A.N. MacLeod (Universiti Laval, Quibec, Canada).
pages cm
Includes bibliographical references and index.
ISBN 978-1-62257-041-6 (hardcover)
1. Language disorders in children. 2. Speech disorders in children. 3. Child development. 4. Children--Language. 5. Language acquisition--Age factors. I. Peter, Beate, 1956- eidotr of compilation. II. MacLeod, Andrea Asenath Nora, editor of compilation.
RJ496.L35C656 2011
618.92'855--dc23

2012018490

Published by Nova Science Publishers, Inc. † New York

For Carol Stoel-Gammon

CONTENTS

PREFACE

From the first cry of a newborn to the science project presentation of a school-age child, the acquisition of speech is an astounding journey. How young children learn to express complex ideas with sequences of speech sounds has been the object of many studies and textbooks, and linguists have built theoretical models around the process of speech acquisition. For some children, the road to mature speech production is rougher than for others and they struggle with various aspects of speech production. To provide the best clinical intervention for them, speech-language pathologists need a thorough understanding of how speech develops typically, how to determine the presence and nature of a speech sound disorder, and how to design and implement treatment.

This innovative textbook offers comprehensive perspectives on speech sound development and disorders from leading experts in the field. Our authors begin with a historical overview of the field, outlining how studies of child speech have influenced various theoretical frameworks that have then found their way into clinical approaches toward remediation of disordered speech. They trace the increasing sophistication of speech production in typical children, following the trajectory from newborn cry to pre-speech vocalizations to the development of segmental and prosodic elements of speech. They present data from cross-linguistic studies and bilingual development and show how adults learn the sound system of a new language. Finally, they describe disordered speech development of various etiologies and provide clinical guidelines for diagnosis and treatment.

With its unique design, this book takes you through time, from the first studies of child speech development using paper and pencil all the way to contemporary techniques such as acoustic analyses and videofluoroscopy and an outlook on the future with promises of creating a catalog of genetic disorder etiologies. It takes you through the range of speech sound acquisition from typically developing children in English and other languages to the perplexing variety of disordered speech and its impact on a child's life. And finally, it takes you through the conceptual worlds of theoretical considerations all the way to the hands-on clinical experience of serving children with speech sound disorders.

This book is unusual not only in terms of the wide scope of topics covered but also because of its many other innovations for the benefit of students and instructors. Rather than merely reading about important features of speech development such as cooing, babble, or disordered speech, you can see and hear examples using the sound and video files that accompany this book. These files can be downloaded from:

www.nova-authors.com/___Encrypted/Book_LINKs/R.ID_8705__B.ID_1914.rar

and we refer to them with symbols in the text for easy reference. We provide practical examples of how to conduct a speech assessment, write an assessment report, design a treatment plan, and select activities for an actual treatment session. In the three appendices, we offer an overview of the International Phonetic Alphabet and its extension for use with clinical population, a systematic summary of phonological processes, and a tutorial on statistical properties of standardized tests and the interpretation of test results. For instructors, a full suite of lecture slides, one set for each chapter, is included and can be modified and individualized.

This book was written for individuals in training for a career in clinical linguistics, an audience comprised of undergraduate and graduate students who are preparing to become speech-language pathologists. We also hope that this text will serve practicing speech-language pathologists as a useful tool to bring their practice up to date with regards to the cutting edge advances in the study of speech sound development. The assumed level of expertise includes basic familiarity with phonetics, phonology, and introductory linguistics. Each chapter ends with a set of review questions to help readers self-assess their understanding of the material. We have also included suggested activities that can enhance the mastery of the materials and guide readers to interact with more complex or advanced facets of the chapter's topic.

Creating a book of such a wide scope and such technical innovation was an ambitious project in many ways. The exquisite expertise of our co-authors made it possible to achieve a cohesive and comprehensive coverage of the selected topics. The video and sound files were contributed by individuals who share our interest in the education of professionals in the field of speech sound development and disorders. The illustrations were created with great dedication and skill by Cara Peter. We are deeply grateful to our family members for their support and cheerleading.

Much of what we know about clinical linguistics, we learned from our doctoral mentor, Carol Stoel-Gammon, Ph.D., who inspired us with her profound insights, energy, and caring. We have been amazed at the range of expertise that Carol has inspired: eleven of our authors, contributing 18 chapters, have had the pleasure to study under her guidance. We have learned a great deal from reading, listening to, and editing this book and we hope that you will as well.

B.P and A.M.

AUTHORS' BIOGRAPHIES

Carol Stoel-Gammon, Ph.D.

Carol Stoel-Gammon is Professor Emerita in the Department of Speech and Hearing Sciences at the University of Washington, Seattle (USA) and an Adjunct Professor in the Department of Linguistics. After receiving an undergraduate degree in History of Art, she went on to study linguistics and was awarded Ph.D. in developmental psycholinguistics from Stanford University under the direction of Professor Charles Ferguson. She was the first research assistant appointed to the Stanford Child Phonology Project; as part of the project, she analyzed phonological acquisition in children acquiring Spanish, which was the topic of her doctoral dissertation.

Dr. Stoel-Gammon's research interests include the study of prelinguistic vocal development, speech and language development in early childhood, cross-linguistic studies of phonological development, and the identification and assessment of speech/language disorders in toddlers. After receiving her doctoral degree, she taught courses in phonology and language acquisition for two years at the State University of Campinas, in Brazil, and then at the University of Colorado, Boulder. She joined the faculty of the Department of Speech and Hearing Sciences at the University of Washington in 1984, has held summer teaching appointments at the University of Calgary and the University of Alberta, and was an Erskine Fellow at Canterbury University, Christchurch, New Zealand.

Dr. Stoel-Gammon is a co-author, with Carla Dunn, of the text *Normal and disordered phonology in children* (1985), a co-author, with Lesley Olswang, Truman Coggins, and Robert Carpenter, of *Assessing prelinguistic and early linguistic behaviors in developmentally young children* (1987), and a co-editor, with Charles Ferguson and Lise Menn of *Phonological development: Models, research, implications* (1992). She wishes to thank colleagues and former students who have contributed to this book.

Martin J. Ball, Ph.D.

Martin J. Ball is Hawthorne-Board of Regents' Support Fund Endowed Professor at the University of Louisiana at Lafayette, having previously held academic positions in Wales and Ireland. He is co-editor of the journal *Clinical Linguistics and Phonetics* (Taylor & Francis), and the *Journal of Interactional Research in Communication Disorders* (Equinox); and of the book series *Communication Disorders across Languages* (Multilingual Matters), and *Language and Speech Disorders* (Psychology Press). His main research interests include sociolinguistics, clinical phonetics and phonology, and the linguistics of Welsh. He is an honorary Fellow of the Royal College of Speech and Language Therapists, and a Fellow of the Royal Society of Arts. He recently received the award of 2012 Distinguished Professor from the University of Louisiana at Lafayette Alumni Foundation. Among his recent books are *Phonology for Communication Disorders* (co-authored with N. Müller and B. Rutter, Psychology Press, 2010), and *Assessing Grammar: The Languages of LARSP* (co-edited with D. Crystal and P. Fletcher, Multilingual Matters, 2012).

(Barbara) May Bernhardt, Ph.D., Registered SLP

(Barbara) May Bernhardt is a Full Professor in the School of Audiology and Speech Sciences at the University of British Columbia in Vancouver, British Columbia, Canada. She is also a registered speech-language pathologist (since 1972). Her areas of specialization in research, teaching and clinical practice are language development, assessment and intervention with a specific focus on phonology and phonetics. The majority of her research time has been in application of nonlinear phonology to phonological assessment and intervention, with a current international crosslinguistic project in 12 languages. Over the past decade she has also focused on ultrasound and electropalatography in speech intervention and early prediction of language impairment. She recently inaugurated the course "Approaches to audiology and speech-language pathology for people of FIrst Nations, Métis and Inuit heritage," the first of its kind in Canadian training programs. She would like to acknowledge the initial source of her interest in phonology, i.e., the Stanford child phonology group, in particular, Drs. Carol Stoel-Gammon, Mary-Louise Edwards and Carolyn Gilbert. She would also like to acknowledge her family for their inspirational love and support and her husband, Joseph Paul Stemberger, for his love, support and deep knowledge of phonology and phonetics.

Eugene H. Buder, Ph.D.

Eugene Buder is an Associate Professor in the School of Communication Sciences and Disorders at the University of Memphis. He was a co-investigator of an NIH-funded project, Bilingual Phonology and Literacy with D.K. Oller (PI) and L. Jarmulowicz (2005-2010), and is currently co-investigator on an NIH-funded project Vocal Exploration and Interaction in the Emergence of Speech with D.K. Oller (PI). Buder directs laboratories for Phonetics, Social Interaction, and Clinical Instrumentation, and teaches in the areas of Speech Science, Acoustic and Perceptual Phonetics, Phonetic Transcription, Clinical Instrumentation, and Digital Signal Processing for Speech and Hearing. He received his undergraduate degree from Harvard University in a special concentration comparing language and music, and obtained a masters degree in Education and Anthropology from the University of Alberta. Buder completed a Ph.D. at the University of Wisconsin-Madison with dual majors in Communication Arts and Communicative Disorders, and conducted post-doctoral studies with Carol Stoel-Gammon at the University of Washington. His longest term interest has been in the rhythmic coordination of speech behaviors in conversational interactions, and his studies have also included acoustic phonetic research on early child language, infant vocalizations, motor speech and voice disorders, and prosimian mother-infant communications.

Carol M. Ellis, Ph.D., CCC-SLP

Carol M. Ellis is an Assistant Professor at Eastern Illinois University. The focus of her research is on applied phonetics and phonology. Her major research interests include speech intelligibility of children with severe speech sound disorders and also speech/language skills of Head Start children. Her specialty areas include applied phonetics and phonology.

Kristina Findlay, B.A.

Kristina Findlay is a Master's in Experimental Medicine - Speech Language Pathology candidate at Université Laval, located in Québec, Québec. Having come to speech-language pathology and research studying after a career in the performing arts, she was fortunate to begin her second career at The Montreal Fluency Centre, supervised by Dr. Rosalee Shenker. Under Dr. Shenker's mentorship, she focused her research on treatment goal transference and best-practice treatment times in bilingual preschool age children with fluency disorders. After the completion of an undergraduate degree at McGill in psychology and linguistics, she moved to Québec and began her Master's in Experimental Medecine under the supervision of Dr. Andrea MacLeod. Concentrating on Québecois francophone and bilingual population, she studies the evolution of phonological representations during language development in preschool-age children

Amber Franklin, Ph.D. , CCC-SLP

Amber Franklin is an assistant professor in the Speech Pathology and Audiology department of Miami University in Ohio. She received her Ph.D. in Speech and Hearing Sciences in 2009 from the University of Washington in Seattle under the direction of Carol Stoel-Gammon. Dr. Franklin's research interests are documenting change in clinical approaches to accent modification; acoustic and articulatory phonetics; cross-language phonetics and phonology; child phonology; and social-cultural aspects of communication.

Daniela Evaristo dos Santos Galea, Ph.D.

Daniela Evaristo dos Santos Galea completed her doctorate in 2008 under the direction of Dr. Haydée Fiszbein Wertzner. In 2006, she spent a semester at the University of Washington in Dr. Carol Stoel-Gammon's laboratory. Her research interests incude typical and disordered phonological development among children who speak Brazilian-Portugese. She is currently works as a consultant for the Brazilian consultant company AFAE that specializes in speech-language and audiology services for schools, and clinicians.

Amy Glaspey, Ph.D., CCC-SLP

Amy Glaspey is Associate Professor in the Department Communicative Sciences and Disorders at the University of Montana. Dr. Glaspey's research interests include phonological disorders, dynamic assessment, and treatment efficacy in preschool-age children. She has developed a measure for assessing phonological change, the Glaspey Dynamic Assessment of Phonology, which she is currently field-testing. Dr. Glaspey received her doctoral degree in Speech and Hearing Sciences at the University of Washington and completed Master's degrees in Communication Disorders and Science, and Early Intervention/Early Childhood Special Education at the University of Oregon.

Megan M. Hodge, Ph.D., Registered SLP, SLP(C), CCC-SLP

Megan Hodge is a speech language pathologist and professor in the Department of Speech Pathology and Audiology at the University of Alberta. She received her B.Sc. in Speech Pathology and Audiology from the University of Alberta, M.Sc. in Speech and Hearing Sciences from the University of Arizona and Ph.D. in Communicative Disorders from the University of Wisconsin-Madison. She has taught graduate level courses in anatomy and physiology of the speech mechanism, speech science and motor speech disorders. Dr. Hodge currently heads the *Children's Speech Intelligibility, Research and Education Laboratory (CSPIRE)* at the University of Alberta. Her research interests include developmental aspects of normal and disordered speech perception and production, perceptual-acoustic correlates of speech intelligibility and linking theory with practice in evaluating and managing children with motor speech disorders.

Barbara Williams Hodson, Ph.D., CCC-SLP

Barbara Williams Hodson is a Professor at Wichita State University in Kansas. Her major teaching and research interests pertain to applied phonetics and phonology, metaphonology, and Spanish phonology. Her professional interests also include mentoring doctoral students.

Linda Jarmulowicz, Ph.D., CCC-SLP

Linda Jarmulowicz is an Associate Professor in the School of Communication Sciences and Disorders at the University of Memphis. She is the director of the Language Acquisition & Analysis Laboratory; was a co-investigor of an NIH-funded project, Phonology and Literacy in Early Bilinguals, with D.K. Oller (PI) and E.H. Buder (2005-2011); and is currently the director of a personnel preparation grant supported by the US Office of Special Education Programs, on training SLP and AuD students to work with interpreters to provide culturally and linguistically appropriate services (2010-2014). Dr. Jarmulowicz received her undergraduate degree in Linguistics and Psychology from the University of Massachusetts. At the City University of New York in New York City, she earned her M.A. in Speech-Language Pathology, and her Ph.D. in Speech and Hearing Sciences. She teaches courses in language development, language-learning disabilities, language disorders in children, and sociocultural bases of communication at the University of Memphis. Dr. Jarmulowicz's research is focused on the development of derivational morphology and linguistic rhythm, especially as they relate to literacy development, and on bilingual language and literacy development.

Margaret Kehoe, Ph.D.

Margaret Kehoe completed her dissertation at the University of Washington in 1995 under the direction of Carol Stoel-Gammon, Ph.D. The title of her dissertation was "An investigation of rhythmic processes in English-speaking children's word productions." Since then, she has conducted research on phonetic and phonological acquisition in English-, German-, Spanish- and French-speaking children as well as in bilingual populations. She currently lives in Geneva, Switzerland, where she teaches at the University of Geneva as well as works as a Speech-Language Pathologist with bilingual children.

Minjung Kim, Ph.D., CCC-SLP

Minjung Kim is an assistant professor in the Department of Human Communication, California State University - Fullerton and is a certified member of the American Speech-Language and Hearing Association. She completed her Ph.D. at the University of Washington under the supervision of Dr. Carol Stoel-Gammon. Her research interests include cross-linguistic and multilingual studies of speech sound development and disorders in children.

Andrea A.N. MacLeod, Ph.D., Registered SLP

Andrea MacLeod is a professor at Université de Montréal, a French-speaking university located in Montréal, Canada. She is a simultaneous bilingual who grew up speaking both English and French. She obtained a clinical master's degree in Communication Science from the University of Vermont. Her interest in phonology was sparked by Dr. Rebecca McCauley who supervised her master's thesis. To pursue her interest in phonology and bilingualism, she moved to Seattle to complete a Ph.D. at the University of Washington under the supervision of Dr. Carol Stoel-Gammon. She studies the acquisition of phonology among monolingual (English and French speakers) and bilingual children with and without speech sound disorders. Her research uses acoustic measures and IPA transcriptions to understand how children attain adult-like speech sound accuracy.

Rebecca J. McCauley, Ph.D. , CCC-SLP

Rebecca McCauley received a B.S. (Psychology) from Louisiana State University, and an M.A. (Social Sciences) and Ph.D. (Psychology: Cognition and Communication) from the University of Chicago. She completed postdoctoral training at the University of Arizona and Johns Hopkins University before joining the faculty at University of Vermont in 1986. During her 23-year tenure at UVM, she achieved the rank of Professor and served in several administrative capacities. In 2008, Rebecca joined The Ohio State University at the rank of Professor and since 2009 has served as chair of the Graduate Studies Committee. Her research/teaching interests focus on assessment and treatment of children's communication disorders, especially speech sound disorders. She has authored and co-edited numerous publications, including 6 books, and is director of the Children's Communications Laboratory. Rebecca holds the ASHA CCC-SLP, is an ASHA Fellow, a Board Recognized Specialist in Child Language, and a former associate editor of *AJSLP*.

Amy E. Meredith, Ph.D., CCC-SLP

Dr. Meredith is a Clinical Associate Professor at Washington State University in Spokane, WA. She received her Ph.D. from University of Washington and her MS in Speech and Hearing Sciences from the University of Arizona. She specializes in the areas of pediatric motor speech disorders and cleft palate. She has been researching childhood apraxia of speech (CAS) for sixteen years, has presented at international conferences on CAS, and has provided over fifty workshops in differential diagnosis and treatment of CAS. She is currently researching the integration of phonologic awareness skills in CAS.

D. Kimbrough Oller, Ph.D

D. Kimbrough Oller received his Ph.D. in Psycholinguistics from the University of Texas in 1971, and is currently Professor and Plough Chair of Excellence at The University of Memphis. He is an External Faculty Member at the Konrad Lorenz Institute for Evolution and Cognition Research, Altenberg, Austria, an affiliate of the Institute for Intelligent Systems at The University of Memphis, and a member of the Scientific Advisory Board of the LENA Research Foundation. Dr. Oller's research focuses on vocal development and acquisition of spoken language. In over 180 articles the work addresses infant vocalizations, early speech production, multilingualism, and evolution of language. His bilingualism research includes *Language and Literacy in Bilingual Children* (edited by D. K. Oller and R. E. Eilers), from Multilingual Matters (2002). His research in evolution and development of language includes The Emergence of the Speech Capacity (2000, Erlbaum), *The Evolution of Communication Systems: A Comparative Approach* (edited by D. K. Oller and U. Griebel, MIT Press, 2004) and in *Evolution of Communicative Flexibility: Complexity, Creativity, and Adaptability in Human and Animal Communication* (edited by D. K. Oller and U. Griebel, MIT Press, 2008). Oller's research has been funded since the 1970's by the National Institutes of Health.

Kiyoshi Otomo, Ph.D.

Kiyoshi Otomo is a professor at the Center for the Research and Support of Educational Practice of Tokyo Gakugei University in Japan, and is currently also serving as the principal of the Special School affiliated with the University, a school for children with intellectual disabilities. Kiyoshi Otomo has assumed an executive board member of the Japanese Association of Communication Disorders, the Japanese Association for the Study of Developmental Disabilities, and the Japan Society of Developmental Psychology, and is the editor in chief of the Japanese Journal of Communication Disorders. Prior to his current position, Kiyoshi Otomo worked at Tokyo Metropolitan Institute for Neurosciences, in which he conducted clinical research in neurogenic speech-language disorders. He received his M.A. in speech and hearing sciences from the University of Illinois, Urbana-Champaign, and Ph.D. in speech and hearing sciences from the University of Washington, where he studied under Carol Stoel-Gammon on early speech development. After obtaining a position at Tokyo Gakugei University in 1992, Kiyoshi Otomo has conducted research on speech-language development in Japanese. His research interests range from the developmental process in typically developing children to atypical processes in children with developmental disabilities. He has developed language assessment scales for young and school-age children learning Japanese as the first language.

Beate Peter, Ph.D., CCC-SLP

Beate Peter is Research Assistant Professor in the Department of Speech and Hearing Sciences at the University of Washington in Seattle. She holds a master's degree in Speech-Language Pathology and a Ph.D. degree in Speech and Hearing Sciences, both completed at the University of Washington under the direction of Carol Stoel-Gammon, Ph.D. Dr. Peter recently completed three years of postdoctoral training in medical and statistical genetics under the mentorship of Wendy Raskind, M.D., Ph.D., in the Division of Medical Genetics at the University of Washington, focusing on the genetics of dyslexia and neurogenic motor diseases. In addition to the Certificate of Clinical Competence, issued by the American Speech-Language-Hearing Association, she holds the Graduate Certificate in Statistical

Genetics, issued by the Department of Biostatistics at the University of Washington. Her research focuses on molecular and statistical genetics of communication disorders, where she identified the first familial speech sound disorder subtype and is applying cutting-edge methods to identify causal genes. Dr. Peter's clinical experience was gained in the public schools, where she was placed in elementary and high schools, and also in a private clinic for children with learning disabilities, where she primarily treated children with deficits in written language.

Karen E. Pollock, Ph.D., Registered SLP, CCC-SLP

Karen Pollock is a professor and chair of the Department of Speech Pathology and Audiology at the University of Alberta. She received a B.A. and M.A. in linguistics and a M.A in speech pathology from the University of Oregon and a PhD in speech-language pathology from Purdue University. Prior to joining the University of Alberta faculty she held academic positions at the University of Northern Iowa and the University of Memphis, where she taught courses in phonetics and children's speech sound disorders. She currently teaches a graduate course in children's phonological disorders and supervises graduate student research. Her research interests include vowel errors in children with phonological disorders, dialect variation and children's speech development, and speech-language development in children adopted internationally.

Alice E. Smith, Ph.D. , CCC-SLP

Dr. Smith specializes in evaluation and treatment of individuals with cleft lip/palate and craniofacial disorders. She received her Ph.D. in Speech Science from the University of Iowa in 1996, and her MA in Communication Sciences and Disorders from the University of Montana in 1987. Dr. Smith has given numerous presentations and workshops in the area of cleft palate. She has taught at The University of Iowa, The University of Arizona, Indiana University of Pennsylvania, and The University of Montana. She is a member of the Ethics Committee for the American Cleft Palate-Craniofacial Society. She is Chair of the Speech Council for Operation Smile International and has volunteered on numerous missions, primarily to Cambodia. She is director of the E&E Speech Education and Therapy Clinic in Phnom Penh, Cambodia where she trains Khmer staff to work with children with both delayed and cleft related speech and language disorders. She has two adopted children with cleft lip and palate.

Anna Sosa, Ph.D., CCC-SLP

Anna Sosa is Assistant Professor of Communication Sciences and Disorders at Northern Arizona University in Flagstaff, AZ, where she supervises graduate student clinicians in the university clinic and teaches courses in phonetics, phonological development and disorders, and communication disorders in infants and toddlers. She is director of the Child Language Lab and her research and clinical interests are focused in the area of pre-linguistic and early phonological development in infants and toddlers with typical and disordered language development, with a specific interest in the relationship between early lexical and phonological development. She received her Ph.D. in Speech and Hearing Sciences in 2008 from the University of Washington in Seattle. Prior to coming to NAU she served as a school-based Speech-Language Pathologist in Washington State.

Anne S. Warlaumont, Ph.D.

Anne S. Warlaumont received her B.A. from Cornell University with a major in Psychology and a concentration in Cognitive Science. She received her Ph.D. in Communication Sciences and Disorders with a certificate in Cognitive Science at the University of Memphis, funded by a U.S. Department of Energy Computational Science Graduate Fellowship. She is currently Acting Assistant Professor of Cognitive Science at the University of California, Merced. Anne's research interests focus on early vocal, speech, and language development, automated analysis of vocal signals, and neural network simulation. Her publications to date have addressed such topics as automated, data-driven analysis of prelinguistic infant vocalizations; neural network modeling of motor and sensorimotor processes in vocalization development; child-caregiver interaction dynamics in typically developing children and children with autism; the role of caregiver input in grammatical suffix acquisition in typical development, late-talking, and specific language impairment; and neural network modeling of brain dynamics in epilepsy.

Krisztina Zajdó, Ph.D.

Krisztina Zajdó, Ph.D., is the Head of the Department of Special Education/Speech-Language Pathology and Associate Professor of SLP at the University of West Hungary, Győr, Hungary. Her current research focuses on the acquisition of speech in monolingual children acquiring Hungarian. She is a native speaker of the Standard dialect of Hungarian. Following the completion of her master's degrees in linguistics and communication at Janus Pannonius University in Pécs, Hungary, she completed her doctoral dissertation on vowel acquisition in monolingual Hungarian-speaking children with Dr. Carol Stoel-Gammon as her adviser at the University of Washington, Seattle in 2002. As a postdoctoral reseracher at the University of Texas at Austin in 2003, she co-edited a book entitled *The Syllable in Speech Production: Perspectives on the Frame Content Theory* (2008; Taylor & Francis), with Dr. Barbara Davis as her mentor. Currently, she collaborates in a cross-linguistic research project headed by Dr. (Barbara) May Bernhardt of The University of British Columbia, Vancouver, B.C. Canada, focusing on speech acquisition in monolingual children from ten different language communities.

I. Background

In: Comprehensive Perspectives …
Editors: Beate Peter and Andrea A. N. MacLeod
ISBN: 978-1-62257-041-6

Chapter 1

CHILD PHONOLOGY, PHONOLOGICAL THEORIES, AND CLINICAL PHONOLOGY: REVIEWING THE HISTORY OF OUR FIELD

Carol Stoel-Gammon and (Barbara) May Bernhardt

INTRODUCTION

This chapter provides a brief overview of the emergence of two related fields of study: child phonology and clinical phonology. Its goal is to provide a framework for the chapters that appear in the book; thus it is not a comprehensive review of speech sound development and disorders. The authors have been active researchers in child phonology since the 1970s, at a time when child phonology and clinical phonology came to be recognized as integral parts of the larger fields of linguistics and speech-language pathology. The chapter has three main sections: a description of the emergence and early period of the study of child phonology; an overview of theories of phonological development; and a more detailed introduction to the field of clinical phonology.

CHILD PHONOLOGY

A Field in its Infancy

Compared to many areas of study, the fields of child phonology, theories of phonological development, and clinical phonology are relatively young, in part because they cross boundaries of more traditional fields, such as theoretical linguistics, cognition, biological foundations of speech and language, and cognitive-social aspects of speech and language. In the 20th century, two strands of research developed in parallel and were then intertwined. One strand was formed by educators and psychologists who were seeking to establish guidelines for speech sound development in children with typical development. Their research was typically based on investigations of large groups of children and looked only at the acquisition of phonemes. Findings yielded norms for the "age of acquisition" or "age of mastery" of each consonant of English; the best known of these studies, by Wellman and colleagues (1931) and Templin (1957), formed the basis for Sander's oft-cited chart (1972) of expected ages for phoneme acquisition, a chart which is still used today. The focus of these norming studies was very narrow: Templin's goal was to "describe the growth of articulation of speech sounds" from 3 to 8 years, whereas Wellman et al. wished to "determine the development" of the ability of children 2-6 years to correctly produce the sounds of the English.

Sidebar 1.1. Some Obsolete Terms Used to Describe Child Speech and Children with Speech Disorders, 1930s to 1960s

Defective articulation
Idiots and imbeciles
Infantile linguistics
Mentally deficient children
Mongoloid speech
Speech defective child
Speech defects

The norms were used to identify children who were not adhering to the "typical" timetable for the acquisition of the phonemes of English. Studies of children identified as having atypical speech development were described with labels that are very different from those of today (see Sidebar 1.1).

Prior to the 1960s, a second set of individuals was also interested in children's speech, from a very different perspective. The focus of this group was to document speech and language development in young children, often using diary studies of their own offspring; the early literature from this group includes the work of Humphreys (1880) and Hills (1914). The diarists were often trained in linguistics, and produced sophisticated and detailed transcriptions of their child's productions; see, for example, Velten (1943); Leopold (1949); Weir (1962); and, more recently, Waterson (1971); Smith (1973); and Labov and Labov (1978). These individuals adopted a variety of theoretical frameworks (see descriptions of theories below) to describe and analyze the data, with Velten testing Jakobson's theory (1941/1968), Waterson using the framework of prosodic phonology (Firth, 1948); and Smith creating "rules" based on Chomsky's framework of generative phonology (Chomsky and Halle, 1968). Within this group, there was no attempt to determine norms or establish order of acquisition. The focus was on *how* children acquired their phonology rather than on *what* they acquired.

Contributions of the Stanford Group

Charles Ferguson, head of Linguistics at Stanford University, played a key role in the emergence of the field of child language acquisition from a linguistically oriented perspective. In 1967, Ferguson offered a course on language acquisition, likely the first linguistically oriented course in the country. An important outcome of his classes was the

Stanford Child Language Research Forum (and the working paper series *Papers and Reports in Child Language Acquisition*), which attracted researchers and academics from around the world. Within the field of language acquisition, Ferguson's primary interest was phonological development and the field of child phonology is one his legacies; in 1968, he obtained a grant from the National Science Foundation to examine aspects of phonological development in English and other languages. The focus of the grant was to explore the core tenets of linguistic theory and their relationship to language acquisition, as noted in the following statement (from the 1967 proposal):

> It seems clear that any general linguistic theory which fails to account for the phenomena of language development is of very limited validity, and it is also clear that the processes of language development offer one of the most fruitful areas for experimental testing of general linguistic hypotheses.

The initial grant proposal was funded, as well as many subsequent proposals, and became known as the "Child Phonology Project" at Stanford University. Many graduate students, research associates, and affiliates with ties to the Child Phonology Project have contributed significantly to our knowledge of phonological development in children with typical and atypical phonological development. These include: Mary Louise Edwards, Carol Farwell, Olga Garnica, Carolyn Johnson, David Ingram, Marlys Macken, Lise Menn, and Marilyn Vihman. The authors of this chapter, Carol Stoel-Gammon and Barbara May Bernhardt, were active members of the Stanford Group. Investigations carried out by the Stanford Child Phonology Project included children from a variety of language backgrounds and used a variety of methodological approaches; the studies extended our understanding of acquisition beyond English, and provided a broader view of phonetic and phonological aspects of acquisition. Languages studied in the early years included Spanish, Japanese, and Swedish as well as English.

Ferguson was also a leader in bringing together individuals interested in child phonology; to this end he was instrumental in organizing two major conferences on the topic, resulting in two important books: *Child Phonology, vols 1 and 2*, published in 1980 (edited by Yeni-Komshian, Kavanagh, and Ferguson) and *Phonological Development: Models, Research, Implications* (edited by Ferguson, Menn, and Stoel-Gammon, 1992).

Major Issues in the Field of Child Phonology

We have learned much about phonological development and disorders since the 1960s, and have broadened the scope of questions and devised new and innovative ways of studying the acquisition of speech and language. In spite of significant advances in many areas, important questions remain unanswered. Three key issues are outlined below and discussed in chapters throughout this book.

Cognitive-Linguistic and Articulatory Aspects of Speech Acquisition

Acquiring the sound system of one's native language requires learning in two domains. First, children must become aware of the sounds and sound patterns of the ambient language; this domain is often referred to as the "cognitive-linguistic" aspect of acquisition. We now know that phonological learning begins in infancy; well before they are able to produce words, infants are capable of distinguishing segmental and prosodic features of their own language from those of other languages. Learning the sound system continues throughout childhood as vocabulary increases and literacy emerges. The second domain, "learning to talk", involves the actual production of words and sounds. Production patterns are linked to pre-speech vocalizations that occur in the first year of life. Over time, the child learns to perform the motor movements needed for the adult-like productions of the words of his language, including the fine phonetic details of place, manner and voicing, for instance the language-specific parameters of voice onset time (VOT) as described in the section on languages beyond English in this volume.

What we do not know much about, as of yet, are the relative contributions of learning in the two domains; we also know little about the interactions between the cognitive and motor aspects of phonological acquisition. One of the major questions for those who work in the area of speech sound disorders centers around the underlying causes of a disorder, and the role played by each of the domains described above. Chapter 15 on disorder subtypes discusses some disorder typologies that posit a differential role of more linguistic vs. more motor-based deficits in different disorder subtypes.

The Search for Universals

The question of "universal" aspects of phonological development, raised by Jakobson in the 1940s and by Ferguson in the 1960s, is still a topic of debate; researchers ask: Can we document patterns of acquisition that occur in all children regardless of the language they are learning? Can we find patterns that occur across all children learning the same language? Research to date has failed to identify a pattern that is truly without exception; there are, however, certain patterns (or tendencies) that have a high probability of occurrence although they are not without exception. These include "tendencies" related to the acquisition of sound classes and word shapes, such as: stop consonants are acquired before fricatives; glides are acquired before liquids; singleton consonants are acquired before consonant clusters; and voiceless unaspirated stops are acquired before stops with other types of voicing (e.g. prevoiced; voiceless aspirated). It has been argued that these "near-universal" patterns are likely associated with universal properties of the human articulatory and perceptual systems. The issue of universal patterns is described in detail in Chapter 9 about universal trends, and specific examples can be found in chapters 10, 11, and 12 on children acquiring French, Brazilian Portuguese, and Korean, respectively.

Although studies have provided some support for universal tendencies in phonological acquisition, they have also highlighted the presence of individual variation. A key paper by Ferguson and Farwell (1975) traced the early productions of three children, each taking different approaches in acquiring words and sounds. A major finding from their study was evidence that children (at least these three children) selected words for their early productive vocabulary based, in part, on the phonological characteristics of the adult form. Other researchers (e.g., Stoel-Gammon and Cooper, 1984; Vihman, 1996) reported the same types of individual differences in the process of acquisition. In light of the substantial variation across children, Ferguson and Macken (1981) proposed that "at least some linguistic universals…derive from the interaction of the learner and a patterned input" (p. 122). In other words, each child plays an active, constructive role in the acquisition process through experimentation and rule discovery based on input. This view of universals differs markedly from the more traditional view that common tendencies in phonetic and phonological learning stem primarily from a shared biological basis for speaking and hearing.

The Nature of Underlying Representations

In order to recognize and produce words, an individual must have some sort of stored representation that provides semantic, syntactic and phonological information for words in the "mental dictionary." These stored representations are referred to as "underlying representations" (URs). In terms of phonology, a UR must have acoustic and articulatory information that is needed for comprehending spoken input and for producing a recognizable form of the word. Word recognition involves the ability to extract and store auditory phonetic information and link it to meaning, whereas word production requires linking a stored form(or forms) with phonatory and articulatory details. Despite decades of discussion, there is little agreement about the number and nature of URs in children (or even in adults). Chomsky and Halle (1968) proposed that the phonological information in a UR was quite abstract, containing only the necessary (unpredictable) elements for production. Under this view, voiceless stops in word-initial position are not coded as aspirated because aspiration of voiceless stops is predictable for English.

In his discussion of URs in children, N. Smith (1973), among others, argued that there is a single UR for both recognition and production of words by young children, based on the adult spoken form. Others have claimed that there are two URs, an auditory representation for recognition of the adult word and an articulatory representation for production (see Menn and Matthei, 1992, for a discussion of two-lexicon models; see Beckman, Munson, and Edwards, 2007; Munson, Edwards, and Beckman, in press, for a different view of a two-lexicon model). In contrast to the single- or dual-entry models of URs, Sosa and Bybee (2008) propose a usage-based account of phonology in which representations are not fixed entities, but emerge "by generalizing over existing forms and extracting patterns of similarity" (p. 484). Within this perspective, a single word may have multiple representations.

A major difficulty in determining the form and nature of URs can be seen in the differences between very young children's ability to detect wo d mispronunciations and their ability to produce words that resemble the adult form. Investigations in the past decade (e.g., Bailey and Plunkett, 2002; Ballem and Plunkett, 2005; Mani and Plunkett, 2007; White and Morgan, 2008) have shown that infants can detect mispronunciations of both vowels and consonants by 14-15 months of age, an age at which the lexicon is very small, and infant productions tend to differ markedly from the adult target forms. Given these findings, the question of URs, and particularly the relationship between representations for perception/comprehension and production, remains open.

The Evolution of Research Methodology

Since the first studies of children's speech, there have been major changes in the databases used for research and the approaches used to analyze the data. The earliest studies were based on data collected from longitudinal studies of individual children or cross-sectional studies of groups of children. Today, a wide variety of data is available to researchers in child phonology. Similarly, the recording of data has changed. Whereas the first studies were based mostly on transcriptions of children's speech done live or from memory, researchers have since moved towards analogue and then digital recordings of speech samples. These recordings can be transcribed and verified for their reliability, and analyzed with acoustic software. Researchers have also studied articulatory movements using kinematography, electropalatography, and ultrasound recordings.

The Databases

As noted above, the earliest studies of phonological development were based on two very different approaches: the large-group investigations by Wellman et al. (1931) and Templin (1957) used cross-sectional data collected from cohorts of children at particular ages; the productions undergoing analysis were typically single-word responses to a set of pictures. In contrast, the early diary studies were based on a single child whose development was followed over time (i.e., longitudinally). The parent observed and transcribed the child's spontaneous productions with no attempt to elicit particular words or sounds. With the advent of linguistic-based investigations, researchers gathered speech samples from small groups of children, using either unstructured or semi-structured approaches to data collection.

At present, a wide range of methods for data collection are used, from single subjects to large groups, and from cross-sectional to longitudinal time frames. In addition, the focus of the research has evolved such that some studies focus on very specific phonetic details (e.g., error patterns of voiceless fricatives, or acoustic features of primary stress), whereas others examine the broader aspects of development (e.g. interactions between phonology and the lexicon, or the relationship between the sounds of babble and the phonology of early words).

One remarkable source of data for current research involves speech samples from the *Child Language Data Exchange System* (CHILDES), a corpus established in 1984 by Brian MacWhinney and Catherine Snow to serve as a central repository for data on first language acquisition (MacWhinney, 2007). The CHILDES database contains transcripts and media data (audio and video) collected from conversations between young children and their playmates and caretakers; the database includes samples from over 20 languages from 130 different corpora (see "PhonBank" in *http://childes.psy.cmu.edu/data/*) and contains many samples from children with speech disorders.

Analyses

The methods used in the analysis of child speech samples vary with the goals of the study. For many years, the most common first step was a phonetic transcription of words in the sample. For diary studies, the transcription was typically done "on-line -- the parent simply listened to the child and transcribed the utterances, without recording them. For more controlled studies, such as those of the Stanford Child Phonology Project, the speech was recorded and then phonetically transcribed. This approach allowed the transcriber to listen to an utterance multiple times, and also allowed more than one individual to make a transcription of the recorded sample.

Prior to the appearance of linguistically based approaches to the study of phonological acquisition, most analyses focused on accuracy. In the norming studies of Wellman et al. (1934) and Templin (1957), for example, the goal was to determine the production accuracy (and age of acquisition) of each phoneme. If a phoneme was produced incorrectly, the error was noted. Thus, an analysis of the productions of a three-year-old child might list the following substitutions:

1) The phoneme /s/ was produced as [t];
2) The phoneme /z/ was produced as [d];
3) The phoneme /f/ was produced as [p]; and
4) The phoneme /v/ was produced as [b].

If we adopt an approach based on phonetic features, rather than single phonemes, the same set errors would be described more simply: target fricatives are produced as stops.

Descriptions of substitutions as *error patterns* affecting classes of phonemes, rather than individual phonemes, brought a major change to our understanding of the nature of speech sound development in young children. It also provided a basis for treating speech disorders, as it more efficient to treat a class of sounds (e.g., fricatives) than to treat individual phonemes (see the discussion of pattern-based approaches in Chapter 22 on treatment design and implementation). A landmark book introducing a linguistic approach to the study of speech development and disorders appeared in 1976: David Ingram's *Phonological Disability in Children.*

This book described error patterns as phonological processes (see theory section below), encompassing several types of errors: substitution of one sound class for another (e.g., fricatives produced as stops; liquids produced as glides); changes in the overall "shape" of a word (e.g., deletion of final consonants; omission of unstressed syllables); and assimilations (e.g., productions in which two consonants become more similar to one another; e.g., non-labial consonants are produced labials when another labial occurs in the word). Phonological processes are described in more detail in Chapter 2 on describing and measuring children's speech abilities, and Chapter 6 on speech development in toddlers, preschoolers, and school-age children; a summary of processes is provided in Appendix 2.

Although phonetic transcription remains the most common first step in the analysis of child speech, additional types of analysis are now available and provide new and exciting ways to examine productions. Acoustic analyses are widely used, sometimes on their own, sometimes to complement phonetic transcription. Acoustic measures are particularly useful in cases in which phonetic transcription is unable to capture some of the nuances in production (e.g., measures of voice onset time or of fundamental frequency). Finally, new technologies, such as ultrasound and electropalatography, provide information that was previously unavailable. See Chapter 2 for a detailed overview of various tools currently used by clinicians and researchers to describe and measure children's speech abilities.

As the field of child phonology received increased attention from linguists and phonologists, a wide range of theories of development were proposed. Each proposal focused on a particular aspect of development and, in most cases, the proposals were derived from phonological theories associated with adult languages. The major theories are described below.

THEORIES OF PHONOLOGICAL DEVELOPMENT: A BRIEF OVERVIEW

Requirements of a Theory

The first publication to seriously address the topic of requirements for a theory of phonological development was authored by Ferguson and Garnica (1975), who worked together at Stanford. Ten years later, the topic was discussed in a text by Stoel-Gammon and Dunn (1985) and then again by Bernhardt and Stemberger (1998), nearly 25 years after the original article. In spite of the extensive time span during which the field of phonological development underwent major changes, views of an adequate theory across the three publications were quite similar, encompassing the tenets described below.

First, a theory of phonological development must account for the facts of both adult and child phonology; for child phonology, it must address not only general patterns of development, but also individual differences across children and variability in word and sound production within a single child. Second, the theory must address relationships between prelinguistic and linguistic development, between perception and production, and acquisition and input. Third, the theory must account for both phonetic (i.e., articulatory) and phonological learning. Finally, it must be compatible with general theories of learning and, as with any well-formed theory, must make testable predictions regarding acquisition. Each of the major theories are summarized below meets some of these requirements but none meets all of them. The second part of this chapter shows how these theories were translated into the clinical field; Chapter 22, on treatment design and implementation, annotates the various approaches by referring back to their theoretical roots.

Theories Associated with Linguistic Analyses of Adult Phonological Systems

In searching for a theory to account for phonological development, researchers have turned towards theories developed to describe adult phonologies. These theories include structural theory, rule and process-based theories, non-linear theories, optimality theory and usage-based theory. Each of these has strengths and weaknesses when applied to the study of child phonology.

Structural Theory

One of the earliest linguistically based theories of phonological acquisition stemmed from the linguist Roman Jakobson (1941/1968) who was a leading figure in the structuralist approach to phonology of the Prague School (Trubetzkoy, 1939). In his 1941 monograph (English translation: 1968), Jakobson proposed that, regardless of the linguistic environment in which they live, children adhere to a universal order of acquisition of phonemic contrasts based on structural principles and implicational hierarchies documented in the phonemic inventories of adult languages. Jakobson not only identified the order of acquisition, but also predicted the types of errors that would occur (e.g., when in error, velar consonants would be produced as alveolars and fricatives as stops). In spite of abundant evidence of individual variability, general patterns of acquisition, across children and across languages, are well documented (e.g., Stokes, Klee, Carson, and Carson, 2005). You can read more about this theory as it has been applied to the cross-linguistic study of child phonology in Chapter 9.

Rule- and Process-Based Theories

In the late 1960's two theories appeared, both proposing that children are born with innate abilities that provide them with the underpinnings needed to acquire language. These were Chomsky and Halle's *generative* phonology and Stampe's *natural* phonology. With the publication of *The sound pattern of English* (Chomsky and Halle, 1968), generative approaches to phonological theory became central to studies of adult phonology. In adult speakers, word productions result from the application of a set of phonological "rules" to abstract underlying forms. In child learners, a basic tenet of generative linguistics is that language acquisition stems from "an innate mental endowment" that allows children to discover the structure of their language with relatively little data from the adult language. In studying children's productions, researchers applied Chomsky's principles and created a set of rules that revealed the nature of differences between the adult pronunciations and the child's (mis-) pronunciations.

Around the same time as the rise of generative phonology, the linguist/phonologist David Stampe proposed a theory of "natural" phonology based on a set of universal and innate "**phonological processes**" that applied to adult and child speech (Donegan and Stampe, 1979; Stampe, 1969). In order to acquire an adult-like phonology, children must learn to suppress, limit, and reorder the processes in accordance with the phonology of their native language. The basic thesis of natural phonology is that phonological systems of both adults and children are influenced by patterns of production and perception. In some cases, phonological processes are in conflict (Stampe, 1969); for example, obstruent consonants tend to be voiceless because they require a strong airflow, and voicing claims much of the outgoing airflow at the level of the vocal folds. When an obstruent consonant occurs between vowels, however, it is easier to keep the vocal folds adducted rather than briefly abduct them, and thus the obstruent ends up being voiced in this environment. These two constraints create a conflict in how to produce the obstruent, with or without voicing. To solve the conflict, one of the two processes can be suppressed, the processes can be limited to a set of contexts, or the processes can be ordered into a hierarchy. Languages differ in the solution that they have adopted.

Stampe's theory continues to be influential as phonological processes are still used to describe the systematic errors observed in typical development and in children with disordered phonological development. Chapter 6 on toddlers and preschoolers provides a more detailed description of these types of errors.

Nonlinear Theories

In the 1970s, there was a shift in phonological theories from linear, segment-based perspectives to nonlinear, hierarchical approaches in which phonological representations were described not as strings of **segments**, but as a hierarchy of phonological "levels", each containing a different type of information (for example, Goldsmith's autosegmental theory, first articulated in his 1976 dissertation; see Goldsmith, 1990). These models include levels of the phrase and **prosodic word**, moving down to the levels of **foot** and **syllable structure**, and then to a hierarchy of features subsumed under the **root node** (also see Bernhardt and Stoel Gammon, 1994; and Bernhardt and Stemberger, 1998, for overviews). Figure 1.1 illustrates the levels from the word to the segments. The hierarchy of features specifies the segments in terms of consonant/vowel, continuancy, nasality, voicing, and place of articulation.

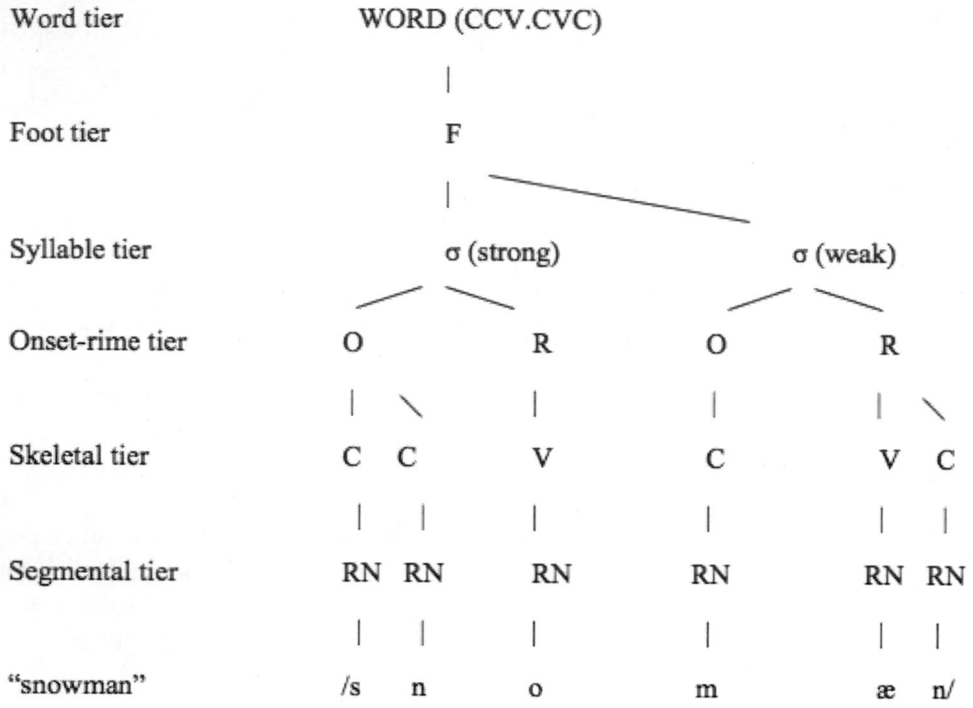

Note: F = foot, σ = syllable, O = onset, R = rime, RN = root node.

Figure 1.1. The word "snowman" from the word tier to the segmental tier.

Optimality Theory

Optimality theory (Prince and Smolensky, 2004; see also Dinnsen and Gierut, 2008) is a "constraint-based" approach that has been applied to the study of phonological development and disorders in recent years. The premise of this approach is that there is a universal set of conflicting "constraints" of two basic types: output constraints, which are based on articulatory and perceptual abilities, and dictate that the output should be minimally costly to the speaker; and faithfulness constraints, which dictate that the output should be as similar to the adult form as possible and thus require a match between the input and output.

Phonological acquisition is viewed as a process of ranking and re-ranking constraints to conform to the constraint patterns of the ambient language (see Bernhardt and Stemberger, 1998, 2008). For example, if a child is first unable to produce word-final consonants (codas), we could say that the markedness constraint Not(Coda) is higher-ranked than faithfulness constraints which ensure the production of a segment, as described in the following notation: Not (Coda) >> Survived (Consonant) or Faith (Consonant). As the child becomes capable of producing codas, Survived (Consonant) and Not (Coda) may be in competition for a while, sometimes one "winning" and sometimes the other. At the end of the developmental process, a final re-ranking is solidified, with Survived (faithfulness) ranked above Not (markedness). However, in rapid speech or different registers, the codas may still be suppressed. Thus, the ranking may never completely solidify.

Usage-Based Theory

A relatively new linguistic theory, "usage-based linguistics" (Kemmer and Barlow, 2000), assumes a close relationship between language use and language structure, with structure seen as both a generator and a product of language use. With specific reference to phonological acquisition, a usage-based approach highlights the roles of language input and use in the instantiation and ongoing modification of the child's phonological system (Bybee, 2001). From this perspective, phonology is not acquired independently of other aspects of grammar, but is intimately linked to the individual words that are present in the lexicon and to the usage characteristics of those words. For more information about the first words period, see Chapter 5 on the transition from babble to first words.

Biological and Cognitive Theories

In addition to theories associated with linguistic analyses of adult phonology, biological and cognitive theories have been proposed to account for phonological development. These theories draw on general biological or cognitive principles and apply them to understanding how a child acquires his speech sound system.

Biological Models

In contrast to the theories summarized above which are based on linguistic theory associated with adult languages, Kent (1992) proposed a theory of early speech development which emphasizes the importance of general principles of developmental biology and the role of anatomical and motor development. In this model, audition and speech motor functions are viewed as genetically determined. Early productions are limited by motor ability, especially by the inability to move the tongue in a precise manner. Kent describes the production of early words as holistic "motor scores" that become more reliable as coordination improves (see Browman and Goldstein, 1992). Productions are rooted in the developing precision of motor performance; over time, a phonemic system emerges through mappings between sensory and motor routines. According to this view, phonological development is "a process in which the child progressively applies available resources in attempting to emulate the mature behavior" rather than "a process in which the child simplifies a fully comprehended version of the mature behavior" (Kent, 1992, p. 85).

Cognitive Theories

Cognitive theories (often referred to as "child centered" theories) arose from the realization that the facts of child phonology, having been tested against the existing linguistic theories, necessitated a more radical departure from adult theory in which child phonology is addressed on its own terms, rather than in relation to the adult system. One of the basic principles of the cognitive theory of phonological development is that children play an *active role* in acquiring the phonology of their language: they choose words to include their productive vocabularies based on their own articulatory abilities; and then formulate, test, and revise hypotheses regarding phonology based on linguistic experience (Menn, 1980; 1983). This theory pays explicit attention to individual patterns of acquisition that are most evident in very earliest stages of development and to the relationship between lexical and phonological acquisition (see Ferguson and Farwell, 1975, for an example).

Appraising the Theories

In summary, it is clear from the above that no one theory of phonological development meets the "requirements of a theory" set out in the in the introduction to this section. Rather, each theory focuses on a specific aspect of development: order of acquisition; nature of errors; individual differences; biological constraints. While each theory has merit on its own, we are still lacking a comprehensive theory or model that integrates across the various domains involved in phonological acquisition. The same problem is apparent when we consider the field of clinical phonology, as described in the following sections.

CLINICAL PHONOLOGY

Introduction to Clinical Phonology

While theories and approaches to investigating child phonology were changing and developing (as sketched above), the discipline of speech-language pathology was also developing, particularly in English-dominant countries. The theories and approaches to describing developmental phonology began to be applied in clinical phonology, following the trends, but usually at a distance of some years or decades. The following discussion provides an outline of the clinical enterprise in child phonology, relating approaches to theories as applicable.

The clinical enterprise concerning child phonology includes the identification, assessment, and treatment of speech difficulties. Speech difficulties in children may primarily concern speech production or be related to other developmental (e.g., general language or cognitive delay) or anatomical or physiological conditions (e.g., motor impairment, hearing loss, cleft palate). The chapters on special populations in this volume address some of these conditions. At each step in the clinical enterprise, the speech-language pathologist (SLP) brings knowledge, skills and evidence to bear, either consciously or unconsciously, on the decision-making process. This decision-making process invokes information and procedures from other more theoretically oriented disciplines, especially linguistics, psychology, education, and health sciences concerning the human body. Overall, the clinical process is essentially based on the scientific method, where aims of assessment or treatment are defined;, methods chosen;, and results observed, analyzed, and interpreted in accordance with the clinician's underlying assumptions, theories, or models. Tools used to describe and measure children's speech abilities are described in Chapter 2, and how these tools are selected and used to generate a clinical profile is the focus of Chapter 20 on the diagnostic process.

Phonological theories in linguistics have provided a rich basis for description, assessment, and treatment of children's speech patterns, from more structural bases early on to more current constraint-based, nonlinear approaches. The linguistic sub-discipline of phonetics has also provided constructs concerning human speech production, with systems for phonetic transcription and different types of objective measures (i.e., acoustic analysis and articulatory analyses). For example, articulatory analyses can be done to study tongue-palate contact patterns using electropalatography; tongue configurations and movement patterns using X-ray, ultrasound, or electromagnetic articulography; nasalance using a nasometer, nasoendoscopy, or videofluoroscopy; and respiratory and vocal characteristics using a respirometer, laryngoscope, or stroboscope.

Clinical phonology has also drawn on constructs and approaches from psychology, including the following areas:

1. Development (e.g., behaviorism, cognitive-interactionist theories, usage-based theories;
2. Information processing (e.g., connectionist theories, dynamic systems models);
3. Perception, memory and attention;
4. Social interaction;
5. Brain and behavior;
6. Assessment tool construction (issues of sampling, reliability and validity); and
7. Treatment methods concerning human conditions (e.g., counseling, interactional methods, evaluation of efficacy).

Other sciences have also provided constructs, theories and evidence concerning perceptual and motor systems (e.g., biology, anatomy, and physiology, as described in Chapter 3 of this volume), brain development and function (neuroscience), computerized methods for data collection, analysis and treatment, and approaches to health and human functioning (International Classification of Function, ICF, World Health Organization, 2001). The degree to which any of the constructs and approaches are invoked in the clinical enterprise will depend on the SLP's knowledge concerning these constructs and approaches, and the individual client being served. Both the student and practicing SLP will find information in this volume to enhance his or her knowledge of clinical phonology.

Clinical Assessment and Selection of Treatment Goals

As noted above, two major aspects of the clinical enterprise concerning child phonology include the identification and assessment of speech difficulties (with identification a sub-component of assessment). There are two factors of paramount importance concerning identification:

1. How the client's speech performance matches those of peers (chronological age or developmental stage); and
2. Possibly most important, whether the client or client's family/community believes there is a problem. In both cases, the SLP takes what is known about developmental norms into account, both to provide information to the client/family/community, and where called-on, to make decisions about the need for treatment (and in some cases, the goals of treatment, given a developmental perspective, e.g., Rvachew and Nowak, 2001, as discussed further below). Reflecting the importance of knowledge concerning phonological development, two major sections of the book (II and III) provide current information on this topic, both for English and other languages, including the bilingual context.

Phonological development studies generally focus on speech production (output) but also on other related aspects of development (perception, phonological awareness and literacy).

The following section highlights major assessment considerations, first for speech production, and secondly for the other related aspects. These are further elaborated in Section V of this volume.

Speech Sample Collection

Generally, a client with a developmental age of less than 3 years of age does not sit for very long to name a set of pictures and/or objects for speech elicitation. The SLP may thus engage a familiar caregiver to interact with the child in a short play session (15-25 minutes), using strategic objects that are designed to elicit both "early-developing" speech sounds (labials, coronals, stops, nasals, glides) across word positions in CV, CVC and CVCV contexts; and some "later-developing" speech sounds and structures (because a chronological mismatch has been noted for children with speech difficulties; Grunwell, 1985). The adult may encourage both spontaneous and imitated productions in as natural a way as possible. The adult may also repeat what she or he believes the child has said, in order to facilitate later transcription. On-line transcription may be possible if the output is limited and simple. Optimally, video and high quality audio signals will be used to capture the babbling sequences and words used, with transcription done by the SLP after the fact, and confirmed with the caregiver. Analysis of the sample will take into account both the child's inventories (e.g., structures of words, speech sounds, features) and comparisons with the adult targets (i.e., relational analyses that includes process or substitution/deletion analyses). Comparison with developmental studies (e.g. Stoel-Gammon, 1991; see the chapter on diagnostic guidelines in this volume) will provide a basis for decision-making on the need for further assessment or treatment.

If a client is developmentally capable of sitting through a standardized speech assessment (articulation or phonology test) there are many options available for English, with fewer for other languages (although this is changing). Two main facts are important to consider when selecting an elicitation tool. First, are developmental norms needed, and if so, does the test have good psychometric properties in terms of items, sampling, and reliability that are relevant and appropriate for the client's cultural and dialectal group (Ball, Bernhardt, and Deby, 2006; McCauley and Swisher, 1984)? Second, does the tool adequately sample the phonology of the language by including not just consonants across word positions, but also vowels, stress and tonal patterns and word shapes in terms of CV sequences (Bernhardt and Holdgrafer, 2001a, b; Bernhardt and Stemberger, 2000)? In addition, Dodd and colleagues suggest that it is important to consider a child's relative consistency in production and that the sampling tool needs to elicit at least a portion of the words multiple times (e.g., Dodd, Holm, Crosbie and McIntosh, 2010). Finally, efficiency may also be a consideration, but efficiency can be viewed in the short-term or long-term: a valid and reliable assessment, even if relatively "long", leads to a well-constructed intervention plan, which will increase treatment efficiency.

Sometimes, a client will have only one speech sound or speech sound group that is not developing as expected. Sibilants or rhotics may be in this category, traditionally the latest-developing speech sounds. Modern technologies (e.g., EPG, ultrasound) are enhancing the assessment of such complex speech sounds in the clinical context (Adler-Bock et al., 2007; Bacsfalvi, 2011; Bernhardt et al., 2005a, b; 2008; Gibbon and Wood, 2010). With images of tongue-palate contacts, or tongue configurations, SLPs are able to better define a client's particular speech difficulties than with transcription or acoustic analysis.

Analysis and Goal-Setting

Once a speech sample is transcribed, in the optimal conditions, the level of analysis needed will reflect the severity of difficulty. The analysis may involve an observation of EPG values, ultrasound image tracings or acoustics, manual calculations (most phonological process and segment-based tests), or scans of the data (Bernhardt and Stemberger, 2000), or more recently, computerized counts of various parameters. See Sidebar 1.2 for examples of computer programs designed for various aspects of speech analysis.

If it is determined that treatment is relevant for the child and wanted by his or her family, the clinician has a number of options to choose from in terms of analysis and goal-setting. The influence of linguistic theories can be seen in this aspect of the clinical enterprise. The theories that appear to have most influenced analysis and goal-setting are structuralist theories, with their focus on single consonants (Van Riper, 1939, 1978) on the one hand, and phonological process or rule-based theories on the other (focusing on general patterns comparing the child's forms with the adult targets, e.g., Dinnsen and Elbert, 1984; Gierut, 1998; Grunwell, 1985; Hodson, 2007; Ingram, 1976, to name a few). In the past two decades, nonlinear phonology and constraint-based theories (Optimality theory) have also been applied, in an expansion and revision of the pattern-based theories of the 1970s (Bernhardt, 1990, 1992a, b, 1994a, b; Bernhardt and Major, 2005; Bernhardt and Stemberger, 2000; Dinnsen and Gierut, 2008; Major and Bernhardt, 1998).

Sidebar 1.2. Selected Computer Programs for Speech Analysis

CAPES ®, Computerized Articulation and Phonology Evaluation System (Masterson and Bernhardt, 2001): *http://www.pearsonassessments.com/HAIWEB/Cultures/en-us/Productdetail.htm?Pid=0158123999andMode=summary.*

LIPP, Logical International Phonetics Program (Oller and Delgado, 1999): *http://www.ihsys.com/site/LIPP.asp?tab=4.*

PHON (Rose and Hedlund, 2011): *http://childes.psy.cmu.edu/phon/.*

PROPH, Profile in Phonology (Long, 2011): www.computerizedprofiling.org.

Phoneme Factory Phonology Screener (Wren, Hughes, and Roulstone, 2006): *http://www.gl-assessment.co.uk/health_and_psychology/resources/phoneme_factory/phoneme_factory.asp.*

When a child produces very few speech sounds that are in error, a segment-based analysis may be sufficient; however, even a single speech sound is complex in its articulatory and acoustic properties. Thus, additional analyses may need to be considered including electropalatography or ultrasound to identify the tongue root, body and tip configurations, or acoustic analyses to identify formants above the second formant (Adler-Bock et al., 2007) for an English /ɹ/. Furthermore, no speech sound occurs in isolation. Thus, the analysis also needs to evaluate the target speech sound(s) in various contexts by phrase, word lengths and stress patterns, word position and other nearby consonants or vowels. Some contexts may show closer approximations to the target than others, affecting the choice and order of treatment items (see below).

When a child produces many speech sounds in error, a segmental analysis is insufficient. Although there have been few randomized control trials in speech therapy, studies suggest that for clients with more significant speech difficulties, a sound-by-sound approach to goal-setting (and consequently treatment) is less efficient than one that addresses patterns, whether based on theories utilizing processes or generative rules (Almost and Rosenbaum, 1998; Gierut, 1998; Hodson, 2004, 2007) or more recently, nonlinear phonology or constraint-based theories (see references above). By targeting broad patterns, a more extensive and rapid generalization across phonemes tends to occur than when working segment by segment. Nonlinear phonology theories show that the phonological system has a hierarchical structure and can be divided into two major components: word structures (phrases, words, syllables, onset-rime, timing units) versus segments (consonants and vowels, with hierarchically organized sets of manner, place and laryngeal features). A systematic analysis of the entire phonological system from the phrase to the feature (as in Bernhardt and Stoel-Gammon, 1994; Bernhardt and Stemberger, 2000; Bernhardt et al., 2010a, b, c, d; Bernhardt and Zhao, 2010) provides a perspective both on the child's developmental needs at various levels of the phonological system, and also on his or her developmental strengths.

For these children, goal selection will optimally target the two broad areas (word structures; segments). It is not yet clear whether the actual targets selected should be developmentally earlier or later, with work by Rvachew and Nowak (2001) and Rvachew and Bernhardt (2010) suggesting that it may be more efficient to target developmentally earlier structures and speech sounds, and work by Gierut (1998) and others (Barlow and Gierut, 1999, 2002; the Learnability Project, *www.indiana.edu/~sndlrng*) suggesting that faster system-wide gains occur when more challenging, marked (later-developing) targets are chosen. Other factors also affect goal selection, as seen in the next section.

Assessment of Related Factors: Contextualizing the Phonology

Children's speech perception skills are also a key part of their abilities in speech production. It is well known that the majority of people with severe hearing impairment will require amplification (hearing aids; cochlear implants) and, usually, speech intervention to become intelligible speakers. Thus, a hearing assessment is always considered an essential part of the phonological evaluation. But even children with intact hearing may have perceptual difficulties. Rvachew and colleagues have shown that assessing and targeting perceptual speech contrasts has a significant and positive impact on intervention outcomes (e.g., Rvachew et al., 1999; Shiller et al., 2010). Furthermore, this impact extends to phonological awareness and literacy (Rvachew et al., 1999). Thus, current evidence suggests the inclusion of speech perception tasks into the assessment and goal setting for children at intermediate and later phases of development.

There is also a rich amount of literature on infant and toddler speech perception in several laboratories (e.g., Juczyk, 2003; Kuhl, 2009; Swingley, 2003; Werker and Stager, 1997). This research suggests that children's early perceptual abilities are linked to later language development (Bernhardt et al., 2007; Werker, Fennel, Corcoran and Stager, 2002). Thus, for children at the early-word stage who require intervention, it may be useful to consider the development of play-based perceptual tasks. These play-based tasks are similar to audiology testing paradigms and require a child to notice the difference by eye gaze, head turn or some other more active means (screen selection) between two items contrasting in some relevant phonological aspect: coda/no coda; cluster/singleton; dorsal/coronal; stop/fricative, etc.

Further to the internal organization of phonology, it has become important for children of 4 years and older to include assessments of their developing phonological awareness skills (segmentation, rhyming, alliteration), because these have been linked to literacy (see Chapter 16 on dyslexia in this volume). Goal selection may also include the incorporation of phonological awareness goals. Bernhardt and Major (2005) note that children in their study who benefited from early phonological awareness training as preschoolers outperformed children who did not, in terms of reading and spelling skills in early grades.

Suprasegmental aspects of a child's speech production can be the focus of assessment as well as treatment. The Prosody-Voice Screening Profile (Shriberg, Kwiatkowski and Rasmussen, 1990) provides a systematic framework for assessing aspects related to prosody and voice production. The development of prosody is the focus of Chapter 7 in this volume.

Links to motor development and biology provide a foundation for oral-motor assessments. The structural integrity of the oral mechanism and the functional characteristics, in terms of articulator movement, stability, and single sound versus sequence repetitions, have been shown to be relevant in the development of goals and treatment strategies at least some of the time, although there is no one-to-one correspondence between the oral mechanism structure/function and speech production (Dworkin and Culatta, 1985).

Finally, and most importantly, the phonological assessment is incomplete without the consideration of the client as a person in his or her environment, both personal-social and physical. Goals and treatment strategies will necessarily reflect the client's interest in the process of change, personality and environment. Assessments utilizing the World Health Organization International Classification of Function (2001) have been suggested by McLeod and Bleile (2004) and others.

Treatment across Various Paradigms

Intervention methods have also followed the theoretical trends in phonology, phonetics, and psychology, with recent innovations in technology enhancing aspects of the treatment process (electropalatrography, ultrasound, nasometry). A recent compendium by Williams, McLeod and McCauley (2010) presents current approaches to treatment, with a split between primarily production-based approaches and approaches in a broader context. Production-based approaches vary in their assumptions from being primarily phonological (linguistically based), focusing on different types of phonologically paired contrasts in production (minimal/maximal/multiple oppositions: Baker, 2010; Baker and Williams, 2010; Williams, 2010), and theories of syllable structure (Bernhardt, 1994a,b; Bernhardt and Gilbert, 1992; Bernhardt et al., 2010a, b, c) to more motorically based approaches. The latter include various visual and motor stimulations and enhancements for oral-motor movements and speech sound productions of various kinds (Clark, 2010; Hayden et al., 2010; Hodge, 2010; Williams and Stephens, 2010) as well as the the use of technologies, such as electropalatography (Gibbon and Wood, 2010) or ultrasound, showing articulatory movements or patterns (Bernhardt et al., 2010c). Production approaches often include imitation and repeating responses at varying levels of intensity and with varying cues as needed from the auditory, visual and tactile-proprioceptive channels of perception. However, even though production approaches lend themselves to repetitive drilling, an approach incorporating "funology" and meaningfulness of phonological contrasts is often used to engage the child (Bernhardt et al., 2010a) during the "drill" practice.

Even though the focus of assessment is often speech production (as noted above), it appears more treatment approaches utilize a broader context, taking, e.g.:

1. A perceptual focus (e.g., Rvachew and Brosseau-Lapré (2010) and Rvachew, Nowak and Cloutier (2004)), where the child is exposed to minimal pair contrasts of the target production and mismatches for that target;
2. A word-based focus (Core Vocabulary) (e.g., Crosbie et al. (2005) and Dodd et al. (2010)), in which key words for the child's life are targeted "sound-by-sound, using cues such as syllable segmentation, imitation and cued articulation" (p. 130, 2010), with the goal of consistent production and intelligibility;
3. A morphosyntactic focus as in Tyler and Haskill (2010) and Tyler et al. (2002), using both focused stimulation and production-based activities (as in narratives or songs) to target morphemes in word-final position (plurals, possessive, past tense, often in clusters);
4. A holistic language focus as in Camarata (2010), Hoffman and Norris (2010), and Hoffman, Norris and Monjure (1996), in play-based contexts with stories, with the "primary conversational focus…on the topic development rather than on the… speech and language goals and performance" (Hoffman and Norris, 2010, p. 346);
5. A phonological awareness focus as in Gillon (2000), Hesketh (2010), and Howell and Dean (1994), in which the child is provided with general information about speech sounds and structures in play-based activities, sometimes focusing on specific units such as onsets or rimes, individual syllables, or segments.

Service delivery also varies in terms of the degree of parent or caregiver input (Bowen, 2009), ordering of goals (cyclically, as in Hodson, 2007; or sequentially), and the amount and frequency of treatment. Comparing outcomes for children in 16-week studies with 2x versus 3x weekly treatments, Bernhardt et al. (2010a) noted equivalent degrees of change in percent consonant match and percent vowel match for the two dosages. However, few studies have examined dosage factors.

Connections

This chapter opens the door to the comprehensive perspectives on child speech development and disorders compiled in this volume. Here, we traced the methodological beginnings of child phonology and clinical phonology; Chapter 2 provides a survey of some contemporary tools for clinicians and researchers. We showcase some of the earliest discoveries about typical speech acquisition of English; Sections II and III provide detailed information on how speech is typically acquired, not only by English-learning children but by children in other linguistic environments as well. We outline some linguistic theories based on adult speech productions and describe how they influenced, and were influenced by, clinical phonology; Sections IV and V provide a clinical compendium of current diagnostic and therapeutic practices, as clinical phonology has become a sophisticated and influential field.

Concluding Remarks

Over the last few decades, there have been rapid changes in technology, enabling deeper analyses of speech production and perception, in both research and clinical realms. In addition, theoretical frameworks in psycholinguistics have started to meld perspectives from information processing and linguistic theory (Bernhardt, Stemberger and Charest, 2010) that can be exploited in speech habilitation. The focus on languages other than English is starting to take off, both in studies and in practice, with researchers around the world contributing data (e.g., see Chapters 10, 11, and 12 describing how children acquire French, Korean, and Brazilian Portuguese, respectively). Political changes in western countries have resulted in an increased respect for the multiplicity of languages in societies of the western world and elsewhere.

At the present time, there is some evidence for certain assessment and treatment practices in clinical phonology, but much more remains to be done. The current textbook provides an opportunity to reflect on phonological development across several languages, and diagnostic and treatment approaches, and provides a basis for future clinical research.

Chapter Review Questions

1. How did the earliest studies of child phonology differ from more current studies in terms of child samples and data formats?
2. What are some similarities in typical speech sound development across all languages?
3. Why is the issue of underlying representations so difficult to study?
4. Describe how each of the linguistic theories was "translated" into clinical practice as a specific type of treatment approach.

Suggestions for Further Reading

Bernhardt, B. M. H., and Stemberger, J. P. (1998). *Handbook of phonological development: From a nonlinear constraints-based perspective.* San Diego: Academic Press.

Bowen, C. (2009). Children's speech sound disorders. *West Sussex*, U. K.: John Wiley and Sons, Ltd.

Ferguson, C. A., L. Menn, L. and Stoel-Gammon, C., Editors (1992). *Phonological development: Models, research, implications.* Timonium, MD.: York Press.

Vihman, M. M. (1997). *Phonological development: The origins of language in the child.* Cambridge, MA.: Blackwell Publsihers, Inc.

SUGGESTIONS FOR STUDENT ACTIVITIES

1. Visit the websites listed in Sidebar 1.2 and determine the functions of the various computer analysis programs for child speech. Describe how you might use each program in clinical practice. Download the free programs and play!
2. Visit the CHILDES website and explore the database, particularly PHONBANK. What types of speech samples are available, and in which formats are they available?
3. Design an experiment that would allow you to determine if a child who regularly says "wed" for "red" can perceive the difference between /w/ and /r/.

ANSWERS TO CHAPTER REVIEW QUESTIONS

1. How did the earliest studies of child phonology differ from more current studies in terms of child samples and data formats?

Some educators and linguists (e.g., Wellman and colleagues (1931), Templin (1957), and Sander (1972)) were interested in discovering at what age typically developing children acquired certain phonemes. Data were collected from large samples of children. A second genre of studies were longitudinal diary studies of individual children, conducted by linguists who chronicled the phonological development of their own children by transcribing child speech samples, often online and without the benefit of recording equipment. These studies were designed to investigate how children went about the acquisition of speech sounds in general, and the authors include Velten (1943), Leopold (1949), Weir (1962), Waterson (1971), Smith (1973), and Labov and Labov (1978). One breakthrough was the discovery that speech sounds were related to each other in terms of production class (e.g., sounds produced by stopping the airflow or constricting the airflow through a narrow opening) and that children tend to acquire sounds as classes rather than as individual sounds. Contemporary studies make use of a full array of sophisticated technologies including ultrasound, electropalatography, and acoustic analysis software. Online databases rich in child speech samples, some glossed, some transcribed, some videotaped, are readily available for downloading.

2. What are some similarities in typical speech sound development across all languages?

Some common trends have been observed across languages regarding sound classes. For instance, stop consonants are acquired before fricatives; glides are acquired before liquids; singleton consonants are acquired before consonant clusters; and voiceless unaspirated stops are acquired before stops with other types of voicing (e.g. prevoiced; voiceless aspirated). Chapter 9 contains a detailed synopsis of many languages where additional crosslinguistic trends are described, for instance, trends regarding vowels. It should be remembered, however, that there are substantial differences not only related to different languages, but also to individual children acquiring the same language.

3. Why is the issue of underlying representations so difficult to study?

An underlying representation is a mentally stored word form that children are thought to rely on when recognizing words spoken to them and when producing words in speech; in terms of phonology, this representation includes articulatory and acoustic properties. Underlying representations are not directly observable; they are inferred on theoretical grounds. It is unknown whether young children have just one set of underlying representations for words or two separate ones, one for recognizing words spoken to them and another one for producing words. Some researchers question whether children even have any specified lexicon at all; usage-based models posit that each instance of a heard or articulated word is evaluated for similarities with previously heard or articulated words. It is puzzling to note that very young children (age 14 to 15 months) can detect mispronunciations in words spoken to them at an age before they can produce these words correctly themselves. It is unknown what factors drive this mismatch.

4. Describe how each of the linguistic theories was "translated" into clinical practice as a specific type of treatment approach.

Structuralist theories have influenced clinical practice with their focus on single consonants (Van Riper, 1939, 1978). Phonological process or rule-based theories have influenced pattern-based treatment approaches (Dinnsen and Elbert, 1984; Gierut, 1998; Grunwell, 1985; Hodson, 2007; Ingram, 1976). Nonlinear phonology and constraint-based theories (Optimality theory) have also found their way into clinical practice (Bernhardt, 1990, 1992a, b, 1994a, b; Bernhardt and Major, 2005; Bernhardt and Stemberger, 2000; Dinnsen and Gierut, 2008; Major and Bernhardt, 1998). Optimality theory has led to approaches that focus on the suppression of phonological constraints and faithfulness to the underlying form. Chapter 22 discusses a variety of treatment approaches and shows how they relate to linguistic theory.

REFERENCES

Adler-Bock, M., Bernhardt, B., Gick, B., and Bacsfalvi, P. (2007). The use of ultrasound in remediation of /r/ in adolescents. *American Journal of Speech-Language Pathology*, 16(2), 128-139.

Almost, D. and Rosenbaum, P. (1998). Effectiveness of speech intervention for phonological disorders: a randomized controlled trial. *Developmental Medicine and Child Neurology*, 40(5), 319-325.

Bacsfalvi, P. (2011). Attaining the lingual components of /r/ with ultrasoundfor three adolescents with cochlear implants. *Canadian Journal of the Association of Speech-Language Pathologists and Audiologists*, 34, 206-217.

Bailey, T. and Plunkett, K. (2002). Phonological specificity in early words. *Cognitive Development*, 17, 1265-1282.

Baker, E. (2010). Minimal pair intervention. In L. Williams, S. McLeod and R. McCauley (Eds.) *Intervention for speech sound disorders in children* (pp. 41-72). Baltimore, MD.: Paul Brookes Publishing.

Baker, E. and Williams, L. (2010). Complexity approaches to intervention. In L. Williams, S. McLeod and R. McCauley (Eds.) *Intervention for speech sound disorders in children* (pp. 95-115). Baltimore, MD.: Paul Brookes Publishing.

Ball, J., Bernhardt, B. and Deby, J. (2006). First Nations English Dialects: Exploratory Project Proceedings. University of Victoria, June 2006.

Ballem, K. and Plunkett, K. (2002). Phonological specificity in 14-month-olds. *Journal of Child Language*, 32, 159-173.

Barlow, J. and Gierut, J. (1999). Optimality Theory in phonological acquisition. *Journal of Speech, Language, and Hearing Research*, 42, 1482–1498.

Barlow, J. A., and Gierut, J. A. (2002). Minimal pair approaches to phonological remediation. *Seminars in Speech and Language* 23, 57-68.

Beckman, M., Munson, B. and Edwards, J. (2007). Vocabulary growth and the developmental expansion of types of phonological knowledge. In J. Cole and J. Hualde (Eds.), *Laboratory phonology* 9, 241–64. New York: Mouton de Gruyter.

Bernhardt, B. (1990). Application of nonlinear phonological theory to intervention with six phonologically disordered children. Unpublished doctoral dissertation, University of British Columbia.

Bernhardt, B. (1992a). Developmental implications of nonlinear phonological theory. *Clinical Linguistics and Phonetics*, 6, 259-282.

Bernhardt, B. (1992b). The application of nonlinear phonological theory to intervention. *Clinical Linguistics and Phonetics*, 6, 283-316.

Bernhardt, B. (1994a). Phonological intervention techniques for syllable and word structure development. *Clinics in Communication Disorders*, 4, 1, 54-65.

Bernhardt, B. (1994b). The prosodic tier and phonological disorders. In M. Yavaş (ed.) *First and second language acquisition* (pp. 149-172). San Diego, CA.: Singular Press.

Bernhardt, B. M., Bacsfalvi, P., Adler-Bock, M., Shimizu, R., Cheney, A., Giesbrecht, N., O'Connell, M., Sirianni, J. and Radanov, B. (2008). Ultrasound as visual feedback in speech therapy: Exploring consultative use in rural British Columbia. *Clinical Linguistics and Phonetics*, 22, 149-162.

Bernhardt, B. M., Bacsfalvi, P., Gick, B., Radanov, B., and Williams, R. (2005a). Exploring electropalatography and ultrasound in speech habilitation. *Journal of Speech-Language Pathology and Audiology*, 29, 169-182.

Bernhardt, B. M., Bopp-Matthews, K., Daudlin, B., Edwards, S., and Wastie, S. (2010a), including D. V. D. section. Nonlinear phonological intervention. In L. Williams, S. MacLeod and R. McCauley (Eds). *Treatment of speech sound disorders* (pp. 315-331). Baltimore, MD.: Brookes Publishing.

Bernhardt, B. M., Gick, B., Bacsfalvi, P., and Adler-Bock, M. (2005b). Ultrasound in speech therapy with adolescents and adults. *Clinical Linguistics and Phonetics*, 19, 605-617.

Bernhardt, B., and Gilbert, J. (1992). Applying linguistic theory to speech-language pathology: the case for nonlinear phonology. *Clinical Linguistics and Phonetics*, 6, 123-145.

Bernhardt, B. H. and Holdgrafer, G. (2001a). Beyond the Basics I: The need for strategic sampling for in-depth phonological analysis. *Language, Speech, and Hearing Services in Schools*, 32, 18-27.

Bernhardt, B. H. and Holdgrafer, G. (2001b). Beyond the Basics II: Supplemental sampling for in-depth phonological analysis. *Language, Speech, and Hearing Services in Schools*, 32, 28-37.

Bernhardt, B. M., Kemp, N. and Werker, J. (2007). Early word-object associations and later language development. *First Language*, 27, 315-328.

Bernhardt, B. and Major, E. (2005). Speech, language and literacy skills three years later: Long-term outcomes of nonlinear phonological intervention. *International Journal of Language and Communication Disorders*, 40, 1-27.

Bernhardt, B. M. H., and Stemberger, J. P. (1998). *Handbook of phonological development: From a nonlinear constraints-based perspective*. San Diego: Academic Press.

Bernhardt, B. H. and Stemberger, J. P. (2000). *Workbook in nonlinear phonology for clinical application*. Austin, T. X.: Pro-Ed. (Copyright reverted to authors: please contact for a digital copy.)

Bernhardt, B. and Stemberger, J. P. (2008). Constraints-based nonlinear phonological theories: Application and implications. In M. Ball (Ed.) *Handbook of clinical linguistics* (pp. 423-438). Oxford, U. K.: Blackwell.

Bernhardt, M., Sirianni, J. and Radanov, B. (2008). Ultrasound as visual feedback in speech therapy: Exploring consultative use in rural British Columbia. *Clinical Linguistics and Phonetics*, 22, 149-162.

Bernhardt, B. M., Stemberger, J. P., Ayyad, H., Ullrich, A. and Zhao, J. (2010b). Nonlinear phonology: Clinical applications for Kuwaiti Arabic, German and Mandarin. In J. Guendouzi (Ed.) *Handbook of psycholinguistics and cognitive processing: Perspectives in communication disorders* (pp. 489-513). London, U. K.: Taylor and Francis.

Bernhardt, B. M., Stemberger, J. P. and Bacsfalvi, P. (2010c). Recent perspectives concerning vowels in phonological intervention: Nonlinear phonology and articulatory visual feedback. In L. Williams, S. MacLeod and R. McCauley (Eds.). *Treatment of speech sound disorders* (pp. 537-555). Baltimore, MD.: Brookes Publishing.

Bernhardt, B. M., Stemberger, J. S. and Charest, M. (2010d). Speech production models and intervention for speech production impairments in children. *Canadian Journal of the Association of Speech-Language Pathologists and Audiologists,* 34, 157-167.

Bernhardt, B., and Stoel-Gammon, C. (1994). Nonlinear phonology: Clinical application. *Journal of Speech and Hearing Research,* 37, 123-143.

Bernhardt, B. M., and Zhao, J. (2010). Nonlinear phonological analysis in assessment of Mandarin speakers. *Canadian Journal of the Association of Speech-Language Pathologists and Audiologists,* 34, 168-180.

Bowen, C. (2009). *Children's speech sound disorders.* Oxford, U. K.: Wiley-Blackwell.

Browman, C., and Goldstein, L. (1992). Articulatory phonology: An overview. *Phonetica*, 49, 155-180.

Bybee, J. (2001). *Phonology and language use.* Cambridge: Cambridge University Press.

Camarata, S. (2010). Naturalistic intervention for speech intelligibility and speech accuracy. In L. Williams, S. McLeod and R. McCauley (Eds.) *Intervention for speech sound disorders in children* (pp. 381-405). Baltimore, MD.: Paul Brookes Publishing.

Chomsky, N., and Halle, M. (1968). *The sound pattern of English.* New York: Harper and Row.

Clark, H. C. (2010). Nonspeech oral motor exercise. In L. Williams, S. McLeod and R. McCauley (Eds.) *Intervention for speech sound disorders in children* (pp. 579-599). Baltimore, MD.: Paul Brookes Publishing.

Crosbie, S., Holm, A., and Dodd, B. (2005). Intervention for children with severe speech disorder: A comparison of two approaches. *International Journal of Language and Communication Disorders*, 40, 467–491.

Dinnsen, D. A., and Elbert, M. (1984). On the relationship between phonology and learning. In M. Elbert, D. A. Dinnsen, and G. Weismer (Eds.), *Phonological theory and the misarticulating child. A. S. H. A. Monographs,* 22, 59-68. Rockville, MD.: A. S. H. A.

Dinnsen, D. A., and Gierut, J. A. (2008). *Optimality theory, phonological acquisition and disorders*. London: Equinox.

Dodd, B., Holm, A., Crosbie, S. and McIntosh, B. (2010). Core Vocabulary Intervention (D. V. D.). In L. Williams, S. McLeod and R. McCauley (Eds.) *Intervention for speech sound disorders in children* (pp. 117-136). Baltimore, MD.: Paul Brookes Publishing.

Donegan, P. J., and Stampe, D. (1979). The study of natural phonology. In D. A. Dinnsen (Ed.), *Current approaches to phonological theory* (pp. 126--173). Bloomington, IN.: Indiana University Press.

Dworkin, J. P. and Culatta, R. (1985). Oral structural and neuromuscular characteristics in children with normal and disordered articulation. *Journal of Speech and Hearing Disorders*, 50, 150-156.

Ferguson, C. A. (1967). Proposal to the National Science Foundation.

Ferguson, C. A., and Farwell, C. B. (1975). Words and sounds in early language acquisition. *Language*, 51, 419-439.

Ferguson, C. A., and Garnica, O. (1975). Theories of phonological development. In E. H. Lenneberg and E. Lenneberg (Eds.), *Foundations of language development: A multidisciplinary approach* (pp. 153-180). New York: Academic Press.

Ferguson, C. and Macken, M. (1981). Phonological universals in language acquisition. *Annals of the New York Academy of Sciences*, 379, 110-129.

Ferguson, C. A., L. Menn, L. and Stoel-Gammon, C., Editors (1992). *Phonological development: Models, research, implications*. Timonium, MD.: York Press.

Firth, J. (1948). Sounds and prosodies. *Transactions of the Philological Society*, 127-152.

Gibbon, F. E. and Wood, S. E. (2010). Visual feedback therapy with electropalatography. In L. Williams, S. McLeod and R. McCauley (Eds.) *Intervention for speech sound disorders in children* (pp. 509-536). Baltimore, MD.: Paul Brookes Publishing.

Gierut, J. (1998). Treatment efficacy: Functional phonological disorders in children. *Journal of Speech, Language, and Hearing Research*, 41, 85-100.

Gillon, G. (2000). Follow-up study investigating the benefits of phonological awareness intervention for children with spoken language impairment. *International Journal of Language and Communication Disorders*, 37, 381-400.

Goldsmith, J. A. (1990). *Autosegmental and metrical phonology*. Oxford: Blackwell.

Grunwell, P. (1985). *Phonological assessment of child speech*. Windsor:NFER-Nelson.

Hayden, D. A., Eigen, J. Walker, A. and Olsen, L. (2010). PROMPT: A tactually grounded model. In L. Williams, S. McLeod and R. McCauley (Eds.) *Intervention for speech sound disorders in children* (pp. 453-474). Baltimore, MD.: Paul Brookes Publishing.

Hesketh, A. (2010). Metaphonological intervention: Phonological awareness therapy. In L. Williams, S. McLeod and R. McCauley (Eds.) *Intervention for speech sound disorders in children* (pp. 247-274). Baltimore, M. D.: Paul Brookes Publishing.

Hills, E. C. (1914). The speech of a child two years of age. *Dialect Notes* 4, 84-100.

Hodge, M. (2010). Developmental dysarthria intervention. In L. Williams, S. McLeod and R. McCauley (Eds.) *Intervention for speech sound disorders in children* (pp. 557-578). Baltimore, MD.: Paul Brookes Publishing.

Hodson, B. (2004). *Hodson Assessment of Phonological Patterns (H. A. P. P.)* (3rd Ed.). Austin, TX.: Pro-Ed.

Hodson, B. (2007). *Evaluating and enhancing children's phonological systems: Research and theory to practice*. Greenville, S. C.: Thinking Publications/Super Duper.

Hoffman, P. and Norris, J. (2010). Dynamic systems and Whole Language intervention. In L. Williams, S. McLeod and R. McCauley (Eds.) *Intervention for speech sound disorders in children* (pp. 333-354). Baltimore, MD.: Paul Brookes Publishing.

Hoffman, P., Norris, J. and Monjure, J. (1996). Comparison of process targeting and Whole Language treatments for phonologically delayed preschool children. *Language, Speech, and Hearing Services in Schools*, 21(2),102-109.

Howell, J. and Dean, E. (1994). *Treating phonological disorders in children*. London, U. K.: Whurr Publishers.

Humphreys, M. W. (1880). A contribution to infantile linguistics. *Transactions of the American Philological Association* 11, 5-17.

Ingram, D. (1976). *Phonological disability in children*. London: Edward Arnold.

Jakobson, R. (1941; English translation: 1968). *Child language, aphasia and phonological universals*. Paris: Mouton.

Jusczyk, P. (2003). The role of speech perception capacities in early language acquisition. In M. T. Banich and M. Mack (Eds). *Mind, brain, and language: Multidisciplinary perspectives* (pp. 61-83). Mahwah, NJ.: US: Lawrence Erlbaum Associates Publishers.

Kemmer, S., and Barlow, M. (2000). Introduction: A usage-based conception of language. In M. Barlow and S. Kemmer (Eds.), *Usage-based models of language* (pp. vii--xxvii). Stanford, CA.: C. S. L. I. Publications.

Kent, R. (1992) The biology of phonological development. In C. A. Ferguson, L. Menn and C. Stoel-Gammon (Eds.), *Phonological development: Models, research, implications* (pp. 65-90). Timonium, MD.: York Press.

Kuhl, P. K. (2009). Early language acquisition: Phonetic and word learning, neural substrates, and a theoretical model. In B. Moore, L. Tyler and W. Marslen-Wilson (Eds.), *The perception of speech: From sound to meaning* (pp. 103-131). Oxford, U. K.: Oxford University Press.

Labov, W. and Labov, T. (1978). The phonetics of *cat and mama. Language* 54, 816-52.

Leopold, W. (1939–1949). *Speech development of a bilingual child.* Evanston, IL.: Northwestern University Press.

Long, S. (2011). P. R. O. P. H. Retrieved from: *http://www.computerizedprofiling.org.*

MacWhinney, B. (2007). The Talk Bank Project. In J. C. Beal, K. P. Corrigan and H. L. Moisl (Eds.), *Creating and Digitizing Language Corpora: Synchronic Databases, Vol.1.* Houndmills: Palgrave-Macmillan.

Major, E. and Bernhardt, B. (1998). Metaphonological skills of children with phonological disorders before and after phonological and metaphonological intervention. *International Journal of Language and Communication Disorders*, 33, 413-444.

Mani, N. and Plunkett, K. (2007). Phonological specificity of vowels and consonants in early lexical representations. *Journal of Memory and Language*, 57, 252-272.

Masterson, J. and Bernhardt, B. (2001). *Computerized articulation and phonology evaluation system (C. A. P. E. S.)*. San Antonio, TX.: Harcourt Assessment. The Psychological Corporation.

McCauley, R., and Swisher, L. (1984). Psychometric review of language and articulation tests for preschool children. *Journal of Speech and Hearing Disorders*, 49, 34-42.

McLeod, S. and Bleile, K. (2004). The I. C. F.: A framework for setting goals for children with speech impairment. *Child Language Teaching and Therapy*, 20, 199-219.

Menn, L. (1980). Phonological theory and child phonology. In G. Yeni-Komshian, J. Kavanagh, and C. Ferguson (Eds.), *Child phonology:* Vol. 1. Production (pp. 23-41). New York: Academic Press.

Menn, L. (1983). Development of articulatory, phonetic, and phonological capabilities. In B. Butterworth (Ed.) *Language production,* vol. 2. (pp. 3-50). London: Academic Press.

Menn, L. and Matthei, E. (1992). The "two lexicon" account of child phonology: Looking back, looking ahead. In C.A. Ferguson, L. Menn and C. Stoel-Gammon (Eds), *Phonological development: Models, research, implications*, 211-247. Timonium, MD.: York Press.

Munson, B., Edwards, J. and Beckman, M. (in press). Phonological representations in language acquisition: climbing the ladder of abstraction. In A. C. Cohn, C. Fougeron and

M. K. Huffman (Eds.), *Handbook of laboratory phonology*. Oxford: Oxford University Press.

Oller, D. K. and Delgado, R. E. (1999). *Logical International Phonetics Program (L. I. P. P.)*. Miami, FL.: Intelligent Hearing Systems.

Prince, A. and Smolensky, P. (2004). Optimality theory: Constraint interaction in generative grammar. Cambridge, MA.: M. I. T. Press.

Rose, Y. and Hedlund, G. (2011). P. H. O. N. Retrieved from *childes.psy.cmu.edu/phon.*

Rvachew, S. and Bernhardt, B. M. (2010). Clinical implications of the dynamic systems approach to phonological development. *American Journal of Speech-Language Pathology*, 19, 34-50.

Rvachew, S. and Brosseau-Lapré, I. (2010). Speech perception intervention. In L. Williams, S. McLeod and R. McCauley (Eds.) *Intervention for speech sound disorders in children* (pp. 295-314). Baltimore, MD.: Paul Brookes Publishing.

Rvachew, S. and Nowak, M. (2001). The effect of target-selection strategy on phonological learning. *Journal of Speech, Language, and Hearing Research,* 44(3), 610-623.

Rvachew, S., Nowak, M. and Cloutier, G. (2004). Effect of phonemic perception training on the speech production and phonological awareness skills of child with expressive phonological delay. *American Journal of Speech-Language Pathology*, 13, 250-263.

Rvachew, S., Rafaat, S. and Martin, M. (1999). Stimulability, speech perception skills and the treatment of phonological disorders. *American Journal of Speech-Language Pathology*, 8(1), 33-43.

Sander, E. (1972). When are speech sounds learned? *Journal of Speech and Hearing Disorders*, 37, 55-63.

Shiller, D. M., Rvachew, S. R. and Brosseau-Lapré, F. (2010). Importance of the auditory perceptual target to the achievement of speech production accuracy. *Canadian Journal of Speech Language Pathology and Audiology,* 34, 181-192.

Shriberg, L. D., Kwiatkowski, J., and Rasmussen, C. (1990). *The Prosody-Voice Screening Profile.* Tucson, AZ.: Communication Skill Builders.

Smith, N. V. (1973). *The acquisition of phonology: A case study.* Cambridge, U. K.: Cambridge University Press.

Sosa, A. V. and Bybee, J. (2008). A cognitive approach to clinical phonology. In M. Ball, M. Perkins, N. Muller and S. Howard (Eds), *The handbook of clinical linguistics* (pp. 480–90). Malden, MA.: Blackwell Publishing Ltd.

Stampe, D. (1969). *The acquisition of phonetic representation.* Paper presented at the Fifth Regional Meeting of the Chicago Linguistic Society, Chicago.

Stoel-Gammon, C. (1991). Normal and disordered phonology in two-year-olds. *Topics in Language Disorders*, 11, 21-32.

Stoel-Gammon, C., and Cooper, J. (1984). Patterns of early lexical and phonological development. *Journal of Child Language*, 11, 247-271.

Stoel-Gammon, C., and Dunn, C. (1985). *Normal and disordered phonology in children.* Austin, TX.: Pro-Ed.

Stokes, S., Klee, T., Carson, C., and Carson, D. (2005) A phonemic implicational feature hierarchy of phonological contrasts for English-speaking children. *Journal of Speech. Language, and Hearing Research,* 48, 817-833.

Swingley, D. (2003). Phonetic detail in the developing lexicon. *Language and Speech*, 46, 265-294.

Templin, M. (1957). Certain language skills in children, their development and interrelationships. *Institute of Child Welfare monographs*, Vol. 26. Minneapolis: University of Minnesota.

Trubetzkoy, N. S. (1939). *Grundzüge der Phonologie*. Prague: Travaux du Cercle Linguistique de Prague.

Tyler, A. A. and Haskill, A. (2010). Morphosyntax intervention. In L. Williams, S. McLeod and R. McCauley (Eds.) *Intervention for speech sound disorders in children* (pp. 355-379). Baltimore, MD.: Paul Brookes Publishing.

Tyler, A. A., Lewise, K. E., Haskill, A. and Tolbert, L. C. (2002). Efficacy and cross-domain effects of a morphosyntax and a phonology intervention. *Language, Speech, and Hearing Services in Schools*, 33, 52-66.

Van Riper, C. (1939, 1978). *Speech correction: principles and methods*. Oxford, England: Prentice-Hall.

Velten, H. V. (1943). The growth of phonemic and lexical patterns in infant language. *Language*, 19, 231-292.

Vihman, M. M., (1996). *Phonological development: The origins of language in the child.* Oxford, U. K.: Blackwell.

Waterson, N. (1971). Child phonology: A prosodic view. *Journal of Linguistics*, 7, 179-221.

Weir, R. (1962). *Language in the crib.* Mouton: The Hague.

Wellman, B., Case, I., Mengert, I., and Bradbury, D. (1931). Speech sounds of young children. *University of Iowa Studies in Child Welfare*, 5, 1-82.

Werker, J. F., Fennell, C. T., Corcoran, K., and Stager, C. L. (2002). Infants' ability to learn phonetically similar words: Effects of age and vocabulary size. *Infancy*, 3, 1-30.

Werker, J. F. and Stager, C. (1997). Infants listen for more phonetic detail in speech perception than in word-learning tasks. *Nature,* 388(6640), 381-382.

White, K.S. and Morgan, J.L. (2008) Sub-segmental detail in early lexical representations. *Journal of Memory and Language*, 59, 114-132.

Williams, L. (2010). Multiple oppositions intervention. In L. Williams, S. McLeod and R. McCauley (Eds.) *Intervention for speech sound disorders in children* (pp. 73-94). Baltimore, MD: Paul Brookes Publishing.

Williams, L., McLeod, and McCauley, R. (2010). *Intervention for speech sound disorders in children*. Baltimore, MD.: Paul Brookes Publishing.

Williams, P. and Stephens, H. (2010). Nuffield Centre dyspraxia programme. In L. Williams, S. McLeod and R. McCauley (Eds.) *Intervention for speech sound disorders in children* (pp. 159-177). Baltimore, MD.: Paul Brookes Publishing.

World Health Organization. (2001). *International Classification of Function, Disability and Health*. Retrieved from *http://www.who.int/classifications/icf/en/.*

Wren, Y., Roulstone, S. and Hughes, A. (2006) Phoneme Factory Phonology Screener. London; NFERNelson.

Yeni-Komshian, G. Kavanagh, J., and Ferguson, C., Editors (1980). *Child Phonology,* vols. 1 and 2. New York: Academic Press.

In: Comprehensive Perspectives …
Editors: Beate Peter and Andrea A. N. MacLeod
ISBN: 978-1-62257-041-6

Chapter 2

DESCRIBING AND MEASURING CHILDREN'S SPEECH SOUND ABILITIES: FROM ARTICULATION TESTS TO ACOUSTIC ANALYSIS FOR CLINICIANS AND RESEARCHERS*

Megan M. Hodge and Karen E. Pollock

INTRODUCTION

During development most children learn to control the actions of respiratory and **vocal tract** structures to produce the sound patterns of the language so that their intended meaning is communicated to listeners through speech. This process involves a dynamic interplay of the child's developing auditory, cognitive, articulatory and sensorimotor mapping capabilities and vocal experiences. As illustrated in the second section of this book, the process of learning to talk has been studied from birth through adulthood. The study of the sounds of human speech is a science referred to as phonetics. Phonetics is a branch of linguistics that includes three basic areas (Ohde and Sharf, 1992). These are *physiologic phonetics,* which is the study of the production of speech sounds by the **articulators** and vocal tract of the talker, *acoustic phonetics*, which is the study of the physical transmission of speech sounds from the talker to the listener and *auditory-perceptual phonetics,* which is the study of the reception and perception of speech sounds by the listener (human auditory nervous system).

Methods from all three areas of phonetics are used to describe and measure children's speech sound abilities; how they develop, and how they conform with or deviate from standard pronunciation.

Most methods used to describe how children produce the speech sounds of their language and the success of their speaking ability are based on perceptual judgments of speech behaviors by trained listeners (for example, speech-language pathologists), often in real time. For example, **articulation testing** is a clinical procedure to determine which speech sounds

* In this chapter, only the masculine form of pronouns is used for efficiency of wording. The masculine form was selected because speech sound delays and disorders occur more frequently in males.

an individual produces correctly and incorrectly, when compared against the standard of correct production, and what type of error has been made when a sound is judged to be incorrect (Goldman and Fristoe, 2000). This requires that the examiner:

1. Knows the standard for correct sound production;
2. Hears and performs a perceptual analysis of the talker's productions of the sound(s); and
3. Compares the result with the standard to decide if the talker's production is correct, that is, falls within the limits of what is considered to be standard pronunciation.

Articulation test results provide a description of speech sounds produced correctly and incorrectly by the talker. They can also be used to determine if a child's acquisition of speech sounds is delayed, compared to his or her peers, and if the observed speech sound error patterns are typical of younger children or atypical. Articulation testing combines methods from articulatory and auditory phonetics.

Audio recordings of the speech sound signal (**waveform**) can be analyzed perceptually (using the human auditory system) and acoustically (using instrumentation that provides visual and numerical descriptions of sound energy patterns in the recordings). A waveform display shows how the amplitude (Y axis) of the signal changes over time (X axis). Amplitude is typically expressed in sound pressure level (SPL) and time is expressed in seconds or milliseconds (ms). Figure 2.1 shows a waveform display of the word "speech." All of the waveform and other acoustic displays in the figures and video files in this chapter were made using TF32 (Milenkovic, 2004), a software program for the time frequency analysis of sound waveforms.

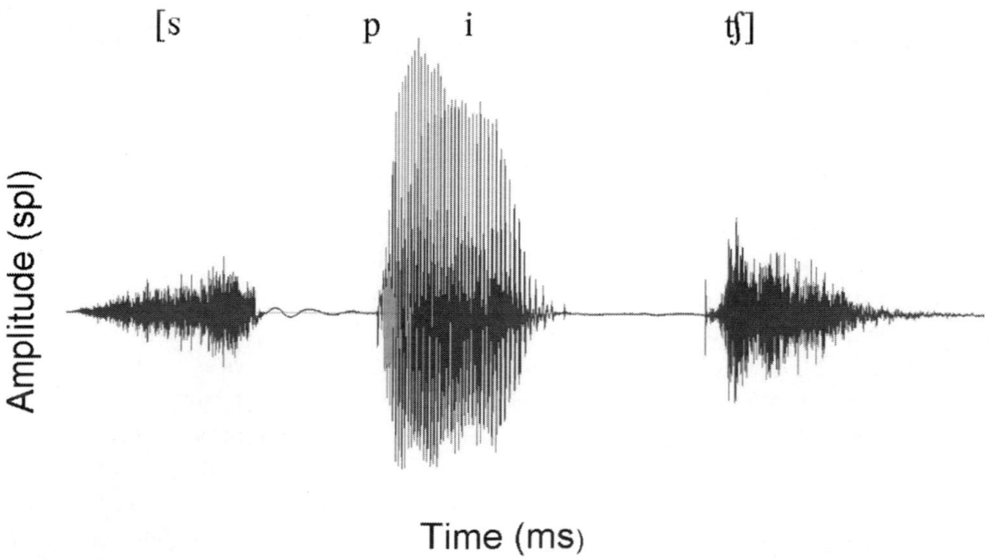

Figure 2.1. Waveform display of the word "speech".

Instrumental acoustic analyses reveal finer grained information about the timing, frequency and intensity characteristics of speech than can be resolved perceptually by the human auditory system. Acoustic analyses provide valuable physical descriptions to supplement perceptual measures of speech behavior. They have been used to study **pre-speech vocalizations** (e.g., Rvachew, Slawinski, Williams and Green, 1999), speech development (e.g., Kehoe, Stoel-Gammon and Buder, 1995; Buder and Stoel-Gammon, 2002), speech disorders (e.g., Higgins and Hodge, 2002; Forrest, Weismer, Hodge, Dinnsen, and Elbert 1990), and more (Kent and Read, 2002). Increased accessibility of digital audio recording and acoustic analysis software means that trained clinicians, as well as speech scientists, can benefit from speech acoustic analyses in their practice.

This chapter reviews how the sounds of speech are produced through the process of **articulation** and illustrates how we sample and describe children's speech sound behaviors using perceptual methods from the field of phonetics. It defines and describes procedures for conducting **independent** and **relational analyses** of children's speech sound systems and addresses how **segmental** and whole word measures and **phonological processes** can be used in relational analyses.

Then it describes measures of related aspects of speech (prosody and voice) and more global aspects of speech behavior (**intelligibility** and **acceptability**) for common clinical and research purposes such as describing the overall severity of speech sound disorders and measuring treatment outcomes.

The chapter concludes with examples of how acoustic measures can be used to supplement our understanding of speech sound production beyond perceptual methods. You will learn about several **acoustic cues** that differentiate speech sounds from each other. After reading this chapter, you will know the basics of how to measure children's speech sound abilities and ways that you can supplement these with fine-grained timing and spectral measures using acoustic analyses. You will be ready to practice applying your knowledge to develop your skills and confidence in measuring children's speech sound behaviors.

How Is Speech Produced? - From Articulation to Speech Acoustics

When we speak, we transform a mental representation of what we want to say (our intention) into a sequence of rapid, coordinated movements of muscles in the torso, neck and upper airway to generate the sound patterns of our language. Speech can be defined as a sound (acoustic) representation of language that is the product of cognitive, linguistic and sensorimotor processes. Speech sounds (consonants and vowels) are produced in sequences that conform to the permissible **syllable shapes** and **word shapes** (**phonotactics**), as well as the stress and intonation patterns, of a particular language. Together, these aspects constitute the language's sound system or **phonology**.

In terms of **speech acoustics**, speech production can be described as a two-part process using **source–filter theory**. The first part of the process involves creating a source of sound. In the second part, the vocal tract acts as a filter to shape sound into the stream of vowels and consonants in the speech signal.

Creating Sound Sources for Speech: "Voice" and "Noise"

Voice. One sound source for speech is "voice." To produce voice, the respiratory system generates and sustains a pressurized air stream from the lungs. The vocal folds adduct and resist the pressurized air stream. The air pressure momentarily overcomes the resistance provided by the adducted vocal folds and blows them apart.

Sidebar 2.1. Segments and Suprasegmental Features: Some Technical Terms

Several terms are used to refer to speech sounds. A phone is a sound produced by the human vocal tract, regardless of a particular language. A phoneme is a class of phonetically similar sounds found in the phonological system of a particular language. Phonemes are the smallest, non-meaningful perceptible units of oral language. They contrast with one another to differentiate the meaning of spoken words. For example, in the word pair "heat" and "hat", /i/ and /æ/ are two different phonemes because they differentiate the meaning of the two words. Allophones, on the other hand, are variations in pronunciation of a phoneme that do not change word meaning. For example, stops can be produced with or without aspiration but are still perceived as the same sound in a word and therefore do not change its meaning. Play file 2S1 to hear an example of an aspirated and unaspirated /t/ in the word "hot".

Access Sound File 1 (Chapter 2)

2S1 The word "hot" with aspirated and unaspirated /t/.

In phonetics, the term "segment" refers to the discrete "units" or consonants and vowel sounds in an utterance. Conversely, the term "**suprasegmental**" refers to features of speech that extend beyond individual segments such as **co-articulation**, syllable and word stress, pause and intonation. In summary, phonetics is the study of speech sounds, and phonemics is the study of speech sounds within a language. Allophones are variations in productions of a phoneme class that do not signal a change in meaning. (Gordon-Brannan and Weiss, 2007). Suprasegmental features describe the auditory patterns of speech beyond the level of individual speech sounds.

The air flowing through the vocal folds causes a momentary pressure drop and they fall back together and the cycle is repeated. In this way, the vocal folds are set into vibration. As the vocal folds snap back to midline during the closing phase of each cycle, they create a complex sound (a sound that has several component frequencies). The periodic recurrence of this sound results in "voice" or "phonation".

The component frequencies of voice include the **fundamental frequency** (f0), defined as the number of vibratory cycles of the vocal folds per second, and whole number multiples (**harmonics**) of f0. Overall length and mass of the vocal folds are the main determinants of, and inversely related to, an individual's f0 range. The smaller the length and mass of the vocal folds, the higher their inherent f0 range. Therefore, as vocal fold length and mass increase with growth, average f0 ranges decrease.

Typical average f0 measures range from 500 Hz at birth to 200 Hz for young women and 150 Hz for young men (Kent and Read; 2002). Perceptually, we hear the f0 of a talker's voice as the pitch of their voice. Voices of higher f0 are perceived as having higher pitch and vice versa. Therefore, the pitch of an infant's voice will be perceived as higher than the pitch of a young man's voice. Play file 2V1 to hear and see the waveforms for a centralized vowel produced by a 3 month-old infant followed by a 21 year-old man. Which do you perceive to have a higher pitched voice? Figure 2.2. shows 30 ms sections from the same infant's and young man's waveforms. Note that the infant's waveform has more cycles of vocal fold vibration (higher fundamental frequency) than the young man's waveform for the same amount of time.

Access Video File 1 (Chapter 2)

2V1 Centralized vowel produced by a 3-month-old infant and a 21-year-old man as depicted in Figure 2.2.

In English, the vowel, glide (/w, j/), liquid (/l, ɹ/) and nasal (/m, n, ŋ/) sounds have voice as the sole sound source (except during whispering). These manners of speech sounds are referred to **as sonorants**.

Noise. A second sound source for speech is "noise". Noise is produced by random disturbances in air pressure that are sufficient to create sound. This sound is referred to as **aperiodic** because there is not a regular pattern in its component frequencies. It is produced during speech in several ways (corresponding to the manners of consonant articulation) by the articulators. The articulators include muscle groups (vocal folds, soft palate, pharynx, tongue root, tongue body, tongue tip, mandible, lips) and passive structures (hard palate, alveolar ridge, teeth). These actions can 1) "stop" the pressurized air stream from the lungs briefly at some location in the vocal tract (place of stop articulation) and then release it suddenly for plosives such as /p, t, k/; 2) force the air stream through a narrow constriction at some location in the vocal tract (place of fricative articulation) for fricatives such as /h, f, s, ʃ, θ/; or combine stopping with release into a fricative for affricates such as /ʧ/. Play file 2V2 to hear and see the waveforms of the words "two", "shoe" and "chew." Observe how the stop, fricative, and affricate consonants differ in the three rhyming words.

Access Video File 2 (Chapter 2)

2V2 Waveforms of the words "two," "shoe," and "chew."

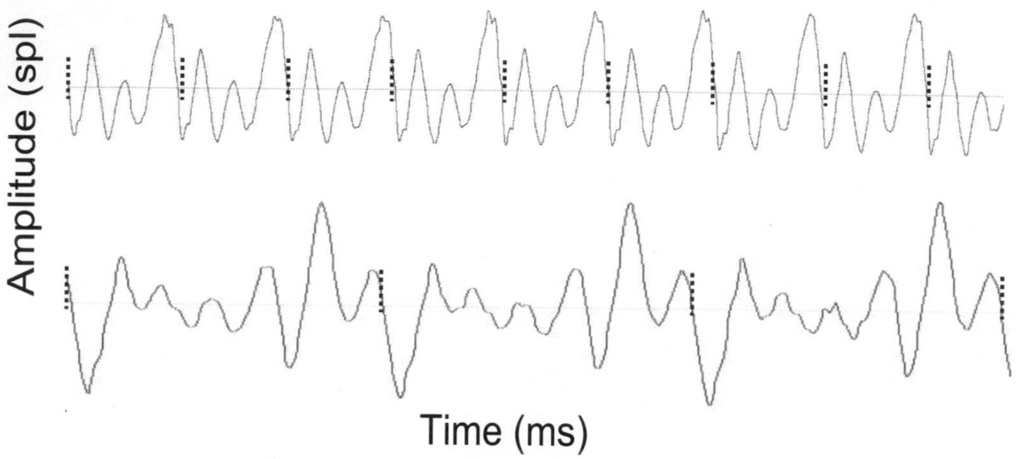

Figure 2.2. 30 ms sections from the waveforms of a centralized vowel as produced by a 3-month-old infant (upper panel) and a 21-year-old man (lower panel). Dashed horizontal bars show approximate individual cycles of vocal fold vibration in each panel.

"Voiced" fricatives (/v, z, ʒ, ð/) and the fricative component of voiced affricates (/ʒ/) have two co-occurring sound sources; one being phonation, created by the vocal folds and the second, noise, created by forcing air through a constriction at the place of articulation. Figure 2.3 shows 30 ms sections taken from the /s/ (upper display) and /z/ (lower display) segments in the words "sue" and "zoo". You will see that only "noise" is visible for /s/ but both noise and "voice" are visible for /z/ (the noise signal appears to be "riding" on regularly occurring cycles of vocal fold vibration). Consonant sounds that have a noise sound source are referred to as **obstruents** and include stops, fricative and affricates.

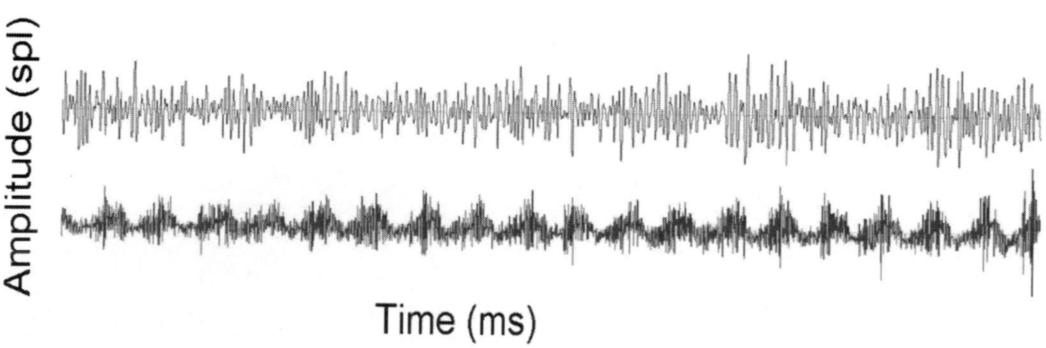

Figure 2.3. 30 ms sections taken from the /s/ (upper display) and /z/ (lower display) segments in waveforms of the words "sue" and "zoo." "Noise" is visible for /s/ but both "noise" and "voice" are visible for /z/.

Vocal Tract as a Sound "Filter" for Speech

In the second part of the speech production process, voice and noise are shaped into the consonant and vowels of the language by how the vocal tract is configured. The actions of the articulators alter the size, shape and number of resonating cavities for a given consonant or vowel. Each vocal tract configuration has different resonant properties that allow some of the frequency components of the sound source to pass through and attenuate others. This is referred to as the "filtering" of sound energy. We refer to the preferred resonating frequencies of the vocal tract for a given configuration as **formants**. Formants are defined by a center frequency and the range of frequencies on either side of the center frequency that fall within 3 dB of the amplitude of the center frequency. Formants change over time as the configuration of the vocal tract changes during speech, for example, during dynamic sounds like glides and **diphthongs** and between adjacent sounds. These changes are referred to as **formant transitions**. Formants are frequency regions that have relatively high amplitudes. The format patterns of a particular speech sound provide important cues to its identity. Figure 2.4 shows a wideband spectrogram of the words "heat" and "hot", spoken by a 6 year-old girl.

Sidebar 2.2. Spectrogram

> A **spectrogram** displays how the frequency components (from low to high, shown on the Y axis) change over time (shown on the X axis). The relative amplitude of the frequency components of the signal are shown in a graded scale (gray or color). The analysis bandwidth can be set to "wide" (> 2x the talker's f0) or to "narrow" (< half the talker's f0). A wide analyzing bandwidth shows formants more clearly than a narrow bandwidth.

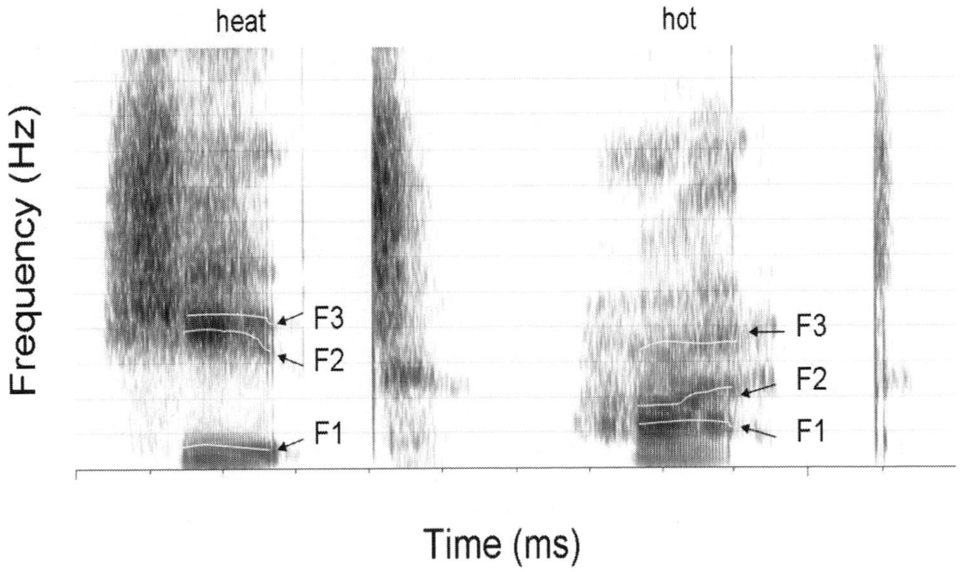

Figure 2.4. Wideband spectrogram for the words "heat" and "hot", spoken by a 6 year-old girl. The formants are numbered consecutively, starting from the one lowest in frequency (F1). Estimated center frequencies of F1, F2 and F3 are indicated by a white line.

The formants are numbered consecutively, starting from the one lowest in frequency (F1, F2, F3, etc.) Observe how the formant patterns differ for the high front vowel /i/ (F1 and F2 are far apart) and the low back vowel /ɑ/ (F1 is higher than in /i/ and F1 and F2 are very close together) in the two words. Estimates of the center frequencies of the first three formants are shown in white. In all of the spectrograms shown in this chapter, the distance between the pale gray horizontal lines on the frequency scale (Y axis) represents 1000 Hz (1 kHz). Also observe the formant transitions as the articulators change position from the vowel to the final consonant. Why are there no formant transitions from the initial consonant to the vowel? See Sidebar 2.3 for a clue.

Sidebar 2.3. The Aspirate /h/ Followed by a Vowel

> The aspirate /h/ is produced at the level of the vocal folds. The articulators are already in position for the following vowel because they are not needed for the aspirate.

In summary, each consonant and vowel has a distinctive pattern of sound (acoustic) energy that reflects its sound source and vocal tract filter characteristics. Articulation is the process by which actions of the vocal tract structures create the distinctive acoustic energy patterns for the sequences of consonants and vowels in the speech signal.

The speech signal is transmitted from talker to listener in the form of sound waves. Sound waves produced by the talker reach the eardrum of the listener, causing it and the organs of the middle and inner ear to vibrate. This activates a complex pathway of neural conduction that results in the perception of sound by the listener (Bess and Humes, 2008). The time-varying patterns of acoustic energy in the sound wave are a physical representation of speech that links talker and listener in communicative interactions (Kent and Read, 2002). When the speech signal contains clear representations of the acoustic patterns of the consonants and vowels of a spoken language, listeners can identify the sounds and words intended by the talker. However, when a child has difficulty controlling the actions of his speech muscles to make clear speech sounds, these may be misidentified by listeners with the result that the child's spoken message is not understood. Play file 2S2 to listen to a short sentence spoken by a six year-old with normal speech motor control and file 2S3 spoken by a child with poor speech motor control resulting from cerebral palsy. For which child are the speech sounds clearer? Which child is more difficult to understand?

Access Sound File 2 (Chapter 2)

2S2 Utterance produced by a 6-year-old child with typically developing speech motor control.

Access Sound File 3 (Chapter 2)

2S3 Utterance produced by a child with impaired speech motor control due to cerebral palsy.

WHAT KINDS OF SPEECH SAMPLES ARE USED TO MEASURE CHILDREN'S SPEECH SOUNDS?

Speech Tasks

How a sample of a child's speech is elicited for measuring and analyzing speech sound behaviors can influence the actual measures that are obtained. There are a number of types of speech samples that have been used to measure children's speech sound behaviors, including samples based on imitation, single word, or spontaneous productions. Selection depends on one's purpose. Options to consider include whether the child's productions will be elicited imitatively (the child is provided with a model of what to say) or not, and if the speech content will be single words or connected speech. When a model is provided to imitate, children may change their typical production to match the model, if they have the capability. Therefore, the sample of their speech that is obtained may not be representative of how they talk in their daily life. However, imitation tasks have the advantage of controlling as much as possible the words that the child says. Single word tasks have the advantages of being relatively easy to elicit either imitatively or spontaneously using a picture or object naming task, and are time-efficient to record and measure. They also ensure that the target word is known. However, children do not typically speak in single words and therefore single words may not provide an accurate representation of their connected speech production. Spontaneous speech samples are thought to be the most representative of children's typical speech (Johnson, Weston, and Bain, 2004). However, spontaneous speech samples of the child's conversation while playing or retelling of a story are time consuming to analyze and the listener may not always know the intended target words in the utterance. They also have the potential for considerable variation from sample to sample in the distribution of phonemes attempted (Flipsen, Hammer and Yost, 2005).

Imitative sentence samples have been investigated as an alternative to spontaneous speech samples because they are more time-efficient to collect and analyze and the target words are not only known, but can be controlled for phonetic and phonemic content. Again, they have the disadvantage of not representing the child's self-generated spoken language. However, Johnson et al. (2004) found similar results when they compared spontaneous speech sampling and sentence repetition tasks. They stated that as long as the imitative sentence set used was scored for all words, included age-appropriate vocabulary and syntax, and ensured all phonemes were sampled, the result should be similar to that obtained with spontaneous speech. Play files 2S4, 2S5, and 2S6 to compare recordings of short samples of 20 imitated single words, 8 imitated sentences and a 60-second spontaneous speech sample during play, respectively, from a 5 year-old child with a speech sound disorder. Which sample is the easiest for you to understand? Why?

Access Sound File 4 (Chapter 2)

2S4 Twenty imitated single words produced by a 5-year-old child with a speech sound disorder.

Access Sound File 5 (Chapter 2)

2S5 Eight imitated sentences produced by a 5-year-old child with a speech sound disorder.

Access Sound File 6 (Chapter 2)

2S6 A 60-second speech sample during play produced by a 5-year-old child with a speech sound disorder.

Another consideration in collecting samples of children's speech is whether the sample will be judged only "on-line" as the child speaks or if it will be judged again "off-line" at a later time from audio or video recordings of the child's speech. Judging samples on-line saves the time needed to listen to the recordings at a later time. In addition, the child's articulatory behaviors and resulting speech signal are not distorted or altered by the recording process. However, a high quality audio or video recording can be played several times to check one's judgments and to compare with similar recordings over time. This can be very useful for children who make speech sound errors. Recording the sample for later transcription is also helpful for beginner clinicians (i.e., not transcribing on-line frees them to focus on test administration and maintaining the child's attention). In addition, audio recordings can be analyzed acoustically to supplement perceptual descriptions of speech sound behaviors. High fidelity audio recordings are needed when recorded speech samples are used to ensure that the recordings recreate the original speech signal as precisely as possible with little or no distortion or background noise. Recommended procedures for obtaining high fidelity recordings include:

1. Use an external microphone that is placed a few inches from the child's mouth (preferably head-mounted so that a constant mouth-to-microphone distance is maintained when the talker moves);
2. Monitor the recording level carefully so it is not too high (to avoid distortion caused by **peak clipping**) or too low (to avoid weak or inaudible signals); and

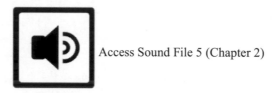

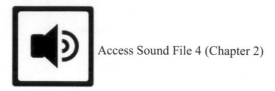

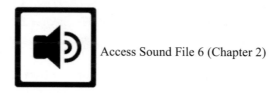

3. Record in a quiet location to avoid extraneous background noise in the recording. The use of headphones is helpful when listening to the recordings. Play files 2S7 and 2S8 to compare the quality of audio recordings. File 2S7 was made using an internal microphone located in a video recorder positioned about 5 feet from the talker. File 2S8 was made using an external head-mounted microphone. Which one sounds better to you?

Access Sound File 7 (Chapter 2)

2S7 Recording obtained with an internal microphone located in a video recorder positioned about 5 feet from the talker.

Access Sound File 8 (Chapter 2)

2S8 Recording obtained with an external head-mounted microphone.

Speech-Like Tasks

Maximum performance tasks such as how long a vowel or a fricative can be sustained or how fast syllables can be repeated are used to measure integrity of the speech motor system in clinical and research protocols (Kent, Kent and Rosenbeck, 1987). These productions are "speech-like" because the speech subsystems are used to generate sounds and sound sequences but they do not meet the criteria for speech because they are not meaningful utterances.

A **maximum phonation duration task** such as sustaining the low back vowel /ɑ/ as long as one can, after inspiring deeply, is measured in seconds. This measure provides information about how efficiently the respiratory subsystem and vocal folds are working to generate voice. Reference values for normative performance on this task are available that differ by age and sex of the talker (e.g., Kent, Kent and Rosenbeck, 1987). As one might expect, values are shorter for children than adults because children have smaller lung volumes.

Diadochokinetic tasks involve rapid alternating movements and are used to examine the accuracy, range, speed and coordination of the oral articulators. Rapid repetition of the syllables [pɑ], [tɑ], and [kɑ] are used to examine movements of the lips, tip of the tongue, and back of the tongue, respectively. These are referred to as monosyllable repetition tasks and are measured in number of syllables repeated per second. Slow, inaccurate or poorly coordinated movements are indicators of motor impairment. Rapid repetition of the syllable sequence [pɑtɑkɑ] is used to examine speech praxis (planning and sequencing) abilities. This is referred to as a tri-syllable repetition task and can be measured in a number of sequences per second or number of syllables per second. Difficulties in maintaining the sounds accurately in the sequence when the talker can produce each syllable accurately in isolation is a potential indicator of apraxia of speech.

Thoonen and colleagues (Thoonen, Maassen, Gabreels and Schreuder, 1999; Thoonen, Maassen, Wit, Gabreels, and Schreuder, 1996) described the application of maximum performance tasks to assist clinicians in identifying the presence and nature of motor speech impairment in younger children (age 6 to 10 years). The tasks used are sustained phonation duration, sustained fricative durations, monosyllable repetition rate for [pɑ], [tɑ], and [kɑ] and tri-syllabic repetition rate for [pɑtɑkɑ]. Children with dysarthria were found to produce short phonation durations (cut-off score of 7.5 seconds) and slow monosyllabic repetition rates (cut-off score of 3.5 syllables per second); children with dyspraxia were not able to produce tri-syllabic repetition tasks accurately or had to use slowed rates to maintain accuracy (cut-off score of 4.4 syllables per second) and had short sustained fricative durations (cut-off score of 11 seconds). Durations and repetition rates can be measured accurately from digital audio recordings of the tasks using waveform editing software. Rvachew, Hodge and Ohberg (2005) provide a tutorial that illustrates how to use audio editing software to obtain the measures for Thoonen et al.'s classification system. Try Activity #1 at the end of the chapter to practice using this classification system using speech from an 8-year-old girl.

Non-word repetition tasks have also been created to measure **phonemic memory** (Dollaghan and Campbell, 1998). The child is presented with recorded auditory models of 1, 2, 3 and 4 consonant-vowel (CV) syllable nonsense words and instructed to repeat exactly what is heard. Examples of 1 and 2 syllable stimuli are /naɪb/ and /teɪvɑk/. The child's consonant and vowel sounds are scored for accuracy in each nonsense word at each syllable length. These scores can then be compared with reference normative data. This measure has been used as a screening measure for language impairment. However, children who have speech sound disorders may do poorly on this measure because of their speech errors, confounding interpretation of the results. To address this problem, Shriberg, Lohmeier, Campbell, Dollaghan, Green, and Moore (2008) created and evaluated a version of a non-word repetition task for children with speech sound errors, referred to as the Syllable Repetition Task. It is an 18-item imitation task containing 2, 3 and 4 syllable CV nonsense words. The only consonants used are /b, d, m, n/ with the vowel /ɑ/. Examples of the stimulus items are /bɑdɑ/, /bɑmɑnɑ/, /bɑmɑdɑmɑ/. Therefore, speech production errors associated with more complex consonants and consonant environments are eliminated. Lower than expected scores on the Syllable Repetition Task have been interpreted as indicating difficulty creating phonological representations. Shriberg and Lohmeier (2008) authored a detailed technical report available at www.waisman.wisc.edu/phonology/ that provides psychometric data, comparison data obtained from 70 children ages 4-to-16 years with typical speech, administration and scoring instructions, and a score form. A PowerPoint presentation of the Syllable Repetition Task that has embedded pre-recorded models of the nonsense word stimuli can also be downloaded from this website. Try Activity #2 to analyze the speech of a 7-year-old boy.

How do we Describe Children's Speech Sounds? From the IPA to Waveform Analysis

In this section you will learn how methods from physiologic (articulatory), auditory-perceptual and acoustic phonetics are used to characterize children's speech sound production.

Perceptual Descriptions of Speech Sounds

Phonetic Transcription. Phonetic transcription by trained listeners is the basic tool used to record the sounds in the speech signal. In the previous section, you saw that some of the symbols used to designate speech sounds look like letters used in the English alphabet but others do not. The **International Phonetic Alphabet (IPA)** is an alphabetic system that was devised by the International Phonetic Association (http://www.langsci.ucl.ac.uk/ipa/) as a standardized way to represent the sounds (phonemes) of spoken language. Foreign language students and teachers, linguists, speech-language clinicians, singers, actors, translators, and artificial language enthusiasts (for example, the Vulcan language of Star Trek fame - see https://webspace.utexas.edu/bighamds/LIN312/Files/Vulcan-guide.pdf), use the IPA. In Appendix 1, you can read how the IPA was created and updated subsequently to accommodate various purposes.

Broad phonetic transcription involves using the IPA base symbols to represent only those aspects of speech that are distinctive in spoken language: phonemes, word boundaries and intonation patterns. For example, standard production of the phrase "speech is my passion" is transcribed in IPA symbols as /spitʃ ɪz maɪ pæʃən/. Slashes, / /, are used to mark off phonemes, all of which are distinctive in the language, without any extra detail. Diacritics are IPA symbols that are used to capture details of pronunciation of speech that may not be used for distinguishing words in the language being transcribed, but which the transcriber wishes to document. Square brackets, [ ], are used for transcribing phonetic details of pronunciation. For example, the symbol [s̪] is used in the phonetic transcription [s̪it] to denote that a young child's pronunciation of /s/ in the word "seat" was dentalized, that is, it was produced with the tongue against the teeth. Play file 2S9 to hear the child's pronunciation of the word.

Access Sound File 9 (Chapter 2)

2S9 Dentalized /s/ in a child's production of the word "seat."

Narrow transcription involves using diacritic symbols with base symbols in the IPA to provide details of a talker's pronunciation. These can be used to capture aspects of how a sound was articulated that are normal variations in pronunciation, that is allophones (for example the use of the aspirated diacritic in [p^{h}ik] for "peak" is used to indicate that the expected allophone of /p/ in this context, [pʰ], was used). Diacritics are also useful when transcribing speech sounds that are recognizable but deviate in some way from standard pronunciation, as in the earlier example of [s̪it] for "seat." A complete list of the base and diacritic symbols used in the IPA can be found on the website of the International Phonetic Association (http://www.langsci.ucl.ac.uk/ipa/) and in Appendix 1.

Table 1 shows the IPA symbols for the consonant phonemes of North American English organized by articulation features of manner, place and voicing. Figure 2.5 shows the IPA symbols for the vowel phonemes of North American English, organized by vowel height and advancements. Stoel-Gammon (2001) provided guidelines for using IPA symbols and diacritics for transcribing the speech of young children. The set of IPA symbols for the consonants of English varies little by geographic region and dialect. However, the set of symbols for the vowels (**monophthongs** and diphthongs) used by speakers of English varies greatly by geographic regions and dialect. This makes phonetic transcription of vowels more challenging (see Pollock and Berni, 2001). As a result, the reliability of vowel transcriptions is often lower than the reliability of consonants when transcriptions of the same speech sample are compared for different trained listeners. How do the vowels shown in Figure 2.5 compare with the English vowels that you use?

Table 2.1. IPA symbols for the consonant phonemes of North American English organized by manner, place and voicing (voiceless consonants are presented first, followed by the voiced consonants) ʔ

	Bilabial	Labiodental	Dental	Alveolar	Postalveolar	Palatal	Velar	Glottal
Plosive	p b			t d			k g	ʔ
Nasal	m			n			ŋ	
Trill								
Tap or Flap				t				
Fricative		f v	θ ð	s z	ʃ ʒ			h
Affricate					tʃ dʒ			
Approximant	w[1]			ɹ		j		
Lateral approximant				l				

[1] /w/ produced with a restriction at the bilabial and velar places of articulation.

An extended set of symbols referred to as Extensions to the IPA (ExtIPA) (Ball and Rahilly, 2002) has been added to represent additional qualities encountered in disordered speech. These include a set of bracket symbols, letter symbols for sounds, diacritics and notations for prosody. See Appendix 2 or http://www.langsci.ucl.ac.uk/ipa/ ExtIPA Chart02.pdf for a description of the ExtIPA symbols that are not part of the IPA. An example of an ExtIPA bracket symbol is double parentheses, (( )), which indicate obscured or unintelligible sounds. (e.g., ((2 syll.)) indicates two audible but unidentifiable syllables). An example of an ExtIPA letter symbol is [fŋ] for a velopharyngeal fricative (snoring sound), which sometimes occurs in children with a cleft palate. Play file 2V3 to hear an example of this sound and see its waveform.

Access Video File 3 (Chapter 2)

2V3. Pharyngeal fricative.

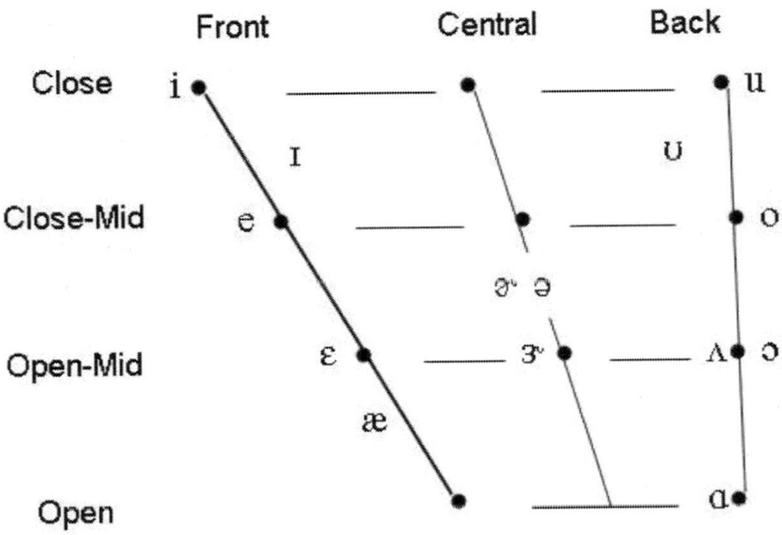

* The following diphthongs are also present in a number of dialects of North American English: /ɔɪ/, /aɪ/, /aʊ/.

Figure 2.5. IPA symbols for the vowel phonemes of North American English. Used with permission.

An example of an ExtIPA diacritic is [s↓]. The downward arrow indicates that the sound was made on ingressive airflow (inspiration) rather than on egressive airflow (expiration). This pattern is sometimes observed in children with cerebral palsy who have poor control of their muscles and run out of air before they have finished saying their words. Play file 2S10 to hear a child with cerebral palsy producing the word "tops" using an ingressive production of /s/. Powell (2001) provides an excellent overview of the issues, challenges, and use of the IPA in transcribing disordered speech.

Access Sound File 10 (Chapter 2)

2S10 The word "tops" produced by a child with cerebral palsy. Note the ingressive airflow during /s/.

Independent Analyses. Once a speech sample has been transcribed, independent and relational analyses can be conducted (Stoel-Gammon and Dunn, 1985). An independent analysis determines what consonants and vowels of the language occur in the child's sample, and in what sequences and word shapes, regardless of their match to standard pronunciation. It provides information about the child's sound and word shape inventory. A speech sound inventory lists all the consonant and vowel types that appeared in the phonetic transcription and a word shape inventory lists all the different shapes of the words based on the number and sequence of component consonants and vowels. For example, the word "bee" has the wordshape CV, indicating a consonant followed by a vowel, whereas the word "bean" has the word shape CVC. Interpreting the results of independent analyses is challenging because normative data are not readily available for comparison. However, research studies that have used these measures can provide valuable information about developmental expectations. For example, Stoel-Gammon (1985) illustrated how independent analyses of meaningful vocalizations recorded from infants between 15 and 24 months were used to describe how their phonetic inventories changed over time.

Relational Analyses. Relational analyses involve a comparison of the phonetic transcription of the child's speech with the presumed adult-like target pronunciation. Note that the "standard" pronunciation could be modified for dialect variation or casual speech modification. A relational analysis requires that the words in the child's utterances are "glossed", meaning that they are written out word by word using orthographic transcription (traditional alphabetic spelling). The child's utterances could be single words, phrases or sentences. Then a phonetic transcription of the target pronunciation of the child's utterances is prepared. The transcription of the child's pronunciation of the utterances is then generated and compared to the transcription of the target pronunciation sound segment by sound segment to identify instances of correct productions and instances of incorrect productions. Incorrect productions may take the form of sound substitutions (another sound is heard in place of the target, as in [tæt] for "cat"), additions (an extra sound or sounds are added to the target, for example, a child's production of the word "blue" (/blu/) is heard as [bəju]), distortions (a variant of the target sound such as a dentalized /s/), or omissions (no sound is produced where the target occurs, as in [si] for "seat."). A relational analysis provides a description of the sounds and word shapes the child is producing accurately and inaccurately. Additional types of relational analyses include segmental and whole word measures and phonological process analyses. Try Activity #3 to create a gloss, a transcription, and an independent and relational analysis of the child's speech.

Segmental and Whole Word Measures. As part of a relational analysis of a speech sample, summary measures of phonetic accuracy can be calculated. Shriberg, Austin, Lewis, McSweeny and Wilson, (1997b) described several phonetic indices of speech accuracy at the level of the segment, based on phonetic transcription of a conversational sample. These included percentage of consonants correct (PCC), percentage of consonants correct-revised (PCC-R), percentage of vowels/diphthongs correct (PVC), percentage of vowels/diphthongs correct-revised (PVC-R), percentage of phonemes correct (PPC) and percentage of phonemes correct-revised (PPC-R). PCC provides a measure of consonant accuracy and scores all consonant omissions, substitutions and distortions as errors. It has been shown to be a reliable and valid measure in numerous studies and to predict severity ratings made by experienced clinicians (Shriberg, Austin, Lewis, McSweeny and Wilson, 1997a). PCC-R differs from PCC in that distortions are scored as correct. Shriberg et al. (1997b) found PCC-R to be the best measure of articulation competence in 3- to 8-year old children as it most accurately distinguished children with normally developing speech from children with a speech disorder. PVC provides a measure of vowel accuracy, which may be compromised in children with developmental dysarthria. PVC scores all vowel omissions, substitutions and distortions as errors while PVC-R counts vowel distortions as correct. PPC provides a combined measure of consonant and vowel accuracy. It is appropriate to use as a single metric to reflect articulation competence on all speech sounds (Shriberg et al., 1997b). PPC-R is similar to PCC-R and PVC-R in that all consonant and vowel omissions and substitutions are scored as incorrect and all distortions are scored as correct. Shriberg et al. (1997b) found PPC and PPC-R to be reliable and valid measures for distinguishing normally developing children from children with speech disorders. However, for the populations studied to date, PPC has not been found to be as sensitive to differences in phonological delay and disorder as PCC because the children studied had high PVC scores. Normative reference data on these measures for ages 2 years through adults are provided in a technical report authored by Austin and Shriberg (1997) available at *www.waisman.wisc.edu/phonology/* and are also described in Shriberg et al. (1997a and 1997b).

Ingram and Ingram (2001) advocated a whole-word approach to phonological assessment, motivated by the assumption that children are word-oriented, not segment-oriented. The correctness of a whole word can be determined by comparing the transcription of the child's word against the standard adult pronunciation. Only a complete match is counted as correct. The number of whole words correct is then divided by the total number of words in the sample and converted to percent whole word accuracy or WWA. Schmitt, Howard and Schmitt (1983) reported WWA for 240 children with age-typical speech between 3 and 7 years of age, based on a 100-word spontaneous speech sample. WWA increased with age from 68.5% for the 3-year-olds to 95.4% for the 7-year-olds.

Proportion of Whole Word Proximity (PWP) (Ingram and Ingram, 2001) provides information about the degree of match between production and target. Ingram's rules for calculating PWP require at least 25 unique words. Only words (e.g., common nouns, verbs, adjectives, prepositions, and adverbs) that are used in adult conversation are counted, compounds are counted if they are spelled as a single word (e.g. "baseball" but not "ice cream"), and each item can only be counted once regardless of the number of productions. PWP is calculated by comparing the phonetic transcription of the child's production with the standard pronunciation of the target word. Each consonant and vowel in the child's production is awarded one point and each correct consonant sound is awarded another point. The score of the child's production is divided by the score of the correct adult target. For example, if the child said "lick" instead of "slick", their PWP score would be 5/7 or .71. Overall PWP is obtained by averaging PWP scores for the 25 words.

Phonological Processes. A phonological process analysis is another type of relational analysis that is used to identify *patterns* of speech sound deviations in a child's sound system. Many of the deviant patterns represent simplifications of sound productions that are systematic deviations of a class of sounds or sound sequences (Gordon-Brannan and Weiss, 2007). In other words, the form produced by the child deviates from the target form in a way that is easier to produce. Examples of this are producing initial fricatives as stops (for example "sock" pronounced as [tɑk]; "zoo" pronounced as [du]), and omitting one or more sounds in a consonant cluster (for example "stop" produced as [tɑp]). Several systems for classifying phonological processes have been described. Gordon-Brannan and Weiss (2007) provide a comprehensive description that consolidates several of these systems into four major categories: syllable structure, assimilation (or harmony), substitution (or feature contrast), and "other." Appendix 2 provides a summary table of phonological processes commonly reported in English phonological development.

Syllable structure processes change the "shape" of the syllables that make up the standard pronunciation of word forms by adding or deleting component consonants and vowels. According to Gordon-Brannan and Weiss, the four most common syllable structure processes are deletion of weak syllables (e.g., "banana" produced as [nænə]), cluster reduction (e.g., "school" produced as [kul]), deletion of final consonants (e.g., "book" produced as [bʊ] and glottal replacement (e.g., "cup" produced as [ʔʌp]). Note that this could also be considered a substitution process as the glottal stop marks the place of a missing consonant and serves to maintain the syllable structure.

In assimilation or harmony deviations, a sound or syllable in the standard pronunciation of the word changes to become more similar to another sound or syllable in the word, such that the sounds or syllables in a word become more alike. In progressive assimilation, a sound in a word is influenced by a preceding sound, for example, when the word "duck" is produced as [dʌt]. In regressive assimilation, which is much more common, a sound is influenced by a later sound in the word, for example, when the word "duck" is produced as [kʌk]. These two examples illustrate consonant assimilation processes. Context-sensitive voicing (e.g., the word "penny" produced as [bɛni] and syllable assimilative processes (e.g., the word "baby" produced as [bibi], also known as syllable reduplication) are also included in this category.

In feature contrast or substitution processes, one sound is replaced by another without being influenced by the surrounding phonemes such that one class of phonemes is replaced by another class of phonemes. Gordon-Brannan and Weiss note that these deviations can affect liquids, stops, fricatives, affricates, nasals and glides and that most of these occur during speech development in children as part of typical development. The name of the particular type of substitution process refers to the class of sounds that is substituted for a sound in the standard pronunciation of a word. For example, in "stopping," stops may be substituted for fricatives, in "fronting," sounds made more anteriorly in the oral cavity are substituted for sounds made more posteriorly (e.g., "cup" produced as [tʌp]), in "backing," the opposite occurs (e.g., the word "tea" is produced as [ki]); in affrication, an affricative sound is substituted, often for a fricative (e.g., the word "shop" is produced as [ʧɑp]) and in gliding, a glide is substituted for another sound, typically a liquid (e.g., the word "lots" produced as [wɑts]).

The "other" processes category includes articulation shifts and idiosyncratic patterns (Gordon-Brannan and Weiss, 2007). In articulation shifts, minimal changes occur in place of articulation, without changes in manner and voicing features. An example of this is substitution of labiodental consonants /f/ and /v/ for the interdental consonants /θ/ and /ð/. Some children use deviations that are unique to their phonological system, such as the use of a preferred sound (e.g., /d/ for all stops, fricative and affricates). This has a significant reduction on intelligibility as the words "two, "goo", Sue", "zoo", and "chew" would all be pronounced as [du]. Gordon-Brannan and Weiss also observed that children may apply more than one phonological process when producing a word. For example, the word "glove" produced as [tʌb] is a result of cluster reduction, velar fronting, and devoicving. Try Activity #4 to practice determining PCC, PVC, and identifying phonological processes for the sample in 2S4.

Articulation Tests

Articulation testing is a clinical procedure to determine which speech sounds an individual produces correctly and incorrectly, when compared against the standard of correct production, and what type of error has been made when a sound is judged to be incorrect. Some tests also include procedures for phonological process analysis. A number of different tests are available. One is described in detail in the following section. Although they share many commonalities, tests differ in overall purpose (e.g., some are designed to assess individual sounds and others, phonological processes), in the set of targeted sounds (e.g., consonants only, or both consonants and vowels) and word positions assessed (e.g., initial, medial, and final, or just initial and final), and in the way in which scores are reported. Tests also differ in the way in which norms were obtained. Some tests exclude children with documented disorders from the normative sample, whereas others use an unselected sample. The size and constitution of the normative sample varies from test to test. Clinicians are therefore highly encouraged to read the test manual carefully and to be aware of the type of cohort against which the tested child is being compared.

One example of a commonly used articulation test is the *Goldman Fristoe 2 Test of Articulation- 2nd Edition* or *GFTA-2* (Goldman and Fristoe, 2000). The *GFTA-2* provides a systematic means of assessing production of the consonant sounds of Standard American English. It samples spontaneous sound production in single words (sounds-in-words section) and in the re-telling of two short picture stories (sounds-in-sentences section). The sounds-in-words section uses pictures to elicit 53 target words that provide 61 opportunities to produce 23 different consonant singletons (/p, m, n, w, h, b, g, k, f, d, ŋ, j, t, ʃ, tʃ, ɹ, l, dʒ, θ, v, s, z, ð/) in the initial, medial, and/or final position as they occur in English (for instance, /ŋ/ does not occur in initial position) and 16 consonant clusters (/bl, bɹ, dɹ, fl, fɹ, gl, gɹ, kl, kɹ, kw, pl, sl, sp, st, sw, tɹ/) in the initial position. Phonetic transcriptions of each test word are provided on the response form beside spaces for the examiner to record the misarticulated (incorrect) productions using the IPA. A discriminative evaluation of the child's production of the target sound(s) in each test word is performed by a person with appropriate training in phonetics and articulation disorders (speech-language pathologist). Sounds identified as being misarticulated are indicated as distortions, omissions, substitutions or additions. On the *GFTA-2*, substitutions are noted by the phonetic symbol of the substituted sound, omitted sounds are noted by using a dash (-), and distortions are noted by "2" if judged to be mild and "3" if judged to be severe. Selected diacritics for nasalization, dentalization, lateralization, prolongation, aspiration, and glottal stops can be used to indicate the type of distortion. Additions are noted by the additional sound plus the correct sound. The errors are entered into a grid on the response form and then counted to determine the total number of articulation errors (range from 0 to 77). This provides the child's raw score on the sounds-in-words section. A similar procedure is used to record the child's responses in the story retell tasks for the sounds-in-sentences section. When the score form is completed for these two sections, the examiner will have a description of the consonant sounds and clusters in each word position that the child produces correctly and incorrectly, in single words and in sentences, and the type of articulation errors made. These can be examined to determine if the child makes more errors on frequently or on less frequently occurring sounds and if errors can be categorized by manner (e.g., gliding of liquids, stopping of fricatives), place (e.g., fronting of velar stops), or voicing features of consonants. Space is provided to note phonological process patterns on the targets. Normative scores that show the child's performance, relative to others of the same age and sex, are available in the test manual for the sounds-in-words section. Raw scores can be converted to standard scores, percentile rank scores and test age equivalents. Appendix 3 reviews test scores and their interpretation for readers' reference.

An example of a test designed to assess the use of phonological processes is the *Khan-Lewis Phonological Analysis* (2nd Ed.) or *KLPA-2* (Khan and Lewis, 2002). The *KLPA-2* provides an opportunity to examine a child's productions of the target words from the *GFTA-2* in order to identify the occurrence of 10 common phonological processes in three broad categories: reduction processes (Deletion of Final Consonants, Syllable Reduction, Stopping of Fricatives and Affricates, Cluster Simplification, Liquid Simplification), place and manner processes (Velar Fronting, Palatal Fronting, Deaffrication), and voicing processes (Initial Voicing and Final Devoicing). After administering the *GFTA-2*, the child's responses are transferred to the *KLPA-2* analysis form where opportunities for each of the 10 processes are examined. The percentage of occurrence of each process is used to determine raw scores, which can then be converted to standard scores, percentile ranks, and test age equivalents.

The *GFTA-2* and *KLPA-2* were not designed to assess vowel production. However, all vowels (except /ʊ/ and /ɔɪ/) are present at least once in the sounds-in-words stimuli so deviations can be observed and noted but are not used to calculate the child's raw score. The test authors provide several reasons for not including vowel assessment. Vowels are less likely to be produced in a deviant manner than consonants; there is dialectical variation in what is considered acceptable production of some vowels; and inter-rater reliability for vowels has been found to be relatively lower than that for consonants. When there are concerns about vowel production, a more complete vowel assessment can be conducted (Pollock, 1994; Stoel-Gammon and Pollock, 2008).

The *GFTA-2* also has a section named "Stimulability." It examines the child's ability to produce each error sound correctly following a model in syllables, words and sentences. Observing the child's responses to strategies to "stimulate" closer approximations of correct sound production when clear models and additional cues are provided about how to make these sounds can help to identify where to start in treatment (sounds for which the child is stimulable) and what approaches may be most appropriate (cues that are effective in shaping more accurate sound productions). Checking the stimulability of untreated speech sound errors periodically provides information about the child's potential readiness to change old patterns for ones that result in accurate sound productions (see also Chapter 20 on diagnostic guidelines for more information on stimulability).

Related Measures

Prosody and Voice

A child's ability to be understood by others is related directly to how clearly the speech sounds of a language are produced but is also influenced by prosody and voice characteristics. As described in Chapter 7, prosodic features cross the boundaries between sound segments and give additional meaning to utterances (i.e., declarative, comment, request, question, emotional coloring, etc.). Shriberg et al. (1992) defined prosody by three parameters: phrasing, rate, and stress. Aspects of phrasing include utterance length, appropriateness of pause locations and rhythmic features. Aspects of rate include the speed of an individual's speech (i.e., too fast, slow, or variable). Aspects of stress include the rate-rhythm patterns of speech (e.g., reduced, excess or equal stress on syllables within a word or across words). Phonetic symbols in the ExtIPA can be used to indicate prosodic characteristics, for example, primary and secondary stress, pause (juncture), rate and intonation.

Shriberg et al. (1992) defined voice by the three parameters of loudness, pitch, and quality. Loudness is observed by noting if a speaker's volume is level, excessive, alternating, or if it decays noticeably over the utterance. Pitch is assessed by observing if it is higher or lower than normal, if there is no pitch change (monopitch), and/or if pitch breaks are present. Shriberg, Kwiatkowski and Rasmussen (1990) classified voice quality into laryngeal and resonance components. Laryngeal features refer to those features generated at the level of the larynx (i.e., breathy, strained-strangled, register breaks) whereas supralaryngeal resonance refers to features generated by articulatory structures above the level of the vocal folds (i.e., nasal, denasal, nasopharyngeal). Phonetic symbols in another extension of the IPA, the Voice Quality Symbols or VoQS (Ball, Esling and Dickson, 1995) can be used to indicate laryngeal and supralaryngeal characteristics, for example, creaky voice, falsetto and nasalized voice.

There are few standardized procedures that have been published to measure prosody and voice using perceptual features. A measure that has been used with children is the *Prosody-Voice Screening Profile (PVSP)* (Shriberg, et al., 1990). The *PVSP* has excellent training and scoring procedures. A reference database is available for speech-normal and speech-delayed children between 3 and 19 years of age in the form of a technical report (Shriberg, Kwiatkowski, Rasmussen, Lof, and Miller, 1992). The *PVSP* assigns codes based on whether or not an utterance is "appropriate" (1) or "not appropriate". If an utterance is deemed "not appropriate" under any of the 3 characteristics of prosody or the 3 characteristics of voice, it is assigned a code that describes what was inappropriate about the utterance. A profile of the child's scores on each of the three prosody and three voice scales is generated to compare with normative cut-off scores.

Acoustic measures of temporal and spectral characteristics of voice and prosody features can be made from audio recordings to supplement and augment perceptual measures. For example, the waveform can be examined to determine if the acoustic correlates of syllable stress (duration, intensity and fundamental frequency) are the same when two syllables have been judged perceptually to have equal stress. Play file 2V4 to hear and see an example of two waveforms of the word "buddy." In one, the word was perceived to have primary stress on the first syllable and secondary stress on the second syllable (standard pronunciation) and in the other, the word was perceived to have equal (primary) stress on each syllable. An example of an acoustic measure for lexical stress is the lexical stress ratio (Shriberg,

Campbell, Karlsson, Brown, McSweeny, and Nadler, 2003). It is reported to have diagnostic significance for children with childhood apraxia of speech.

Access Video File 4 (Chapter 2)

2V4 The word "buddy" with standard lexical stress on the first syllable and with equal stress on both syllables.

Speech Intelligibility and Acceptability

Speech sound accuracy, prosody and voice characteristics contribute to how well a child's speech can be understood by listeners (intelligibility) and how well it conforms to what is expected for a child of the same age and sex (acceptability). Speech intelligibility and speech acceptability are referred to as global or integrative measures because they reflect multidimensional aspects of speech. They also provide a more functional estimate of the impact of a speech sound disorder on a child's spoken communication than articulation tests or percent phonemes correct scores. Weiss (1980) stated that by age four years, audio recordings of children's conversational speech should be close to 100 percent intelligibility to unfamiliar listeners who are asked to write what the child said, word-by-word, and do not know what the child is attempting to say. This is referred to as a word identification task. The child may still have some age-appropriate speech sound errors but these do not interfere with listeners' ability to understand what he is saying. Note that this is orthographic (alphabetic), not phonetic transcription. Play file 2S11 to listen to four utterances of a child with speech sound disorder of unknown origin. His three utterances have a total of 20 words. How many of them can you understand?

Access Sound File 11 (Chapter 2)

2S11 Four utterances (20 words) produced by a child with a speech sound disorder of unknown origin.

Figure 2.6. compares his word identification scores on single word, imitated sentences on the *Test of Children's Speech (TOCS+)* Intelligibility Measures (Hodge and Gotzke 2010; 2011; also see www.tocs.plus.ualberta.ca) and 100 contiguous words from a spontaneous speech sample. It is apparent that the type of sample influences his intelligibility scores.

Hodge and Whitehill (2010) provide detailed information about the issues, challenges and methods of intelligibility measurement. Gordon-Brannan and Hodson (2000) compared the intelligibility scores of 4 – 5-year-old children with a range of speech production proficiency on several types of speech samples. Based on their results, they recommended that the preferred sample type was spontaneous speech using word transcription tasks by unfamiliar listeners. In many cases, direct measures of intelligibility are not made because of time constraints and instead estimates or ratings are made of how intelligible a child's speech is.

For example, a rating scale by Morris, Wilcox and Schooling (1995) ranged from "conversational speech reflects adult patterns" to "conversational speech is intelligible only with knowledge of context and familiarity with the child and child's sound system." However, identification measures of intelligibility are preferred because they are more reliable and more sensitive than estimates and ratings. Examples of word identification intelligibility measures for children include the *Children's Speech Intelligibility Measure* (Wilcox and Morris, 1999) and the *TOCS+ Intelligibility Measures* (Hodge and Gotzke 2010; 2011).

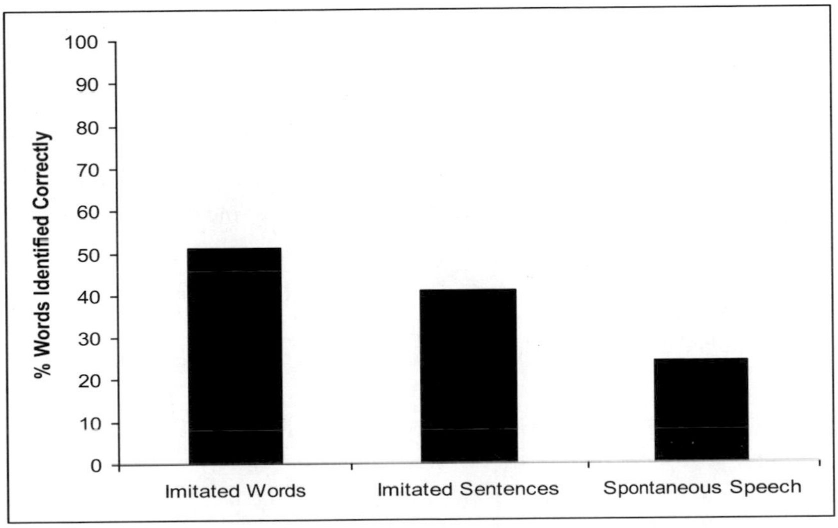

Figure 2.6. Comparison of word identification intelligibility scores on an imitated word and imitated sentence tasks and a 100-word contiguous spontaneous sample recorded during play.

Acceptability is a less well-understood and less common measure of speech function than intelligibility. Definitions of acceptability range from subjective impressions of the pleasingness of speech (Witzel, 1995) to the potential for a person to experience social, educational, or vocational problems because of speech (Lang, Starr, and Moller, 1992). Rating scales are used typically to indicate listeners' judgments about perceived "acceptability".

Files 2S12 and 2S13 are recordings of an 8-year-old girl obtained before and following treatment to correct consonant and vowel articulation errors, increase overall vocal pitch and improve intonation and stress patterning. Using the scale in Figure 2.7, rate her acceptability for each recording. Which recording do you think was made post-treatment? Why?

Access Sound File 12 (Chapter 2)

2S12 Recordings of a child pre- and post-treatment.

Access Sound File 13 (Chapter 2)

2S13 Recordings of a child pre- and post-treatment.

1 2 3 4 5 6 7

Acceptable Unacceptable

Figure 2.7 Acceptability scale. Circle the number that represents your perception of the recorded samples in 2S12 and 2S13, based on your expectations for an 8-year-old girl.

How Can we Use Acoustic Analyses to Supplement Descriptions of Children's Speech Sound Production?

The physical speech signal represented in recorded acoustic waveforms can be examined, measured and analyzed to describe timing, frequency, and intensity characteristics of speech sounds. The frequency components of a speech signal and their relative amplitude are referred to as its "spectral" characteristics that change over time.

For some speech sounds, such as stop consonants, spectral characteristics change very rapidly. For others like monophthong vowels and fricatives, spectral characteristics are relatively stable while for others like diphthongs and glides, spectral changes occur but at a slower rate than for stops. The details of timing and spectral characteristics that can be resolved in the acoustic waveform and in further analyses of these to produce **spectrograms** and **spectra** surpass that of the human nervous system.

Sidebar 2.4. Spectrum

A **spectrum (plural = spectra)** is a display that is usually made of a short section of a sound segment (e.g., a section from a vowel or a fricative). The display shows the relative amplitude (SPL shown on Y axis) of the frequency components (shown on X axis) of the section of the signal that has been selected.

Therefore, it can be very useful to supplement perceptual descriptions of speech sounds with acoustic ones. Free downloadable acoustic software (www.fon.hum.uva.nl/praat/) called Praat (Boersma and Weenink, 2005) can be used to record and measure waveforms of speech audio recordings and create spectrograms and spectral displays. It is fun to make recordings of your speech and then "see" what it looks like. The process of relating speech sounds to their visual representation is referred to as "segmenting" a spectrogram. Examples of segmented spectrograms (with waveforms above) for the authors' first names appear in Figure 2.8. Activity #5 provides a chance to try this out for yourself.

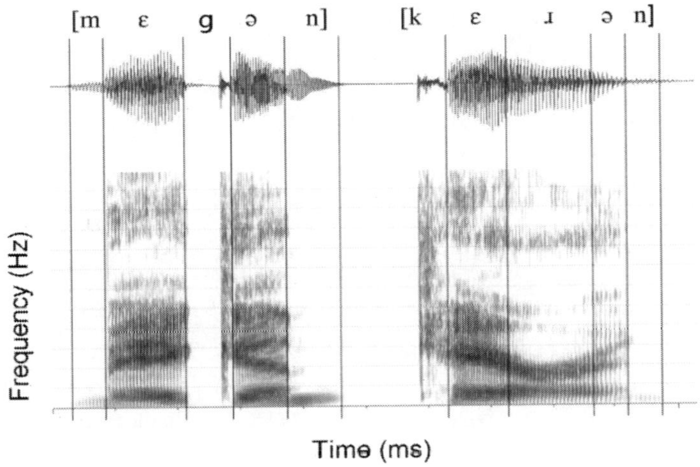

Figure 2.8. Segmented spectrograms and waveforms for the authors' first names.

Spectral-temporal characteristics have been identified that are "*acoustic cues*" to the recognition of articulatory features of obstruent and sonorant sound classes. These include cues for voicing, place and manner features of obstruents (stops, fricatives and affricates), cues for manner and place for sonorants (nasals, liquids and glides) and cues for height, place, rounding, length, and manner (monophthong vs. diphthong) for vowels.

The following sections provided examples of acoustic cues for articulatory features of various sound classes and how they may provide insights about a child's speech sound productions beyond those obtained from perceptual methods.

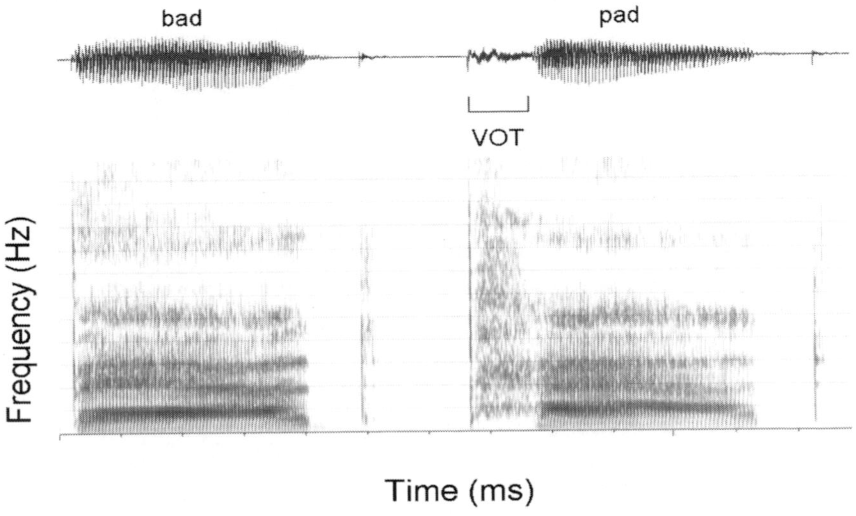

Figure 2.9. Waveform above and wideband spectrogram below of a recording of the words "bad" and "pad" that were perceived as accurate productions.

Obstruents. One of the most common measures of timing is **voice onset tim***e* or VOT. This is the duration in milliseconds between the release of a stop burst and the onset of vocal fold vibration for the following vowel. Figure 2.9 shows a waveform above and spectrogram below of a recording of the words “bad” and “pad”. Note that VOT is longer for /p/ than /b/ and that the stop burst has greater amplitude for /p/ than /b/. In addition, aspiration “noise” is visible during the VOT interval for /p/. VOT, burst amplitude and presence/absence of aspiration noise in the VOT interval are three cues to the voiced-voiceless feature contrast, with VOT being the “primary” cue.

Sidebar 2.5. Aspiration

Aspiration is the noise produced by airflow through the constricting vocal folds following the release of a voiceless stop. The vocal folds are still separated when the occlusion is released. This results in air flowing through the closing glottis for a short period of time after the release. The singleton /t/ in “top” is aspirated but not the cluster member /t/ in “stop.”

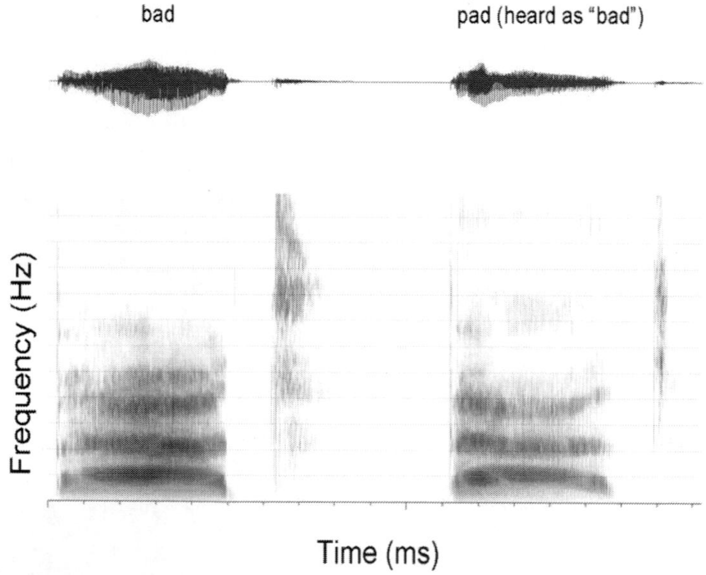

Figure 2.10. Waveforms and spectrograms for the words “bad” and “pad” produced by a 5-year-old child. Both words were transcribed as [bæd] by an experienced transcriber.

In general, VOTs that are shorter than 20 ms are typically perceived as voiced stops and VOTs longer than 20 ms are typically perceived as voiceless stops. When voicing errors are perceived, acoustic descriptions of VOT provide more detailed information about the child’s articulatory timing for voiced and voiceless stops. Figure 2-10 shows the waveforms and spectrograms for the words “pad” and “bad” produced by a 5 year-old child with a speech sound disorder. An experienced listener transcribed each of these words as [bæd]. Why do you think this is? Looking at the spectrograms and waveforms, do you think the child is using the same VOT when making /b/ and /p/? If not, is the difference in the direction that you expect for voiced and voiceless consonants? More information about acoustic cues for stop voicing in children with phonological disorders can be found in Forrest and Rockman (1988). Chapters 12 and 14 describe how VOT is used in different languages by monolingual children learning Korean and bilingual children learning English and Spanish.

As was shown in Figure 2.3, voiced fricatives can be distinguished from voiceless fricatives by the presence of phonation (voice) combined with noise in the fricative segment. Which fricative segment shown in 2V5 has both **periodic** and aperiodic sound?

Access Video File 5 (Chapter 2)

2V5 Voiced and voiceless fricatives before the vowel /i/.

Acoustic cues for stop place of articulation include spectral characteristics of the stop burst and the onset of the second formant frequency in the transition from the release of the stop to the following vowel (F2 locus). During occlusion for a stop, there is little or no acoustic energy, but upon rapid release of the constriction, the transient burst of air escaping from the oral cavity creates noise.

Although the noise burst is of short duration (usually no more than 40 ms), its spectrum holds important acoustic cues that can be used to identify the place of articulation. For example, acoustic cues that have been found to distinguish alveolar from velar word-initial stops are the mean frequency and shape of the burst spectra (Kent and Read, 2002). Alveolar stop bursts have higher mean frequencies (e.g., 2500-400 Hz for adults) and the shape of their spectra appears to "fall" over time, while velar stop bursts have relatively lower mean frequencies (1500-2500 Hz for adults) and have a more "compact" shape. In addition, the F2 locus for alveolar stops is around 1800 Hz for adults. In contrast, the F2 locus for velar stops can be in two regions depending on the place of the following vowel (around 1300 Hz before back vowels and around 3000 Hz before front vowels). Figure 2.11 shows the waveforms and spectrograms for the words "tea" and "key" produced by the first author and judged to be accurate. Estimates of the F2 loci are marked with a white lines. The burst spectra for a 20 ms segment of the initial consonants, centered on the stop burst, are shown below each word.

Compare Figure 2.11 with Figure 2.12, which shows the same displays for these words produced by a child who was described as having a "fronting" error pattern. How do the acoustic cues differ for the production of "key" in Figure 2.11 and 2.12s? Does this fit with what you now know about what acoustic cues distinguish velar from alveolar place?

To learn more about the acoustic characteristics of voiceless stops that differ in place of articulation /p, t, k/ in adults' and children's (aged 3-5 years) productions, see Nissen and Fox (2009). These same authors also studied the acoustic characteristics of fricatives that differ in place (/s, ʃ/) (Nissen and Fox, 2005).

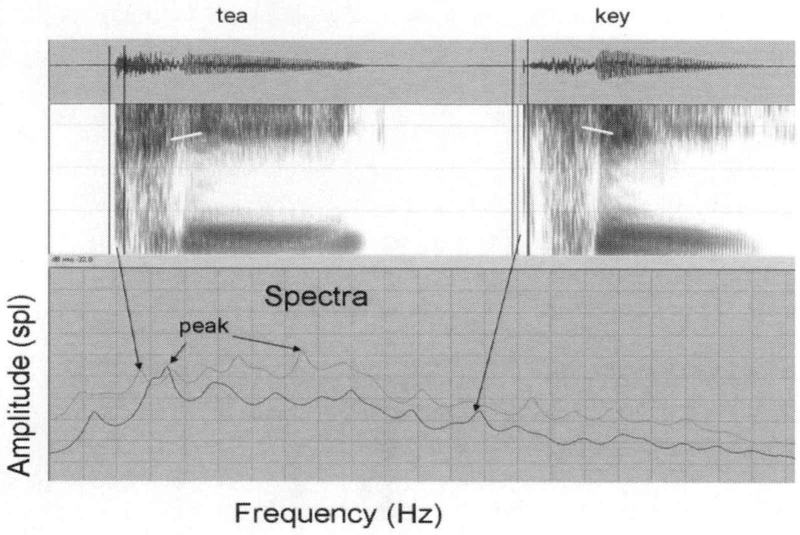

Figure 2.11. Waveforms and spectrograms for the words "tea" and "key" produced by the first author. Estimated F2 loci are indicated with a white line. Burst spectra for a 20 ms segment of the initial consonants, centered on the stop burst are shown in the lowest panel below the respective words. Note that the burst spectrum for [t] (gray trace) has a higher peak frequency than the burst spectrum for [k] (black trace).

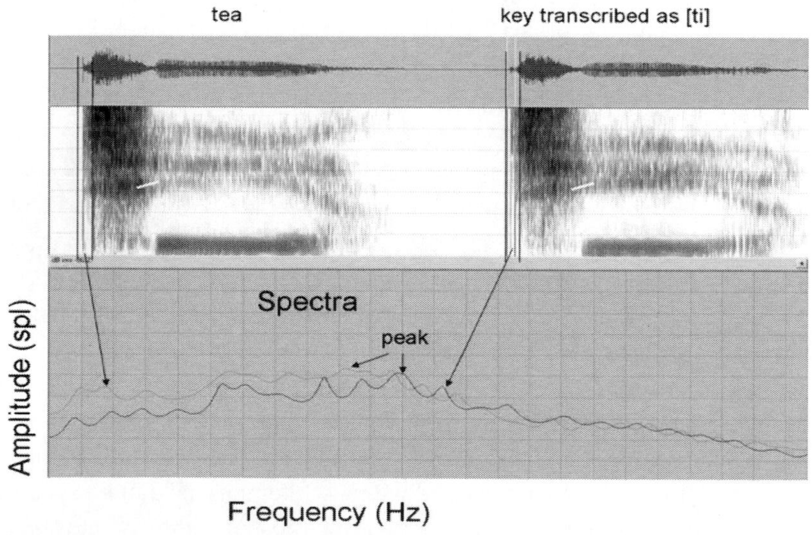

Figure 2.12. Waveforms and spectrograms for the words "tea" and "key" produced by a 5-year-old child with a "fronting" error pattern. Estimated F2 loci are indicated with a white line. Burst spectra for a 20 ms segment of the initial consonants, centered on the stop burst are shown in the lowest panel below the respective words. Note that the burst spectrum for [t] (gray trace) is very similar in shape to the burst spectrum for the first sound in the child's attempted production of "key."

Acoustic cues that distinguish stop, fricative and affricate manners of articulation are noise duration and noise rise time (Kent and Read, 2002). Longer duration (greater than 130 ms) and high-frequency noise is a hallmark of fricatives compared to stops (duration less than 75 ms). An affricate combines the acoustic cues for a stop followed by a fricative at the same place of articulation but the duration of the fricative portion in the affricate is shorter than in fricatives. Figure 2.13 shows the waveforms and spectrograms for the words "two" and "sue" produced by the first author and judged to be accurate. The slower noise rise time and longer noise duration is apparent for the fricative /s/. Noise rise time is the time it takes the amplitude envelope to reach its maximum value (Kent and Read, 2002). Stops and affricates have more rapid rise times (< 33 ms) than fricatives (>76 ms). Figure 2.14 shows the waveforms and spectrograms for the words "two" and "sue" produced by a child but were both transcribed as [tu]. Why do you think the child was perceived to "stop" the fricative /s/? Replay media file 2V2 to see waveforms for a word initial voiceless stop, fricative and affricate.

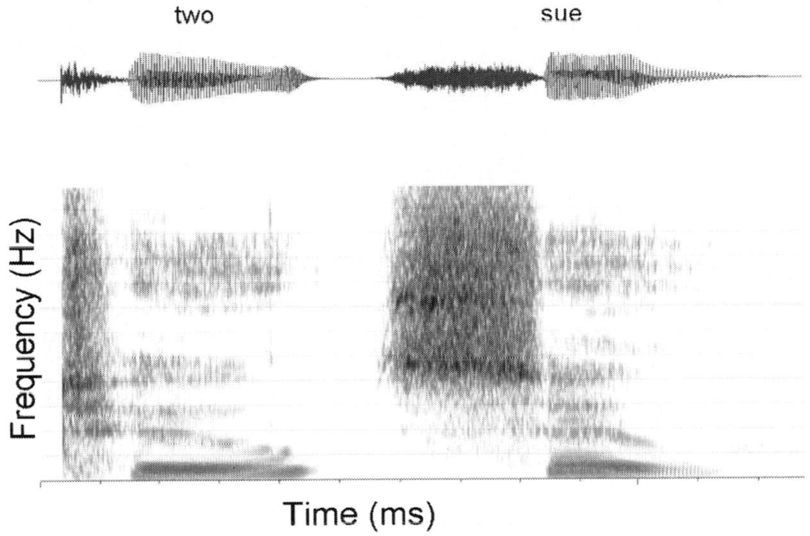

Figure 2.13. Waveforms and spectrograms for the words "two" and "sue" produced by the first author and judged to be accurate.

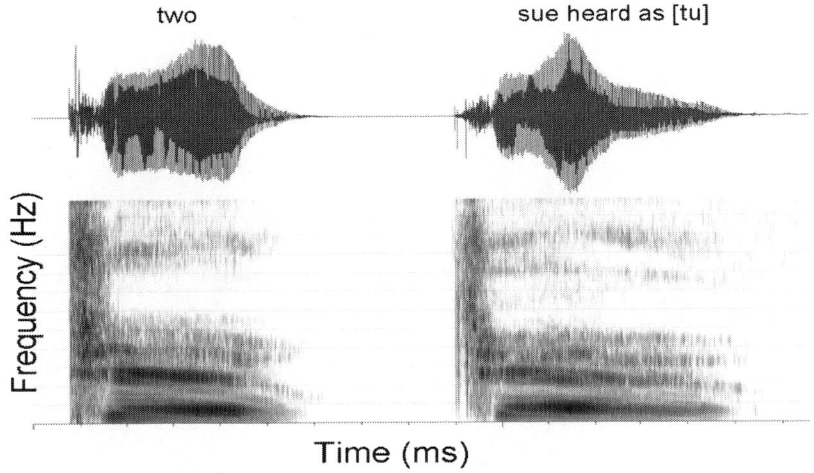

Figure 2.14. Waveforms and spectrograms for the words "two" and "sue" produced by a child but were both transcribed as [tu].

Vowels. As described in the section on source-filter theory, vowels are distinguished by their formant frequencies that reflect resonating frequencies of the vocal tract cavities. The relative frequencies and distance between formants provides the distinctive acoustic identity of speech sounds. Vowels can be identified from spectrograms using knowledge of the principles that relate articulatory parameters (how the tongue, lips and mandible change the relative length and cross-sectional area of the resonating cavities of the vocal tract) to the relative location and spacing of their respective first two formants. The first formant frequency (F1) is related to the degree of vocal tract constriction. The more open the vocal tract (i.e., the lower the vowel), the higher is F1. As vowel height increases, F1 frequency decreases. Therefore, F1 is relatively lower for high vowels than low vowels.

The second formant frequency (F2) is related to the site of vocal tract constriction. The more anterior the site of vocal tract constriction, the higher is F2. As site of major vocal tract constriction moves from back to front, F2 frequency increases. Therefore, front vowels have relatively higher F2 frequencies than back vowels. Principles that relate higher formants to articulation are more complex and less well understood. As the degree of lip rounding/protrusion increases, all formants decrease, with the greatest effect on the second formant (F2).

Figure 2.15 shows waveforms and wideband spectrograms of the words "heat," "hat," "hut," "hot," and "hoot" produced by a 6-year-old girl with typical speech production. Does the pattern of F1 and F2 across the five vowels fit with the articulatory principles relating formants to vowel place and height? For the vowel /u/, is there acoustic evidence that the child was increasing lip rounding during the vowel? (Hint: Does F2 decrease during /u/ or is it stable?)

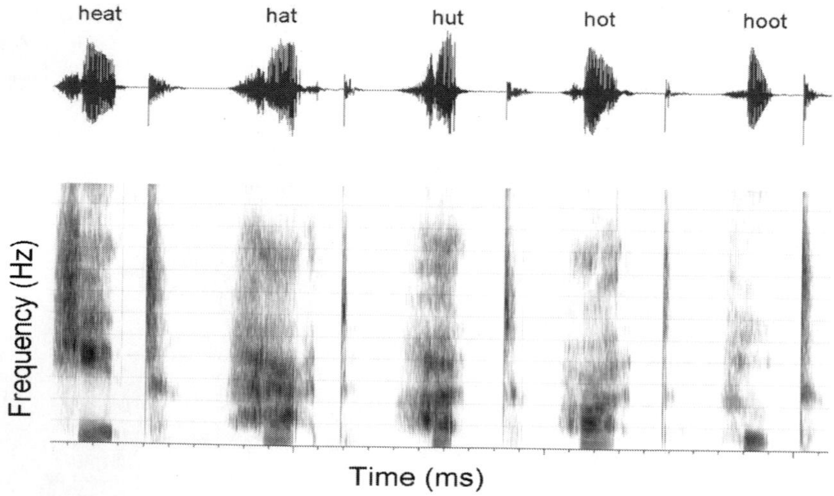

Figure 2.15. Waveforms and wideband spectrograms of the words "heat," "hat," "hot," and "hoot" produced by a 6-year-old girl with typical speech production.

Figure 2.16 shows waveforms and wideband spectrograms for the words "shot" and "shut" recorded from a 5-year-old boy with a speech sound disorder. An experienced listener transcribed both these words as [ʃʌt]. Is this what you might expect from examining F1 and F2 for the two vowels shown in the spectrogram?

Sidebar 2.6. Corner Vowels

Corner or "point" vowels are the ones that are found at the extremes of the classic vowel height and place chart. In western Canadian English, the dialect of the first author and her research population, these include the highest, front vowel /i/, the lowest front vowel /æ/, the highest back vowel /u/ and the lowest back vowel /ɑ/. A vowel "quadrilateral is created when the F1 and F2 center frequencies are measured and plotted on an X-Y plot (F1 on the X axis and F2 on the Y axis). The lines are connected between the points to form a four-sided figure. The area enclosed by this quadrilateral is sometimes referred to as the "vowel" area or space. Several studies have shown that size of vowel area is correlated positively with a child's speech intelligibility (e.g., Higgins and Hodge, 2002). Try Activity #6 to create a vowel quadrilateral of your corner vowels.

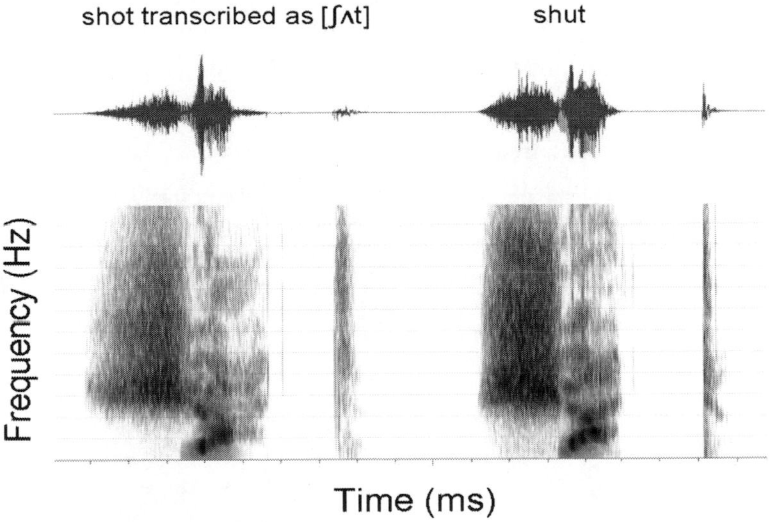

Figure 2.16. Waveforms and wideband spectrograms for the words "shot" and "shut" recorded from a 5-year-old boy with a speech sound disorder.

Diphthongs are characterized by formant transitions as vocal tract configuration changes from the onset to offset. Figure 2.17 shows spectrograms of a 4-year-old's production of the words "top" and "type". Observe that for the monophthong vowel in "top", the formants are relatively stable while in the diphthong in "type," formant transitions are obvious as vowel place shifts forward (F2) and vowel height increases (F1). If a child has slow and limited tongue and jaw movements, how do you think the formants of this diphthong would be affected?

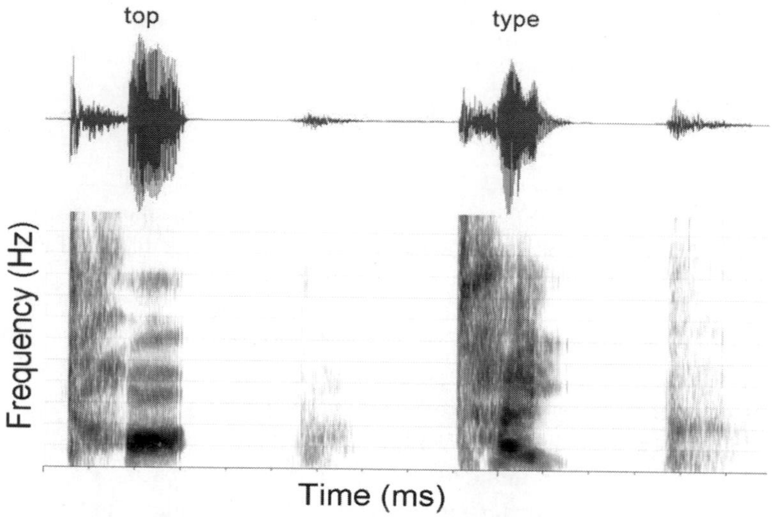

Figure 2.17. Spectrograms of a 4-year-old's production of the words "top" and "type" judged to be accurate.

Glides and Liquids. These consonants are also sonorants. Glides are like diphthongs in that they involve a change from one vocal tract configuration to another. However, the rate of change from one vocal tract configuration to the next is faster so resonant frequencies change more rapidly in glides than diphthongs (i.e., formant transition rates are greater in glides than diphthongs). Glides /w/ versus /j/ can be distinguished by their relative F2 values and the direction of their F2 formant transitions to and from adjacent sounds. Their perception depends primarily on F1 and F2. F1 is low in both due to high tongue position at the start: /w/ like /u/; /j/ like /i/. For /w/: F2 rises as lips unround and tongue moves from /u/ position, except when /u/ follows, as in /wu/. For /j/, F2 falls as tongue position moves from /i/ position, except when /i/ follows, as in /ji/.

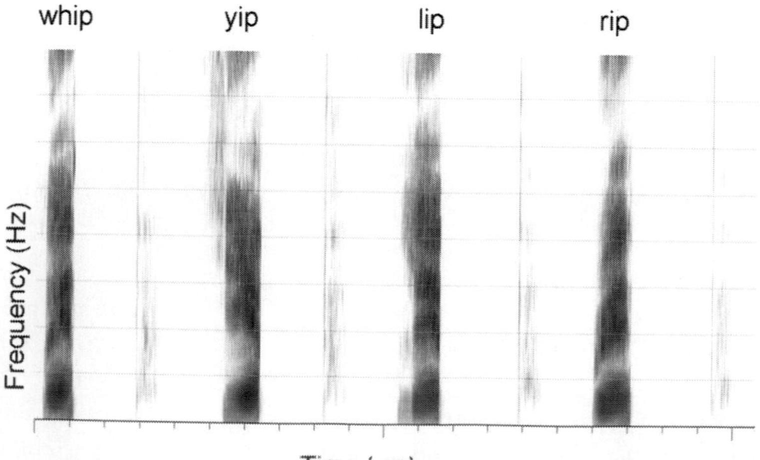

Figure 2.18. Wideband spectrograms of the words "whip", "yip", "lip" and "rip" produced by the first author.

For liquid /l/ versus /ɹ/, F1 and F2 frequencies are similar for both; transition to the following vowel is slower for /ɹ/ (e.g., 300 ms), and faster for /l/ (e.g., 70-100 ms). Their perceptual distinction is based on F3. For /ɹ/: F3 is very close to F2, with a separation of F2 and F3 into the following vowel. Figure 2.18 shows wideband spectrograms of the words "whip", "yip", "lip" and "rip" produced by the first author. Observe how the F1, F2 and F3 patterns change for the glides and the liquids.

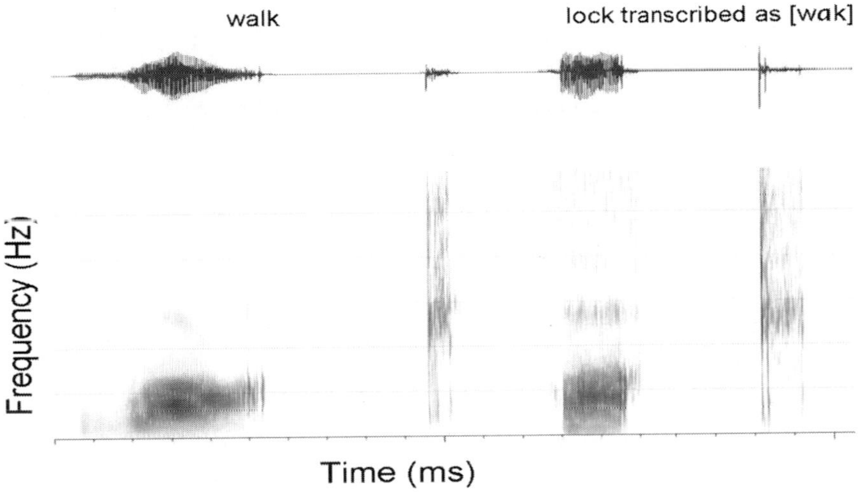

Figure 2.19. Wideband spectrograms of the words "walk" and "lock" produced by a child before treatment.

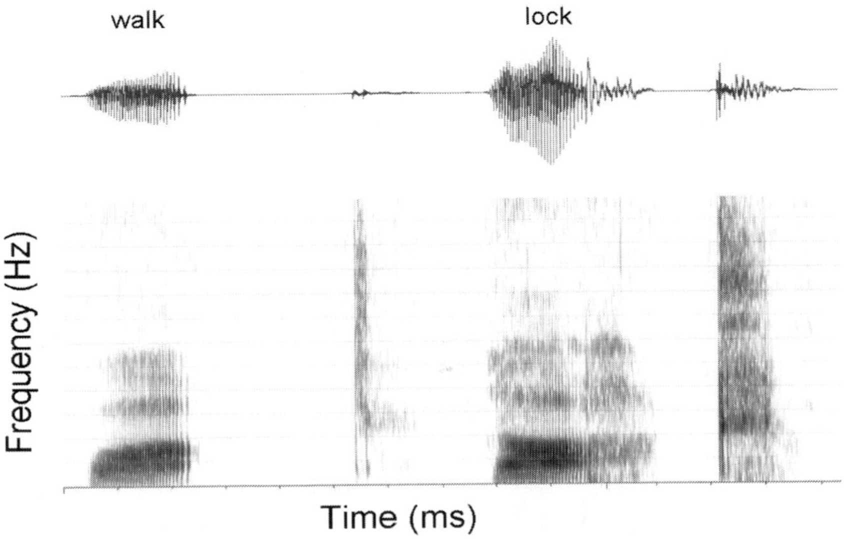

Figure 2.20. Wideband spectrograms of the words "walk" and "lock" produced by the same child in Figure 2.19 after treatment.

Figure 2.19 shows wideband spectrograms of the words "walk" and "lock" produced by a child with a speech sound disorder. An experienced listener transcribed both words as [wɑk]. Do the formant patterns for the initial sounds in each word appear similar? Figure 2.20 shows the same child saying these words after articulation treatment. In this case, a listener not involved in treatment transcribed these words as [wɑk] and [lɑk], respectively. Does the spectrogram support what the listener heard?

Syllable Structure. Acoustic analyses can also provide insights into children's syllable structure errors. For example, Figure 2.21, shows the waveform and spectrogram of the words "stop" and "top" produced by a child with cerebral palsy. Both words were transcribed as [tɑp] (i.e., described as cluster reduction on "stop"). However, examination of the waveform reveals a shorter VOT, smaller burst amplitude and minimal aspiration in the child's production of the word "stop" compared to "top". These differences suggest that the child is not producing these two words in the same way even though they were perceived to be the same word.

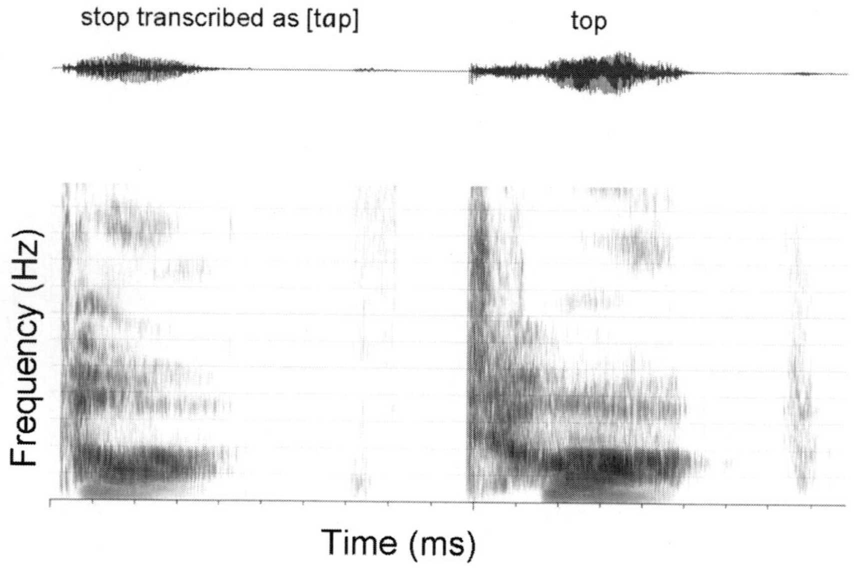

Figure 2.21. Waveforms and spectrograms of the words "stop" and "top" produced by a child. Both words were transcribed as [tɑp].

Figure 2.22 shows a child's production of the word "bad" that was transcribed as [bæ] (i.e., described as final consonant deletion). However, examination of the waveform reveals that F2 is moving upward to the locus for /d/. This suggests that the child is actually marking the final consonant but not in a way that can be perceived. Productions such as these, in which the child is perceived to neutralize a contrast in the adult language, but upon closer inspection (for example, of a waveform and/or spectrogram) is found to produce a contrast, is known as a **covert contrast**.

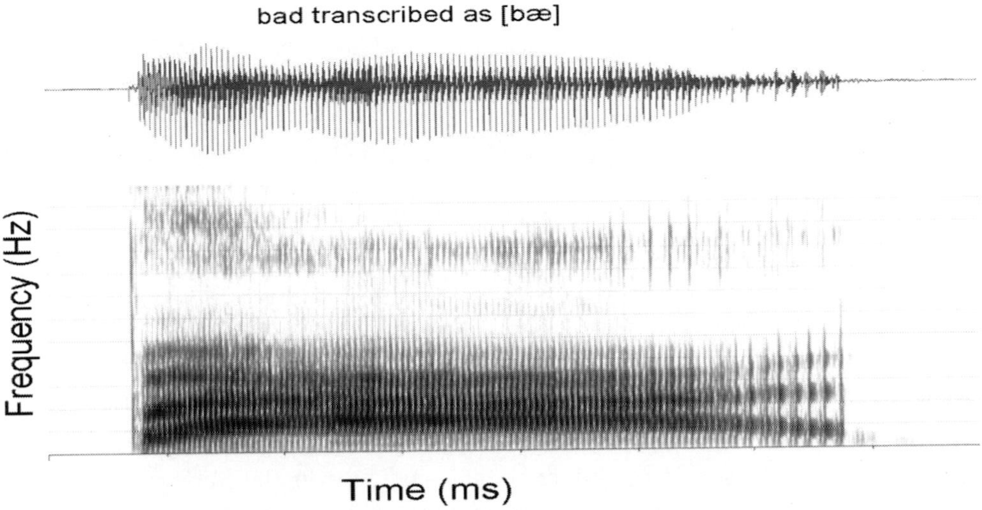

Figure 2.22. Waveform and spectrogram of a child's production of the word "bad" where the final consonant was not perceived but the formant patterns at the end of the vowel are moving in the direction expected for /d/.

This section has provided examples of acoustic cues that distinguish the sound classes of English. When children are perceived to make speech sound errors, acoustic analyses can be used to examine these in more detail and capture differences between sounds that are not perceptible. This information may assist in selecting treatment goals and determining treatment effectiveness.

CONNECTIONS

The science of speech behavior and its development draws on multiple fields of study. Chapter 3 describes the biological substrates of speech. The present chapter illustrates how theories from the fields of acoustics, linguistics (phonology and phonetics), and psychology have been applied to describe and measure speech behaviours. These methods and measures are integral to collecting and interpreting data to describe and classify types of speech sound disorders, the topic of Chapter 15. You will revisit them again in Chapter 20 when considering guidelines for assessment and in Chapter 21, when you learn about measures that are evaluated for "evidence" of the effectiveness of therapy. Many of the remaining chapters illustrate how perceptual and acoustic descriptions have been used to investigate speech development and disorders, for instance, Chapter 4 on pre-speech development. We hope that you find this chapter to be a useful reference that stimulates you to learn more about children's speech behaviors and how they can be measured.

CONCLUDING REMARKS

In this chapter you have learned that source-filter theory explains the relationships among articulatory, acoustic and auditory phonetics. In other words, it explains how actions of the speech muscles create the sound patterns of speech and the acoustic cues that distinguish the consonants and vowels of a language that are perceived by listeners to understand what has been said. Methods from these inter-related areas of phonetics are used to describe and measure children's speech sound production abilities. The primary method is phonetic transcription, a skill that requires extensive training and practice to master for children, especially with speech sound disorders. Phonetic transcription of children's speech samples provides the "raw material" for various analyses that are used to describe children's speech development at a given time, compare descriptions over time, and make decisions about the existence, nature and severity of a speech sound disorder. Therefore, it is important to ensure that a sample appropriate for the measurement purpose is obtained. It is recommended that a high fidelity recording be made of the child's speech sample to check the reliability of the transcription. Acoustic analyses can be used to augment phonetic transcription because they reveal fine-grained timing and spectral details in the speech signal that may not be discernable by the human ear. Independent and relational analyses can be performed on the "raw material" generated through phonetic transcriptions to describe a child's speech sound inventory, individual speech sound errors, patterns of speech sound deviations (phonological processes) and measure speech sound accuracy. Speech sound accuracy and prosody and voice characteristics contribute to a child's speech intelligibility and acceptability. These are global measures of speech production competence that are challenging to measure reliably but provide important information about the functional impact of a speech sound disorder on a child's life. By completing the suggested learning activities, you will gain skill and confidence in applying and extending your new knowledge to describe and measure speech production abilities in children with and without speech sound disorders.

Chapter Review Questions

1. The source-filter theory describes speech production as a two-part process. Describe how the two "sound sources" are generated for speech. How does the vocal tract act like a "filter" to produce the distinctive sound patterns of individual consonants and vowels?
2. Deciding what type of speech sample to collect depends on the purpose of your assessment. What are some of the factors that should be considered? Discuss the advantages and disadvantages of imitated versus spontaneous samples and single word versus connected speech samples.
3. What is the purpose of speech-like tasks? How do they differ from speech tasks? Give two examples of speech-like tasks and explain what information they provide regarding children's speech abilities.
4. Phonetic transcription using the International Phonetic Alphabet (IPA) is a basic tool used by speech-language pathologists and others to represent the speech sounds produced by a speaker. Provide a rationale for collecting high quality audio recordings of the speech samples to be transcribed. Then list three ways to ensure that that the audio recording has high fidelity.

5. What is the difference between independent and relational analyses of speech samples? Give one example of each. What type of analysis does an articulation test provide?
6. Calculate PCC and PCC-R for the following brief speech sample:

teach	[t̪iʃ]
clock	[təlɑk]
clown	[k̬waʊn]
fish	[fɪʃ]
balloon	[bəwum]
broom	[bwʌm]
thumb	[s̪ʌm]
yellow	[lɛloʊ]
rose	[woʊs]
rain	[wẽɪ]

7. Using the sample provided in question 6 above, calculate WWA and PWP.
8. Define the three parameters of prosody and of voice according to Shriberg et al. How might prosody and voice influence the intelligibility of a child's speech?
9. Intelligibility and acceptability are global measures of children's speech. How do intelligibility and acceptability differ from each other and how can they be measured?
10. What acoustic cues could you examine to support a perceptual judgment that a child was making voicing errors on initial stops? What acoustic cues could you examine to support a perceptual judgment that the child was also "centralizing" vowel productions?

SUGGESTIONS FOR FURTHER READING

Review of Articulatory Phonetics and Phonetic Transcription

Small, L.H. (2005). Phonetics: *A practical guide for students* (2nd Ed). Boston: Allyn and Bacon. (includes exercises and audio CD)

Bauman-Waengler, J. (2009*). Introduction to Phonetics and Phonology: from Concepts to Transcription.* Boston: Pearson. (includes workbook and DVD.)

http://web.uvic.ca/ling/resources/ipa/charts/IPAlab/IPAlab.htm - provides audio examples of all IPA sounds - the full interactive version is only available to registered users and U. Victoria students, but the limited version is freely accessible.

http://www.yorku.ca/earmstro/ipa/index.html similar site from York U - nice addition is flash animation demo of diphthongs.

Pollock, K.E., Berni, M.B. (2001). Transcription of vowels. *Topics in Language Disorders*, 21, 22-40.

Powell, T.W. (2001). Phonetic transcription of disordered speech. *Topics in Language Disorders*, 21, 52-72.

Stoel-Gammon, C. (2001). Transcribing the speech of young children. *Topics in Language Disorders*, 21 (4), 12-21.

Phonological Assessment

AJSLP (2002) special forum on phonology – *American Journal of Speech-Language Pathology,* Volume 11(3), pp. 211-263. (contains 11 brief articles by various authors).

Other Languages

McLeod, S. (2007). The International Guide to Speech Acquisition. Clifton Park, N. Y.: Thomson Delmar Learning. This resource covers 24 different languages and many dialects of English and includes information on articulation and phonology assessment tools in that language.

Intelligibility and Acceptability

Flipsen, P. (2006). Measuring the intelligibility of conversational speech in children. *Clinical Linguistics and Phonetics*, 20(4), 303-312.

Gordon-Brannan, M., Hodson, B.W. (2000). Intelligibility/Severity measurements of prekindergarten children's speech. *American Journal of Speech-Language Pathology,* 9, 141-150.

Hodge, M.M., Whitehill, T. (2010). Intelligibility impairments. In J. S. Damico, M. J. Ball, and N Müller (Eds.) *Handbook of Language and Speech Disorders*. pp 99-114. Blackwell Publishers.

Hodge, M.M., Gotzke, C. L. (2011). Minimal pair distinctions and intelligibility in preschool children with and without speech sound disorders. Clinical Linguistics and Phonetics, 25(10), 853–863.

Speech Acoustics

Reetz, H., Jongman, A. (2009). *Phonetics: Transcription, production, acoustics, and perception* p. 105. Chichester, West Sussex: Wiley-Blackwell.

Kent, R.D and Read (2002). *The acoustic analysis of speech* (2nd ed). Albany, N. Y.: Singular/Thompson Learning.

Suggestions for Student Activities

1. Read the article by Rvachew et al. (2005) and then use the recordings for the tasks that are provided with this chapter for an 8-year-old girl to classify her performance as showing signs of dysarthria, apraxia of speech, or neither.

   Access Sound Files 14 - 43 (Chapter 2)

2. Read the Syllable Repetition Task Technical (SRT) Report (Shriberg and Lohmeier, 2008) available at *www.waisman.wisc.edu/phonology/technical report* and then follow the directions to obtain the scores for a 7-year-old boy whose recordings for the task are provided with the chapter. (Note that a revised reference database for the SRT has been published (Lohmeier and Shriberg, 2011) and is posted on the same website.)

   Access Sound File 44 (Chapter 2)

3. Create a "gloss" for the single word speech sample in file 2S4 and generate a phonetic transcription of the standard adult production underneath each word, leaving space below each standard transcription for a transcription of the child's utterances. Next, generate a phonetic transcription of the child's production below each word's standard transcription. Use your transcriptions to create a sound and wordshape inventory (independent analysis) for the child's word productions in the sample. Then conduct a relational analysis to identity the sounds and word shapes that the child produced incorrectly at least once in the sample words.
4. Determine PCC and PVC scores for the words produced by the child in file 2S4. Then determine percent WWA for the words produced by the child in file 2S4. Identify phonological processes that could account for the errors produced by the child in file 2S4.
5. Use Praat to make a recording of yourself saying your name and then create a spectrogram of the recording. See how well you are at "reading" the changing spectral patterns over time to find the sections of the spectrogram that match each of the consonant and vowel sounds in your name. This process is referred to as "segmenting" a spectrogram.
6. Use Praat to make a recording of yourself saying the words "heat", "hat", "hot" and "hoot." Measure the first and second formants at the midpoint of each vowel segment. Then plot the F1 and F2 coordinates for each vowel segment on a graph to create a "vowel quadrilateral". Refer to Higgins and Hodge (2002) for more instructions about procedures.

7. Use Praat to examine the pre and post treatment recordings in files 2S12 and 2S13. Based on what you have learned about speech acoustics, can you find acoustic "evidence" that her vocal pitch and production of vowels and /ɹ/ improved in the post-recording?

ANSWERS TO CHAPTER REVIEW QUESTIONS

1. Describe how the two "sound sources" are generated for speech. How does the vocal tract act like a "filter" to produce the distinctive sound patterns of individual consonants and vowels?

Voice is produced by the interaction of the adducted vocal folds resisting the pressurized air stream that results in regularly occurring open-close cycles of the vocal folds. The air flowing through the vocal folds causes a momentary pressure drop and they fall back together and the cycle is repeated. In this way, the vocal folds are set into vibration. As the vocal folds snap back to midline during the closing phase of each cycle, they create a **complex sound**. The periodic recurrence of this sound results in "voice" or "phonation". Noise is produced by random disturbances in air pressure that are sufficient to create sound. This sound is referred to as aperiodic because there is not a regular pattern in its component frequencies. It is produced during speech in several ways (corresponding to the manners of consonant articulation) by the articulators. These actions can 1) "stop" the pressurized air stream from the lungs briefly at some location in the vocal tract (place of stop articulation) and then release it suddenly for plosives such as /p, t, k/; 2) force the air stream through a narrow constriction at some location in the vocal tract (place of fricative articulation) for fricatives such as / h, f, s, ʃ, θ/; or combine stopping with release into a fricative for affricates such as /ʧ/.

The actions of the articulators alter the size, shape and number of resonating cavities for a given consonant or vowel. Each vocal tract configuration has different resonant properties that allow some of the frequency components of the sound source to pass through and attenuate others. This is referred to as "filtering" of sound energy.

2. Deciding what type of speech sample to collect depends on the purpose of your assessment. What are some of the factors that should be considered? Discuss the advantages and disadvantages of imitated versus spontaneous samples and single word versus connected speech samples.

When collecting a speech sample, there is often a trade-off between obtaining the most representative sample of the child's typical speech and controlling the phonetic and phonemic content of the sample in order to evaluate specific abilities. Imitative samples allow for control over the phonetic/phonemic content of the sample and may provide an indication of a child's ability to change their production when a model is provided, but they are not representative of everyday abilities. Spontaneous samples are considered to be more representative of a child's typical speech, but the phonetic/phonemic content will vary from sample to sample and listeners may not always be able to accurately "gloss" the child's utterances, especially if the child has limited intelligibility. Single word tasks, such as picture naming tasks, are easy to administer and analyze and the intended target or "gloss" is known. However, children don't typically speak in single words and thus such samples are not as representative of their typical speech abilities. Connected speech samples are generally more time consuming to collect and analyze but are more representative of typical speech. It is important to remember that single word samples can be spontaneous (for example, naming pictures of objects) or imitative ("repeat after me"). Connected speech samples can also be spontaneous (for example, recording a child's conversation while playing) or imitative (for example, repeating a set of sentences with controlled content).

3. What is the purpose of speech-like tasks? How do they differ from speech tasks? Give two examples of speech-like tasks and explain what information they provide regarding children's speech abilities.

Speech-like tasks are used to measure the integrity of the speech perceptual-motor system and can assist in the identification of different types of speech impairment. They are different from speech tasks in that the utterances are not meaningful (that is, they involve the production of sounds, syllables, and longer sequences that do not contain recognizable words in the child's language). Examples of speech-like tasks include:

- Maximum phonation duration – sustained /a/ after deep inspiration, measured in seconds – provides information about how efficiently the respiratory subsystem and vocal folds are working to generate voice.
- Diadochokinetic task – rapid repetition of monosyllables or multisyllable sequences – measured in syllables per second (or sequences per second) – provides information about the accuracy, range, speed, and coordination of movements of the lips, tongue tip, and back of tongue, with poor performance indicative of motor impairment.
- Non-word repetition – repetition of nonsense words of varying lengths – provides information about phonological memory and is sometimes used as a screening for language impairment.

4. Phonetic transcription using the International Phonetic Alphabet (IPA) is a basic tool used by speech-language pathologists and others to represent the speech sounds produced by a speaker. Provide a rationale for collecting high quality audio recordings of the speech samples to be transcribed. Then list three ways to ensure that that the audio recording has high fidelity.

Having a high quality audio recording of the speech sample allows the transcriber to listen to the child's production several times to check one's judgments. This may be particularly useful when transcribing children who make speech sound errors. In addition, recordings can be analyzed acoustically to supplement the phonetic transcriptions. High fidelity recordings are necessary to ensure that the recordings recreate the original speech signal as precisely as possible with little or no distortion or background noise. Three ways to ensure high fidelity recordings include using an external microphone (preferably head-mounted), monitoring the recording level to avoid peak clipping or weak/inaudible signals), and recording in a quiet location to avoid extraneous background noise.

5. What is the difference between independent and relational analyses of speech samples? Give one example of each. What type of analysis does an articulation test provide?

An independent analysis describes the child's productions without comparison to the presumed adult target. Examples of independent analyses include a speech sound inventory or word shape inventory. A relational analysis involves a direct comparison of the child's production to the target form. Examples of relational analyses include segmental measures of phonetic accuracy such as PCC, PVC, and PPC, whole word measures such as WWA or PWP, and phonological process analyses. An articulation test provides a relational analysis.

6. Calculate PCC and PCC-R for the following brief speech sample:

teach	[t̪iʃ]
clock	[təlɑk]
clown	[k̬waʊn]
fish	[fɪʃ]
balloon	[bəwum]
broom	[bwʌm]
thumb	[s̪ʌm]
yellow	[lɛloʊ]
rose	[woʊs]
rain	[wẽɪ]

PCC = 42% (10/24); PCC-R = 50% (12/24). The difference is that [t̪] in *teach* and [k̬] in *clown* are considered "incorrect" in PCC, but "correct" in PCC-R.

7. Using the sample provided in question 6 above, calculate WWA and PWP.

WWA = 1/10 (fish is the only word that is produced with full accuracy); PWP = .78 (3/5 + 6/7 + 6/7 + 5/5 + 6/8 + 6/7 + 4/5 + 5/6 + 3/5 + 3/5 = 47/60). Note however, that PWP is typically calculated on 25 words, not just 10 words.

8. Define the three parameters of prosody and voice according to Shriberg et al. How do you think that prosody and voice might influence the intelligibility of a child's speech?

Shriberg et al. define prosody by the three parameters of phrasing (e.g., appropriateness of pause locations and rhythm), rate (e.g., too fast, too slow, variable), and stress (e.g., reduced, excess or equal stress on syllables within a word or across words). Voice is defined by the three parameters of loudness (e.g., level, excessive, alternating, decaying over utterance), pitch (e.g., too high, too low, monopitch, or breaks in pitch), and quality (including both laryngeal features such as breathy or strained-strangled and supralaryngeal features such as nasal or nasopharyngeal). Poor prosody can affect a child's intelligibility, even if all of the speech sounds are produced correctly, because prosodic information gives additional meaning to utterances by indicating word stress and utterance boundaries for the listener. When the voice is not loud enough, a listener will have difficulty hearing the speech signal and when voice quality is poor, the voice sound source for sonorant sounds will be distorted.

9. Intelligibility and acceptability are global measures of children's speech. How do intelligibility and acceptability differ from each other and how can they be measured?

Intelligibility refers to how well a child's speech can be understood by listeners and acceptability refers to how well a child's speech conforms to what is expected for a child of similar age and sex. Intelligibility can be measured directly through word identification tasks such as the Children's Speech Intelligibility Measure or the TOCS+ Intelligibility Measures, or estimated indirectly through rating scales. Acceptability is typically measured using listener rating scales.

10. What acoustic cues could you examine to support a perceptual judgment that a child was making voicing errors on initial stops? What acoustic cues could you examine to support a perceptual judgment that the child was also "centralizing" vowel productions?

Voice onset time (VOT), burst amplitude and presence/absence of aspiration noise are cues to initial stop consonant voicing. In "voiced" stops, VOT is shorter, burst amplitude is weaker and aspiration noise is negligible. "Centralized" vowels would have formant frequencies that are more similar to the central vowel /ʌ/ rather than the characteristic formant frequency pattern of the target vowel. For example, if the low back vowel /ɑ/ is centralized, F1 and F2 are further apart than in a non-centralized production.

REFERENCES

Austin, D., Shriberg, L.D. (Revised 1997). Lifespan reference data for ten measures of articulation competence using the Speech Disorders Classification System (SDCS.) (Tech. Rep. No. 3). Phonology Project, Waisman Center, University of Wisconsin-Madison. Accessed at *www.waisman.wisc.edu/phonology/bib/tech.htm*.

Ball, M.J., Esling, J., Dickson, B.C. (1995). The VoQS system for the transcription of voice quality. *Journal of the International Phonetic Association,* 25, 71-80.

Ball, M., Rahilly, J. (2002). Transcribing disordered speech: The segmental and prosodic layers. *Clinical Linguistics and Phonetics*, 16(5), 329-344.

Bess, F.H., Humes, L.E. (2008). *Audiology: The fundamentals* (4th Ed.). Philadelphia: Lippincott Williams and Wilkins.

Boersma, P., Weenink, D. (2005). Praat Version 4.3.12 [Computer software]. Institute of Phonetic Sciences, University of Amsterdam. Accessed at *www.fon.hum.uva.nl/praat/.*

Buder, E.H., Stoel-Gammon, C. (2002). American and Swedish children's acquisition of vowel duration: Effects of vowel identity and final stop voicing. *Journal of the Acoustical Society of America*, 111(4), 854-1864.

Dollaghan, C., Campbell, T. (1998). Non-word repetition and child language impairment. *Journal of Speech, Language and Hearing Research*, 41, 1136-1146.

Flipsen, P., Jr., Hammer, J.B., and Yost, K.M. (2005). Measuring severity of involvement in speech delay: Segmental and whole-word measures. *American Journal of Speech-Language Pathology*, 14(4), 298-312.

Forrest, K., Rockman, B.K. (1988). Acoustic and perceptual analysis of word-initial stop consonants in phonologically disordered children. *Journal of Speech and Hearing Research*, 31, 449-459.

Forrest, K., Weismer, G., Hodge, M., Dinnsen, D.A., Elbert, M. (1990). Statistical analysis of word-initial /k/ and /t/ produced by normal and phonologically disordered children. *Clinical Linguistics and Phonetics*, 4(4), 327-340.

Goldman, R. Fristoe, M. (2000). *Goldman Fristoe Test of Articulation* (2nd Ed.). Circle Pines, MN: American Guidance Service Inc.

Gordon-Brannan, M.E.. Hodson, B.W. (2000). Intelligibility/severity measurements of prekindergarten children's speech. *American Journal of Speech-Language Pathology*, 9, 141-150.

Gordon-Brannan, M. E., Weiss, C.E. (2007). *Clinical management of articulatory and phonologic disorders* (3rd Ed). Baltimore, MD: Lippincott, Williams and Wilkins.

Higgins, C. M., Hodge, M.M. (2002). Vowel area and intelligibility in children with and without dysarthria. *Journal of Medical Speech-Language Pathology*, 10(4), 271-277.

Hodge, M.M., Gotzke, C.L. (2010). Stability of intelligibility measures for children with dysarthria. *Journal of Medical Speech-Language Pathology*, 18(4), 61-65.

Hodge, M.M., Gotzke, C.L. (2011). Minimal pair distinctions and intelligibility in preschool children with and without speech sound disorders. *Clinical Linguistics and Phonetics*, 25(10), 853–863.

Hodge, M.M., Whitehill, T. (2010). Intelligibility impairments. In J.S. Damico, M. Ball, N. Müller (Eds.) *Handbook of Language and Speech Disorders* (pp 99-114). Oxford, UK: Blackwell Publishers.

Ingram, D., Ingram, K.D. (2001). A whole-word approach to phonological analysis and intervention. *Language, Speech, and Hearing Services in Schools*, 32(4), 271-283.

Johnson, C.A., Weston, A.D., Bain, B.A. (2004). An objective and time-efficient method for determining severity of childhood speech delay. *American Journal of Speech-Language Pathology*, 13(1), 55-65.

Kehoe, M., Stoel-Gammon, C., Buder, E. (1995). Acoustic correlates of stress in young children's speech. *Journal of Speech and Hearing Research*, 38, 338-350.

Khan, L., Lewis, N. (2002) *Khan-Lewis Phonological Analysis* (2nd Ed.). San Antonio, TX: Pearson.

Kent, R.D., Kent, J.F., Rosenbeck, J.C. (1987). Maximum performance tests of speech production. *Journal of Speech and Hearing Disorders*, 52, 367-387.

Kent, R.D., Read, C. (2002). *The acoustic analysis of speech* (2nd Ed). Albany, NY: Singular/Thompson Learning.

Lang, B.K., Starr, C.D., Moller, K. (1992). Effects of pubertal changes on the speech of persons with cleft palate. *Cleft Palate-Craniofacial Journal*, 29(3), 268-270.

Lohmeier, H.L., Shriberg, L.D. (2011). Reference Data for the Syllable Repetition Task (SRT) (Tech. Rep. No. 17). Phonology Project, Waisman Center, University of Wisconsin-Madison. Accessed at *www.waisman.wisc.edu/phonology/bib/tech.htm.*

Milenkovic, P.H. (2004). TF32. Department of Electrical Engineering, University of Wisconsin-Madison, Madison, WI.

Morris, S., Wilcox, K., Schooling, T. (1995). The preschool speech intelligibility measure. *American Journal of Speech-Language Pathology*, 4, 22-28.

Nissen, S.L., Fox, R.A. (2005). Acoustic and spectral characteristics of young children's fricative productions: A developmental perspective. *Journal of the Acoustical Society of America*, 118(4), 2570-2578.

Nissen, S.L.., Fox, R.A. (2009). Acoustic and spectral patterns in young children's stop consonant production. *Journal of the Acoustical Society of America*, 126(3), 1369-1378.

Ohde, R., Sharf, D. (1992). *Phonetic analysis of normal and abnormal speech.* New York, NY: MacMillan Publishing Co.

Pollock, K.E. (1994*), Assessment and remediation of vowel misarticulations, Clinics in Communication Disorders*, 4, 23-37.

Pollock, K.E., Berni, M.B. (2001). *Transcription of vowels. Topics in Language Disorders*, 21, 22-40.

Powell, T.W. (2001). Phonetic transcription of disordered speech. *Topics in Language Disorders*, 21, 52-72.

Rvachew, S., Hodge, M., Ohberg, A. (2005). Obtaining and interpreting Maximum Performance Tasks from children: A tutorial. *Journal of Speech-Language Pathology and Audiology*, 29(4), 145-157.

Rvachew, S., Slawinski, E.B., Williams, M., Green, C. (1999). The impact of early onset otitis media on babbling and early language development. *Journal of the Acoustic Society of America*, 105, 467-475.

Schmitt, L.S., Howard, B.H., Schmitt, J.F. (1983). Conversational speech sampling in the assessment of articulation proficiency. *Language, Speech, and Hearing Services in Schools*, 14, 210-214.

Shriberg, L.D., Austin, D., Lewis, B.A., McSweeny, J.L., Wilson, D.L. (1997a). The percentage of consonants correct (P. C. C.) metric: Extensions and reliability data. *Journal of Speech, Language, and Hearing Research*, 40, 708-722.

Shriberg, L.D., Austin, D., Lewis, B.A., McSweeny, J.L., Wilson, D.L. (1997b). The speech disorders classification system (SDCS): extensions and lifespan reference data. *Journal of Speech, Language, and Hearing Research*, 40(4), 723-740.

Shriberg, L.D., Campbell, T.F., Karlsson, H.B., Brown, R.L., McSweeny, J.L., Nadler, C.J. (2003). A diagnostic marker for childhood apraxia of speech: the lexical stress ratio. *Clinical Linguistics and Phonetics*, 17, 549–574.

Shriberg, L.D., Kwiatkowski, J., Rasmussen, C. (1990). Prosody-Voice screening profile (P. V. S. P.) scoring forms and training materials. Tucson, AZ: Communication Skill Builders.

Shriberg, L.D., Kwiatkowski, J., Rasmussen, C., Lof, G.L., Miller, J.F. (1992). The Prosody-Voice Screening Profile (P. V. S. P.): Psychometric data and reference information for children (Tech rep. No. 1). Phonology Project, Waisman Center on Mental Retardation and Human development, University of Wisconsin-Madison, Madison, WI. Accessed at *www.waisman.wisc.edu/phonology/bib/tech.htm.*

Shriberg, L.D., Lohmeier, H.L. (2008). The Syllable Repetition Task (Tech. Rep. No. 14). Phonology Project, Waisman Center, University of Wisconsin-Madison. Madison, WI. Accessed at *www.waisman.wisc.edu/phonology/bib/tech.htm.*

Shriberg, L.D., Lohmeier, H.L., Campbell, T.F., Dollaghan, C.A., Green, J.R., Moore, C.A. (2008). A Non-word Repetition Task for Speakers with Misarticulations: The Syllable Repetition Task (S. R. T.). *Journal of Speech, Language and Hearing Research*, 52, 1189-1212.

Stoel-Gammon, C. (1985). Phonetic inventories, 15-24 months: A longitudinal study. *Journal of Speech and Hearing Research*, 28 (4), 505-512.

Stoel-Gammon, C. (2001). *Transcribing the speech of young children.* Topics in Language Disorders, 21 (4), 12-21.

Stoel-Gammon, C., Dunn, C. (1985). Normal and disordered phonology in children. Austin, TX: Pro-Ed.

Stoel-Gammon, C., Pollock, K. (2008). Vowel development and disorders. In M.J. Ball, M.R. Perkins, N. Muller, S. Howard (Eds.), *The Handbook of Clinical Linguistics*. Oxford, UK: Blackwell Publishing (pp. 525-548).

Thoonen, G., Maassen, B., Gabreels, F., Schreuder, R. (1999). Validity of maximum performance tasks to diagnose motor speech disorders in children. *Clinical Linguistics and Phonetics*, 13, 1-23.

Thoonen, G., Maassen, B., Wit, J., Gabreels, F., Schreuder, R. (1996). The integrated use of maximum performance tasks in differential diagnostic evaluations among children with motor speech disorders. *Clinical Linguistics and Phonetics*, 10, 311-336.

Weiss, C. (1980) Weiss Comprehensive Test of Articulation. Hingham, MA: Teaching Resources Corporation.

Wilcox, K., Morris, S. (1999). Children's Speech Intelligibility Measure. Toronto: The Psychological Corporation, Harcourt Brace and Company.

Witzel, M.A. (1995). Communicative impairment associated with clefting. In: Shprintzen, R.J., Bardach, J., eds. *Cleft palate speech management: A multidisciplinary approach* (pp. 137-166). St. Louis: Mosby.

II. Chronological Development: The First Cry and Beyond

In: Comprehensive Perspectives …
Editors: Beate Peter and Andrea A. N. MacLeod
ISBN: 978-1-62257-041-6

Chapter 3

Biological Substrates of Speech Development: A Brief Synopsis of the Developing Neuromuscular System

Beate Peter

Introduction

Speech is, simply put, the finishing stage of transducing a thought into sound waves. Producing speech is by its nature a physical act, fundamentally involving air movement: To generate speech, the airstream, whether flowing in or out of the lungs, must be constricted in various places along the laryngeal and articulatory system and to various degrees of closure. The product is an exquisitely complex string of sounds and silences with a rich tapestry of spectral and temporal characteristics, intended to be re-transduced into a thought in the perception of a listener.

Much like the sounds in a symphony are generated by an orchestra of players and their instruments, the aerodynamics of speech require a coordinated set of structures and systems, consisting, at a minimum, of these: the central and peripheral nervous systems (CNS and PNS), the respiratory system, the larynx, the articulators, and the auditory system. Each of these plays a distinct role in the speech production process: The brain, part of the CNS, is the site where the cognitive and linguistic content of the message is generated and translated into motor commands. The brain also receives and interprets acoustic and **kinesthetic** feedback regarding the utterances being produced. The spinal cord, part of the CNS, and the nerves, part of the PNS, communicate motor commands and sensory feedback between the brain and the speech producing organs. The respiratory system powers the speech output by producing the airflow necessary to generate an acoustic signal. The larynx serves as a site of air constriction that generates the voicing component of the speech signal. The articulators add air constriction to generate various other types of acoustic signals, for instance the hissing sound in /f, s, ʃ/ as the air is forced through narrow channels, or the popping sound in /p, t, k/ as the airflow is briefly stopped, then released. The articulators further add critical acoustic information by providing the required shape of the oral and pharyngeal cavities to generate vowel sounds and by shunting the airflow through the nasal cavity to create the nasal resonance required for certain vowels and consonants. The auditory system picks up the speech sounds as they are being produced, providing the speaker with immediate feedback and allowing for modification and correction of various aspects of the speech signal, for instance sound intensity, voice quality, and misarticulations.

Most of these structures and systems are essentially fully formed at birth, although not adult-like in size and orientation, but it will typically take several years before a child can use them in such a way that even an unfamiliar listener can understand clearly what was said. This chapter describes some general principles of human development and traces the developmental trajectories of the structures and systems involved in speech production. A detailed treatment of anatomical and physiological substrates of speech is the subject of various other sources and, hence, beyond the scope of this chapter.

Developmental Trajectories

General Principles of Prenatal Development and Beyond

From a single egg cell, fertilized by a single sperm cell, a mature human develops over time. During the first week after fertilization, the single fertilized cell divides several times, forming a cluster of cells called blastocyst. During the second week after fertilization, the blastocyst attaches to the uterine wall. In the middle of the third week, it differentiates into three distinct cell layers called endoderm ("inner layer"), mesoderm ("middle layer"), and ectoderm ("outer layer"), all arranged as flat layers on an oval shaped disk approximately 1.5 **millimeters** (mm) long. The endoderm gives rise to most of the epithelium of the digestive tract, the epithelium of the respiratory system, structures of the digestive tract, and other epithelial layers. The mesoderm gives rise to the different types of muscle tissue, connective tissue, most of the cardiovascular system, skeleton, and the reproductive and excretory organs. The ectoderm gives rise to the epidermis, the central and peripheral nervous systems, and the lens of the eye.

Early in the fourth week, when the embryo is less than 4 mm long, the heart begins to beat and by the end of the eighth week, when the embryo is approximately 30 mm long, all major organs and structures are formed. Between the ninth week and birth, a developmental stage referred to as the fetal period, the structures grow further and become more refined. Birth typically occurs at 35 to 38 weeks after fertilization. As early as 22 weeks after fertilization, a fetus can survive if born prematurely, although the actual chances of survival, even up to 28 weeks after fertilization, depend on various factors including weight and the maturational stage of the nervous system and the lungs (Moore, Persaud, and Torchia, 2008).

At the moment of birth, the infant's metabolism undergoes a drastic change from umbilical oxygen and nutrient supply to airborne oxygen delivery and oral feeding. Other maturational changes, not nearly as dramatic, continue to unfold across the lifespan, affecting the various organ systems in different and specific ways and following different time courses. For instance, the growth of the cranium and brain volume progresses rapidly after birth and is considered essentially complete by approximately 6 years of age, whereas skeletal growth of the face and other structures continues until completion in adolescence or even adulthood (Melsen and Melsen, 1982). The growth of the larynx is an example of **sexual dimorphism** in humans, as the growth rates of males and females begin to diverge at approximately age 9 years, resulting in a substantially larger larynx and lower fundamental vocal frequency in male adults, compared to female adults (Kent, 1994). The integrity of **white matter** in the brain is an example of nonlinear development across the lifespan, increasing in children and adults, then declining again as a function of age (Bartzokis et al., 2010).

Central and Peripheral Nervous Systems (CNS and PNS)

The CNS consists of the brain and the spinal cord, in other words, those parts of the nervous system that are encased in bone (cranium and spinal column). One small exception to this general definition is the retina of the eye, technically considered part of the CNS but not fully encased in bone. The PNS consists of all nervous system components that lie outside of the bony encasement. The PNS can be subdivided into two components: The somatic PNS contains efferent nerves innervating the skin, muscles, and joints that are under voluntary control as well as the afferent sensory neurons that convey information back to the CNS, whereas the visceral PNS, also called autonomic nervous system, regulates the involuntary action of the internal organs, glands, and blood vessels and also transfers visceral afferent information. In this chapter, the focus is on the somatic PNS, not the visceral PNS.

The Central Nervous System

As mentioned, the CNS and PNS both arise from the embryonic ectoderm layer. Early in the fourth week after fertilization, a neural tube forms, giving rise to the CNS structures. At the center of the neural tube is a neural canal, to differentiate later into the central canal of the spinal cord and the ventricles of the brain. The **rostral** end of the neural tube differentiates into three bulges called primary brain vesicles from which the brain structures arise. From rostral to **caudal**, the vesicles are labeled forebrain, midbrain, and hindbrain. By the end of the fifth week, the forebrain further differentiates into the telencephalon ("end brain"), from which the cerebral hemispheres arise, visible by the seventh week after fertilization, and the diencephalon ("interbrain"), from which the thalamus, hypothalamus, and epithalamus arise. By this same time, the hindbrain also differentiates and develops the metencephalon ("afterbrain"), from which the pons and the cerebellum arise, and the myelencephalon ("spinal brain"), giving rise to the medulla. The midbrain does not differentiate further into separate structures and develops into the adult midbrain. The remainder of the neural tube becomes the spinal cord.

The major brain structures are distinct in terms of **morphology** and function. The two cerebral hemispheres account for over 80% of total brain volume. Their surface, called cortex, has six distinct layers of neurons and contains areas crucial for the perception and interpretation of visual, auditory, and tactile information and also for cognitive, linguistic, and motor functions. The exact composition of cell types varies among the cortical regions. Deep in each cerebral hemisphere are structures important for motor, memory, and emotional functions. The thalamus is a relay center for general sensory information, whereas the hypothalamus regulates many of the autonomic functions related to emotions, hormones, and body temperature as well as food and water intake, and the epithalamus regulates the sleep/wake cycle. The cerebellum (Latin for "little brain") accounts for approximately 10% of total brain volume and consists of two hemispheres, similar to the cerebral hemispheres. It is crucial for coordinated and smooth motor functioning including for speech production. Together with the pons and the medulla, the midbrain forms the brainstem. The midbrain serves various functions including passing information between the spinal cord and the cerebral hemispheres and contributing to motor control and sensory perception. The pons (Latin for "bridge") passes information between the cerebellum and the motor cortex as well as between the higher brain centers and the spinal cord. The medulla contains many populations of cells serving specific purposes, for instance monitoring the bloodstream for oxygenation and toxins, regulating the heart rate, and relaying auditory and vestibular information. Figure 3.1 illustrates the developmental stages of the major brain structures.

The cells in brain tissue fall essentially into two categories, neurons and glial cells. Neurons receive electrical and chemical inputs from their environment and send their responses to other neurons along their axons, which are long and extremely thin extensions protruding out from their gray cell bodies. In that sense, neurons are the information processing system in the brain. A neuron's job is to integrate the input from many other neurons that are connected to its input structures via **synapses**, and if the combined input energy exceeds a certain threshold, an electrical response is triggered causing the neuron to send a signal to all neurons that synapse with its output structure. Glial cells support the work of the neurons by providing structural scaffolding, nourishment, and waste disposal. One type of glial cell in the CNS is called oligodendrocyte. Its function is to wrap the axons of neurons in a layer of insulation, which speeds up the information transfer along the axons. Oligodendrocytes and the analogous cells in the PNS called Schwann cells contain myelin, which is white in color. Areas of the brain that are dense in neuron cell bodies appear gray in dissection, whereas areas dense in myelin-wrapped axons appear white. The terms "**gray matter**" and "white matter" refer to these two types of brain tissue, respectively.

As mentioned, the cerebral cortex consists of six layers of neuron bodies and has highly specialized regions that differ in function and in their cell composition. Its prenatal development is a fascinating story. During the first three to four weeks after fertilization, precursor brain cells are generated in a region deep in the brain called ventricular zone. The precursor cells result from cell division (**mitosis**), causing an exponential increase in number of these cells. After this period, for each two daughter cells of a cell division process, one becomes a migratory cell, traveling outward to its destination in the cortex along special guide cells called radial glia, whereas the other daughter cell remains in the ventricular zone to undergo additional cycles of mitosis. The earliest migrating cells end up in the lowest cortical layers and the later migrating cells pass them by, forming the outer cortical layers, so that the cortex is built from the inside out. As the prenatal cortex continues to assemble new neurons, it folds into the characteristic pattern of gyri (bulges) and sulci (valleys). If the cortex could be peeled off an adult human brain and spread out on a flat surface, it would cover a surface of roughly .75 **meter** $(m)^2$ to 1 m^2 (8.1 to 10.8 square feet). This impressive amount of cortical surface relative to the size of the brain reflects the fact that among mammals, humans have the most deeply wrinkled brain surface.

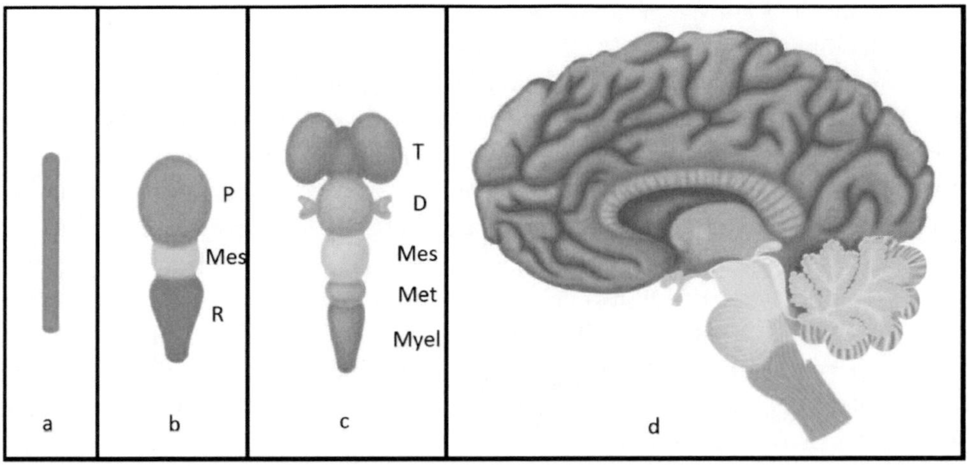

Figure 3.1. Differentiation of the neural tube into the structures of the adult brain (not drawn to scale). a. Neural tube, 2 weeks post fertilization. b. Primary brain vesicles, 3 weeks post fertilization. c. Secondary brain vesicles, 4 weeks post fertilization. d. Adult brain structures. D = diencephalon, Mes = mesencephalon, Met = metencephalon, Myel = myelencephalon, P = prosencephalon, T = telencephalon.

By the time a baby is born, the brain has essentially all the structures, cortical layers, and surface convolutions of an adult brain. One exception is the amount of white matter insulating the axons of the neurons, which will continue to develop throughout childhood and early adulthood, depending on sex, brain region, and environmental factors. In a sample of healthy adult males, maximum integrity (measured as lowest water content) in white matter occurred at age 39, then declined as a function of age (Bartzokis et al., 2010). In addition to an increase of white matter cells in the developing brain, other glial cells are being generated, together accounting for the rapid growth of total brain volume by age 6 years (Giedd et al., 1999).

It was thought for many years that the process of neurogenesis (formation of new neurons by mitosis) is complete by the time a child is born. This assumption turned out to be incorrect. The adult human brain generates new neurons throughout life, specifically in two brain structures deep in the cerebral hemispheres, the caudate nucleus and the dentate gyrus of the hippocampus, both crucial for encoding new memories, particularly the hippocampus. This was discovered by researchers investigating the brain tissue of deceased cancer patients who, prior to their deaths, had agreed to receive injections of a labeling substance called bromodeoxyuridine that is taken up by cells during mitosis. The caudate nuclei and hippocampi in these brains showed evidence of newborn neurons created by mitosis (Eriksson et al., 1998). More evidence of adult neurogenesis was found in the brain scans of taxi drivers in London, who are required to commit the highly complex city map to memory. The taxi drivers had larger hippocampi, compared to the general population, and the more experienced taxi drivers had larger hippocampi, compared to those with less experience (Maguire et al., 2000). When mitosis is curbed as part of cancer treatment to prevent the tumor cells from dividing, the memory dysfunctions often observed in cancer patients following chemotherapy are thought to reflect the fact that neurogenesis in the caudate nucleus and the hippocampus has been curtailed as a side effect from the cancer treatment (Dietrich, Monje, Wefel, and Meyers, 2008).

To function, the cortical neurons must communicate with each other and with other neurons in the brain. As mentioned, their points of contacts are their synapses. Long before birth, before the 27th week after fertilization, neurons begin to establish synapses. Not all these synapses will be used, however, and many of them are eliminated in early childhood in a process called synaptic pruning. The process of creating and eliminating synapses follows a different time course in different cortical regions. For instance, a peak density of synapses is reached at 3 months of age for the auditory cortex but at 15 months of age in frontal cortex areas (Huttenlocher and Dabholkar, 1997). The prenatal human brain not only creates an excess of synapses among neurons but actually also an excess number of neurons. In the course of normal brain development, many of these extra neurons die in a process called apoptosis. All neurons have a built-in program for self-destruction. Why do most neurons survive despite this program? It is now known that the protective effect of certain proteins including nerve growth factor (Cohen and Levi-Montalcini, 1956; Cohen, Levi-Montalcini, and Hamburger, 1954) involves switching off the expression of genes programmed for apoptosis (Horvitz, Shaham, and Hengartner, 1994).

Generally, the sensory and motor centers of the left hemisphere are connected to body regions on the right side, and vice versa. This explains why brain injuries in one hemisphere's motor regions can cause weakness, paralysis, or numbness in the opposite side of the body.

The human cerebral hemispheres are not entirely symmetrical in structure. For instance, an area of cortex called insula, buried in a deep fissure on the lateral surface, is typically larger in the left hemisphere than in the right, and this asymmetry is evident as early as 16 to 17 weeks post fertilization (Afif, Bouvier, Buenerd, Trouillas, and Mertens, 2007). A similar asymmetry, also developing prenatally, has been observed for the planum temporale, a small area of cortex located near an area crucial for speech comprehension. A lack of this asymmetry in the planum temporale has been observed in individuals with dyslexia (Galaburda, Sherman, Rosen, Aboitiz, and Geschwind, 1985) and language impairment (Jernigan, Hesselink, Sowell, and Tallal, 1991). The two hemispheres differ also in terms of function. Research in individuals with focal brain damage and with surgically disconnected hemispheres, as well as functional brain imaging in a variety of individuals, shows that speech and language functions are primarily processed in the left hemisphere, as summarized in a number of reviews (Crinion and Leff, 2007; Hickok, 2009). This is even true for sign language, even though it is encoded in body gestures and perceived in the visual modality (Gordon, 2004). It is not yet clear how this distinctly human structural and functional lateralization of speech and language to the left hemisphere is related to the fact that 90% of humans are right-handed and, hence, have finer motor control in the left hemisphere.

The Peripheral Nervous System

While the neural tube forms during the third week after fertilization, a small part of the ectoderm moves to a position parallel to the neural tube and forms the neural crest, which gives rise to the PNS. Neural crest cells move to each side of the neural tube and differentiate to become, among other structures, the sensory neurons of the spinal nerves and of some of the cranial nerves. During the fourth week after fertilization, spinal motor nerve fibers begin to protrude from the spinal cord and spinal sensory neurons assemble into ganglia. The motor and sensory nerves become longer and grow into the developing limbs.

During the fifth and sixth week, the twelve cranial nerves, grouped into three embryological origins, begin to appear. The first group consists of the somatic **efferent** cranial nerves, originating in the brainstem and including the trochlear (cranial nerve, CN IV), abducens (CN VI), hypoglossal (CN XII), and most of the oculomotor (CN III) cranial nerves. These nerves resemble the spinal motor nerves in their somatic motor function but differ from them in that their origins lie in the brainstem, not in the spinal column. The second group consists of the cranial nerves originating in the pharyngeal arches, which are precursor regions for the face, mouth, and anterior neck. In this group are the trigeminal nerve (CN V), the facial nerve (CN VII), the glossopharyngeal nerve (CN IX), the vagus nerve (CN X), and the accessory nerve (CN XI). The third group consists of the special sensory nerves related to smell, vision, hearing, and balance and includes the olfactory nerve (CN I), the optic nerve (CN II), and the vestibulocochlear nerve (CN VIII).

For purposes of speech production, several of the cranial nerves play a crucial role. The hypoglossal nerve has mostly efferent functions, carrying motor commands to the muscles inside and underneath the tongue during speech movements as well as chewing and swallowing. It also carries **proprioceptive** information from the tongue back to the brain. The trigeminal nerve is a major sensory nerve of the face and carries sensory information from the anterior tongue and other facial structures to the brain. The glossopharyngeal nerve carries motor commands to, and sensory information from, the posterior areas of the tongue and throat. It also picks up taste sensations from these regions. Taste sensations from the anterior part of the tongue are picked up by the facial nerve, a mixed nerve that also provides the muscles of the face with motor commands. The vagus nerve provides motor commands to the pharynx and larynx. The accessory nerve joins some of the vagus fibers to supply motor control of the pharynx and larynx and also controls movement of the soft palate. The vestibulocochlear nerve conveys auditory and balance information to the brain. Figure 3.2 is a schematic drawing of those cranial nerves that are crucially important for speech. The nerves are shown from their point of exit from the cranium to their motor and/or sensory endpoints. Intracranially, they are attached to the CNS at the level of the brainstem and upper spinal cord.

Respiratory System

As mentioned, air movement is a fundamental requirement for speech production. Immediately following birth, the baby inhales air for the first time and lets out the legendary first cry. In the months prior to birth, the lungs have undergone many changes. From a tracheal bud, appearing in the fourth week after fertilization, two bronchial buds develop during the fifth week and consecutive subdivisions create a system of 17 orders of branches by 24 weeks. After birth, an additional seven rounds of subdivisions develop. By 16 weeks, all lung components have essentially formed except for those that process the air exchange. Between weeks 16 and 26, the lung tissue continues to become more vascularized and develops tiny bulges called terminal saccules. Between week 26 and birth, the epithelial lining of the saccules thins out substantially and becomes covered with surfactant. The presence of surfactant is crucial for breathing because it prevents the walls of the membranes to stick together from tension forces. From week 32 through age 8 years, saccules develop

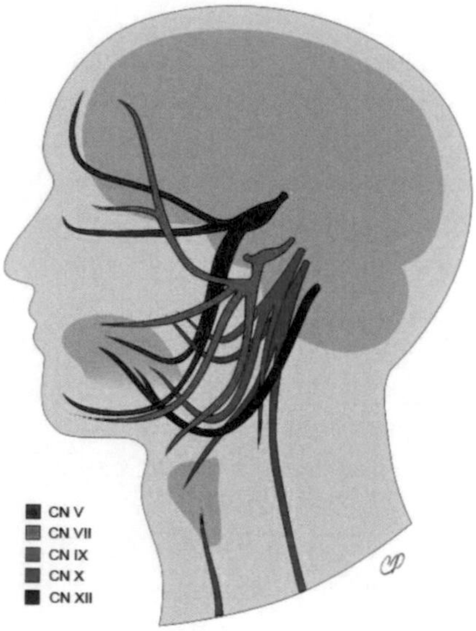

Figure 3.2. Cranial nerves V (trigeminal), VII (facial), IX (glossopharyngeal), X (vagus), and XII (hypoglossal).

tiny pits called alveoli where oxygen and carbon dioxide are exchanged during breathing. By the time a child is 8 years old, 300 million alveoli have formed, the same number as present in an adult lung.

The relative size and maturational stage of the respiratory system control its function. For instance, breathing rates in terms of breaths per minute are highest in children under 2 years of age and decline gradually into adulthood, and in all age groups, breathing rates are higher when awake, compared to when asleep. An awake child under age 2 years takes 48 breaths per minute when awake and 40 when asleep. An adult between 30 and 36 years of age takes 27 breaths per minute when awake and 22 when asleep (Rusconi et al., 1994). These changes reflect differences in oxygen needs as well as in lung size and capacity. Another measure of lung function is vital capacity, defined as the amount of air measured in L (**liters**) that can be inhaled after a maximal exhalation. Vital capacity increases in children and young adults, peaking at approximately 5.3 L, then decreases with age in older adults to approximately 3.5 L (Gaultier and Zinman, 1983; Tobin, Chadha, et al., 1983; Tobin, Jenouri, et al., 1983). The published vital capacity data shows that vital capacity is substantially greater in males compared to females and is correlated with body height (Gaultier and Zinman, 1983; Zapletal, Samanek, and Paul, 1987). A similar developmental trajectory is seen in maximum phonation time, the maximum duration of a phonated vowel after a maximal inhalation. Girls age 3;6 (years;months) to 3;11 were able to sustain a vowel for an average of 6.3 seconds (s) and boys at that age averaged 7.7 seconds. Durations for females at age 17 years averaged 22.0 seconds and for males, 28.7 seconds (Finnegan, 1984). In older adults, phonation times decrease as a function of age (Raymond D. Kent, 1997).

Larynx

The larynx is the first site of possible constriction for air flowing out from the lungs, and if constricted with just the right amount of closure, an audible buzz is generated that is perceived as voicing. The larynx sits in the anterior neck, directly above the trachea, and consists of an outer rigid frame of cartilage and an inner system of muscles and joints. The epiglottis is a cartilaginous structure that moves to cover the upper opening of the larynx during the swallowing process. Inside the larynx, two paired muscles, the thyroarytenoids, are an essential part of the vocal folds. They are suspended horizontally in the larynx like two curtains that originate in the front of the larynx and can be moved to an open or closed position in the back. Depending on how closely the two muscles are drawn together toward the midline, no voice, a whispered sound, or audible voice is produced.

As evident from a newborn's first cry, the larynx is functional at birth. Its cartilages arise from neural crest cells, originating in the ectoderm, whereas the laryngeal muscles arise from mesoderm and its epithelial lining, from endoderm. A laryngeal opening and the epiglottis are visible at six weeks after fertilization. Laryngeal cartilages are visible by week 10. Following birth, the larynx grows rapidly. At approximately 9 years of age, the growth rate diverges for males and females, resulting in a much larger larynx in adult males than in females. A newborn's vocal folds are less than 4 mm long. By age 1, they measure approximately 5.5 mm. By age 16, males have undergone a laryngeal growth spurt and their vocal folds are over 17 mm to 20 mm in length while measuring approximately 12.5 mm to 17 mm in females at that age (Zemlin, 1998). The sound file 3S1 is an example of the cry of a one-day-old newborn baby. Listen for the high fundamental frequency and the rapid breath cycles.

Access Sound File 1 (Chapter 3)

3S1 Newborn crying.

The fundamental frequency at which the vocal folds vibrate is perceived as vocal pitch and depends on a variety of parameters including the length, tension, and mass of the vocal folds. A speaker can vary these parameters considerably and at will, for instance to create a rising pitch when asking a question or when singing. In general, however, average fundamental frequency in conversation or when reading out loud is largely influenced by the anatomical length of the vocal folds. This explains why infants under age 1 have fundamental frequencies between 400 Hz and 500 Hz, children between 3 and 5 years have a fundamental frequency of approximately 300 Hz, and by young adulthood, females have fundamental frequencies of approximately 200 Hz and males, approximately 110 Hz (Kent, 1976; Robb and Saxman, 1985). With advancing age, physiologic changes cause the fundamental frequency to rise slightly in males (Hollien and Shipp, 1972).

Articulators

Speech production involves acting on the airstream to or from the lungs in such a way that sound is generated and modified to produce sequences of speech sounds. The articulators consist of stationary structures such as the hard palate and teeth as well as of moveable structures such as the velum, tongue, and lips. Producing the word "development" requires the involvement of all of these structures – try it!

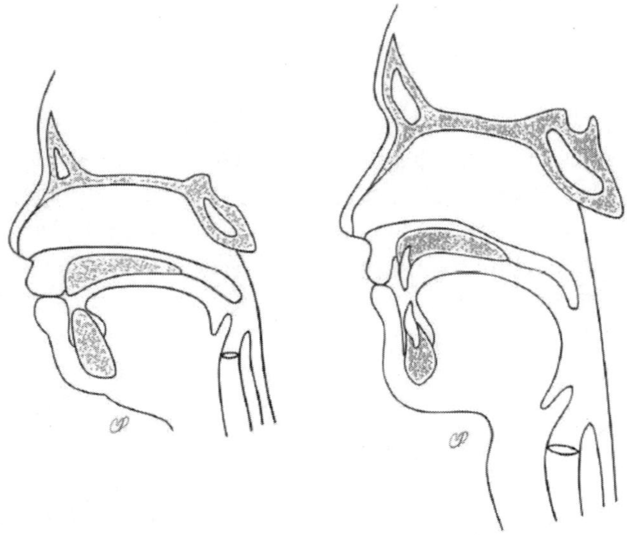

Figure 3.3. Relative positions of craniofacial structures at birth and in adults (not drawn to scale).

The articulators, along with other structures of the head and neck, arise from the **pharyngeal arch apparatus**, a set of bulging structures that are visible in the fourth week after fertilization. By the sixth week, five primitive swellings, also called processes, start fusing to form the face. The frontonasal process descends from the forebrain to form the internal and external components of the nose. Two maxillary processes grow forward and toward the midline to form the upper lips and palate, with the central portion of the anterior upper palate derived from the frontonasal process. Two mandibular processes fuse to form the mandible and lower lip. When the two maxillary processes do not fuse properly with the frontonasal profess, cleft lip and/or cleft palate can result. Chapter 17 in this volume focuses on clefting and its effects in speech development. By the 9th week, the hard palate has fused and by the 12th week, the soft palate has fused as well. Also by the 12th week, the velopharyngeal muscles and the tongue have formed.

At birth, the relative position of the articulators differs from that in adults (Figure 3.3). In the newborn, the tongue fills up the oral cavity almost completely. The epiglottis sits so high in the vocal tract that it almost touches the velum, and the larynx also sits higher in the vocal tract than in older children and adults. A newborn's lips are round in shape, compared to the more lateral spread in older children and adults. The first primary teeth, usually incisors, do not appear until 6 or 7 months after birth and the last primary molars appear between ages 2 and 3 years. The primary teeth last until approximately age 6 years, when they start to fall out and the permanent teeth begin to erupt. The last set of molars, the wisdom teeth, do not erupt until adulthood and in some cases not at all. Figure 3.3 shows the relative positions of the craniofacial structures at birth and in adults (not drawn to scale).

Auditory System

The auditory system consists of an external component made up of the auricle and the ear canal where sound is funneled into the head, the middle ear with its tympanic membrane and chain of tiny bones called ossicles that convert sound into mechanical vibrations, the cochlea where the mechanical vibrations are transduced into neural impulses, the vestibularcochlear nerve (CN VIII) that carries the neural signal to the brainstem, several relay stations in the brain that process and organize the neural signal, and the auditory cortex where the neural signal is further processed and integrated. The frequencies that a the healthy adult at the peak of auditory sensitivity can perceive range from approximately 20 Hz to over 20,000 Hz. Sounds produced by the articulatory system arrive in the auditory system of the speaker via two pathways, air conduction and bone conduction. Bone conduction delivers sound from the articulatory sound sources to the cochlea by acoustic vibrations in the bones of the head. The quality of the perceived sound is different from air conducted sound, and this difference may account for the many anecdotal comments that one's own voice, as played from a recording, sounds "strange."

At the beginning of the fourth week after fertilization, a precursor of the cochlea appears on the surface of the myelencephalon, deepens into a pit and forms a vesicle that becomes detached from the surface. Between 20 and 22 weeks after fertilization, the cochlea reaches its adult size and form. Precursors for the ossicles in the middle ear begin to appear in the fourth week after fertilization. By the 16th week, the ossicles have formed as cartilage that begins to be replaced by bone, a process that is complete by the 24th week. The middle ear continues to grow in size, along with the rest of the skeleton, except the cranium, through puberty. At six weeks after fertilization, small bulges called auricular hillocks begin to appear on the sides of the embryo's neck. The hillocks grow and move up into their position at the side of the head by the tenth week after fertilization. Differentiation into the folded structure of the auricle is complete by week 32. The ear canal starts out as a plate of epithelium, forming a cavity by week 8. By week 26, the canal is fully formed but continues to grow in size until age 9 years.

Midway through prenatal development, the fetus shows first evidence of responding to sound. In a landmark study of prenatal hearing development in 450 fetuses between 17 weeks after fertilization and full term (Hepper and Shahidullah, 1994), pure tones were introduced to the maternal abdomen and fetal movements were recorded using ultrasound imaging. At 17 weeks post fertilization, responses to the lowest presented frequencies at 100 Hz, 250 Hz, and 500 Hz were noted. At 27 and 29 weeks after fertilization, fetuses responded to 1,000 Hz and 3,000 Hz, respectively.

It should be remembered that the prenatal environment is filled with fluid and, unlike in life after birth, the sound received by the cochlea does not involve air conduction. The acoustic environment surrounding the fetus includes sounds generated by the maternal organs, the mother's voice during speech and song, and external sounds. High-frequency sounds undergo substantial attenuation inside the fluid environment while low-frequency sounds at and below 200 Hz are even slightly enhanced. Because of this environmental filtering, fetuses are mostly exposed to sounds < 500 Hz. This implies that, in the fetal environment, vowels and the voicing components of consonants in maternal speech signals are transmitted more than the voiceless sound components of consonants. It should be mentioned here that much of the prosody in the speech signal, e.g., intonation and lexical stress, is generated using variations in fundamental vocal frequency. There is evidence that the prenatal exposure to maternal speech contributes to prenatal processing of speech sounds: At birth, newborns show a strong preference for their mother's voices, compared to other female voices, and also a preference for their mother's voices with natural prosodic features, compared to their mother's voices lacking intonational contours (Mehler, Bertoncini, and Barriere, 1978). Newborns also can reliably distinguish between the language to which they were exposed before birth and a language with different prosodic characteristics (Mehler, Lambertz, Jusczyk, and Amiel-Tison, 1986). Their cry patterns show similarities to the prosody of the prenatally ambient language (Mampe, Friederici, Christophe, and Wermke, 2009). See Chapter 7 for a detailed account on the development of prosody.

Regardless of the specific prenatal exposure to one woman's speech signal, infants are born with the ability to distinguish between many of the world's speech sounds (Werker and Tees, 1983). By the first birthday, this astonishing ability is lost, and speech sound discrimination is retained only for those sounds present in the ambient language (Kuhl, Williams, Lacerda, Stevens, and Lindblom, 1992; Werker and Tees, 1992).

ALL PLAYERS IN CONCERT: THE ORCHESTRATION OF SPEECH

On June 26, 1963, John F. Kennedy, the 35th President of the United States, addressed a large crowd of people in what was then West Berlin. The political climate was dominated by the Cold War. President Kennedy's speech was an emphatic expression of support for democracy.

Toward the end of his speech, President Kennedy said, "Two thousand years ago the proudest boast was *civis Romanus sum* (I am a Roman citizen). Today, in the world of freedom, the proudest boast is '*Ich bin ein Berliner*!'"

Historic recordings of his speech show that President Kennedy had written notes in front of him as he spoke but only looked down at them occasionally. From historical records, it is apparent that he had practiced his speech ahead of time. In most naturalistic contexts, a speaker formulates his or her utterances mentally, often while still producing the sounds of the phrase previously formulated. Whether pre-planned or formulated spontaneously, speech production is preceded by a cognitive and linguistic encoding process that translates an idea into a sequence of words.

President Kennedy spoke in short phrases, as many public speakers do, especially when delivering a speech through an amplification system that produces echoes in large spaces surrounded by buildings. Each short phrase was preceded by a brief inhalation. In spontaneous speech and reading, a close correlation between the volume of air inhaled prior to speech onset and the length of the subsequent breath group has been observed in adults (Hixon, 1973; Huber, 2008; Sperry and Klich, 1992; Winkworth, Davis, Adams, and Ellis, 1995). This shows that the respiratory system is programmed for the breath demands of the utterance while it is still in its linguistic planning stage. It is unknown whether children adjust their inhaled air volumes for utterance length as well, although in general, their speech breathing parameters resemble those of adults by age 10 years (Hoit, Hixon, Watson, and Morgan, 1990). Both adults and children inhale more air before producing louder speech tokens, compared to medium loudness levels (Hixon, 1973; Stathopoulos and Sapienza, 1997).

Several times during his speech, President Kennedy repeated a word or phrase. For instance, he said, "I uh... I ... I appreciate ... I appreciate my interpreter translating my German." The large audience was very responsive to his statements, breaking into loud applause and cheers on several occasions just as President Kennedy was about to start a new sentence. Feedback from listeners is not the only auditory feedback modifying the flow of speech production. As we speak, we hear our own speech via air conduction as well as via bone conduction directly to the cochlea. This type of self-feedback allows us to regulate many aspects of our speech including speed, volume, and intonation. Together with other feedback mechanisms such as kinesthetic input, it also allows us to monitor for speech errors and to repair them, as a radio announcer did as soon as he realized he just misspoke: "Wall Streek's ... Wall Street's most recent winning streak [...]", or as a university instructor did in his electrical engineering course lecture: "This is just a sinkle ... a single, simple acoustic tube" (examples taken from the author's collection of observed speech errors). Both of these examples, incidentally, illustrate speech planning errors resulting from anticipating salient aspects of the speech sounds in a word further ahead in the planned utterance and merging it with the speech sound sequence of the word currently being produced.

President Kennedy had not studied German formally but prior to delivering his speech, he had practiced the phrase that became famous: "*Ich bin ein Berliner*" (I am a Berliner). The German word "*ich*" (/ɪç/) contains a consonant not found in English, the palatal fricative /ç/. Many second language learners of German substitute the [ʃ] sound for this sound, perhaps because it is acoustically similar and because it is part of their native phoneme inventory. President Kennedy's production of this sound was slightly fronted as well. (Chapter 8 focuses more in detail on adult learners of a language.)

Experienced speakers show evidence of **coarticulation**, where articulatory features of one sound are evident in the preceding or subsequent sound(s). In part, this phenomenon can be explained by the fact that the tongue and the lips are separate articulators and can be programmed to function somewhat independently of each other (Daniloff and Moll, 1968). This leads to lip spreading during the /fr/ segments of the word "free" in anticipation of the vowel /i/ and in lip rounding during the /tr/ segments of the word "true" when the vowel /u/ is anticipated, as seen in President Kennedy's speech. Coarticulation can even cross word boundaries. For instance, in the phrase "if you," the /f/ might be executed with rounded lips but with spread lips in the phrase "if he" in anticipation of the vowel in the subsequent word. In an experiment designed to compare children with typical development and children with language impairment to adults, both groups of children showed evidence of adult-like coarticulation by age 4 to 5 years (Smith, 2006).

Another aspect of speech production that develops in children over time is the ability to sequence oral movements efficiently. "Freedom is indivisible," said President Kennedy. "Indivisible" is a five-syllable word with a VC.CV.CV.CV.CVC structure (V = vowel, C = consonant), where four of the five V segments remain the same across the word but the C segments vary in place and manner, requiring considerable skill in sequencing the articulators. Diadochokinetic tasks are designed to test for motor sequencing, using single syllables such as /pa/, /ta/, and /ka/ as well is two- and three-syllable combinations such as /pata/ and /pataka/. A meta-analysis of published norms (Fletcher, 1972) shows that syllable durations decrease in children as a function of age, indicating increasingly rapid speeds. Of interest, at approximately 10 years, the syllable durations in the disyllables become shorter than the monosyllables (Figure 3.4). Why might this be? To produce a series of monosyllables such as /papapapa …./ or /tatatata …/, the jaw and lips repeat an oscillatory cycle of opening and closing over and over. To produce a rapid series of /pata …/, however, two different oscillations, one for /pa/ and one for /ta/, are overlaid and interleaved in time. As mentioned, the lips and tongue can be programmed fairly independently.

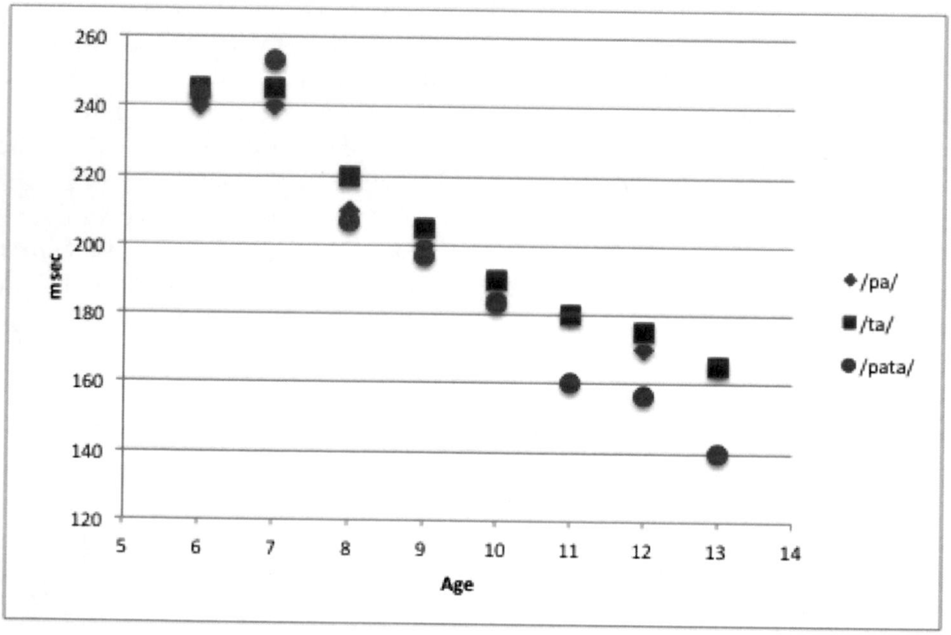

Figure 3.4. Meta-analysis of syllable durations (msec) in child productions of diadochokinetic tasks as a function of age (Fletcher, 1972).

To achieve the shorter durations in disyllables, the two oscillatory cycles for the monosyllables must be synchronized in time, an ability that children develop with age. We found that a speed advantage for alternating movements extends to finger movements as well and that deficits in alternating movement speeds run in families with familial speech sound disorder consistent with childhood apraxia of speech (CAS) (Peter and Raskind, 2011). CAS is a proposed subtype of speech sound disorder characterized by planning and/or programming spatiotemporal parameters of motor sequences, as outlined in a recent position statement published by the American Speech-Language-Hearing Association (*http://www.asha.org/docs/html/PS2007-00277.html*). For more information on CAS, consult Chapters 15 and 18.

Sidebar 3.1. Did Speech Evolve from Grunts around the Cave Fire?

When we speak, we use some of the same structures and systems that are used for the elementary and life-sustaining functions of airway protection, chewing, and swallowing. Does this mean that these functions came first and speech is a relatively recent human trait? If so, how did humans first represent meaning by making sounds with their vocal tracts? Let's review some speculations on this intriguing but ultimately unprovable topic.

According to the gestural theory, early *Homo Sapiens* communicated using hand gestures and eventually switched to oral articulation. This view is held by Michael Corballis (Corballis, 2002), who explains that the idea goes back to the 18th Century philosopher Condillac. Corballis believes that vocal languages emerged roughly 60,000 to 100,000 years ago, concurrent with a presumed explosion in cultural sophistication evident in human artifacts in Africa prior to migrations out of Africa. As outlined by William Stokoe, the recognition that the sign languages used by deaf communities are true languages is compatible with this view (Stokoe, 2001). In this context, it is interesting to note that infants are capable of representing meaning with simple hand signs long before they produce their first word (Acredolo and Goodwyn, 1988; Acredolo and Goodwyn, 1996).

A contrasting view is that language evolved in the spoken modality without manual gestures as a precursor. This view is held by Stephen Pinker (Pinker, 1995), who proposes that spoken language evolved as such by natural selection. Pinker claims that individuals with more advanced verbal skills had an advantage that translated into higher survival rates and greater reproductive success, so that their genetic heritage became more prevalent in the population. Pinker and others speculate that the human version of the *FOXP2* gene is the result of a mutation that equipped its carriers with the characteristically fine orofacial muscle control that distinguishes humans from nonhuman primates and other mammals. Note that this gene is only one of several, if not many, that are required for speech and language development.

Exactly how humans got the idea to use their vocal apparatus to communicate has been the object of speculation. One possibility is that social bonds, originally formed by mutual grooming, came to be nurtured with spoken language instead (Dunbar, 1996). Another view is that the rhythmic opening and closing movements of the jaw while chewing food provided the motor template for speech syllables, so that speech is a derivative of eating (MacNeilage and Davis, 2001). Perhaps vocal communication had a nonverbal but oral, more music-like precursor, as described in Mithen's (Mithen, 2006) "Hmmm" hypothesis, where Hmmm stands for holistic (not composed of meaningful subunits), multimodal (both vocal sound and hand gesture), manipulative, and musical (see Sidebar 3.2 for additional information).

As mentioned, there is no way to answer the question of how our linguistic communication evolved in an empirical way. Nonetheless, curiosity about the **phylogeny** of speech is just as legitimate as curiosity of the **ontogeny** of speech, which is the subject of this book.

Sidebar 3.2 Singing

Have you ever wondered why all cultures of the world have developed music, both instrumental and vocal? To sing is to overlay speech on a given musical rhythm and pitch, where the rhythm and pitch form a melody and the speech component forms a linguistic message. This is as true of rap as it is of Bach's cantatas.

If verbal communication provides an adaptive advantage, what are the advantages of singing? Since Charles Darwin asked this question (Darwin, 1871), many possibilities have been proposed.

As reviewed by W. Tecumseh Fitch (Fitch, 2006), music may have preceded oral language as a form of protolanguage. One proponent of this hypothesis is Steven Mithen (Mithen, 2005). He claims that this protolanguage was holistic (not composed of segmented elements), manipulative (influencing the emotional states and behaviors of oneself and others), multimodal (using both sound and movement), musical (temporally controlled, rhythmic, and melodic), and mimetic (utilizing sound symbolism and gesture), resulting in the whimsical "Hmmm" acronym (p. 172).

Male birds and whales sing to attract a mate. The idea that humans who sing well have better options of finding a mate has been considered (Miller, 2001). Choral singing could have evolved as a form of social bonding within larger groups. The use of lullabies is found in all cultures and may represent a special form of mother-child bonding.

Alternatively, it is possible is that music has absolutely no adaptive function. According to Steven Pinker (Pinker, 1997), music is "auditory cheesecake " that evolved as a byproduct of other, more adaptive behaviors such as walking and speech. Music could simply be a form of play that serves no immediate purpose.

Regardless of their respective adaptive functions, speech and music share some biological substrates, for instance the auditory system. In music, two tones that are separated by whole octaves are perceived as being highly similar (Burns, 1999). The octave is a basic building block of musical scales in all cultures of the world (Burns & Ward, 1978). Is the octave-related similarity in music also found in the fundamental frequency of the speech signal? In a recent study, young children imitating nonwords produced by an adult male adjusted their fundamental frequency to match the pitch in the adult's voice at a frequency an octave above the adult male's fundamental frequency (Peter, Larkin, & Stoel-Gammon, 2009). This implies that the children, whose vocal range did not overlap with that in the male adult's voice, were sensitive to the octave-related similarity in vocal pitch and used it to make their spoken imitations sound even more like the stimulus.

CONNECTIONS

Skilled use of several structures, including the larynx, contributes to the expression of prosody, as described in Chapter 7. Adults acquiring the phonetic and phonemic features of a second language already have a fully developed and coordinated speech production system that was trained on their first language. Given this established set of speech production skills, does their speech acquisition process differ substantially from that seen in infants learning to produce speech? This interesting question is discussed in Chapter 8. Around the world, millions of infants are in the process of acquiring the speech features of their ambient language. Do the speech sounds in different languages impose motoric challenges that tax the developing system in similar ways? This volume's section on languages beyond English sheds light on cross-linguistic aspects of speech acquisition. How structural and functional deficits in the developing speech system interfere with the acquisition of speech is described in the chapters on special populations.

CONCLUDING REMARKS

Although, as mentioned in the Introduction, all the major structures and systems necessary for speech are fully formed at birth, newborns are two to four years away from using their biological substrates to produce completely understandable speech. One reason is that the proportions of tongue size and oral cavity do not yet allow for substantial movement in space, and teeth do not erupt until later in the first year of life. Another aspect is that speech production is one of the most complex activities we humans engage in, not only in terms of coordinating multiple moving structures in a precisely timed sequence but also in terms of determining the exact spatial excursion and force of each articulator, always monitoring for acoustic and kinesthetic feedback.

In addition, we must generate new semantic and syntactic content to be translated into motor commands while being busy executing the motor commands generated a fraction of a second ago. All this parallel activity requires a tremendous amount of integration on multiple levels (cognitive, linguistic, motor, kinesthetic, auditory). It is not surprising that the production of the first word, at approximately one year of age, is preceded by many stages of vocalization. Imagine that your task is to perform an improvised toccata for organ by operating two full keyboards, a set of foot pedals, and a full compliment of register settings.

To be able to do this successfully, you may need to take organ lessons and practice daily for many years, even though you may have listened to organ music all your life. The analogous is true for human children learning to talk, except that they typically master the task without formal lessons. To them, it's child's play, so to speak.

CHAPTER REVIEW QUESTIONS

1. How is symmetry between the cerebral hemispheres related to language development?
2. What effect does the ambient acoustic environment during prenatal development have on the fetus?
3. Describe the sexual dimorphism of the vocal folds.
4. What is one physical indication that motor planning for an entire utterance takes place before the first word is spoken?
5. How can you explain speed differences in monosyllabic and multisyllabic diadochokinetic tasks from a motor control perspective?

SUGGESTIONS FOR FURTHER READING

Bear, M. F., Connors, B. W., and Paradiso, M. A. (2007). *Neuroscience: Exploring the brain.* Philadelphia: Lippincott Williams and Wilkins.

Deutsch, D. E. (1999). *The psychology of music.* 2nd Edition. San Diego: Academic Press.
Kent, R. D., and Vorperian, H. K. (1995). *Development of the craniofacial-oral-laryngeal anatomy: A review.* San Diego: Singular.

SUGGESTIONS FOR STUDENT ACTIVITIES

1. Whether humans are hard-wired to acquire speech or whether they figure out how to speak by trial and error is the subject of a debate that has been going on for many decades. According to the behaviorist view, the use of spoken language is learned like any other behavior. According to the nativist view, humans have an innate ability to acquire spoken language. Based on the reviews cited here or any others you encounter, create a list of arguments for each of these views and formulate your own position.

   Hegde, M. N., and Weitzman, R. (2010). Language and grammar: A behavioral analysis. *Journal of Speech-Language Pathology and Applied Behavior Analysis*,5(2), 90 - 113.
   Anderson, S. R., and Lightfoot, D. W. (2000). The human language faculty as an organ. *Annu Rev Physiol*, 62, 697-722.

2. Is the use of language unique to humans, or do animals have a linguistic capacity as well? Read the reviews cited here or any others you find and create a list of arguments for each of these two positions, then formulate your own position.

   Hauser, M. D., Chomsky, N., and Fitch, W. T. (2002). The faculty of language: what is it, who has it, and how did it evolve? *Science,* 298(5598), 1569-1579.
   Fitch, W. T., Huber, L., and Bugnyar, T. (2010). Social cognition and the evolution of language: constructing cognitive phylogenies. *Neuron,* 65(6), 795-814.
   Pinker, S., and Jackendoff, R. (2005). The faculty of language: what's special about it? *Cognition,* 95(2), 201-236.

ANSWERS TO CHAPTER REVIEW QUESTIONS

1. How is symmetry between the cerebral hemispheres related to language development?

In typical development, the insula and the planum temporale are larger in the left hemisphere, compared to the right. A lack of this asymmetry has been observed in the brains of individuals with language impairment and dyslexia.

2. What effect does the ambient acoustic environment during prenatal development have on the fetus?

We know that fetuses respond to sound by the 17th week post fertilization, indicating that the auditory system functions by this time. Newborn babies can distinguish not only their mother's voice from that of another female adult voices, but also the language to which they were exposed prenatally from other languages.

3. Describe the sexual dimorphism of the vocal folds.

Infants have very short vocal folds, resulting in a high fundamental frequency. The vocal folds grow commensurate with body growth in boys and girls, resulting in a slowly decreasing fundamental frequency. In adolescence, the vocal folds of boys, but not girls, undergo a growth spurt that causes a rapid drop in fundamental frequency.

4. What is one physical indication that motor planning for an entire utterance takes place before the first word is spoken?

The volume of inhaled air prior to an utterance is commensurate with the length of the planned utterance.

5. How can you explain speed differences in monosyllabic and multisyllabic diadochokinetic tasks from a motor control perspective?

In older children and adults, multisyllabic sequences are produced faster than monosyllabic sequences. Multisyllabic sequences can be modeled as separate repetitive cycles of opening/closing movements. For instance, to produce /pata/, the lips are programmed for one repetitive cycle to produce /papapa… / and the anterior tongue is programmed to produce /tatata …/. These two cycles are interleaved in time to produce /pata/. In older children and adults, the lips and the tongue can be programmed independently of each other, resulting in a speed advantage for this type of task. Younger children and individuals with motor programming deficits do not show this speed advantage.

References

Acredolo, L., and Goodwyn, S. (1988). Symbolic gesturing in normal infants. *Child Dev.*, 59(2), 450-466.

Acredolo, L., and Goodwyn, S. W. (1996). *Baby signs: How to talk with your baby before your baby can talk.* Chicago: Contemporary Books.

Afif, A., Bouvier, R., Buenerd, A., Trouillas, J., and Mertens, P. (2007). Development of the human fetal insular cortex: study of the gyration from 13 to 28 gestational weeks. *Brain Struct. Funct.,* 212(3-4), 335-346. doi: 10.1007/s00429-007-0161-1.

Bartzokis, G., Lu, P. H., Tingus, K., Mendez, M. F., Richard, A., Peters, D. G., Mintz, J. (2010). Lifespan trajectory of myelin integrity and maximum motor speed. *Neurobiol.*

Aging, 31(9), 1554-1562. doi: S0197-4580(08)00302-3 [pii]. 10.1016/j.neurobiolaging. 2008.08.015.

Burns, E. M. (1999). Intervals, scales, and tuning. In D. Deutsch (Ed.), *The psychology of music.* 2nd Ed. (pp. 215 - 264). San Diego: Academic Press.

Burns, E. M., and Ward, W. D. (1978). Categorical perception--phenomenon or epiphenomenon: evidence from experiments in the perception of melodic musical intervals. *J. Acoust. Soc. Am.*, 63(2), 456-468.

Cohen, S., and Levi-Montalcini, R. (1956). A Nerve Growth-Stimulating Factor Isolated from Snake Venom. *Proc. Natl. Acad. Sci. US,* 42(9), 571-574.

Cohen, S., Levi-Montalcini, R., and Hamburger, V. (1954). A Nerve Growth-Stimulating Factor Isolated from Sarcom as 37 and 180. *Proc. Natl. Acad. Sci. US*, 40(10), 1014-1018.

Corballis, M. C. (2002). *From hand to mouth: the origins of language*. Princeton: Princeton University Press.

Crinion, J. T., and Leff, A. P. (2007). Recovery and treatment of aphasia after stroke: functional imaging studies. *Curr. Opin. Neurol.*, 20(6), 667-673. doi: 10.1097/WCO.0b013e3282f1c6fa. 00019052-200712000-00012 [pii].

Daniloff, R., and Moll, K. (1968). Coarticulation of lip rounding. *J. Speech Hear Res.*, 11(4), 707-721.

Darwin, C. (1871). *The descent of man, and selection in relation to sex*. New York: D. Appleton and Company, 549 and 551 Broadway.

Dietrich, J., Monje, M., Wefel, J., and Meyers, C. (2008). Clinical patterns and biological correlates of cognitive dysfunction associated with cancer therapy. *Oncologist*, 13(12), 1285-1295. doi: theoncologist. 2008-0130 [pii]. 10.1634/theoncologist.2008-0130.

Dunbar, R. I. M. (1996). *Grooming, gossip, and the evolution of language*. Cambridge, Mass.: Harvard University Press.

Eriksson, P. S., Perfilieva, E., Bjork-Eriksson, T., Alborn, A. M., Nordborg, C., Peterson, D. A., and Gage, F. H. (1998). Neurogenesis in the adult human hippocampus. *Nat. Med.,* 4(11), 1313-1317. doi: 10.1038/3305.

Finnegan, D. E. (1984). Maximum phonation time for children with normal voices. *J. Commun. Disord.*, 17(5), 309-317. doi: 0021-9924(84)90033-9 [pii].

Fitch, W. T. (2006). The biology and evolution of music: a comparative perspective. *Cognition*, 100(1), 173-215. doi: S0010-0277(05)00225-8 [pii]. 10.1016/j.cognition.2005.11.009.

Fletcher, S. G. (1972). Time-by-count measurement of diadochokinetic syllable rate. *J. Speech Hear Res.*, 15(4), 763-770.

Galaburda, A. M., Sherman, G. F., Rosen, G. D., Aboitiz, F., and Geschwind, N. (1985). Developmental dyslexia: four consecutive patients with cortical anomalies. *Ann. Neurol.*, 18(2), 222-233. doi: 10.1002/ana.410180210.

Gaultier, C., and Zinman, R. (1983). Maximal static pressures in healthy children. *Respir Physio.l*, 51(1), 45-61.

Giedd, J. N., Blumenthal, J., Jeffries, N. O., Castellanos, F. X., Liu, H., Zijdenbos, A., Rapoport, J. L. (1999). Brain development during childhood and adolescence: a longitudinal MRI study. *Nat. Neurosci.,* 2(10), 861-863. doi: 10.1038/13158.

Gordon, N. (2004). The neurology of sign language. *Brain Dev.*, 26(3), 146-150. doi: 10.1016/S0387-7604(03)00128-1. S0387760403001281 [pii].

Hepper, P. G., and Shahidullah, B. S. (1994). Development of fetal hearing. *Arch. Dis. Child*, 71(2), F81-87.

Hickok, G. (2009). The functional neuroanatomy of language. *Phys. Life Rev.*, 6(3), 121-143. doi: 10.1016/j.plrev.2009.06.001.

Hixon, T. J. (1973). Kinematics of the chest wall during speech production: volume displacements of the rib cage, abdomen, and lung. *J. Speech Hear Res.*, 16(1), 78-115.

Hoit, J. D., Hixon, T. J., Watson, P. J., and Morgan, W. J. (1990). Speech breathing in children and adolescents. *J. Speech Hear Res.*, 33(1), 51-69.

Hollien, H., and Shipp, T. (1972). Speaking fundamental frequency and chronologic age in males. *J. Speech Hear Res.*, 15(1), 155-159.

Horvitz, H. R., Shaham, S., and Hengartner, M. O. (1994). The genetics of programmed cell death in the nematode Caenorhabditis elegans. *Cold Spring Harb. Symp. Quant. Biol.*, 59, 377-385.

Huber, J. E. (2008). Effects of utterance length and vocal loudness on speech breathing in older adults. *Respir. Physiol. Neurobiol.*, 164(3), 323-330. doi: S1569-9048(08)00219-X [pii]. 10.1016/j.resp.2008.08.007.

Huttenlocher, P. R., and Dabholkar, A. S. (1997). Regional differences in synaptogenesis in human cerebral cortex. *J. Comp. Neurol.*, 387(2), 167-178. doi: 10.1002/(SICI)1096-9861(19971020)387:2<167:AID-CNE1>3.0.CO;2-Z [pii].

Jernigan, T. L., Hesselink, J. R., Sowell, E., and Tallal, P. A. (1991). Cerebral structure on magnetic resonance imaging in language - and learning -impaired children. *Arch. Neurol.*, 48(5), 539-545.

Kent, R. D. (1976). Anatomical and neuromuscular maturation of the speech mechanism: evidence from acoustic studies. *J. Speech Hear Res.*, 19(3), 421-447.

Kent, R. D. (1994). *Reference manual for communicative sciences and disorders: Speech and Language*. Austin: ProEd.

Kent, R. D. (1997). *The speech sciences*. San Diego: Singular Pub. Group.

Kuhl, P. K., Williams, K. A., Lacerda, F., Stevens, K. N., and Lindblom, B. (1992). Linguistic experience alters phonetic perception in infants by 6 months of age. *Science*, 255(5044), 606-608.

MacNeilage, P. F., and Davis, B. L. (2001). Motor mechanisms in speech ontogeny: phylogenetic, neurobiological and linguistic implications. *Curr. Opin. Neurobiol.*, 11(6), 696-700. doi: S0959-4388(01)00271-9 [pii].

Maguire, E. A., Gadian, D. G., Johnsrude, I. S., Good, C. D., Ashburner, J., Frackowiak, R. S., and Frith, C. D. (2000). Navigation-related structural change in the hippocampi of taxi drivers. *Proc. Natl. Acad. Sci. US*, 97(8), 4398-4403. doi: 10.1073/pnas.070039597. 070039597 [pii].

Mampe, B., Friederici, A. D., Christophe, A., and Wermke, K. (2009). Newborns' cry melody is shaped by their native language. *Curr. Biol.*, 19(23), 1994-1997. doi: S0960-9822(09)01824-7 [pii]. 10.1016/j.cub.2009.09.064.

Mehler, J., Bertoncini, J., and Barriere, M. (1978). Infant recognition of mother's voice. *Perception*, 7(5), 491-497.

Mehler, J., Lambertz, G., Jusczyk, P., and Amiel-Tison, C. (1986). [Discrimination of the mother tongue by newborn infants]. *C. R. Acad. Sci. III*, 303(15), 637-640.

Melsen, B., and Melsen, F. (1982). The postnatal development of the palatomaxillary region studied on human autopsy material. *Am. J. Orthod.*, 82(4), 329-342.

Miller, G. F. (2001). The mating mind: How sexual choice shaped the evolution of human nature. *Psycoloquy*, 12(8), 1-15.

Mithen, S. J. (2005). *The Singing Neanderthals: The Origins of Music, Language, Mind and Body*. London: Weidenfeld and Nicolson.

Mithen, S. J. (2006). *The singing neanderthals : the origins of music, language, mind, and body*. Cambridge, Mass.: Harvard University Press.

Moore, K. L., Persaud, T. V. N., and Torchia, M. G. (2008). *Before we are born: essentials of embryology and birth defects* (7th ed.). Philadelphia, P. A.: Saunders/Elsevier.

Peter, B., Larkin, T., and Stoel-Gammon, C. (2009). Octave-shifted pitch matching in nonword imitations: the effects of lexical stress and speech sound disorder. *J. Acoust. Soc. Am.*, 126(4), 1663-1666. doi: 10.1121/1.3203993.

Peter, B., and Raskind, W. H. (2011). Evidence for a familial speech sound disorder subtype in a multigenerational study of oral and hand motor sequencing ability. *Topics in Language Disorders*, 31(2), 145-167. doi: 10.1097/TLD.0b013e318217b855.

Pinker, S. (1995). *The language instinct* (1st HarperPerennial ed.). New York: Harper Perennial.

Pinker, S. (1997). *How the mind works*. New York: Norton.

Robb, M. P., and Saxman, J. H. (1985). Developmental trends in vocal fundamental frequency of young children. *J. Speech Hear Res.*, 28(3), 421-427.

Rusconi, F., Castagneto, M., Gagliardi, L., Leo, G., Pellegatta, A., Porta, N., Braga, M. (1994). Reference values for respiratory rate in the first 3 years of life. *Pediatrics*, 94(3), 350-355.

Smith, A. (2006). Speech motor development: Integrating muscles, movements, and linguistic units. *J. Commun. Disord.*, 39(5), 331-349. doi: S0021-9924(06)00062-1 [pii]. 10.1016/j.jcomdis.2006.06.017.

Sperry, E. E., and Klich, R. J. (1992). Speech breathing in senescent and younger women during oral reading. *J. Speech Hear Res.*, 35(6), 1246-1255.

Stathopoulos, E. T., and Sapienza, C. M. (1997). Developmental changes in laryngeal and respiratory function with variations in sound pressure level. *J. Speech Lang Hear Res.*, 40(3), 595-614.

Stokoe, W. C. (2001). *Language in hand: Why sign came before speech*. Washington, D. C.: Gallaudet University Press.

Tobin, M. J., Chadha, T. S., Jenouri, G., Birch, S. J., Gazeroglu, H. B., and Sackner, M. A. (1983). Breathing patterns. 1. Normal subjects. *Chest,* 84(2), 202-205.

Tobin, M. J., Jenouri, G., Lind, B., Watson, H., Schneider, A., and Sackner, M. A. (1983). Validation of respiratory inductive plethysmography in patients with pulmonary disease. *Chest,* 83(4), 615-620.

Werker, J. F., and Tees, R. C. (1983). Developmental changes across childhood in the perception of non-native speech sounds. *Can. J. Psychol.*, 37(2), 278-286.

Werker, J. F., and Tees, R. C. (1992). The organization and reorganization of human speech perception. *Annu. Rev. Neurosci.*, 15, 377-402. doi: 10.1146/annurev.ne.15.030192.002113.

Winkworth, A. L., Davis, P. J., Adams, R. D., and Ellis, E. (1995). Breathing patterns during spontaneous speech. *J. Speech Hear Res.*, 38(1), 124-144.

Zapletal, A., Samanek, M., and Paul, T. (1987). *Lung function in children and adolescents: Methods, references values*. Basel: Karger.

Zemlin, W. R. (1998). *Speech and hearing science: anatomy and physiology* (4th ed.). Boston: Allyn and Bacon.

In: Comprehensive Perspectives …
Editors: Beate Peter and Andrea A. N. MacLeod
ISBN: 978-1-62257-041-6

Chapter 4

AN ACOUSTIC PHONETIC CATALOG OF PRESPEECH VOCALIZATIONS FROM A DEVELOPMENTAL PERSPECTIVE

Eugene H. Buder, Anne S. Warlaumont and D. Kimbrough Oller

INTRODUCTION

From a newborn's cry to a child's first word at approximately 12 months of age, a wide variety of sounds is produced. Many of these have much in common with sounds produced by other mammals, for example vegetative sounds such as coughing and burping, or "fixed signals" (Lorenz, 1951) such as crying due to hunger or other discomfort, or laughter in response to being tickled. Other sounds are clearly more volitional in nature, and are often termed babbling or, following Oller (2000), "**protophones**."

There are many reasons to believe the protophones are precursors to speech: because only humans produce them, because all normally developing infants produce them before speaking, because they occur in a rough developmental sequence, becoming more speech-like across the first year, and because disruption of the normal pattern for age at onset is associated with a variety of developmental disorders (for review see Oller, 2000). Protophones that emerge earliest differ greatly from speech in terms of phonatory, articulatory, and acoustic characteristics. This fact compels us to utilize a special methodology capable of illustrating the relations between protophones and speech. Instead of describing the protophones *as* speech sounds, we address them on their own terms as special pre-speech categories and features. This chapter offers a catalog of protophones from the first months of life to the onset of meaningful speech. State-of-the-art spectrograms and accompanying sound files illustrate each of these protophones, along with a rough outline of orders of occurrence (empirically verified or presumed based on the infrastructural theory) of different protophone groups.

HISTORY OF THE PROTOPHONE APPROACH TO STUDYING INFANT VOCALIZATIONS

The linguist Jakobson asserted that infant babble was random and purposeless behavior unrelated to the development of speech sounds. His "discontinuity theory" (Jakobson, 1941, 1968) was later shown to be incorrect. For instance, the phonological characteristics of canonical babble (e.g., [ba], [ma]. [baba], [dada]) and early words are very similar with respect to syllable types and shapes (Nakazima, 1962; Oller, Wieman, Doyle, and Ross, 1975; Stoel-Gammon and Cooper, 1984; Stoel-Gammon and Dunn, 1985; Vihman, Macken, Miller, Simmons, and Miller, 1985). Moreover, most children produce babbling for several months after the emergence of first words, at least up until age 18 to 20 months (Stoel-Gammon and Dunn, 1985).

Prior to the late 1970s, scientists interested in studying infant vocalizations took one of two approaches. They either transcribed infant vocalizations phonetically, using the same phonetic categories as would be used for transcribing adult speech (Irwin, 1947, 1948), or they measured the acoustic properties of infant vocalizations, using acoustic measurements designed for adult speech (Lynip, 1951). While both methods have their place and continue to sometimes be used by scientists and clinicians alike, in the late 1970s and early 1980s a new way of understanding and measuring infant vocalizations was developed (Koopmans-van Beinum and van der Stelt, 1986; Oller, 1980, 1986; Stark, 1980). This approach focuses on the precanonical protophones, recognizing that these early prelinguistic sounds are more primitive than, and quite distinct from, later sounds that can appropriately be characterized within the International Phonetic Alphabet (IPA). The protophone categories are generally recognizable intuitively by adult listeners (where caregivers are deemed to be the key listeners). Within each infant, the protophone categories that are produced regularly can be thought of as the infant's infraphonological repertoire, representing the infant's capabilities to produce contrastive sounds volitionally.

Taking a protophone-based approach to the study of infant vocalizations, rather than a phonetic transcription approach or pure acoustic measurement approach, has allowed researchers to discover what appear to be fairly universal developmental trends in infant vocalizations across the first year. Researchers have tended to describe these trends in terms of stages. Similar stages have been independently identified by a variety of research groups. A typical characterization is provided below (see "Comments on order of development and ages of onset in protophones").

It is interesting that while there seems to be no dispute about the idea that there are consistent universal patterns, there has been considerable effort to try to determine possible effects differing ambient languages may have on very early vocalizations. Although no one disputes that there are also major similarities in babbling across infants from all language groups that have been studied, there are a number of reports that contend that by the end of the first year there are specific language effects (de Boysson-Bardies, 1999; Levitt and Wang, 1991; Vihman and de Boysson-Bardies, 1994). At the same time there have been a number of failures to determine ambient language effects in the first year (Atkinson, MacWhinney, and Stoel, 1970; Eady, 1980; Navarro, Pearson, Cobo-Lewis, and Oller, 1998). Because the methodology of such research is difficult at best, the matter of whether or not there are ambient language effects on prelinguistic vocalizations remains, in our opinion, unresolved.

The one issue that seems clear is that much of infant vocal development, and presumably the basic scheme of protophone stages, is universal.

Other research on protophone use has focused on infants with hearing impairment or autism (Ertmer and Iyer, 2010; Paul, Fuerst, Ramsay, Chawarska, and Klin, 2011; Sheinkopf, Mundy, Oller, and Steffens, 2000), on patterns of repetition and coordination of vocalizations between child and caregiver (Buder, Warlaumont, Oller, and Chorna, 2010; Warlaumont, Oller, Dale, Richards, Gilkerson, and Xu, 2010), on the influence of social reinforcement on protophone productions (Goldstein and Schwade, 2008), and on automatic classification of protophones (Warlaumont, Oller, Buder, Dale, and Kozma, 2010).

In the glossary below, we describe the major protophone categories currently used in our infant vocalization research. They constitute the kinds of sounds that, in accord with our findings, most infants produce during the first year or so of life as they progress from simple, primitive sounds in the months right after birth to sophisticated sequences of sounds that resemble adult speech to a much greater extent. We focus on the most commonly occurring features of the most commonly occurring protophone categories in infancy.

Guidelines for Coding Protophone Categories

Protophone categories are those primitive categories of sounds that are thought to be speech-related, or precursors to mature speech. Thus we exclude fixed, species-specific signals such as crying or laughter, and vegetative sounds, produced as byproducts of purely physiological events such as feeding, moving the torso, lifting, or sneezing. As speech-related sounds, protophones can generally be divided into two categories: those related to phonation and those related to syllabification and/or articulation.

Three issues regarding our system of coding (and corresponding guidelines) need to be taken into account in order to understand how we intend the term protophone to be understood and how we go about categorization. These concern:

1. Coding at the utterance-level
2. Forced-choice coding
3. The focus on volitionally produced sounds

First, we generally code at the "utterance" level, where utterances are taken to be "breath-groups" (Lynch, Oller, Steffens, and Buder, 1995); that is, an utterance consists of the vocalization occurring on a single egress of the breathing cycle. We have of course coded and analyzed infant sounds at other levels as well (from sub-segmental to super-clusters of utterances), but the protophone terminology applies primarily to the utterance level.

The second issue concerns the fact that in keeping with utterance-level coding, we generally impose a forced choice on coders for both phonatory and syllabification/articulation judgments of protophones—only one code (though sometimes it consists of the combination of two features as in for example squeal-yells or growl-yells) may be used to describe the phonation and one code to describe the syllabification/articulation for each utterance. This approach forces the listener to ignore many characteristics of utterances and to focus instead on only the most salient features of utterances, despite the fact that it is often clear that multiple features are recognized by the listener. Especially for long utterances the forced choice is often difficult, because, for example, infants may vary their phonation, as well as types of syllabification/articulation, considerably within the utterance. The justification for this coding approach is partly theoretical: parents and other caregivers, the most important listeners in children's lives, tend to focus on global features of infant utterances and to ignore details within utterances. The justification is also partly practical: the time cost of coding is often prohibitive if details are taken into account. As children get older we consider much more syllabic or even phonetic detail for each utterance, because (among various reasons) it is clear that by that time syllabic and phonetic details play important roles in parent-infant communication (see Chapter 5 by Anna Sosa for a description of early speech).

To exemplify this whole-utterance categorization approach, consider that an utterance can contain, in sequence, both a squeal portion and a vowel-like or "**vocant**" portion (in the phonatory realm), but coders are required to indicate one or the other. Similarly an utterance can consist of both a glottal stop syllabification and a canonical syllabification (in the articulation/syllabification realm), but coders are required to choose one of the two. The coder's choice (in accord with our protocol) is guided by a combination of intuition about saliency of the competing features of the utterance, infraphonological theory, and lessons learned from evaluating inter-observer reliability of coding for protophones. For example, if squeal and vocant features co-occur within an utterance, the listener chooses squeal, which is often very salient because it represents a substantial departure from the infant's most common phonatory mode. However, if the squeal portion is deemed by the listener to be very low in saliency, it can be ignored and the utterance can be treated as a vocant. If a glottal stop syllable co-occurs in the same utterance with a canonical one, the listener chooses canonical because canonical syllables are deemed, theoretically, to be more advanced developmentally.

However, this sort of mutual exclusivity in using the coding categories is not an irreversible requirement for the future—it is certainly possible to envision protophone coding procedures where multiple protophone codes are involved (perhaps weighted by their saliency). Such complex coding seems ultimately desirable especially if we wish to characterize fully the relations between protophones and the more advanced forms of real speech. As greater control over the protophones develops, their characteristics gradually become integrated as features of a more elaborate scheme of vocalization. For example, within a single utterance, phonatory and pitch-related features (first seen as squeals, growls and vocants) can come to serve as prosodic accompaniments of richly differentiated syllabic sequences—in adult speech, well-formed sentences or parts of sentences are sometimes produced in a squeal or growl register.

The final issue is that protophone coding focuses on volitionally produced sounds, and because humans can produce any kind of sound volitionally on some occasions (even vegetative sounds such as coughing!), the coder is forced also to make an intuitive judgment about the volitional nature of infant vocalization. This requirement forces the coder to simulate the natural judgment style of caregivers, whose task it is to nurture the infant's well-being and who interpret infant sounds as indicators of state, need and fitness. Caregivers' judgments are taken to be the most important reference point in coding because it is the caregivers who negotiate with infants over the functions and ultimately the meanings of their vocalizations. The volitional nature of vocalization is clearly an important indicator of the progression toward speech in and of itself, and caregivers appear to have a sense of the extent to which infants vocalize intentionally. They naturally recognize the difference between playful, exploratory sounds and sounds that are motivated by pain or fear, for example, and they understand that the former are more volitional. Further, no other primate shows volitional vocalization to nearly the extent that the human infant does (Cheney and Seyfarth, 1999; Hauser, 1996; Owren and Goldstein, 2008). The extent of volitional control appears, however, to vary continuously across utterances rather than representing a binary (on-off) characteristic of utterances. For example, it is often observed that a single infant utterance may contain both fuss and vowel-like elements. Again, a forced choice is required (in accord with our protocol) in coding to differentiate among the more reflexive sounds of infants (the ones that resemble more the sounds of other primates' warning calls, vocal threats or vegetative sounds) and the more volitional ones, the ones that form more important foundations for speech.

Glossary of Protophone Categories

In this section, we introduce the key protophone categories for coding infant vocalizations. We begin by describing reflexive sounds not included among the protophones. Then we describe protophones in two realms: phonation and syllabification/articulation.

Reflexive Sounds

As noted above, the protophone coding scheme focuses on volitional sounds and excludes reflexive sounds. The latter include cries, fusses, laughs, and vegetative sounds as described below.

Cries and **fusses**. Cry and fuss sounds are present as reflexive, species-specific vocalizations from birth. They are always associated with negative emotional valence and are not considered speech-related. Sound file 4S21 included with Suggested Activities below is an example of the cry of a one-week-old infant.

Laughs. Although they do not emerge until about four months of age, laughs, like cries, are species-specific vocalizations that are strongly associated with a fixed set of social and emotional contexts, in this case positive contexts (Sroufe and Wunsch, 1972). When they are produced in an apparently reflexive way they are considered to be similar to sounds of other mammals and thus to be less speech-related than the protophones.

Vegetative sounds. These sounds include burps, sneezes, coughs, hiccups, grunts, and yawns. Vegetative sounds are unintentional side-effects of various behaviors such as feeding or postural control, and they are not specialized as (that is, naturally selected to be) communicative signals (Hockett and Altmann, 1968). It is worth noting that grunts often require visual (as opposed to just audio) information in order to distinguish them from certain protophones, especially quasivowels or growls. A grunt (as we use the term) is deemed to be produced reflexively (as an accompaniment of movement or physical straining), while the protophones are deemed to be produced volitionally.

Phonation-Related Protophones

Phonation-related protophones are defined in terms of how they are produced at the glottis. These include **eggresive** vocants, squeals and growls, whispers and yells, and ingressive or ingressive-egressive vocalizations. These phonation-related protophones are described below.

Quasivowels and **full vowels**. Both of these are types of vocants. Quasivowels are the more primitive vocants. The characteristic differentiating them from full vowels is the auditory impression that they are produced with the vocal tract in a neutral or "unpostured" configuration. They tend to be acoustically short and quiet, and often include the muffled quality associated with nasality, though they do not necessarily always have all these characteristics. Full vowels tend to be longer and louder. A defining characteristic of full vowel quality is the auditory impression that the vocal tract *is* postured, with deliberate positioning of the mouth and tongue in a speech-like way, yielding a vowel quality distinct from that corresponding to an at rest position of the tract.

The vocants, both quasivowels and full vowels, are also defined by the auditory impression of normal speech-like phonation and pitch (in contrast with the phonation and pitch characteristics of squeals and growls). The phonatory and pitch characteristics of vocants must be within the infant's "habitual" range.

Squeals and **growls**. Squeals differ from vocants in that they have extreme high pitch, beyond the range of the infant's habitual voice (typically twice as high or higher than the mean habitual pitch) and may also be associated with falsetto or "loft" voice. Growls differ from vocants primarily in that they either have very low pitch, below that of the infant's habitual voice, or that they are within the habitual pitch range but have a harsh or noisy quality. The growls that are not harsh or noisy are often associated with pulse register, in phonatory patterns usually dubbed "fry" or "creak," and these tend to be well below the habitual pitch range. It is critical to emphasize that growls are sometimes *within* the habitual pitch range, and can even exceed the perceived mean pitch if they have a harsh, rough or noisy phonatory quality (but do not reach the pitch range of squeals). Squeals can also have vocal qualities departing from normal phonation but (in our definition) always have above-typical pitch and usually quite a bit of pitch variability. Thus, squeals and growls are protophones that are marked by differences from vocants with regard to phonation in terms of pitch and phonatory quality.

If a vocalization contains both a vocant and either a squeal or a growl (occurring in sequence within the vocalization), the listener is encouraged to make a judgment as to whether the squeal or growl characteristic is "salient." If the auditory impressionistic answer is yes, the vocalization is categorized as squeal or growl, not vocant. This judgment depends on the overall auditory impression rather than exclusively on either the relative amplitude or the relative duration of the squeal or growl portion of the sound. Similarly, if a vocalization includes both squeal and growl characteristics, the observer is encouraged to categorize the sound in terms of which characteristic seems more salient, squeal or growl. Some utterances present a relative balance of the features and can thus be difficult to code with high interjudge agreement.

Whispers and **yells**. Whispers and yells are also phonation-related protophones. Whispers are quiet and not voiced, though the air can be heard passing through the laryngeal cavity. Importantly a sound is not judged to be a whisper if it is deemed to be the mere byproduct of breathing. It must instead be perceived as a volitional sound. Yells are notably loud sounds, and usually have a pressed quality, but the defining quality with yells is that they are produced with amplitude that is beyond the habitual range of the producer's voice.

Ingressive vocalizations and ingressive-egressive sequences. Phonatory protophones with a sound source that is produced somewhere within the larynx (or possibly trachea) by air flowing inward toward the lungs, as opposed to the typical case of phonation in speech which occurs as air is flowing out of the lungs, are termed ingressive. Ingressive vocalizations can occur in isolation, but some infants produce regular coherent sequences of ingressive and egressive vocalization in rapid alternation, where the rate of each ingress and egress is near that of syllabic timing, and where there are scarcely any silences between ingresses and egresses—these sequences are not categorized as multiple utterances (though we use a breath-group criterion to define utterance boundaries in all other cases), but as ingressive-egressive sequences.

Syllabification and Articulation-Related Protophones

Some infant protophones include significant supraglottal activity. When the articulatory tract is constricted sufficiently, a consonant-like sound ("**closant**") emerges. In some cases the supraglottal activity constitutes a sound source that may occur in the absence of phonation or completely concurrent with it. In other cases supraglottal activity can break utterances up into syllable-like chunks. In addition the glottis itself can be used to break up phonatory sequences into syllables. These syllabification/articulation-related protophones include raspberries, clicks, goos, glottal sequences, and both marginal and canonical babbling and are described below.

Raspberries. Raspberries are trills or vibrants formed most often with the lips or the tongue and lips, and occasionally by the tongue body against the toothless alveolar ridge. Such non-phonatory sound sources are associated with certain consonants in a very few languages, but in infancy they are often also produced as extended sounds, with or without concurrent voicing.

Clicks. Clicks are sounds that involve creating a supraglottal sub-cavity that has negative pressure. When the pressure is released, it forms a non-phonatory sound source that is considered in our scheme to be an articulation-related protophone.

Goos. Goos are vocalizations with very primitive articulation where a tongue closure articulation in the back of the oral cavity is superimposed upon phonation, usually normal phonation. While goos do include articulation, the product usually does not yield clear syllabification, but rather seems only to hint at the infant's emerging potential for syllabification by articulation. Typically goos are variable in timing, and thus usually seem disorganized or erratic and inconsistent with the features of well-formed syllabification. However, occasionally, as if by chance, they do show well-timed movements consistent with more mature syllabification. We will return to goos in the following sections on marginal and canonical babbling to provide a few additional tips on how to distinguish goos from those other protophones.

Glottal stop sequences. Interruption of phonation at the larynx can be thought of as the most primitive mechanism of syllabification, because it requires no supraglottal movement. Glottal stop sequences in our coding system always consist of at least two perceived syllables broken up by one or more glottal interrupts. The coding of glottal stop sequences does not take account of glottal stop onsets or offsets to utterances. Repetitive glottal stop sequences occur when phonation and glottal stops alternate within an utterance and when the phonatory periods are long enough to be deemed "syllables" and the glottal stops are deemed long enough to be syllable margins (that is to have at least the duration that stop consonants have in mature speech). On many occasions the auditorily perceived glottal interruptions actually consist of phonation that merely dips into pulse register (yielding the vocal quality often termed creaky voice or fry), without an extended stop *per se*. The ear seems to interpret this pulse interrupt in much the same way as a full glottal stop.

Marginal babble and **canonical babble**. These are the most advanced of the protophones. They are sounds with syllable-like patterns generated by supraglottal articulation. Marginal babble is distinguished from canonical babble in one of two ways. The first is timing: canonical babble has speech-like speed of timing of the transitions (nominally <120 ms) between consonant-like and vowel-like portions of the syllable, whereas marginal babble does not include such speech-like timing of C to V or V to C. The key factor here is that the listener should judge a syllable as a marginal babble if the transition itself can be directly perceived, that is to say "auditorily tracked," but the listener should judge a syllable as a canonical babble if the transition is so quick that it becomes an integral part of the syllable whole, not auditorily recognizable *as* a transition. Even syllables with glide onsets ([wa], for example) can be (and in real speech usually are) pronounced with rapid transitions (i.e., <120 ms), and such onsets are by this criterion deemed canonical. However, if transitions are drawn out (regardless of the type of consonant-like element) to the point of being slow enough to be perceived as transitions, the syllable is classified as a marginal babble. For example, it is possible to "auditorily track" a 200 ms formant transition starting with lip approximation and rounding and concluding in a low vowel-like sound—such a transition can be variously interpreted auditorily as a sequence of a vowel-like sound resembling [u] followed gradually by a vowel-like sound resembling [a], or as a single unified transition between an initiating glide-like element and a low vowel. Either way, if the transition itself is perceived, we categorize the sound as a marginal babble. The second way that a syllable can be "marginal" is by possessing no full vowel as a nucleus and possibly thus having no substantial transition to track—a quasivowel nucleus adjacent to most consonant-like gestures produces relatively little formant movement and is thus unlike distinctively well-formed CV or VC syllables occurring in natural languages. It should be added however, that quasivowel nuclei can appear in reduced, unstressed syllables in adult speech. Canonical syllables must, then, have a full vowel as a nucleus along with a rapid transition from margin to nucleus.

A note of clarification is in order regarding gooing. In essence gooing is an early developing form of marginal babbling (very often with quasivowel nuclei) and with consonant-like articulations that are predominantly produced in a relatively disorganized way in the back of the vocal tract, probably with the dorsum of the tongue against the soft palate, although this has not been physiologically verified. As infants mature in the first year, the back articulation predominance gives way to more frequent use of anterior articulations and full vowel nuclei become more common. Consequently marginal babbling in 5 and 6 month olds often seems much more well-organized from the standpoint of syllabicity than gooing, which is very common in two and three month olds but becomes rare after four months.

Within canonical babbling, there are subtypes of protophones: isolated syllables, where the infant produces a CV or VC alone in an utterance; **reduplicated babble**, where syllables repeat as in [mama]; and **variegated babble**, where perceived syllables change notably across the sequence, as in [mami] or [mana]. Importantly, we require that reduplicated babbling includes at least one clearly canonical syllable. Usually there are more, but as long as the remaining syllables are perceived to be of similar form, they may in fact be marginal syllables, and the utterance as a whole will still qualify as a reduplicated babble. Again this is a case of utterance-level forced-choice coding. The most advanced (canonical) syllables in the sequence are used as the basis for the overall judgment. Variegated babble requires at least two canonical syllables, and they must be deemed different by the listener. This is another case of required intuitive judgment by the listener, who is encouraged to react as a caregiver might. A sequence of similar syllables is deemed reduplicated and minor details of articulation are ignored as long as the overall impression is that the infant intends the syllables (at least one of which is canonical) to be the same category. A sequence of syllables is deemed variegated if the overall impression of the listener is that at least *two different* canonical syllables were intentionally produced by the infant. Reasoning supporting this intuitive approach to differentiation of syllable types in canonical babbling has been presented in Oller and Griebel (2008) and Ramsdell (2009).

A question that often arises in the context of research on canonical babbling is, "What kinds of phonetic elements occur?" We prefer to focus this discussion at the syllabic level, because we find little reason to believe that infants in the first year possess a segmented syllabic structure, that is, we presume they possess no distinction between consonants and vowels, but rather produce syllabic wholes (MacNeilage, 1998). Further, it appears that the most accurate way to portray early syllables is in underspecified phonetic terms focusing at the syllabic level. Using this approach, it can be said that common canonical syllables of the end of the first year of life, the syllables that appear to be intentionally produced by infants and consistently recognized by caregivers, are very few in number. They virtually always include a CV-like structure where the offset portion is usually perceived as a relatively low or central vowel-like element, and where the onset is typically a labial or alveolar stop or nasal, or a glide-like onset, either labial or lingual. Less frequently velar stop onsets or fricative-like onsets are seen. Thus the number of syllabic contrasts that commonly occur in infants in the first year represents a mere handful of the global patterns that appear to occur across a wide variety of ambient languages.

Comments on Order of Development and Ages of Onset in Protophones

There have been numerous publications addressing stages of development of protophones (e.g., Elbers, 1982; Holmgren, Lindblom, Aurelius, Jalling, and Zetterstrom, 1986; Koopmans-van Beinum and van der Stelt, 1986; Stark, 1981). While the stage models that have been proposed are far from identical, they tend to agree on a series of key points. Here is a summary of stages consistent with a review by Oller (2000), who sought to encapsulate key points of agreement among the published models:

1. Crying and vegetative sounds are present from the first day of life, but laughter (even though it is considered a fixed signal) shows an onset at around four months.
2. The earliest protophones, including quasivowels and occasional glottal stop sequences, occur right after birth (the phonation stage).
3. At one to four months of age gooing occurs, usually in face to face interaction with caregivers (the primitive articulation stage).
4. By three months many new protophones begin to appear, especially full vowels, raspberries, squeals, growls, yells and whispers (the expansion stage). During this period marginal babbling also emerges.
5. Usually in the second half year of life canonical babbling appears (the canonical stage). It has not been empirically proven that reduplicated canonical babbling precedes variegated babbling (Mitchell and Kent, 1990; Smith, Brown-Sweeney, and Stoel-Gammon, 1989), even though other authors have presumed that it does (Elbers, 1982; Oller, 1980). It may be that the lack of confirmation thus far regarding the presumed ordering is due to reliance on traditional phonetic transcription as a means of trying to determine whether infant utterances should be deemed reduplicated or variegated. That method may obscure global patterns because of focus on phonetic details that may be of little relevance to the infant's intended syllabic categories (or the caregiver's perception of the infant's intended categories). In other words, phonetic transcription in such cases may cause a failure to see the forest for the trees. Our expectation is that as more infrastructurally sensitive methods of coding come into play—methods that emphasize global patterns presumably intended by infants and recognized by caregivers—it may be possible to confirm the presumed ordering of reduplicated babbling preceding variegated (see again (Oller and Griebel, 2008; Oller and Ramsdell, 2008, July; Ramsdell, 2009)).

Infant vocalization research has shown clearly that late onset of canonical babbling (after 10 months of age) is grounds for clinical concern (Eilers and Oller, 1994). Infants with severe or profound hearing impairment show such late onset, and hearing infants with similar delays are at risk for late onset of talking. Considerable research is focused on a variety of clinical groups (including autism, Down syndrome, and William's syndrome) to try to determine other characteristics of early protophone development that may be of clinical significance (Lynch, Oller, Steffens, Levine, et al., 1995; Masataka, 2001; Paul et al., 2011).

An Acoustic Phonetic Catalog of Selected Protophone Examples

The following pages review 20 examples of protophones, displaying waveforms, spectrograms, and occasionally amplitude-by-frequency spectra of the sound files associated with this chapter. To duplicate a typical coding experience, the reader may wish to first listen to the sound files, and then consult the displays and commentaries for guidance. The emphasis is on audible and visible acoustic correlates of the defining characteristics of primary protophone types as reviewed in the Glossary section of this chapter above. Note that protophone coding is essentially based on auditory impressions and does not require spectrography in our standard approach. However, consultation of acoustic visualizations, such as waveforms and spectrograms, can be helpful in learning and making protophone judgments, can be useful for expository purposes, and may lead to more detailed evidence for the mechanisms of production (and may even lead to a systematically "infraphonetic" level of classification). In our examples, we have focused on the characteristics that we believe require additional guided practice; thus, we have omitted examples of the non-protophone categories and protophones whose characteristics are relatively obvious, such as whisper and click. We include only a few examples of canonical babbling, because canonical syllables are relatively easily recognized (Oller, Eilers, and Basinger, 2001). We also include only one episode of reduplicated babbling, and do not present examples differentiating reduplicated babbling, variegated babbling, and **gibberish**, because the definitional issues related to these categories are less well resolved than in other cases. The examples are arranged roughly in order of the ages at which they tend to first appear, but exceptions are made to emphasize contrasts and to point out that there is extensive overlap amongst the stages of vocal development, especially as protophone characteristics developing earlier are typically available, and utilized, by older infants (or even adults).

It is hoped that simply listening and reading the labels and basic definitions will give readers the core experience needed to build skills and to achieve a basic level of reliability in coding infant vocalizations. Many technical terms used to describe the spectrogram and waveform have been introduced in Chapter 2. There is also much technical "subtext" in the discussion of these examples, which may presume familiarity with more advanced speech-scientific theories and methods; we encourage motivated readers to consult references listed with the examples below to achieve a deeper understanding of the technical aspects of the displays and source-filter mechanisms underlying vocal production. For additional general support the reader may benefit from consultation of textbooks in acoustic phonetic theory and instrumentation (e.g., Baken and Orlikoff, 2000; Johnson, 2003; Kent and Read, 2002; Stevens, 1998). Note, finally, that we do not restrict ourselves to focusing purely on the features that would determine the forced-choice coding of the utterances in our formal coding procedure for the phonatory and syllabification/articulation realms; we provide considerable additional detail about the vocalizations *per se*.

Access Sound Files 1 - 20 (Chapter 4)

4S1 through 4S20 Protophone Examples 1 through 20.

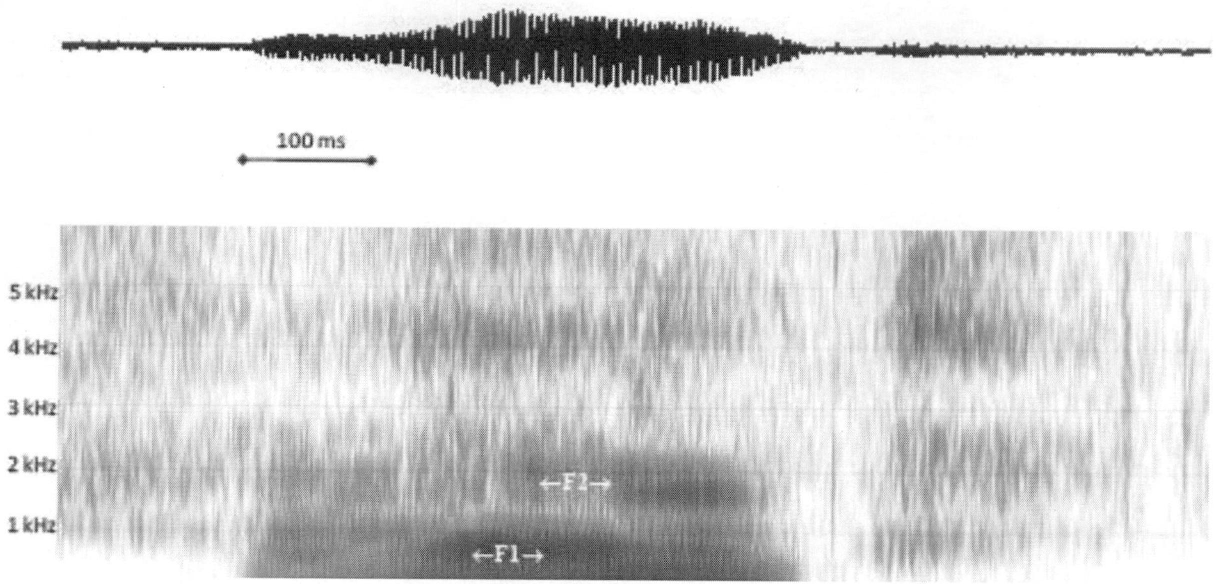

Example 1. A quasivowel, produced by an infant aged 3½ months. Quasivowels are produced with a neutral vocal tract configuration and are typically quiet and short. In this and all other spectrogram displays to follow, horizontal grid lines mark 1 kHz frequency intervals, frequency scales will be provided, and a 100 ms duration reference line will be placed at utterance onset to indicate the time scale.

What we can learn from careful listening: This quasivowel is fairly brief (at approximately 450 ms), it is audibly quiet, and the vowel quality is relatively neutral and stationary.

What we can learn from the acoustic analysis: First of all some technical notes for orientation to formant observations—the bandwidth of analysis in this particular spectrogram is 600 Hz. Normally such a wide analyzing filter renders formant frequencies clearly and obscures harmonics. However, because the fundamental frequency of this infant is quite high compared to an adult (i.e., 400 Hz), this interacts with the analyzing filter to produce a horizontal texture that obscures the formant frequencies somewhat (Buder, 1996)—see also some notes at the end of this paragraph regarding the 'muffled' appearance of formant structure. Nonetheless, F1 appears to be around 800 Hz (especially salient in the middle) and F2 appears to be around 1800 Hz (especially salient at the end). The faint band of energy around 4 kHz is probably F3. It is important to recognize that the "neutral" vocal tract posture characteristic of quasivowels is not the central vowel schwa, which would produce more even formant frequency spacing, and the relatively low F2 of this production is consistent with a slightly back tongue position that seems likely for an infant 'resting' oral anatomy. Several other common characteristics of the quasivowel are visible here: softness and breathiness of phonation accounts for the dominance of low energy and an absence of any harmonics above 2.5 kHz, and it is likely that a slightly open velo-pharyngeal port introduces nasality. Nasality damps (i.e., muffles or reduces) the overall sound energy, broadening the formant bandwidths and making them difficult to discern both spectrographically and audibly, and coupling to the nasal cavities also can introduce anti-resonances that disrupt the clarity of more basic vowel formant structure (Buder, 2005). In addition to overall quietness, evidenced by the sound energy being not much above the background noise level, these phonatory source and upper vocal tract filter characteristics combine to create the overall muffled energy distribution (wider band resonances) and low frequency emphasis in this sound.

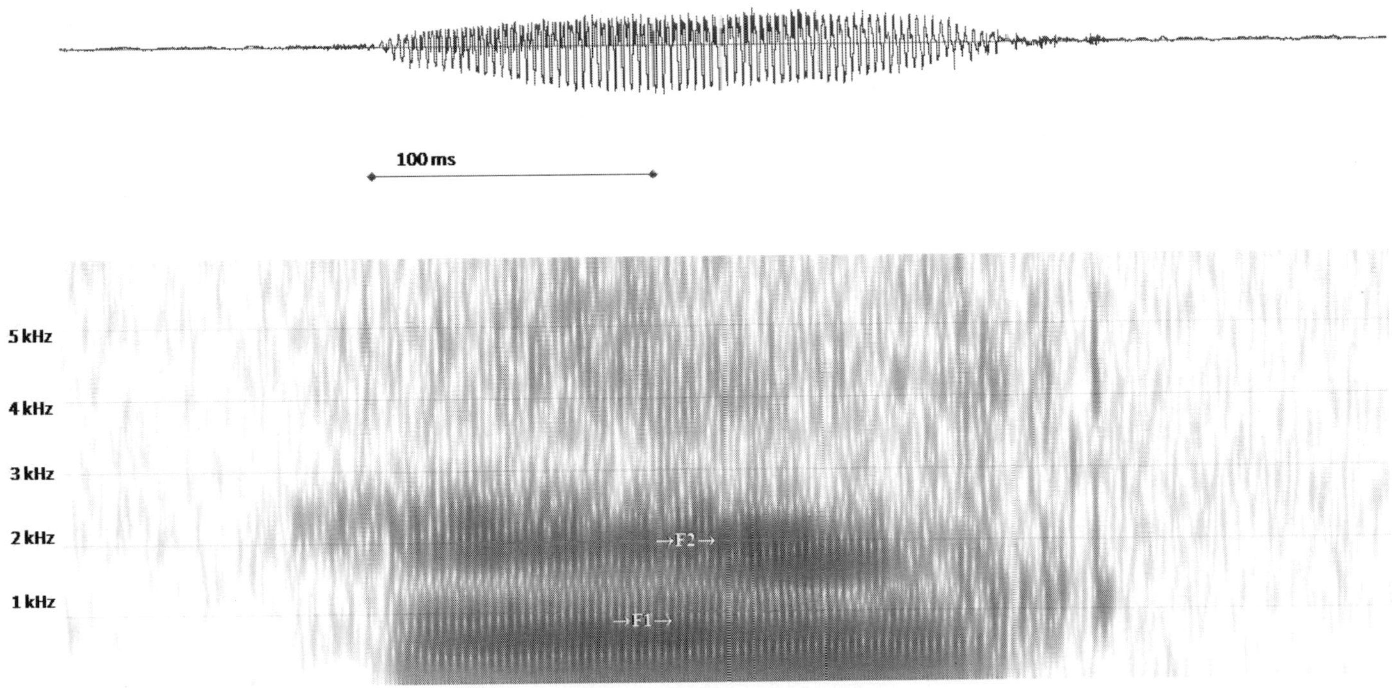

Example 2. Another quasivowel, produced by the same infant at the same age (3½ months) as Example 1.

What we can learn from careful listening: This vocalization was produced with just slightly more phonatory energy and perhaps less nasalization than Example 1. It may be heard to have a slightly different resonance quality but it is still impressionistically unarticulated (unpostured) as a vowel and thus has the neutral sound characteristic of quasivowels.

What we can learn from the acoustic analysis: The same waveform scale and spectrogram range and bandwidth settings from Example 1 have been used. Formants 1 and 2 are more visible in part because there is less damping due to nasal resonance. F1 and the F2 do not shift during the production—note the complete absence of any significant formant movement in the nucleus of this sound. When no obstruent turbulence source energies occur at the onsets or offsets of vocalizations, they would be coded as quasivowels only. In this example, it is possible to hear some turbulence at the end possibly resulting from frication. Thus, this particular example might also be coded as a goo if it is perceived that the frication is based on constriction of the tongue dorsum. The vertical striations following Example 2 are likely glottal in origin, but some audible and visible impression of slight formant movement at the very end of this example suggests the possibility of vocal tract movement towards closure.

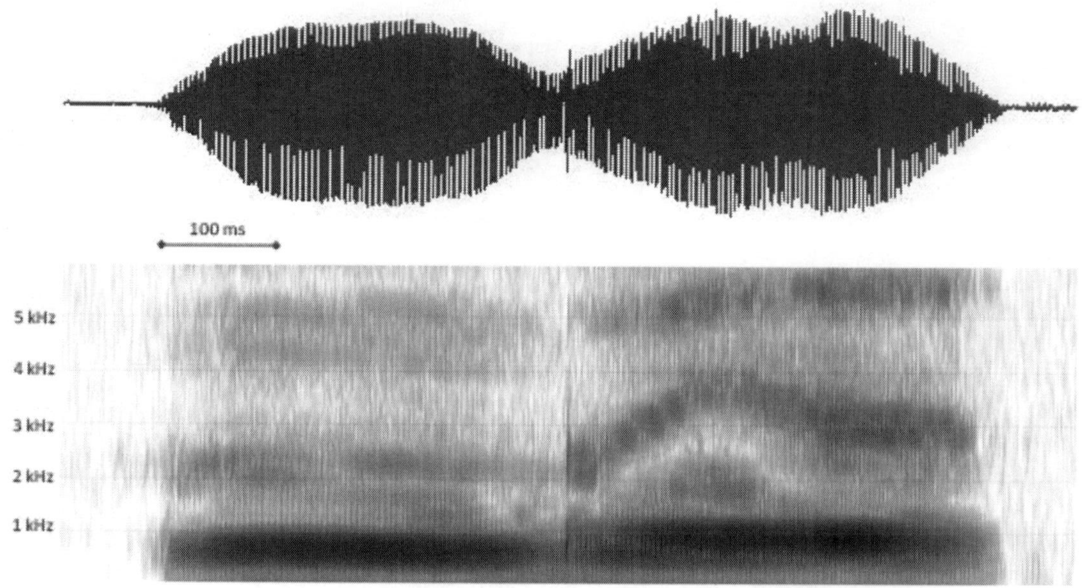

Example 3. A goo, preceded by a quasivowel, and followed by a full vowel, produced by the same infant at the same age as the two preceding examples.

What we can learn from careful listening: We hear stronger phonation and most importantly articulation. Characteristic of the typical goo, this articulation can be heard as involving dorsal tongue contact probably to the soft palate.

What we can learn from the acoustic analysis: The same display settings as Examples 1 and 2 are again used here. We see stronger phonation evidenced by the greater amplitude as well as the greater excitation of the higher frequency resonances and clearer formant structure. We also see articulation, which can be heard as involving dorsal tongue contact probably to the soft palate. It is likely that the velo-pharyngeal port is acoustically and aerodynamically closed for at least the second half of this production. Evidence for this closure can be found in the sharp closing and release-like event that is visible about half-way through the vocalization, caused by some other oral valve. This stop-gap and pressure release would only manifest itself if the VP port is closed; the closure is also evident in the attenuation of the waveform and reduced higher frequency energy in the spectrogram during the closure, and in the faint appearance of a plosive-like burst following this evidence of closing. Aerodynamically no such events can occur if significant air is leaking through the nasal cavity. We can also hear and see evidence of this closure in the relative clarity of the formants which would result from relatively more sharply-tuned resonances that should occur when there is reduced acoustic damping by the nasal cavity, but there is also stronger phonation and a somewhat lower fundamental frequency, which also helps to render those formants more visible. The clear formants also help to display formant movement quite clearly in the latter half of this vocalization, characterizing the full vowel as having been produced with a non-neutral vocal tract position. As we will see in other examples, movement is not necessary for this characterization, but here it audibly and visibly involves an anterior gesturing with the tongue (seen in F2 movement) and some lowering of the jaw (seen as F1 elevation). Goos can have only slow transitions and thus do not include canonical syllables. The slow transitions imply that goos can be thought of as a type of marginal babble that tends to occur particularly early in life and generally includes back articulation.

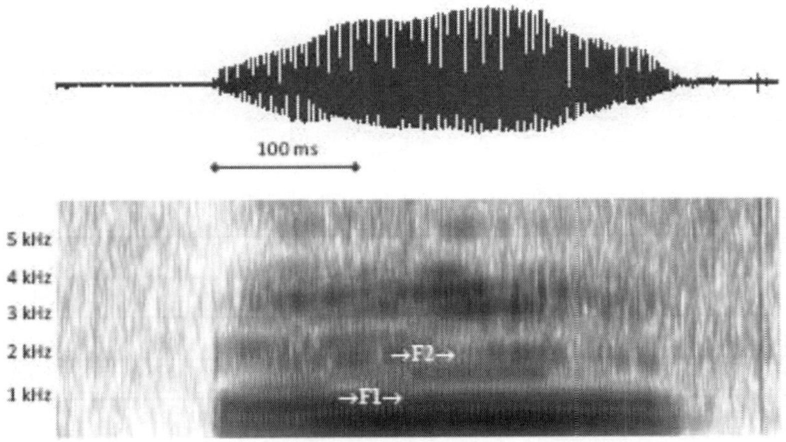

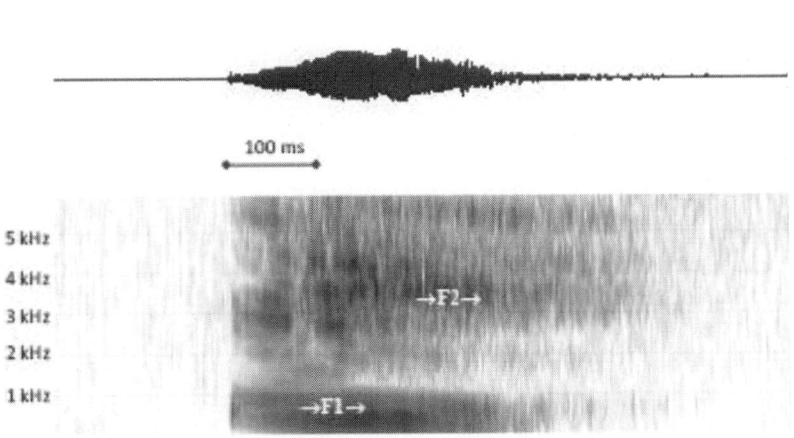

We categorized Example 4 on the left as a quasivowel, and Example 5 on the right as a full vowel. These examples are displayed here side by side to reinforce some additional principles and distinguishing characteristics regarding quasivowels and full vowels as isolated types of vocalizations (i.e., as nucleus-only vocalizations lacking syllabic margins).

While Example 5 has been coded as a full vowel, rather than as a quasivowel, it is not the most unambiguous of cases. Examples 4 and 5 were produced by a much older infant, aged approximately 11 months, which reinforces the fact that early-emerging protophones may still occur later in development even though infants this age will normally also be producing fully articulated canonical syllables.

What we can learn from careful listening: The pitch of the two examples is lower than in previous examples. The quasivowel of Example 4 has no clearly non-neutral vowel, but in Example 5 it is possible to hear a sudden onset (hard glottal attack) and a relatively clear non-central vowel articulation.

What we can learn from the acoustic analysis: The formants are generally a bit lower than in previous examples, consistent with elongation of the vocal tract that will have occurred by this age. Also note that the full vowel on the right, unlike that previously seen in Example 3, is produced without marginal articulations (although it audibly and visibly does begin with a hard glottal attack), or with much change in vocal tract shape, and therefore it has mostly steady formant frequencies. Example 4 on the left, classified as a quasivowel, illustrates a more neutral formant pattern and can therefore be viewed as a baseline against which the full vowel example can be seen and heard as having a postured vocal tract. It is also noteworthy in these examples that the full vowel is in fact produced more quietly, with soft and breathy phonation, and is shorter in duration than the quasi-vowel on the left. Quasivowels are often produced as relatively quiet and short protophones, occurring most often in younger infants whose respiratory and phonatory mechanisms are less well developed, but Example 4 is an exception. Finally, note that there is also less evidence of nasality in these older infant's productions.

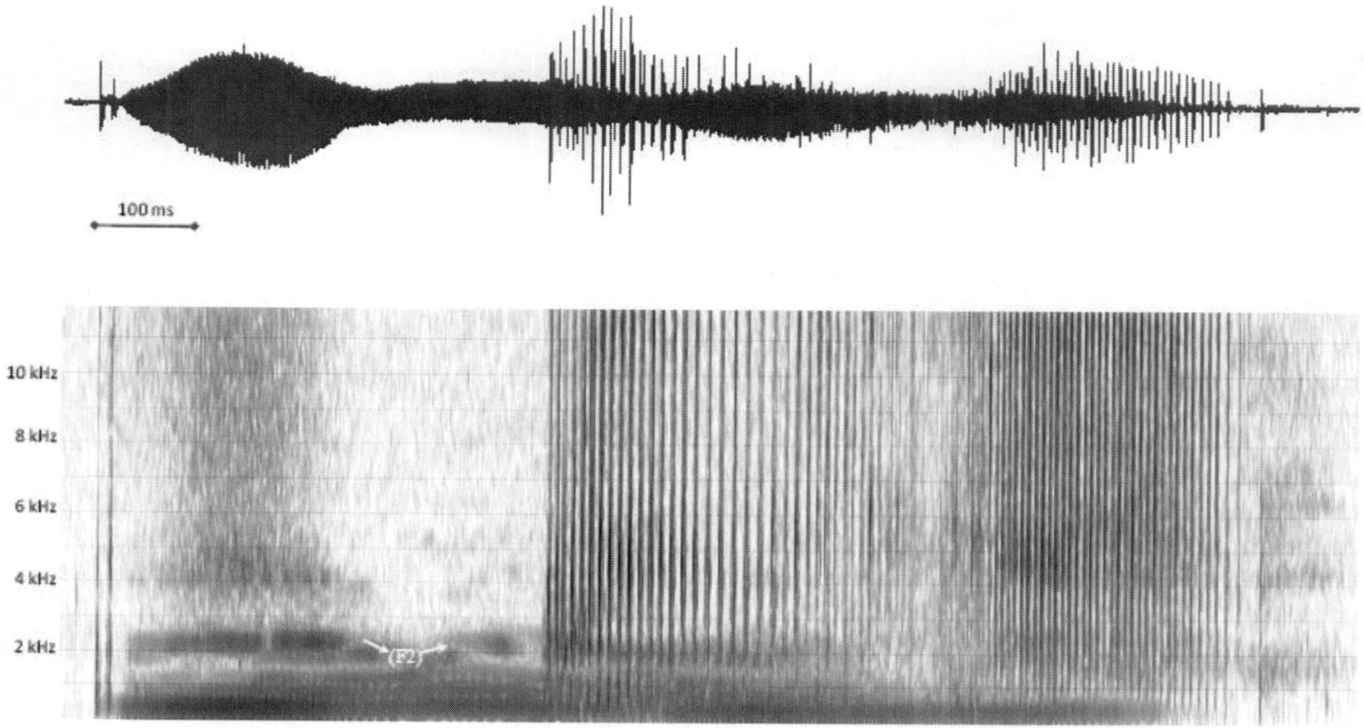

Example 6 returns to the younger infant from previous examples (aged 3½ months), and illustrates a more complex sequence that includes a new protophone type, the raspberry.

What we can learn from careful listening: The first portion begins with a burst at the onset which sounds labial followed by some vowel articulation. The second portion has rapid vibration that is characteristic of a raspberry. It is interesting to note that although most infants produce raspberries, as noted in the glossary above they correspond to a phoneme that is rare in adult languages.

What we can learn from the acoustic analysis: For this display the spectrogram frequency range has been expanded to illustrate some of the higher frequency components that occur with "closant" types of sources like trilling/vibrating at the lips, as seen in the latter 3/5 of this vocalization. The first portion of this vocalization is a goo, with bursting at the utterance onset (that sounds velar), followed by a vowel nucleus, and then by a quieter and somewhat higher pitch segment with evidence of formant movement in the resonance near 2kHz, which is probably F2 (see label in spectrogram). The latter portion of this vocalization is a raspberry; acoustic manifestations of rapid vibrating of the lips are clearly evident in the spectrogram. Phonation continues during this raspberry, and while phonation often occurs in raspberries, it is not a defining characteristic of this protophone type.

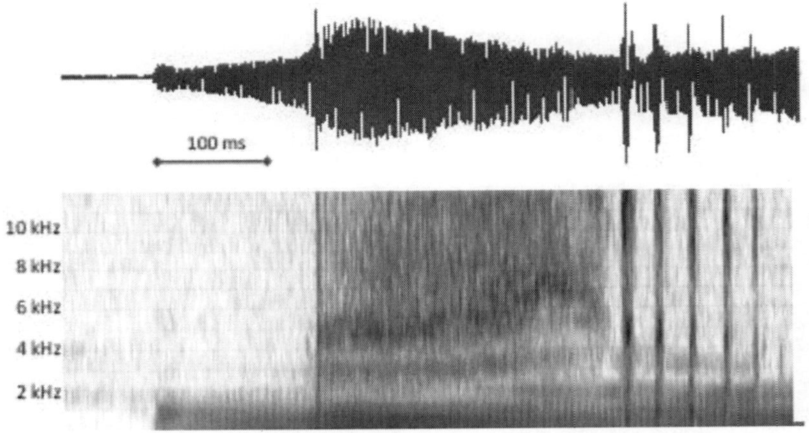

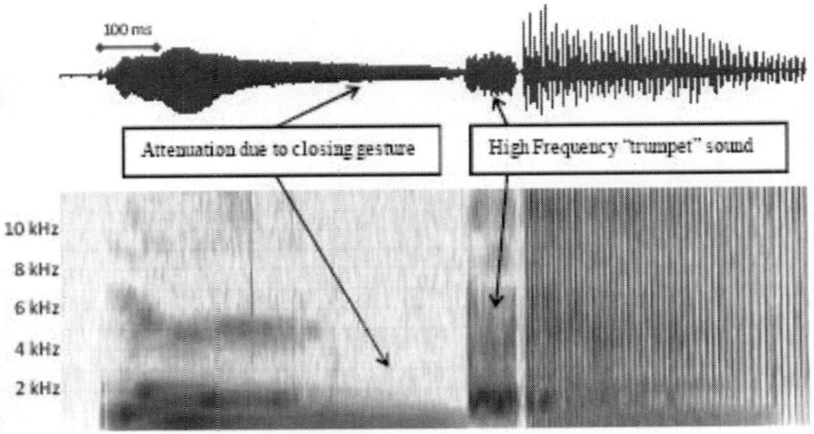

Examples 7 and 8 are presented here side by side to compare varieties of raspberry. All the raspberries presented in examples 6-8 were produced by the same 3½ month old infant during one 20 minute recording session. One possible interpretation of this phenomenon is that the infant was exploring her ability to produce sounds by controlling pressures and airflows with a valving mechanism other than at the glottis (i.e., at the lips). Depending on the speed of labial vibration a raspberry may be a *trill*, a *vibrant* with salient roughness (as in Example 6), or even a very high frequency vibrant that produces a tonal characteristic, like the lip action used in playing a trumpet.

What we can learn from careful listening: In Example 7 there is first voicing during bilabial closure, then bilabial frication concurrent with phonation, then bilabial trilling with phonation (this is especially visible during the trilling in this example). In Example 8 the full vowel phonation is followed by a raspberry characterized by rough vibration, i.e., a vibrant type of raspberry.

What we can learn from acoustic analysis: The spectrograms displayed on this page were obtained with an extremely broad analyzing bandwidth of 1000 Hz, which helps to resolve the fine temporal details of these productions (see basic acoustic phonetic resources for more on the topic of "time/frequency" tradeoffs in spectrography). Measurements of the periodicity in the labial vibrations may help provide acoustic phonetic bases for auditory classifications of trill vs. vibrant type. The raspberry segment at the end of Example 7 is classified as a trill, with a frequency of about 30 Hz. There are actually at least two raspberry-type phenomena at the end of Example 8: a fast vibrant type is evident through the last third, with vibrations occurring at approximately 100 Hz. Prior to this, after the initial phonated full vowel segment becomes fully attenuated, there seems to be an extremely high frequency vibrant lasting about 85 ms. Note that in Example 7 there is first voicing during bilabial closure, then bilabial frication concurrent with phonation, then bilabial trilling with phonation (this is especially visible during the trilling in Example 7). In Example 8 the full vowel phonation is marked by falling formant frequencies (beginning about midway through the full vowel) associated with attenuation of the output, which are both clear correlates of closing at the lips, followed by the tonal vibrant which must be produced with very high pressure behind a tight closing, which then yields to a rough vibrant probably associated with a slight reduction in the resistance of the bilabial valve (with a very brief complete closing in between).

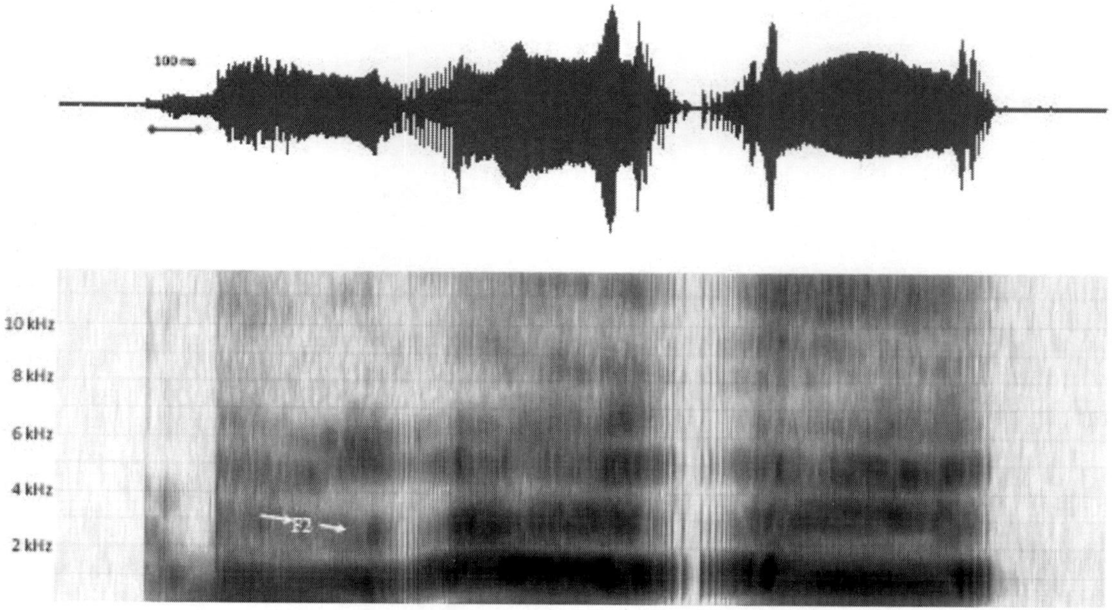

Example 9 introduces a *glottal* sequence. This vocalization is one of many produced in a single 20 minute session by an infant nearly 4 months of age who, similarly to the previous infant, seemed to be practicing with valving operations, but here, glottaly. Because the beginning of the utterance includes a presumably velar closure, the utterance would best be characterized within the forced choice system as a goo (the most advanced protophone category to which the utterance pertains), but here we focus on the characteristics of glottal stop sequencing as another kind of articulatory feature.

What we can learn from careful listening: This example begins with an oral closure, then a full vowel that is interrupted by short silences heard auditorily as glottal gestures that rapidly suppress phonation.

What we can learn from the acoustic analysis: The spectrogram is again very wideband to emphasize temporal structure. The two interruptions of phonation dividing this vocalization into three segments are produced by glottal gestures that decelerate phonation, clearly visible as glottal pulses between the segments. The first glottal interruption is essentially a continuous yet brief dip of fundamental frequency in and out of pulse register, while the second effectively stops phonation for an instant and so might be considered a full glottal stop—see Buder, Oller, Chorna and Robinson (2008) for further details on these and other types of vibratory regimes found in infant phonation. The initial segment of this sequence is a goo, with a presumably velar onset transitioning slowly into a full vowel; some articulatory movement continues during this vowel, visible as a slowly falling F2 (labeled). The second and third segments which are broken up by the glottals are also full vowels: even though the formants appear to be evenly spaced, the audible vowel qualities that justify the full vowel categorization in both cases reinforce the fact that even spacing does not characterize the neutral posture in infant vocants. These spectrographic images also lack the lower frequency emphasis and broadband hallmarks of typical quasivowels. The second and third "syllables" here provide the most unambiguous full vowels (as opposed to quasivowels) to this point in our examples.

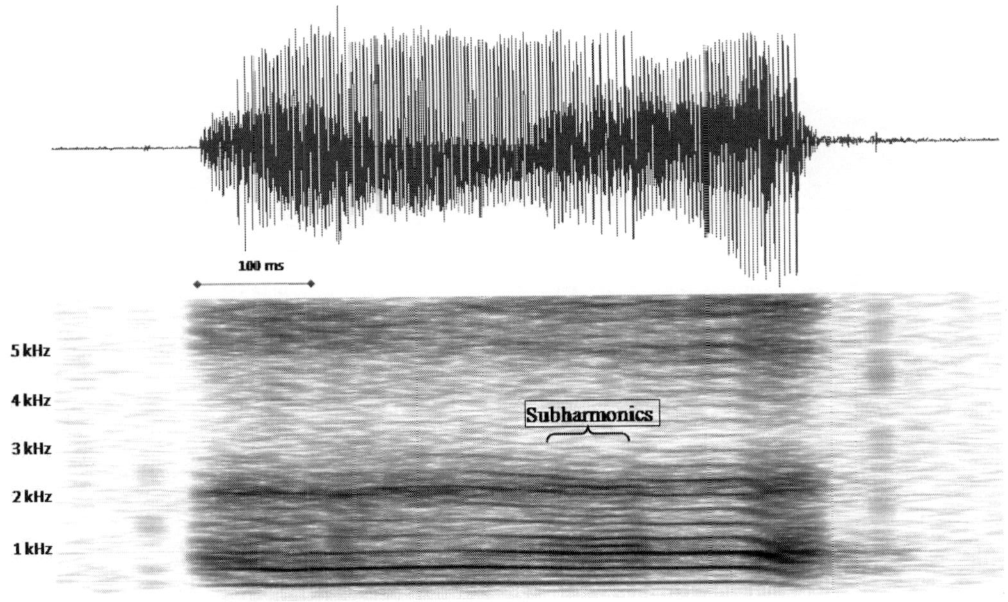

Example 10 is a *growl*, produced by a different infant than example 9 but again at about 4 months of age.

What we can learn from careful listening: Fairly low pitch and rough phonation is maintained throughout the utterance. It is not necessary for growl characteristics to last for an entire utterance to mark it as a growl vocalization; the requirement is substantial salience of the growl characteristic.

What we can learn from acoustic analyses: This display is our first example of an extremely narrowband spectrogram (10 Hz bandwidth) which is useful for discerning the frequency detail of harmonic structure, and therefore the types of vibratory dynamics that characterize distinct *regimes* used by Buder et al. (2008) to classify types of infant phonation. Fairly low frequency and rough phonation is maintained throughout the utterance and three additional features characterize the current example as a clear growl: A. There is interharmonic noise throughout, giving the sound a harsh characteristic. B. Due to this interharmonic noise and/or variations in periodicity affecting the harmonics themselves, harmonic structure is not always clear—note the instability especially at the onset and the lack of patterning above the 7th harmonic in most of the first half. C. There is an episode of subharmonics about 2/3 of the way through the utterance, marked by the appearance of distinct but relatively lower intensity harmonics appearing in between the main harmonics. During this episode there is resemblance to the pulsing waveform to the previous example of glottal interrupts, which results from the appearance of a dramatically low reduction in fundamental frequency in both cases, and both productions can be heard to involve medial compression at the glottis. Unlike pulsed phonation due to glottal interruption, however, in which the voice drops more or less smoothly to just one very low fundamental frequency, subharmonics in phonation can be perceptually noted as a distinct kind of roughness created by the concurrent presence of two sets of harmonics that appear abruptly (at octave relationships in this "period-2" type of subharmonic regime); this leads to some ambiguity regarding the 'true' fundamental frequency.

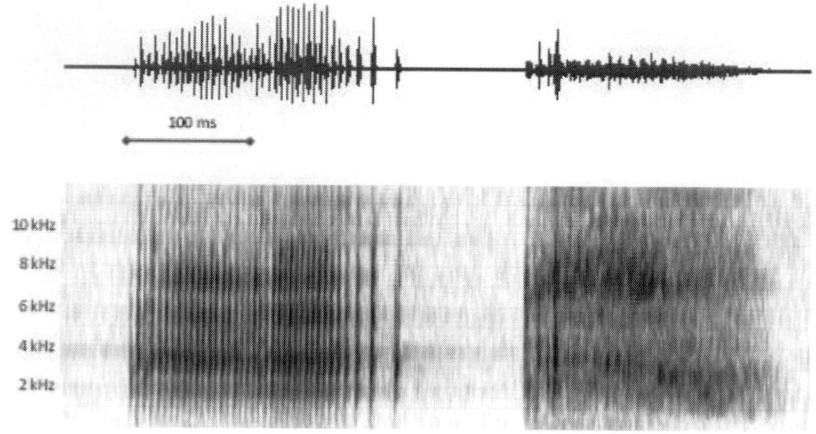

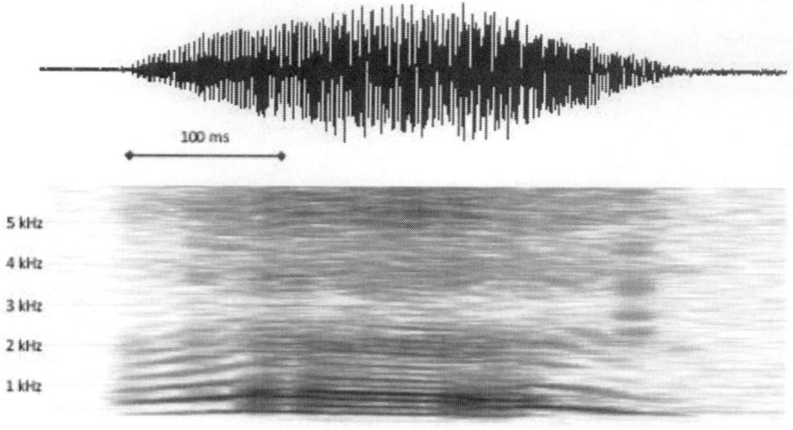

Examples 11 and 12 above are two more examples of growls and help illustrate that the term encompasses quite a range of possible variations from normal phonation. The growl on the left was produced by an older infant at about 10 months of age, and the growl on the right by a different infant at about 4 months of age.

What we can learn from careful listening: Both examples have rough vocal quality that characterizes them as growls. Example 11 can be compared with the glottal sequence of Example 9 to illustrate the principle that pulse phonation can be sustained and salient enough in an utterance to justify the growl categorization (there is a also a full glottal stop in this utterance, followed by an expiratory release, like a "glottal plosive").

What we can learn from acoustic analysis: Example 11's spectrogram is wideband for temporal resolution of pulses, but Example 12 on the right is again displayed with 10 Hz bandwidth analysis to reveal the complex harmonic patterning that dominates the central portion of the utterance. The utterance begins with modal phonation and ends with a higher frequency loft sound as the amplitude is dropping, and these portions include relatively little complexity or interharmonic noise. In contrast, the central portion of example 12 is extremely unstable, with alternating patterns of period-2 and period-3 subharmonics and ending with virtually chaotic vocal fold vibration just before jumping into the loft register. This central portion is the most salient auditorily and thus marks the vocalization as a growl. Note that there is an audible click near the end of the phonation (marked on the spectrogram), which causes some irregular bands of energy to appear in the higher frequencies (2.5 kHz and higher) of the spectrogram; this is almost certainly an environmental sound not produced by the infant.

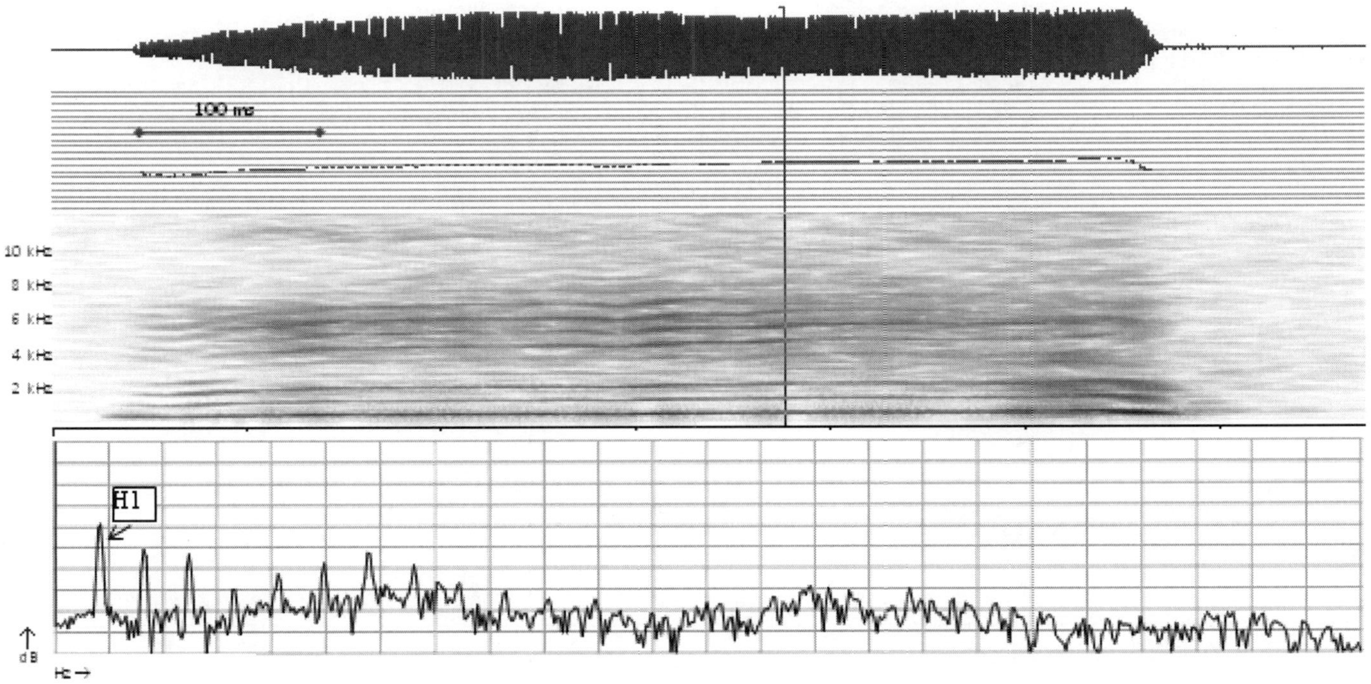

Example 13 is a squeal, produced by the same 4-monther who produced the growl of Example 12 (and recorded in the same session).

What we can learn from careful listening: Most definitively, this squeal is produced loudly with a very high pitch. This high pitch clearly marks the example as a squeal.

What we can learn from acoustic analysis: We have provided a fundamental frequency (f_0) trace between the waveform and narrowband spectrogram; the grid marks in the f_0 panel are at 100 Hz intervals, and at the point where the vertical cursor has been placed it can be seen that the f_0 is above 800 Hz. From this trace, it is clear that the f_0 is far above this infant's (or any typical infant's) modal f_0, a hallmark of squeal. Acoustic analysis of f_0 in infant squeals may be difficult for some analyzing software's algorithms, especially if they are not designed to accommodate such high frequencies through adaptive algorithms or parameter controls that allow the algorithm to be tuned to the appropriate range. Narrowband spectrographic or spectral displays shown above can be used to further validate the f_0. In the bottom spectrum panel of this figure (with intensity in dB on the vertical axis (10 dB grid) and frequency in Hz on the horizontal axis (1 kHz grid)), the first harmonic is f_0 and this can be seen to occur just below 1 kHz. Examination of its higher harmonics help to confirm that the f_0 is about 800 Hz (in voiced sounds, harmonics appear at both odd and even integer multiples of the first harmonic). Another reason that the spectrum is displayed in this example is to illustrate a typical aspect of the "loft" regime, which is an audible characteristic of this particular squeal: the first harmonic is much stronger in amplitude than any of the successive harmonics. In modal voice the first harmonic may be equal to or even weaker than the second (but upper harmonics should show an overall general decline in amplitudes for all voices).

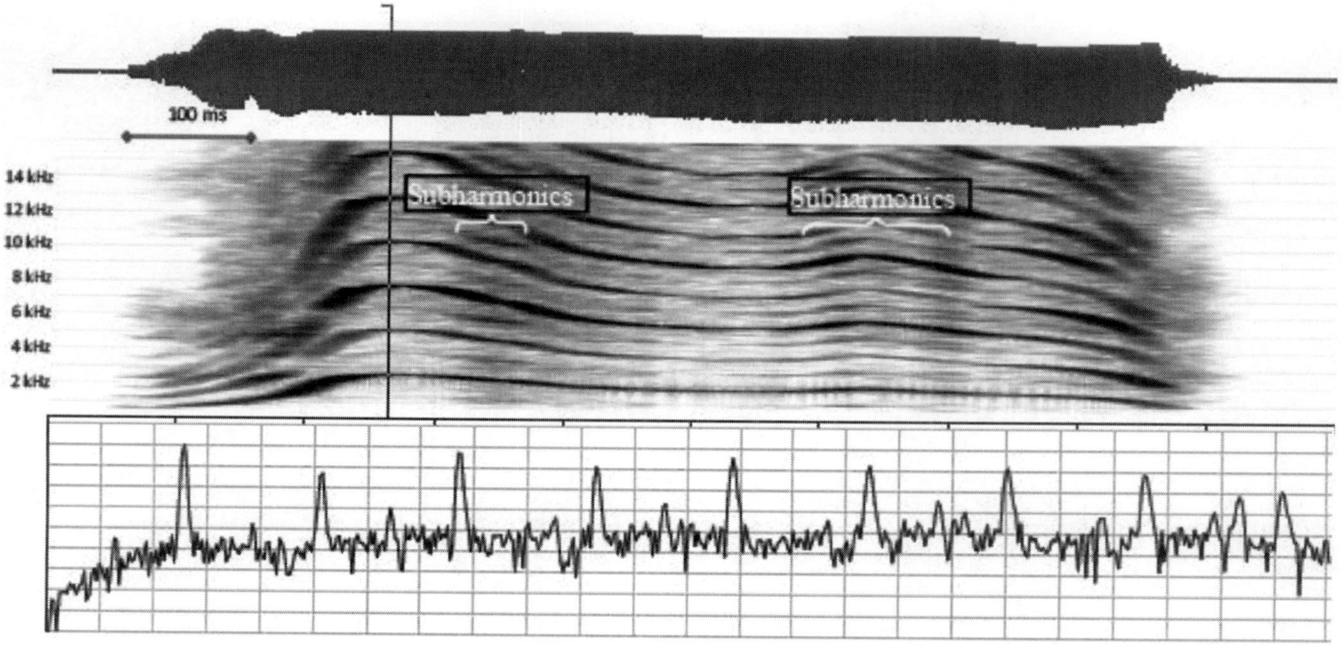

Example 14 is another squeal, produced by the same infant in Example 13, but at 6 months.

What we can learn from careful listening: Watch out! This impressive vocalization is very loud, even after scaling it down from its original recorded level. It is also very high-pitched. Thus, this vocalization may be considered to be both a "squeal" and a "yell."

What we can learn from acoustic analysis: The default algorithm of the commercially available TF32 program could not track this squeal, which is why there is no f_0 contour displayed here. Instead we have presented the spectrum taken at the cursor, where the harmonic time contours in the spectrogram peak. The spectrum reveals that the harmonics are more than 2500 Hz apart and the seventh harmonic at 18 kHz, so the f_0 is approximately 2600 Hz (18000/7 = 2570) at its peak. Still, we have observed even much higher f_0 produced by infants of this age. In comparison to Example 13, it can also be seen that the energies of the harmonics decline only slightly; even though this is an extremely high-pitched phonation it is also quite pressed-sounding, and is definitely not in loft register. It is primarily the high f_0, typically accompanied by extensive f_0 movement, that characterizes squeals. Inspection of the spectrogram reveals incipient subharmonics in this phonation of period-2 just past the first peak and apparently even period-4 during the second pitch peak. However, they are not audible as the double-pitched kind of roughness associated with fully developed subharmonics. These patterns might even be related to the fact that the intensity of this phonation exceeded the linear range of the microphone used to record it, causing analog amplitude clipping which accounts for the strange flatness of the waveform contour; the concomitant distortion may have exacerbated the appearance of subharmonics. This is a known issue in obtaining and interpreting infant vocalizations: in order to pick up reasonably salient quiet vocalizations (cf. Quasivowel in Examples 1 and 2), one must allow for distortions at the higher end of infants' amazing range.

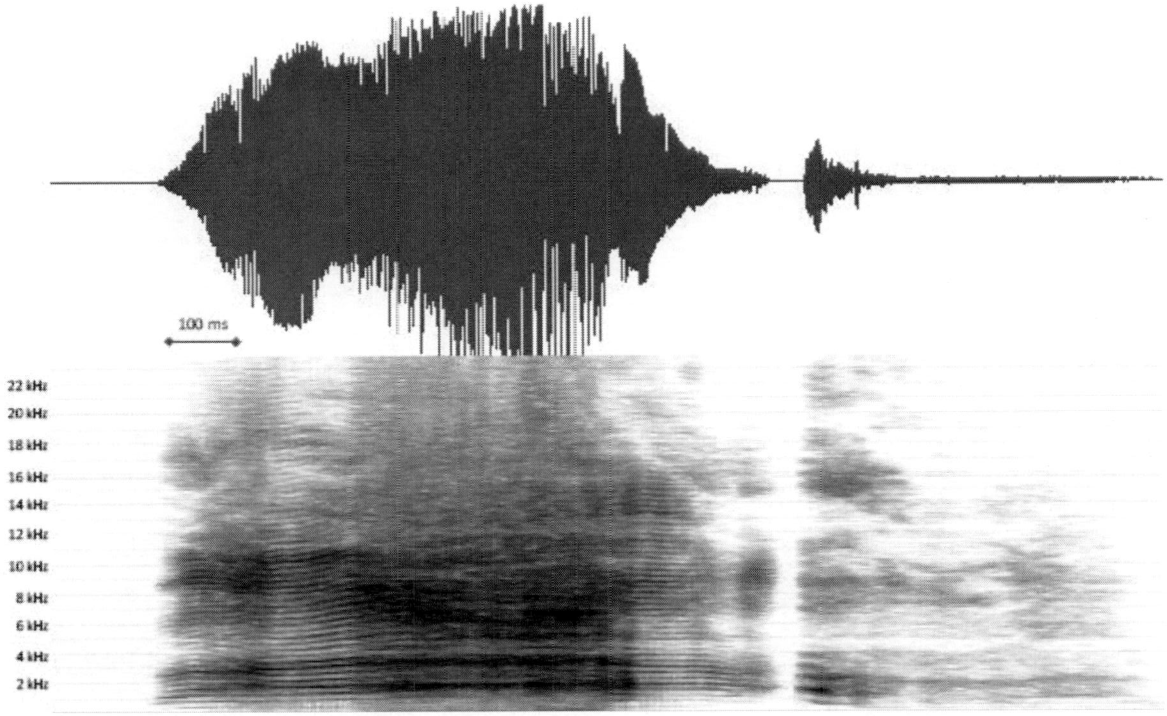

Example 15 is a *yell*, produced by a 10 month old infant.

What we can learn from careful listening: Similar to Example 14, there is a pressed quality to this loud phonation, but its pitch is only slightly higher than the infant's normal pitch and it is not perceived as a squeal. It is loud and has rough qualities that also justify a "growl" classification.

What we can learn from the acoustic analysis: Note that in this spectrogram, as in the display of Example 14, a full 16 kHz is displayed, so the harmonics are much more closely spaced than in many of the previous examples. A very salient aspect of this vocalization is its loudness but also its vocal quality—again very pressed, with relatively flat harmonic energies extending many multiples up through the spectrum. The utterance should also be categorized as a growl due to the rough qualities in the middle and highest amplitude portion. Closer inspection of this segment reveals subharmonics which so deeply modulate the basic rate of vibration that they develop a primary pulse-like form that can be seen and heard to be as low as 100 Hz in fundamental frequency (those details are not perspicuous in the image above). This sample also has some clipping, and in this case the amplitude of the recorded signal also exceeded the range of the digitizing hardware; the waveform peaks touch the edges of the displayed range. This may again somewhat exacerbate the rough perception of the loudest portion, but it does not fully account for the phonatory roughness yielding the *growl-yell* categorization.

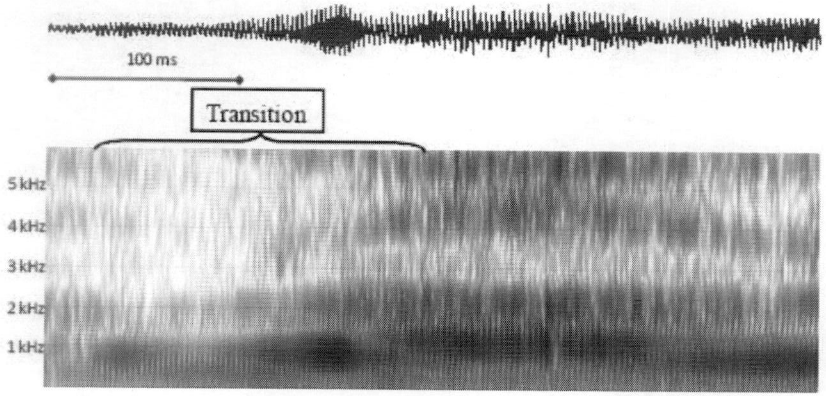

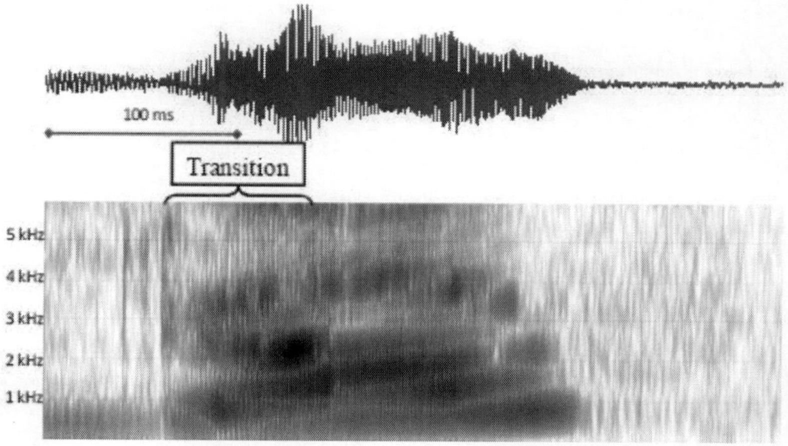

Example 16 on the left is a *marginal babble* produced by a 12 month old infant, and Example 17 on the right is a *canonical babble* produced by the same infant in the same recording session.

What we can learn from careful listening: Both examples have an audible syllable structure, with full vowels and articulated onsets. The transition from the onset into the vowel in Example 16 is slow, and, thus, this syllable is classified as "marginal babble." In contrast, Example 17 is a well-formed syllable with a rapid transition from the consonant to the vowel (it is also produced in squeal register).

What we can learn from the acoustic analysis: The spectrograms are 800 Hz bandwidth analyses to highlight the formant structure (although the rise in pitch at the end of Example 17 causes some visual resolution of harmonic patterning even at this large bandwidth). It is also important to know that the time intervals displayed here are exactly the same—just under 400 ms—to help compare some important temporal aspects of the formant and amplitude dynamics. Most importantly, visual and segment-specific auditory examinations suggest that the onset of the marginal babble develops over an interval of 150 ms or more before reaching a stable vowel nucleus, while the onset of the canonical babble is complete within 60-90 ms. These onsets are defined primarily in terms of formant movement: in theory, when the oral cavity is closed and then opens, F1 always rises (Stevens, 1998). The marginal babble in Example 16 does not seem to begin with a full closure, so this principle does not specify a necessary rise in F1. Further, the full vowel in the syllable may be relatively high, resulting in a low F1 with relatively little rise in F1 across the utterance. In accord with speech acoustic theory, F2 transitions will be more or less evident depending on place of consonant closure—none seems to occur here—and/or place (front/back tongue position) of vowel. These formant-frequency-determining factors are complex and interact in ways that do not always yield straightforward measurability of formant transitions, especially in infant utterances. Thus we often cannot distinguish easily between canonical and marginal syllables based on formant transition measurements alone. However, the rapid formant movements of Example 17 are evident enough, and the transition patterns of this example are visibly different than the much more gradual rise in overall amplitude and very slowly developing F2 amplitude discernible in the marginal babble of Example 16. These factors, especially with the slow amplitude rise in Example 16, support the auditory judgment that 16 is a marginal syllable while 17 is canonical. Example 17 can also be categorized as a squeal in the phonatory domain, given its very high frequency ending.

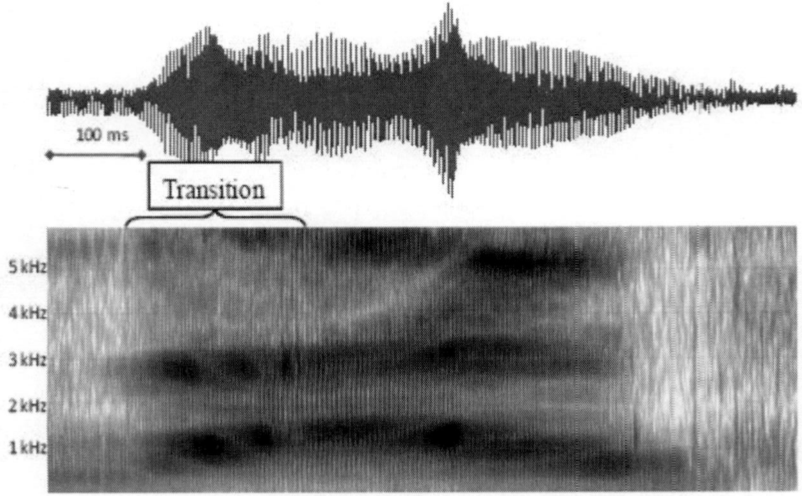

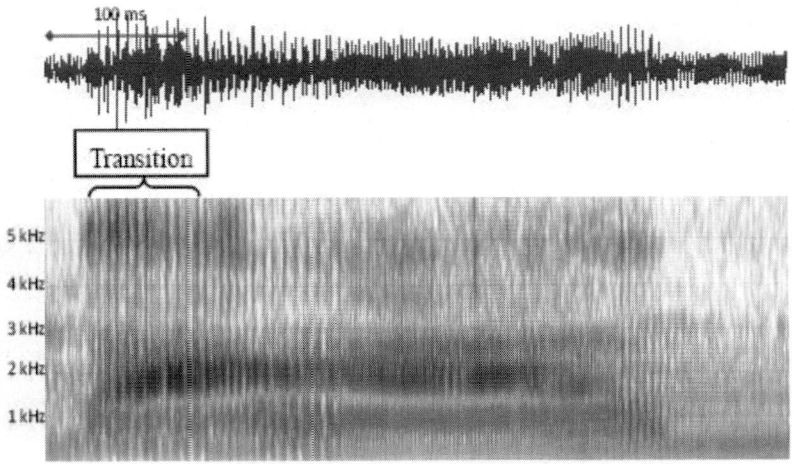

Example 18 on the left is another marginal babble produced by a 10 month old infant, and Example 19 on the right is a canonical babble produced by the same child in the same recording session.

What we can learn from careful listening: Again, both examples could be said to have audible syllable structure, with articulated onsets and an open nucleus, but only Example 19 is deemed a well-formed syllable, with an onset that is articulated rapidly enough into the nucleus to have canonical status. Example 19 is also audibly a growl.

What we can learn from the acoustic analysis: Unlike the previous marginal babble in Example 16, Example 18 has very clear formant visibility and a strong voice, but again the transition is slow enough to be "audibly tracked" (lasting at least 130 ms). In this particular example the overall difference between the amplitude at the beginning of the opening gesture and at the vowel nucleus is also small over the transition interval, and there is barely any F2 frequency change. The canonical babble in Example 19 may seem a bit ambiguous in at least two respects: (1) There is no turbulence event associated with an obstruent release, but note that this is not necessary for a well-formed adult canonical syllable. (2) The utterance is also a growl, which illustrates again the fact that growls and squeals can occur as the phonatory qualities of articulated syllables (also possible in adult connected speech!). Notable positive features characterizing Example 19 as a canonical syllable include a rapid transition from opening into a stable vowel nucleus (c. 65 ms), a rapid rise in amplitude over this interval, and an F2 which (though faint) falls rapidly in frequency.

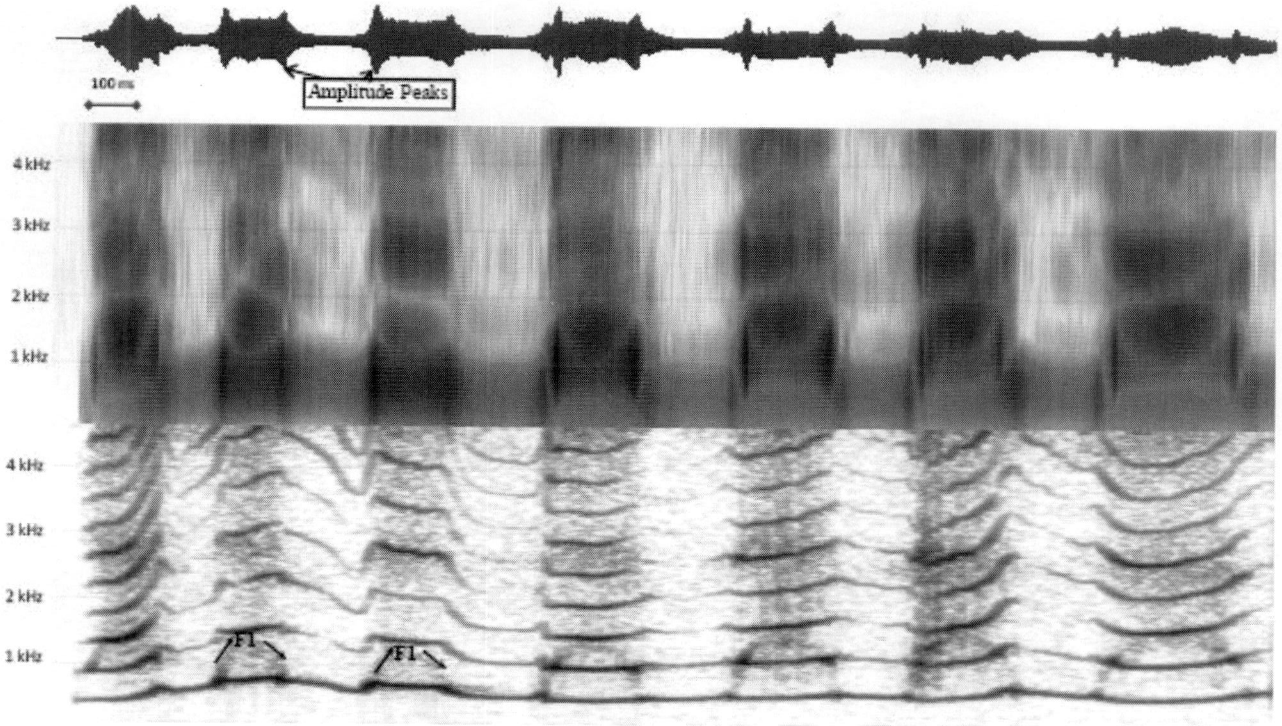

Example 20 is a single breath group sequence of reduplicated canonical syllables, a kind of celebration of babbling that adult listeners recognize as truly speech-like and to which they are usually therefore tempted to ascribe meaning. The infant producing this example was 10½ months old.

What we can learn from careful listening: In this example, we can hear seven clearly produced CV syllables with full vowels (or squeals) in each nucleus.

What we can learn from the acoustic analysis: Two spectrograms are presented, a very wideband (900 Hz) spectrogram is displayed on the top and a very narrowband (10 Hz) spectrogram on the bottom. The rate of production of these syllables is just under 3 per second (average duration 370 ms per syllable); adults generally produce about 4 or 5 syllables per second in conversation. Some acoustic curiosities are worth explaining here as babbling often includes such features: the odd peaks in amplitude at syllable margins are caused by the passing of F1 through the first and second harmonics, as can be seen quite clearly in the narrowband spectrogram. This concurrence of specific source energies with vocal tract resonance may occur in adults as well but is far more likely in infant vocalizations due to especially high f_0 in proportion to vocal tract resonances. More to the point of characterizing canonical syllabicity, the clear and relatively rapid traversal of F1 from low to high frequencies and back verifies that these sounds are produced by rapid closing-opening gestures. Finally, note that at least some of the higher pitch syllables in this sequence, like those for which F1 movement has been marked, would also be squeals in their phonatory feature coding.

Connections

The preceding chapter describes anatomical substrates for sound production that are essentially in place at birth. In this chapter, we considered the great variety of pre-speech vocalizations typically produced by infants as they progress towards first words. We show how these vocalizations attain increasing similarity with speech in terms of timing, articulation, and complexity.

Chapter 5 describes how, around their first birthdays, young children produce first words, how first words not only resemble characteristics of babbling but also coexist with it for a few months, and how word productions become less variable and also become increasingly sophisticated in terms of segmental content and word shape. As infants mature, their pre-speech vocal development relies on sensory feedback. Chapter 19 describes pre-speech development of infants who have hearing impairments or other developmental disabilities.

Concluding Remarks

The focus of this chapter was on the speech-related sounds infants produce starting at birth. These sounds were described in terms of protophone categories and features, including quasivowels, full vowels, squeals, growls, whispers, yells, ingressives, raspberries, clicks, glottal stops, goos, marginal syllables, canonical syllables, reduplicated babble, and variegated babble.

The historical and theoretical underpinnings of the categories as well as guidelines for applying the protophone categorizations were discussed. As infants mature, the categories build on each other, leading to increasing phonatory and articulatory sophistication and increasing resemblance to speech. This direct correspondence to observed stages of prelinguistic vocal development is at the heart of the protophone-based approach.

Chapter Review Questions

1. The discontinuity theory held that early vocalizations were unrelated to speech. We now know the theory to be false. What are some ways that babbling and speech are related?
2. How are protophones different from vegetative sounds and fixed signals such as cry and laughter?
3. What are the differences between marginal and reduplicated or variegated canonical babbling?

Suggestions for Further Reading

Oller, D. K. (2000). The emergence of the speech capacity. Mahwah, N. J.: Laurence Erlbaum.

Suggestions for Student Activities

1. Listen to sound file 4S22. Alternatively, make your own recording of an infant, preferably one between 2 and 12 months old, during a time when he/she is vocalizing. Identify the protophones from this chapter that are present in the recording, excluding any reflexive sounds. Also note the frequency with which each protophone occurs.

Access Sound File 22 (Chapter 4)

4S22 Recording of a 9-week-old infant (this example, and 4S21 below, were provided by Beate Peter).

2. Compare and contrast the cries in sound file 4S21 with those from 4S22. Do you sense a difference in the volitional nature of the vocalizations in the two sound files? Do you hear any evidence of supraglottal articulations in 4S21?

Access Sound File 21 (Chapter 4)

4S21 Cries of a one-week-old infant.

3. Interview a person who is a primary caregiver for an infant between the ages of two and twelve months of age. Describe the protophone categories to them and ask them which ones their infant currently produces, and how frequently.
4. Observe a caregiver/infant interaction. What protophones does the infant produce, and how does the caregiver respond to them?
5. Conduct a literature review on the differences in protophone development across different populations, such as infants with hearing impairment, those with Down syndrome, and those of varying socioeconomic status. Address both differences and similarities in protophone emergence across these populations.

Answers to Chapter Review Questions

1. The discontinuity theory held that early vocalizations were unrelated to speech. We now know the theory to be false. What are some ways that babbling and speech are related?

While protophones are mostly not speech-like in the sense of having identifiable phonemic characteristics, they are infraphonological in the sense that they are contrastive. For example, squeals and growls are quite distinctive in their phonatory characteristics. Another way in which babbling is related to speech is that it is clearly volitional. Together, these characteristics strongly support the notion that infants are actively exploring the ways in which sounds can be structured. Additionally, children's vocalizations come to have more speech-like characteristics as they progress from birth to first words. For example, they come to have fully resonant nuclei and syllabic timing (as in canonical babbling).

2. How are protophones different from vegetative sounds and fixed signals such as cry and laughter?

Protophones are produced volitionally, whereas vegetative sounds and fixed signals are produced reflexively. Sometimes, however, the difference can be a little difficult to discern as the boundaries may be a bit fuzzy. For example, fuss or whimper may be perceived as somewhat volitional compared to full blown cry, and chuckling can also be somewhat volitional in comparison to reflexive laughter.

3. What are the differences between marginal and and reduplicated or variegated canonical babbling?

The essential feature distinguishing canonical babbles is the closant-vocant transition. In a fully developed canonical syllable, the transition between the consonant-like and vowel-like portions of the speech are typically less than 120 ms. In a marginal syllable, this transition is typically longer than 120 ms. Another way to distinguish canonical and marginal syllables is by listening. If the transition between consonant and vowel can be directly tracked as a gradual movement, then the syllable is marginal. If the transition is fast enough that the transition between consonant and vowel sounds immediate, it is canonical. Canonical syllables are the prototypical syllables of adult speech. Canonical babble may consist of a single syllable or of sequences of syllables. In a sequence, if at least one syllable in the sequence is clearly canonical then the sequence is said to be canonical.

REFERENCES

Atkinson, K., MacWhinney, B., and Stoel, C. (1970). An experiment in the recognition of babbling. *Papers and Reports on Child Language Development*, No. 1. Stanford, CA.

Baken, R. J., and Orlikoff, R. F. (2000). *Clinical measurement of speech and voice*. San Diego: Singular Publishing Group.

Buder, E. H. (1996). Experimental phonology with acoustic phonetic methods: Formant measures from child speech. In D. Ingram (Ed.), *Proceedings of the UBC international conference on phonological acquisition* (pp. 254-265).

Buder, E. H. (2005). The acoustics of nasality: Steps towards a bridge to source literature. *Perspectives on Speech Science and Orofacial Disorders*, 15(1), 4-8.

Buder, E. H., Chorna, L., Oller, D. K., and Robinson, R. (2008). Vibratory regime classification of infant phonation. *Journal of Voice,* 22, 553-564.

Buder, E. H., Warlaumont, A. S., Oller, D. K., and Chorna, L. B. (2010). Dynamic indicators of mother-infant prosodic and illocutionary coordination. In *Proceedings of Speech Prosody 2010*. Chicago, IL.

Cheney, D. L., and Seyfarth, R. M. (1999). Mechanisms underlying vocalizations of primates. In M. D. Hauser and M. Konishi (Eds.), *The design of animal communication* (pp. 629-644). Cambridge, MA: MIT. Press.

de Boysson-Bardies, B. (1999). *How language comes to children: From birth to two years.* Cambridge, MA: MIT Press.

Eady, S. J. (1980). *The onset of language-specific patterning in infant vocalization.* (Master's thesis), University of Ottawa, Ottawa, Canada.

Eilers, R. E., and Oller, D. K. (1994). Infant vocalizations and the early diagnosis of severe hearing impairment. *Journal of Pediatrics*, 124, 199-203.

Elbers, L. (1982). Operating principles in repetitive babbling: A cognitive continuity approach. *Cognition,* 12, 45-63.

Ertmer, D. J., and Nathani Iyer, S. (2010). Prelinguistic vocalizations in infants and toddlers with hearing loss: Identifying and stimulating auditory-guided speech development. In M. Marschark and P. E. Spencer (Eds.), *The Oxford handbook of deaf studies, language, and education, Vol. 2* (pp. 360–375). Oxford: Oxford University Press.

Goldstein, M. H., and Schwade, J. A. (2008). Social feedback to infants' babbling facilitates rapid phonological learning. *Psychological Science,* 19(5), 515-523.

Hauser, M. (1996). *The evolution of communication*. Cambridge, MA: MIT Press.

Hockett, C. F., and Altmann, S. A. (1968). A note on design features. In T. A. Sebeok (Ed.), *Animal communication: Techniques of study and results of research* (pp. 61-72). Bloomington, IN: Indiana University Press.

Holmgren, K., Lindblom, B., Aurelius, G., Jalling, B., and Zetterstrom, R. (1986). On the phonetics of infant vocalization. In R. Zetterstrom (Ed.), *Precursors of early speech* (pp. 51-63). New York: Stockton Press.

Irwin, O. C. (1947). Infant speech: consonant sounds according to manner of articulation. *Journal of Speech and Hearing Disorders*, 12, 402-404.

Irwin, O. C. (1948). Infant speech: development of vowel sounds. *Journal of Speech and Hearing Disorders,* 13, 31-34.

Jakobson, R. (1941). *Kindersprache, Aphasie und allgemeine Lautgesetze*. Uppsala: Almquist and Wiksell.

Jakobson, R. (1968). *Child language, aphasia and phonological universals* (A. R. Keiler, Trans.). Den Haag: Mouton.

Johnson, K. (2003). *Acoustic and auditory phonetics* (2nd ed.). Malden, MA: Blackwell Publishing.

Kent, R. D., and Read, W. C. (2002). *The acoustic analysis of speech* (2nd ed.). Albany, N. Y.: Delmar.

Koopmans-van Beinum, F. J., and van der Stelt, J. M. (1986). Early stages in the development of speech movements. In R. Zetterstrom (Ed.), *Precursors of early speech* (pp. 37-50). New York: Stockton Press.

Levitt, A. G., and Wang, Q. (1991). Evidence for language-specific rhythmic influences in the reduplicative babbling of French- and English-learning infants. *Language and Speech*, 34(3), 235-249.

Lorenz, K. (1951). Ausdrucksbewegungen höherer Tiere. *Naturwissenschaften*, 38, 113-116.

Lynch, M. P., Oller, D. K., Steffens, M. L., and Buder, E. H. (1995). Phrasing in prelinguistic vocalizations. *Developmental Psychobiology*, 28, 3-23.

Lynch, M. P., Oller, D. K., Steffens, M. L., Levine, S. L., Basinger, D. L., and Umbel, V. M. (1995). Development of speech-like vocalizations in infants with Down syndrome. *American Journal of Mental Retardation*, 100(1), 68-86.

Lynip, A. W. (1951). The use of magnetic devices in the collection and analysis of the preverbal utterances of an infant. *Genet Psychol Monogr,* 44(2), 221-262.

MacNeilage, P. F. (1998). The frame/content theory of evolution of speech production. *Behavioral and Brain Sciences*, 21(4), 499-546.

Masataka, N. (2001). Why early linguistic milestones are delayed in children with Williams syndrome: Late onset of hand banging as a possible rate-limiting constraint on the emergence of canonical babbling. *Developmental Science*, 4(2), 158 164.

Mitchell, P. R., and Kent, R. D. (1990). Phonetic variation in multisyllabic babbling. *Journal of Child Language,* 17, 247-265.

Nakazima, S. (1962). A comparative study of the speech development of Japanese and American English in childhood. *Studia Phonologica*, 2, 27-39.

Navarro, A., Pearson, B. Z., Cobo-Lewis, A. B., and Oller, D. K. (1998). Identifying the language spoken by 26-month-old monolingual- and bilingual-learning babies in a no-context situation. In H. Walsh (Ed.), *Proceedings of the 22nd Annual Proceedings of the 22nd Boston University Conference on Language Development* (Vol. 2, pp. 557-568). Somerville, MA: Cascadilla Press.

Oller, D. K. (1980). The emergence of the sounds of speech in infancy. In G. H. Yeni-Komshian, J. F. Kavanagh and C. A. Ferguson (Eds.), *Child phonology* (Vol. 1: Production, pp. 93-112). New York: Academic Press.

Oller, D. K. (1986). Metaphonology and infant vocalizations. In R. Zetterstrom (Ed.), *Precursors of early speech* (pp. 21-35). New York: Stockton Press.

Oller, D. K. (2000). *The emergence of the speech capacity.* Mahwah, N. J.: Lawrence Erlbaum Associates.

Oller, D. K., Eilers, R. E., and Basinger, D. (2001). Intuitive identification of infant vocal sounds by parents. *Developmental Science*, 4(1), 49-60.

Oller, D. K., and Griebel, U. (2008). The origins of syllabification in human infancy and in human evolution. In B. Davis and K. Zajdó (Eds.), *The syllable in speech production* (pp. 29-62). New York: Lawrence Erlbaum Associates.

Oller, D. K., and Ramsdell, H. L. (2008, July). *The creation of phonological categories and the negotiation of word meanings in early lexical development.* Paper presented at the XI International Congress for the Study of Child Language, Edinburgh.

Oller, D. K., Wieman, L., Doyle, W., and Ross, C. (1975). Infant babbling and speech. *Journal of Child Language*, 3, 1-11.

Owren, M. J., and Goldstein, M. H. (2008). Scaffolds for babbling: Innateness and learning in the emergence of contextually flexible vocal production in human infants. In D. K. Oller and U. Griebel (Eds.), *Evolution of communicative flexibility: Complexity, creativity and adaptability in human and animal communication* (pp. 169-192). Cambridge, MA: MIT Press.

Paul, R., Fuerst, Y., Ramsay, G., Chawarska, K., and Klin, A. (2011). Out of the mouths of babes: Vocal production in infant siblings of children with ASD. *Journal of Child Psychology and Psychiatry*, 52, 588-598.

Ramsdell, H. (2009). *The emergence of phonological categories in human infancy: A study of methodologies*. (Doctoral dissertation), The University of Memphis. ProQuest database.

Sheinkopf, S. J., Mundy, P., Oller, D. K., and Steffens, M. (2000). Vocal atypicalities of preverbal autistic children. *Journal of Autism and Developmental Disorders*, 30(4), 345-353.

Smith, B. L., Brown-Sweeney, S., and Stoel-Gammon, C. (1989). A quantitative analysis of reduplicated and variegated babbling. *First Language*, 9, 175-190.

Sroufe, L., and Wunsch, J. (1972). The development of laughter in the first year of life. *Child Development*, 43, 1326-1344.

Stark, R. E. (1980). Stages of speech development in the first year of life. In G. H. Yeni-Komshian, J. F. Kavanagh and C. A. Ferguson (Eds.), *Child phonology* (Vol. 1: Production, pp. 73-92). New York: Academic Press.

Stark, R. E. (1981). Infant vocalization: A comprehensive view. *Infant Medical Health Journal*, 2(2), 118-128.

Stevens, K. N. (1998). *Acoustic Phonetics*. Cambridge, MA: The MIT Press.

Stoel-Gammon, C., and Cooper, J. A. (1984). Patterns of early lexical and phonological development. *Journal of Child Language*, 11(2), 247-271.

Stoel-Gammon, C., and Dunn, C. (1985). *Normal and disordered phonology in children*. Austin, TX: Pro. Ed.

Vihman, M. M., and de Boysson-Bardies, B. (1994). The nature and origin of ambient language influence on infant vocal production and early words. *Phonetica*, 51, 159-169.

Vihman, M. M., Macken, M. A., Miller, R., Simmons, H., and Miller, J. (1985). From Babbling to Speech - a Re-Assessment of the Continuity Issue. *Language*, 61(2), 397-445.

Warlaumont, A. S., Oller, D. K., Buder, E. H., Dale, R., and Kozma, R. (2010). Data-driven automated acoustic analysis of human infant vocalizations using neural network tools. *The Journal of the Acoustical Society of America*, 127, 2563-2577.

Warlaumont, A. S., Oller, D. K., Dale, R., Richards, J. A., Gilkerson, J., and Xu, D. (2010). Vocal interaction dynamics of children with and without autism. In S. Ohlsson and R. Catrambone (Eds.), *Proceedings of the 32nd Annual Conference of the Cognitive Science Society*, Austin, TX: Cognitive Science Society, 121-126.

In: Comprehensive Perspectives …
Editors: Beate Peter and Andrea A. N. MacLeod
ISBN: 978-1-62257-041-6

Chapter 5

Transitions to First Words

Anna Sosa

Introduction

"She said 'mommy'"! These words, proclaimed with delight by parents, suggest the onset of a new stage of development, a stage eagerly anticipated by parents of young children around the world. Near the time of their first birthday, children begin to attach meaning to the sounds they have been practicing to produce true words. By their second birthday, their vocabulary has grown to about 300 words. This chapter addresses topics related to the development of speech during the transition from babble, discussed in Chapter 4, through the "first words period," which is generally defined as the period from the onset of the child's first word through the development of a 50-word expressive vocabulary, which for many children is attained by about 18 months of age.

Defining True Words

But how do we know that she really said "mommy"? How do we know that it's really a word? As described in Chapter 4, children begin producing sounds and syllables that sound very speech-like sometime between 6 and 9 months of age. These canonical syllables contain consonants and vowels that may be combined in ways that sound very much like real *words*. For example, the 8-month-old who babbles the string "dada" may produce something that is acoustically almost identical to what the 15-month-old squeals when his father walks into the room. So, what is the difference between these two utterances? The generally accepted understanding of a true word is that it must have a stable semantic reference together with a (relatively) stable phonetic form that in some way resembles the phonetic characteristics of the adult target word. Thus, a child who regularly produces the phonetic form [ba] every time he sees a ball would be credited with a true word. While the child's production is not exactly like the adult form because of the missing final /l/, the form is sufficiently similar to the target and used consistently enough in reference to a ball in the environment to convey the child's intent to say "ball." Of course, caregivers may differ in their interpretation of their child's utterances. Some parents may be quite liberal in accepting their child's babbles as words, resulting in reports of children who began "talking" at 7 or 8 months. Other parents may be slower to accept their child's attempts at words if their production is quite different from the target form.

During this transition from babble to words, children may produce sound sequences that are relatively stable and are used consistently in a given context, but do not fit the full definition of a true word. The most common term for these productions is *protoword.* Protowords differ from true words in that they are not phonetically similar to an identifiable target form and the interpretation of their meaning is highly context-dependent. Some protowords may even include an accompanying communicative gesture as part of the production pattern. For example, production of the syllables [mamamam] while using a reaching gesture toward a desired object with opening and closing of the fingers may be interpreted to mean "give me" or "I want that," but would not be considered a true word. Most parents are extremely good at recognizing their child's transition from babbled strings of syllables with no intended target to the use of true words that have both a semantic referent and a phonetic target.

Relationship between Babble and First Words

Overlap between Babble and Words

The task of accurately identifying the onset of true words would be even easier had early assertions regarding the relationship between pre-linguistic babble and language proved true. Roman Jakobson, perhaps the first child phonologist, claimed that the child "loses all of his ability to produce sounds in passing over from the pre-language stage to the first acquisition of words" (Jakobson, 1941/1968, pp.21), implying, perhaps, a period of silence that would indicate the transition to first words. A great body of work demonstrates, however, that this is not the case. First of all, there appears to be an extended period of overlap between babble and language use during which time the relative proportion of linguistic utterances to babble increases until babble is no longer observed and all utterances produced are interpreted as meaningful speech. The duration of this period of overlap varies from child to child, but babble and meaningful speech may coexist for many months (Stoel-Gammon, 1998). Furthermore, the sounds and syllable shapes that are reported to occur frequently in babble are the very same sounds and syllables that make up the child's first words.

During babble, babies can both hear and feel the sounds they are producing and can begin to link their articulatory patterns with a specific acoustic output, creating an *auditory-articulatory feedback loop* (Stoel-Gammon, 1998). In addition to kinesthetic and acoustic feedback, they also receive social feedback from caregivers when their babbled productions are interpreted as meaningful utterances. The mother of a 10-month-old, for example, who babbles [dædæ] may encourage the repetition of the utterance in specific contexts by interpreting the child's babble as a production of the word "daddy." Gros-Louis, West, Goldstein and King (2006) found that caregivers were more likely to interpret babble that contained consonants (i.e. CV syllables) as a meaningful utterance, compared to vocalic babble, thereby reinforcing the production of vocalizations with consonants. These babbled syllables form the building blocks for words and children are encouraged, both internally via the feedback loop and externally via caregiver responsiveness, to take these practiced motor patterns and use them in their first attempts at producing words.

General Phonetic Characteristics of First Words

Typically, children produce their first word between 11 and 13 months and continue producing one-word utterances until they have assembled an expressive vocabulary of approximately 50 words. While there is certainly a great deal of variation in the production of early words during this *first words period*, both across individual children and across languages, there are also common tendencies in the observed phonological properties of these first words that are quite striking. Consonants used in early words tend to come from a restricted range of manner classes, primarily stops or plosives (e.g. /b, d, ɑ), nasals (e.g. /m, n/), and glides (i.e., /w, j/). As described in Chapter 4, these are the same classes of sounds that occur most often in babble. Consonants that are often notably absent from these first words include fricatives (e.g. /s, ʃ, θ/), affricates (i.e., / ʧ, ʤ/), and liquids (i.e. /l, r/). Children's first words are also quite limited in terms of syllable structure; the most frequent syllable structures produced by English-speaking children include CV (as in "bye"), CVC (as in "mom"), and CVCV (as in "baby"). In general, children tend to have a larger number of consonants in initial position of syllables than in final position and there are some differences in terms of manner and voicing that may occur depending on the position. For example, initial consonants during the first words period include primarily voiced stops (e.g. /b, d/) and nasals, whereas voiceless stops (e.g. /t/) and voiceless fricatives (e.g. /s/) are somewhat more common in final position, if final consonants exist at all (Robb and Bleile, 1994; Stoel-Gammon, 1985). One might suggest two possible explanations for the observation that children's early productions of words are limited in terms of words shapes and consonants used. One is that children systematically simplify the target consonants and word shapes of adult words so that they fit within their limited articulatory abilities. The other is that children actually choose to say words that consist of simple syllable shapes and a restricted set of consonants while avoiding words with more complex phonetic targets. The former is certainly true; children regularly produce target consonants in a manner that may be somehow easier for them to achieve motorically (e.g. target /v/ produced as [b]). They also frequently simplify the syllable structure of words by omitting final consonants (e.g. [dɑ] for "dog") or by deleting entire syllables (e.g. [næna] for "banana"). There is, however, also evidence for the second explanation. If we examine the first ten words acquired by English speaking children as determined by the normative data for the MacArthur-Bates Communicative Development Inventory (CDI), a parental checklist of vocabulary words commonly acquired by young children (see Sidebar 5.1), we see some obvious patterns.

Sidebar 5. 1. Earliest Words.
The first ten words acquired by English-speaking children according to normative data from the Communicative Development Inventory

daddy, mommy, bye, ball, hi, dog, no, baby, kitty, book

First, all of the words are either one or two syllable words with CV, CVC, or CVCV syllable structure. Additionally, with only two exceptions (i.e. final /l/ in "ball" and initial /h/ in "hi"), all of the target consonants are either stops or nasals. Given the restricted phonological characteristics of the target words, children do not have to do much in the way of simplification to produce these words; these are syllable shapes and sounds that they have been practicing since they started producing canonical babble and that become the *canonical syllables* in the first words. Given this lack of phonetic complexity in these first words, early attempts at words may actually be quite accurate relative to the adult target form.

Even beyond these first few words, similar patterns are observed. Stoel-Gammon (1998) looked carefully at the phonological characteristics of the target forms of early acquired words (words acquired between 11 and 19 months of age) and later acquired words (words acquired between 20 and 30 months of age). A comparison of the two sets showed that the earlier acquired words were more restricted in terms of syllable shapes and consonants present than the later acquired words, suggesting that articulatory complexity of the target word is a factor that influences which words children will include in their early productive vocabulary. The early words had very few initial or final consonant clusters and a full 57% of the words had stop consonants in initial position. The most frequent initial consonant in the earliest acquired words was /b/, representing 22% of all of the words. Similarly, Stoel-Gammon and Peter (2008) showed that /b/- initial words but not /p/- initial words were highly prevalent in the expressive lexicon of young toddlers, decreasing in proportion as a function of age, whereas words beginning with a later developing sound, for instance /s/, were rare in the expressive lexicon of young toddlers, increasing in proportional prevalence as a function of age. There appears to be something about the /b/ sound that makes it easily accessible to young children as they are learning to talk; perhaps it is because it is more visual than consonants produced with the tongue so the child is able to see what the adult is doing to produce the sound and is not relying solely on acoustic cues. A child's preference for words with sound patterns that are easy to produce is called *lexical selection.*

An analysis of early and later acquired words by Cantonese-speaking children demonstrates that it's not just English-speaking children who choose their first words based on phonetic properties. Using normative data from the Cantonese adaptation of the MacArthur-Bates Communicative Development Inventory, similar results were found (Fletcher, Chan, Wong, Stokes, Tardif and Leung, 2004); the earlier-acquired words had primarily stops, nasals, and glides in initial position, with the unaspirated voiceless stop /p/ (which is acoustically very similar to an English /b/) accounting for approximately 11% of all words and /m/ accounting for 16%. Similar to the English analysis, these strong preferences were not observed for the later acquired words, suggesting that the influence of the "phonetic factor" in children's selection of words diminishes as children approach their second birthday.

Preferred Patterns and Lexical Selection in Individual Children

While children as a group are observed to select their first words from a phonologically restricted subset of the adult vocabulary, individual children may have even more specific preferences for individual sounds or sound patterns. Observational studies have shown that children display patterns of choices in their acquisition of early words that reflect their own phonological abilities and preferences. Specific sound pattern preferences in babble are seen to carry over into meaningful speech, forming the building blocks for an individual child's early lexicon. One consequence of this preference for specific sound patterns or *vocal motor schemes*, as they have been called (Vihman, 1992), is that children in the earliest stages of speech development may end up with many words in their nascent productive vocabulary that are nearly *homophonous*. For example, one child studied by Ferguson and Farwell (1975) showed a marked preference for acquiring words with *sibilant consonants* (i.e. /s/-like consonants). The words "see," "shoes," "ice," "eyes," "cheese," "sit," and "juice" were all included in her early vocabulary, resulting in several words that may have sounded quite similar in her speech. Another child, described by Stoel-Gammon and Cooper (1984), had a preference for words with velar stops. For this child, 11 of his first 50 words (22%) had a velar stop in final position of the target form. These findings indicate that the specific words a child produces early in the process of lexical acquisition are determined not only by semantic and social/pragmatic influences, but also by a child's productive phonological ability.

In addition to the evidence from these observational examples, experimental evidence for the phenomenon of lexical selection based on phonological preferences was found. A series of studies was conducted to evaluate young children's ability to learn novel words with phonological characteristics that were either "IN" the individual child's productive repertoire or "OUT" of the repertoire. In a pair of studies by Leonard, Schwartz, and colleagues (Leonard, Schwartz, Morris and Chapman, 1981; Schwartz and Leonard, 1982), young children in the first words period were found to be more likely to produce novel real or nonsense words with syllable structures and consonants that were consistent with their own productive phonology, even after controlling for semantic factors and input factors (i.e. frequency of exposure to the new words). Again, this provides evidence that children don't just select their early words based on semantic or pragmatic importance, but also based on phonological factors.

The importance of the phonetic component in starting to say words has been offered as an explanation for why children around the world are often observed to say the word for the male parent before they acquire the word for the female parent, in spite of the tendency for the mother to be the primary caregiver. Locke (1985) notes that, cross-linguistically, many terms for "father" (e.g., *dada, papa)* have oral stops while most terms for "mother" (e.g. *mama, mami*) have nasal sounds. Since oral stops are more frequent than nasal stops in babble, the child would be able to use this frequently practiced motor routine to produce his first word, "daddy," which is often reported as the first word acquired by English-speaking children, with an average age of acquisition of approximately 11 ½ months (Fenson, Dale, Reznick, Thal, Bates, Hartung, Pethick and Reilly, 1993).

An Emerging Phonological System

The Word as The Minimal Unit of Production

Information stored in the mental lexicon about the sound structure of words is called the *phonological representation*. The phonological representations of adults are thought to contain information about the individual sounds that make up a word. In other words, adults are assumed to "know" that the word *cat* comprises three unique sounds and that these sounds can be combined in other ways and with different sounds to create new meanings. During the earliest stages of speech development however, children are not necessarily thought to have adult-like phonological representations. While some phonological theories have attributed adult-like representations to children from the onset of language production (e.g. Smith, 1973; Bernhardt and Stemberger, 1998), other child phonologists have hypothesized that the unit of representation for the very young child may be larger than the individual sound, perhaps the whole word (e.g. Ferguson and Farwell, 1973; Vihman and Croft, 2007; Waterson, 1971).

Several hallmarks of early speech production support the word as the basic unit of representation. Young children are often highly variable in their production of sounds and words; they may produce a sound accurately in one word but not in another (*inter-word variability*), or they may produce the same word in different ways (*intra-word variability*). This observed variability has been taken to indicate that the underlying phonological representations of young children may not be as detailed as those of adults and that these "fuzzy" representations may allow for more variability in production. For example, Ferguson and Farwell (1973) describe a young girl who uses 10 different productions of the word "pen" during a short period of time. They describe the productions as reflecting general knowledge of the articulatory features present in the target word (e.g.. lip closure, voicelessness, nasalization), but lacking detailed information regarding the organization of each of those features within the word as a whole, resulting in variable production. They conclude that the young child's phonological system is best described as a "phonic core of remembered lexical items and articulations which produce them" (Ferguson and Farwell, 1973, p. 437], as opposed to consisting of adult-like phonemic representations. Other examples of intra-word variability (adapted from Sosa and Stoel-Gammon, 2012) include the following productions of the word "juice" by a child, age 24 months: [dus, dʊst, ʤʊs, dʊʃ, ʤʊʃ], and the word "frog" was variously produced as [bwʌk, wʌk, fwʌt, fwʌ, fwʌk] by another child, also age 24 months. Video clip 5V1 shows examples of variable productions recorded during a play session with a boy, age 20 months. Sidebar 5.2 is a schematic representation of intra-word variability.

Access Video File 1 (Chapter 5)

5V1 Play session with a boy, age 20 months.

Sidebar 5.2. Intra-Word Variability

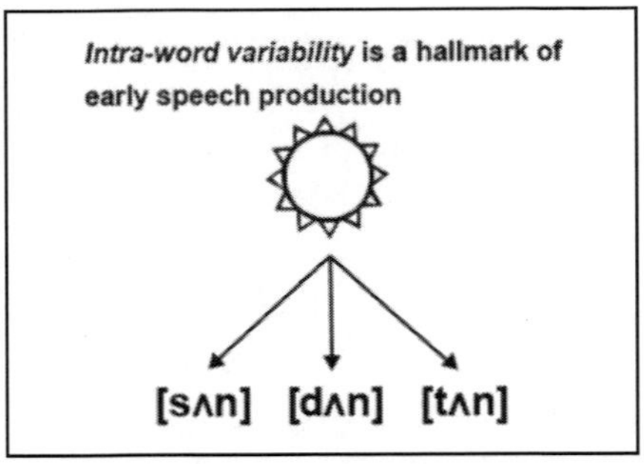
Intra-word variability is a hallmark of early speech production
[sʌn] [dʌn] [tʌn]

Any clinician or researcher attempting to analyze the speech patterns of children during the first words period would likely agree that it can be very difficult to describe their productions in terms of consistent simplifications of target phonemes (i.e. *phonological processes*). While the speech errors of slightly older children can often be described on a segment-by-segment basis (e.g. a target fricative is produced as a stop), it is often very difficult to identify consistent error patterns in the speech of the youngest talkers. Furthermore, those error patterns that are identifiable typically operate at the level of the whole word rather than at the level of the individual phoneme. For example, very young children may use the phonological process of *reduplication*, which is the exact or partial repetition of a syllable (e.g. [baba] for "bottle"). They may also exhibit patterns of *harmony*, also referred to as assimilation, across an entire word, whereby all consonants or vowels are produced using similar articulatory features; harmony may include producing the individual sounds with the same place, manner, and/or voicing. For example, a child who produces the word "duck" as [gʌkgʌk] is using both reduplication and consonant harmony.

Observations of early word forms in a variety of different languages have led some researchers to suggest that the organizational unit of early phonological representations is an articulatory template (Piske, 1997; Vihman and Croft, 2007; Waterson, 1971), which is described as a whole-word phonotactic or metrical pattern that a child can use for the production of multiple words. For example, one Estonian-speaking child described originally by Vihman (1981) and adapted by Vihman and Croft (2007) had a "nasal template" that he used to produce a variety of words that had nasal consonants in the adult target. The template took the form of the consonant /n/ followed by a vowel and then any other nasal consonant (e.g. [næŋ], [nɪŋ], and [nɪn] for target /kiŋ/ meaning "shoe" and [nən] for adult target /rind/ meaning "breast"). Similarly, Waterson (1971) described a young boy who had many words that fit a "sibilant template", which consisted of an optional stop consonant followed by a vowel and the sound /ʃ/ (e.g. [ʊʃ] for both "fish" and "vest"). As the child learns new words, he may approach the production of a word by "fitting" it into an existing template based on some degree of phonetic or acoustic similarity. The assumption is that these templates are formed on the basis of the individual child's preferred production patterns or vocal motor schemes in combination with acoustic features of the adult target that are most salient for the child. As seen in the examples above, the phonetic structure of the templates may be defined quite loosely, thereby allowing for a certain degree of variability in production. These patterns, again, suggest that the minimal unit of linguistic representation for the young child in the earliest stages of language may best be described in terms of units larger than the individual phoneme.

Transition to a Phonemic System

At what point do children transition from this hypothesized holistic representation of the sounds of speech to a more segmental representation? The general assumption is that as the child's lexicon grows, more segmental phonemic representation emerges (Lindblom, 1992; Nittrouer, Studdert-Kennedy and McGowan, 1989; Vihman, 1996). Several researchers have suggested that phonemic representation emerges at the end of the first words period, as the child approaches a 50-word expressive vocabulary (e.g., Vihman, 1996). Recent evidence suggests that this transition is most likely a very gradual process that may occur on a word-by-word basis and that the development of phonemic representation may begin somewhat later than was earlier hypothesized. Sosa and Stoel-Gammon (2006) investigated intra-word variability in four children between 12 and 24 months to explore whether patterns of intra-word variability might shed light on the hypothesized transition from whole-word to phonemic representation. High rates of variability throughout the period were found and in contrast to the anticipated general decline in variability as the productive vocabulary grew, three of the four children observed displayed variability peaks corresponding to the onset of two-word combinations, which occurred between 21 and 24 months. At these points, the children had between 139 and 236 words in their expressive vocabularies according to the parent report. These peaks in variability were interpreted as indicative of a general reorganization of the linguistic system, including the beginning of reorganization from a holistic to a more segmental type of phonological representation.

Other studies of both speech perception and speech production suggest that the process of reorganization may not be complete until much later, perhaps even as late as age 7 or 8 years (Charles-Luce and Luce, 1990; Garlock, Walley and Metsala, 2000). Most child phonologists seem to agree that children during the first words period are not operating with underlying phonological representations that are exactly the same as the adult representations (see Sidebar 5.3). What is not entirely agreed upon, however, is exactly when or how these representations become adult-like. As you will see in the next chapter, the speech patterns of children approaching their 3rd year of life are often described in terms of consistent phonological patterns operating at the level of the individual segment, suggesting that toddlers and preschoolers have developed at least some knowledge of the individual sounds that make up the words they are saying.

Sidebar 5.3. Perception vs. Production

Some aspects of speech perception and production in early childhood make for a puzzling mix of seeming contradictions. Based on characteristics of early speech production, children are often thought to lack phonetic detail in their phonological representations and are described as using more holistic or "whole-word" representations. Conversely, infants by 4 months of age have demonstrated remarkable sensitivity to subtle phonetic distinctions (e.g., Eimas, Siqueland, Jusczyk and Vigorito, 1971) and older children who produce errors on certain speech sounds often reject an adult's production of a word that demonstrates the same error, suggesting that they are able to perceive the mistake when produced by someone else. Due to these inconsistencies, the debate regarding the nature of young children's phonological representations persists.

CONNECTIONS

The information provided in this chapter about the speech characteristics of children as they transition from babble and begin to use words has focused on typical development. Absent obvious sensory, structural, or motor impairments (see Chapters 17, 18, and 19 for information about speech development in special populations), children in the very earliest stages of language development are rarely, if ever, diagnosed as having speech or articulation disorders. If a child is delayed in the acquisition of an expressive vocabulary, it is extremely difficult to know whether the rate-limiting factor is more speech-based (i.e. actual difficulty producing the sounds and sound combinations necessary to make words) or whether it reflects a general language delay or disorder. We do know, however, that abilities in these two areas are typically commensurate. That is, children with small vocabularies have more limited speech production abilities than children with larger vocabularies; in fact, phonological ability has been found to be more closely related to the size of a child's expressive vocabulary than it is to the child's chronological age (Paul and Jennings, 1992; Rescorla and Ratner, 1996; Smith, McGregor and Demille, 2006; Stoel-Gammon and Dale, 1988). Causal factors can be difficult to tease out, however. Is the child's expressive vocabulary limited because they are not able to produce a variety of speech sounds, or is the phonetic repertoire limited because the child has not yet begun to say very many words, so he or she can "get by" with just a few sounds and syllable shapes?

While general information about speech production should be gathered as part of a comprehensive evaluation of a child for whom concerns regarding language development exist, there are currently no norm-referenced clinical tools available to "diagnose" a speech disorder in children this young. Speech and language assessment instruments usually include a few questions about the nature of the child's vocalizations. For example, the *Preschool Language Scale – 4th Edition* (PLS-4) has two questions for children between 12 and 17 months that specifically address speech production. One item is passed if the child "babbles two syllables together (e.g., [mama], [bada])" and the second item is passed if the child has been observed to use at least five different consonant sounds. Yes or no answers to these questions do not provide much detailed information regarding the speech production patterns of the child. Clinicians must therefore rely on informal assessments of speech production and a detailed knowledge of expected production patterns during the first words period in order to adequately assess a child's speech production abilities. Examples of assessments and analyses appropriate for children during this period include *phonetic inventory* (i.e. a list of all consonants, vowels, and syllable shapes produced by the child), frequency of vocalizations during a given time period, and ratios of utterances containing consonants to all utterances produced. There are also a handful of more formal analysis procedures that have been proposed. These include phonological mean length of utterance (PMLU; Ingram, 2002), syllable structure level (SSL; Paul and Jennings, 1992), index of phonetic complexity (IPC; Jakielski, Maytasse and Doyle, 2006), and the word complexity measure (WCM; Stoel-Gammon, 2010b). Each of these measures is intended to assess the breadth of a child's phonological system, rather than focusing on whether individual sounds are produced correctly or incorrectly in relation to an adult target, as formal articulation tests are designed to do (Stoel-Gammon, 2010b). Without the availability of normative data to which results of these analyses can be compared, accurate interpretation continues to depend on the clinician's in depth knowledge of typical patterns of speech production during this period.

Concluding Remarks

This chapter presents information about the speech production characteristics of children during the first words period, defined as the period from the onset of the first word to the acquisition of an expressive vocabulary of about 50 words. Beginning in the 1970s, a handful of researchers began to refute previously held beliefs regarding the relationship between babble and later language. Specifically, repeated observations that the sounds produced during babble are the same sounds used in early words, and that children seem to have individual preferences for specific sounds and sound patterns that span the period from babble to first words, have lead to the conclusion that pre-linguistic vocalizations, specifically canonical babble, form the articulatory building blocks for language production.

This chapter also summarizes information suggesting that children's knowledge regarding the sound structure of the words they produce may be more global and less specified on a segmental level than that of adults.

Variable production of individual sounds in different words as well as variability in the production of the same word, use of preferred articulation patterns or *word templates*, and the observation of whole word rather than segmental simplification processes suggest that the minimal unit of phonological representation for children may be at the level of the word rather than something smaller like the phoneme. A number of attempts to apply what we have learned regarding typical speech production abilities in young children to the clinical assessment of children with delays in speech and/or language development have been made.

Nonetheless, we are still limited in our ability to use what we have learned about the nature of typical speech development during the first words period for early diagnosis of possible speech disorders.

Future work should focus on developing clinical applications that will allow us to identify children with early signs of speech production disorders and perhaps to predict which children will require intervention related directly to limitations in speech production abilities.

Chapter Review Questions

1. Which consonant classes and syllable shapes are most common in children's productions of early words?
2. What differentiates a true word from babble?
3. How do a baby's pre-linguistic vocalizations influence the composition of her early vocabulary?
4. Why should the definition of a true word be qualified to include the phrase "relatively stable phonetic form", rather than just "stable phonetic form"?
5. What evidence refutes earlier claims that babble and meaningful speech are unrelated?

6. What factors influence a child's selection of words to include in their early productive vocabulary? In other words, why do children try to say some words but not others?
7. Why do some researchers believe that the minimal unit of phonological representation for young children is the whole word rather than the individual phoneme?

SUGGESTIONS FOR FURTHER READING

Ertmer, D.J., Inniger, K.J. (2009). Characteristics of the transition to spoken words in two young cochlear implant recipients. *Journal of Speech, Language, and Hearing Research*, 52, 1579-1594.

Ferguson, C.A., Farwell, C.B. (1975). Words and sounds in early language acquisition. *Language*, 51, 419-439.

McCleery, J.P., Tully, L., Slevc, L.R., Schreibman, L. (2006). Consonant production patterns of young severely language-delayed children with autism. *Journal of Communication Disorders*, 39, 217-231.

Stager, C.L., Werker, J.F. (1997). Infants listen for more phonetic detail in speech perception than in word-learning tasks. *Nature*, 388 (6640), 381-382.

Stoel-Gammon, C. (2010a). Relationships between lexical and phonological development in young children. *Journal of Child Language*, First View Articles.

Vihman, M., Croft, W. (2007). Phonological development: toward a radical templatic phonology. *Linguistics*, 45, 683.

SUGGESTIONS FOR STUDENT ACTIVITIES

1. Research the 1st 10 words acquired by children in two different languages using adaptations of the CDI. What do you notice about the phonological characteristics of the target words?
2. Using the provided video clip 5V1 of a 20-month-old boy, answer the following questions.
   a) What is his phonetic inventory? What consonants does he produce? What vowels does he produce? What syllable shapes does he produce?
   b) Are there any examples of the following speech phenomena: 1. intra-word variability, 2. inter-word variability, 3. consonant harmony, 4. reduplication, 5. homophonous forms? If so, provide an example for each.

ANSWERS TO CHAPTER REVIEW QUESTIONS

1. Which consonant classes and syllable shapes are most common in children's productions of early words?

Stops, nasals, and glides are the most frequent consonants in early words and early words tend to consist of simple syllable structures, including CV, CVC, and CVCV.

2. What differentiates a true word from babble?

While the phonetic characteristics of babble and early words are very similar, true words include a relatively stable phonetic form paired with a semantic referent.

3. How do a baby's pre-linguistic vocalizations influence the composition of her early vocabulary?

Many babies have preferred production patterns that are used in babble. These same patterns are also observed in their early words and may influence which words they choose to include in their productive vocabulary.

4. Why should the definition of a true word be qualified to include the phrase "relatively stable phonetic form", rather than just "stable phonetic form"?

Children are often quite variable in their production of early words. Intra-word variability, which may result in a single word being produced in multiple ways, is quite common. This type of instability in production does not mean that the child is not actually producing a real word.

5. What evidence refutes earlier claims that babble and meaningful speech are unrelated?

Studies of children's production patterns during the transition from babble to speech have found that there is often an extended period of overlap between babble and speech, that the sounds used in babble are the same sounds that are used in early words, and that children often have individual preferences for specific sounds and sound patterns and that these patterns are used both in babble and in meaningful speech. There is no evidence of a period of silence during the transition from babble to speech and there are no major differences in terms of the phonetic characteristics of late babble and early speech, suggesting that canonical syllables used in babble form the building blocks for early speech.

6. What factors influence a child's selection of words to include in their early productive vocabulary? In other words, why do children try to say some words but not others?

In addition to semantic and pragmatic reasons for attempting a specific word (e.g., the family has a beloved dog, the child hears the word 'dog' frequently, and the child really likes the dog), there is also evidence suggesting that children choose words based on phonetic or phonological factors. They may choose words that are made up of consonants and syllable shapes that they have been practicing during babble and are somehow "easier" for them to produce and they may avoid words that contain later developing sounds (e.g., affricates and liquids) and syllable shapes (e.g., initial and final consonant clusters).

7. Why do some researchers believe that the minimal unit of phonological representation for young children is the whole word rather than the individual phoneme?

Children's productions of early words are often very difficult to describe on a segment-by-segment basis. Observed speech production phenomena, including inter- and intra- word variability, the use of phonological templates, and use of whole-word rather than segmental phonological processes (e.g., reduplication, consonant harmony, etc…), suggest that children's phonological representations may not contain the same degree of segmental information as those of adults.

REFERENCES

Bernhardt, B., Stemberger, J. (1990). *Handbook of phonological development: From the perspective of constraint-based non-linear phonology*. San Diego, C. A.: Academic Press.

Charles-Luce, J., Luce, P.A. (1990). Similarity neighborhoods of words in young children's lexicons. *Journal of Child Language*, 17, 205-215.

Eimas, P.D., Siqueland, E.R., Jusczyk, P.W., Bigorito, J. (1971). Speech perception in infants. *Science*, 171, 303-306.

Fenson, L., Dale, P., Reznick, S., Thal, D., Bates, E., Hartung, J., Pethick, S., Reilly, J. (1993). MacArthur communicative development inventories. San Diego, C. A.: San Diego State University.

Ferguson, C.A., Farwell, C.B. (1975). Words and sounds in early language acquisition. *Language*, 51, 419-439.

Fletcher, P., Chan, C.W., Wong, P.T., Stokes, S., Tardif, T., Leung, S.C. (2004). The interface between phonetic and lexical abilities in early Cantonese language development. *Clinical Linguistics and Phonetics*,18, 535-545.

Garlock, V.M., Walley, A.C., Metsala, J.L. (2001). Age-of-acquisition, word frequency, and neighborhood density effects on spoken word recognition by children and adults. *Journal of Memory and Language*, 45, 468-492.

Gros-Louis, J., West, M., Goldstein, M., King, A. (2006). Mothers provide differential feedback to infants' prelinguistic sounds. *International Journal of Behavioral Development*, 30, 509-516.

Ingram, D. (2002). The measurement of whole-word productions. *Journal of Child Language*, 29, 713-733.

Jakielski, K.J., Maytasse, R., Doyle, E. (2006). Acquisition of phonetic complexity in children 12-36 months of age. Poster session presented at the annual convention of the American Speech-Language-Hearing Association, Miami, F. L.

Jakobson, R. (1941/1968). Child language, aphasia and phonological universals (A. R. Keiler, Trans.). The Hague, Netherlands: Mouton.

Leonard, L., Schwartz, R.G., Morris, B., Chapman, K. (1981). Factors influencing early lexical acquisition: Lexical orientation and phonological composition. *Child Development*, 52, 882-887.

Lindblom, B. (1992). Phonological units as adaptive emergents of lexical development. In Ferguson, C.A., Menn, L.,Stoel-Gammon, C. (Eds.), *Phonological development: Models, research, implications* (pp. ??). Timonium, M. D.: York Press.

Locke, J.L. (1985). The role of phonetic factors in parent reference. *Journal of Child Language*, 12, 125-220.

Nittrouer, S., Studdert-Kennedy, M., Mcgowan, R.S. (1989). The emergence of phonetic segments: Evidence from the spectral structure of fricative-vowel syllables spoken by children and adults. *Journal of Speech and Hearing Research*, 32, 120-132.

Paul, R., Jennings, P. (1992). Phonological behavior in toddlers with slow expressive language development. *Journal of Speech, Language and Hearing Research*, 35, 99-107.

Piske, T. (1997). Phonological organization in early speech production: Evidence for the importance of articulatory patterns. *Speech Communication*, 22, 279-295.

Rescorla, L., Ratner, N. (1996). Phonetic profiles of toddlers with Specific Language Impairment. *Journal of Speech and Hearing Research*, 39, 153-169.

Robb, M., Bleile, K. (1994). Consonant inventories of young children from 8 to 25 months. *Clinical Linguistics and Phonetics*, 8, 295-320.

Schwartz, R.G., Leonard, L.B. (1982). Do children pick and choose? An examination of phonological selection and avoidance in early lexical acquisition. *Journal of Child Language*, 9, 319-336.

Smith, B.L., McGregor, K. K., DeMille, D. (2006). Phonological development in lexically-precocious two-year-olds. *Applied Psycholinguistics*, 27, 355-375.

Smith, N.V. (1973). The acquisition of phonology: A case study. Cambridge, M. A.: University Press.

Sosa, A.V., Stoel-Gammon, C. (2012). Lexical and phonological effects in early word production. *Journal of Speech, Language and Hearing Research, 55,* 596-608..

Sosa, A.V., Stoel-Gammon, C. (2006). Patterns of intra-word phonological variability during the second year of life. *Journal of Child Language*, 33, 31-50.

Stoel-Gammon, C. (1985). Phonetic inventories, 15-24 months: A longitudinal study. *Journal of Speech and Hearing Research*, 28, 505-512.

Stoel-Gammon, C. (1998). Sounds and words in early language acquisition. In Paul, R. (Ed.), *Exploring the speech-language connection* (pp. 25-52). Baltimore, M. D.: Paul H. Brookes Publishing Co.

Stoel-Gammon, C. (2010a). Relationships between lexical and phonological development in young children. *Journal of Child Language*, FirstView Articles.

Stoel-Gammon, C. (2010b). The word complexity measure: Description and application to developmental phonology and disorders. *Clinical Linguistics and Phonetics*, 24, 271-282.

Stoel-Gammon, C., Cooper, J. (1984). Patterns of early lexical and phonological development. *Journal of Child Language*, 11, 247-271.

Stoel-Gammon, C., Dale, P. (1988). Aspects of phonological development of linguistically precocious children. Paper presented at Child Phonology Conference, University of Illinois, Chapaign-Urbana.

Stoel-Gammon, C., Peter, B. (2008). Syllables, segments, and sequences: Phonological patterns in the words of young children acquiring American English. In: Davis, B., Zajdó, K. (Eds.) *Syllable development: The Frame/Content Theory and Beyond.* Mahwah, N. J.: Lawrence Erlbaum Associates, Inc.

Vihman, M.M. (1981). Phonology and the development of the lexicon: Evidence from children's errors. *Journal of Child Language*, 8, 239-264.

Vihman, M.M. (1992*). Early syllables and the construction of phonology. In Phonological development: models, research, and implications* (Ferguson, C.A., Menn, L. Stoel-Gammon, C. Eds.). Timonium, M.D.: York Press, pp. 393-422.

Vihman, M.M. (1996). Phonological development: The origins of language in the child. Cambridge, M. A.: Blackwell.

Vihman, M.M., Croft, W. (2007). Phonological development: Toward a radical templatic phonology. *Linguistics*, 45, 683.

Waterson, N. (1971). Child phonology: A prosodic view. *Journal of Linguistics*, 7, 179-211.

In: Comprehensive Perspectives …
Editors: Beate Peter and Andrea A. N. MacLeod
ISBN: 978-1-62257-041-6

Chapter 6

THE TRAJECTORY TOWARDS MASTERY OF THE PHONOLOGICAL SYSTEM: FROM TODDLERS TO SCHOOL-AGED CHILDREN

Andrea A. N. MacLeod

INTRODUCTION

Around age 11 to 12 months, children begin to produce their first words. As children practice producing these words, they receive feedback through their own senses and from people around them. This practice and feedback begins the process of fine-tuning that leads to increasingly adult-like speech-sound production by the onset of puberty. By understanding typical phonological development, a speech-language pathologist (SLP) can identify delayed and disordered phonological development at an early age. In this chapter, my goal is to provide an understanding of the different facets of typical phonological development based on research that has focused on children's productions. To this end, I have provided a summary of research that reports on English monolingual children's phonetic and phonological development from the age of two to thirteen. I focus on the production of English since phonological development in this language has been thoroughly studied across a broad age range. The choice of studies included in this review was guided by two criteria: (1) studies that provide a description of typical phonological production in monolingual English-speaking children between the ages of 2 and 13 years; and (2) studies published in English scientific journals.

A total of 31 studies were analyzed and summarized for this chapter. These studies cover a wide age-range, include longitudinal, cross-sectional, and group study designs, and vary with regards to the type of speech samples and the targeted measures. In Table 6.1, I have summarized key information about each of these studies, including the variety of English studied, the age range studied, the methodological approach, and the type of speech sample used. Throughout the chapter, references to these studies are made in the text using superscript number that corresponds to the reference number of each study listed in Table 6.1.

Table 6.1. Summary of studies of phonological development in English monolingual children aged 2;0 to 13;0

Reference Number	Study	Age	Variety of English	N (typical children)	Approach	Speech Sample	Focus
1	James, D. G. H. (2001).	2;0-7;11	Australia	50	Cross-sectional	Picture naming (199 words)	Error patterns
2	Otomo, K., and Stoel-Gammon, C. (1992).	1;10-2;6	USA	6	Longitudinal	Target words elicited in play	Vowels
3	Kehoe, M., and Stoel-Gammon, C. (1997).	1;10-3;10	USA	18	Cross-sectional	Target words elicited in play	Weak syllable deletion
4	Selby, J. C., Robb, M. P., and Gilbert, H. R. (2000).	1;3-3;0	USA	4	Longitudinal	Spontaneous speech	Vowels
5	Kirk, C., and Demuth, K. (2005).	1;5-2;7	USA	12	Cross-sectional	Target words elicited in play	Cluster
6	Pollock, K. E., and Berni, M. C. (2001).	1;6-2;11, 2;6-6;0	USA	165	Cross-sectional	Picture naming (140 words)	Vowels
7	Preisser, D. A., Hodson, B. W., and Paden, E. P. (1988).	1;6-2;5	USA	60	Cross-sectional	Picture naming (24 words)	Phonological patterns
8	Stoel-Gammon, C. (1987).	2;0	USA	33	Cross-sectional		Consonant acquisition and syllable shapes
9	Wyllie-Smith, L., McLeod, S., and Ball, M. J. (2006).	2;0-2;11	Australia	16	Cross-sectional	Spontaneous speech	Cluster production
10	Dyson, A. T. (1988).	2;0-3;0	USA	20	Cross-sectional	Spontaneous speech	Consonant acquisition
11	Watson, M. M., and Scukanec, G. P. (1997).	2;0-3;0	USA	12	Longitudinal	Spontaneous speech	Consonant acquisition and phonological patterns and accuracy (PCC) and syllable shape
12	Prather, E. M., Hedrick, D. L., and Kern, C. A. (1975).	2;0-4;0	USA	147	Cross-sectional	Picture Naming (44 words)	Consonant acquisition and feature acquisition

Reference Number	Study	Age	Variety of English	N (typical children)	Approach	Speech Sample	Focus
13	Roulstone, S., Loader, S., Northstone, K., and Beveridge, M. (2002).	2;1	UK	1127	1 group	Picture Naming (16 words)	Phonological patterns and intelligibility
14	Stokes, S. F., Klee, T., Carson, C. P., and Carson, D. (2005).	2;1	USA	40	1 group	Spontaneous speech	Feature acquisition
15	Bland-Stewart, L. M. (2003).	2;1-2;11	USA	8	Longitudinal	Spontaneous speech	Consonant acquisition and phonological patterns and syllable shapes
16	Dodd, B., and McIntosh, B. (2010).	2;1-2;11	UK	62	Cross-sectional	Picture Naming (32 words)	Accuracy, typical errors
17	McIntosh, B., and Dodd, B. J. (2008).	2;1-2;11	UK	62	Cross-sectional	Picture Naming (32 words)	Consonant acquisition and phonological patterns and accuracy (PCC, PVC, PPC)
18	Haelsig, P. C., and Madison, C. L. (1986).	2;10-5;2	USA	50	Cross-sectional	Picture Naming (144 words)	Phonological processes
19	Schwarz, I. C., Burnham, D., and Bowey, J. A. (2006).	2;6-3;0	New Zealand	60	Longitudinal	Picture Naming (22 words)	Initial C accuracy
20	Roberts, J. E., Burchinal, M., and Footo, M. M. (1990).	2;6-8;0	USA	145	Cross-sectional	Picture naming (41 words)	Phonological patterns
21	Lowe, R. J., Knutson, P. J., and Monson, M. A. (1985).	2;7-4;6	USA	1048	Cross-sectional	Word repetition (9 words)	Fronting
22	Shriberg, L. D. (1993).	3;0-5;11	USA	117	Cross-sectional	Spontaneous speech	Accuracy (PCC)
23	Arlt, P. B., and Goodban, M. T. (1976	3;0-6;0	USA	240	Cross-sectional	Picture naming (48 words)	Consonant acquisition
24	Dodd, B., Holm, A., Hua, Z., and Crosbie, S. (2003).	3;0-6;11	UK	684	Cross-sectional	Picture naming (80 words)	Consonant acquisition and phonological patterns and accuracy (PCC, PVC, PPC)

Table 6.1. (Continued)

Reference Number	Study	Age	Variety of English	N (typical children)	Approach	Speech Sample	Focus
25	James, D. G., van Doorn, J., McLeod, S., and Esterman, A. (2008).	3;0-7;11	Australia	283	Cross-sectional	Picture naming (199 words)	Consonant deletion
26	Smit, A. B., Hand, L., Freilinger, J. J., Bernthal, J. E., and Bird, A. (1990).	3;0-9;0	USA	979	Cross-sectional	Picture naming (80 words)	Consonant acquisition
27	Flipsen, P. (2006).	3;1-8;1	USA	320	Cross-sectional	Spontaneous speech	Intelligibility
28	Robb, M. P., and Gillon, G. T. (2007).	3;2	USA and New Zealand	20	Cross-sectional	Spontaneous speech	Rate
29	Wells, B., Peppe, S., and Goulandris, N. (2004).	5;6-13;9	UK	120	Cross-sectional	Standard task	Intonation
30	MacLeod, A.A.N., Laukys, K., Rvachew, S. (2011).	1;6 and 3;0	Canada	19	Cross-sectional	Spontaneous speech	Consonant accuracy
31	Dyson, A. T., and Paden, E. P. (1983).	1;11-2;11	USA	40	Longitudinal	Picture and object naming (36 words)	Error patterns

The 31 studies analyzed in this chapter were published over a 35-year time span from 1975 to 2010. The majority of studies describe phonological development during the preschool years. Although only data from English speaking children were included in the search, these children were living in a variety of English-speaking countries: Australia, Canada, New Zealand, and the United States of America. The studies that targeted children under the age of 3 years tended to focus on longitudinal descriptions of a small number of children; in contrast, studies that targeted older children tended to focus on cross-sectional descriptions of large groups of children. Similarly, longitudinal studies tended to sample spontaneous speech, whereas cross-sectional studies tended to use picture naming to obtain a speech sample. Finally, these studies covered a broad range of sub-areas of phonology.

In order to summarize the results across these studies, I will focus on three facets of phonological development: accuracy, inventory, and error patterns. The measures used to study these three facets are described in detail in Chapters 2 and 20 and thus only a brief summary is provided here.

Accuracy. Accuracy of speech production can be measured using a variety of measures. Some measures focus on phoneme accuracy by calculating the number of phonemes correctly produced and dividing by the total number of consonants, vowels, or phonemes produced (e.g., *Percent Consonants Correct* (PCC), *Percent Vowels Correct* (PVC), and *Percent Phonemes Correct* (PPC)).

Other measures take into account accuracy and distortion by calculating the percentage of consonants produced accurately and the percentage of consonants in error due to a distortion (e.g., Articulation Competency Index (ACI), Shriberg, 1993). In contrast to PCC, ACI is sensitive to consonant errors due to distortions in older age groups where few children or adults make frank consonant errors (Shriberg, 1993). Intelligibility Index (II) reflects the percentage of words judged intelligible by a trained transcriber for a given speech sample (Shriberg, 1993).

Finally, some measures focus on both consonant accuracy and the production of consonants and vowels (e.g., Phonological Mean Length of Utterance (PMLU) and Percent Whole-Word Proximity (PWP), Ingram and Ingram, 2001). In general, measures of accuracy provide a quantitative summary of a child's phonological production but they do not provide qualitative information about the type of error patterns, the phonemes in error, or the consistency of the errors; thus, they cannot be used alone to describe the developmental process.

Inventory. Measures of inventory provide a more qualitative description of phonological development by listing the consonants, vowels and syllable structures that children can produce. Inventory measures can be divided into three broad categories: *phonetic inventory, phonological inventory* (also referred to as *phonological or relational* inventory), and *phonotactic inventory*.

A *phonetic inventory* is a list of the consonants and vowels that a child produces, even if they are not the correct phoneme for the target word. Other terms for phonetic inventory are segmental inventory or absolute inventory. Criteria for including a consonant or a vowel in a phonetic inventory vary: for example, a child may need to produce at least two examples of the consonant or vowel in question in the same position (Stoel-Gammon, 1987), or two examples regardless of the context (Dinnsen et al., 1990).

A *phonemic inventory* makes reference to consonants and vowels that are used by the child to contrast words in an adult-like manner. In other words, a phonemic inventory is a list of the consonants and vowels that a child correctly produces in the correct position in the word. Criteria for including a consonant or a vowel in a phonemic inventory also vary. In cross-sectional group studies, a baseline for creating a phonemic inventory is often set at one of two levels: a phoneme is included if 75% and 90% of the group correctly produces the target phoneme (Prather Hedrick and Kern, 1975; Smit et al., 1990). Some studies consider all places of articulation together, while others describe accuracy by place of articulation. As with segmental inventories, it is possible to provide an inventory of consonant clusters produced and of clusters that are produced accurately.

A *phonotactic inventory* provides an overview of the syllable and word shapes produced by children. It may include syllable and word shapes that are produced accurately or ones that are produced but that do not match the adult target.

In the reviewed studies, descriptions of phonetic, phonemic and phonotactic inventories provided a qualitative and quantitative picture of what children are able to produce. For each age group, the phonetic, phonemic, and phonotactic inventories are provided. In cases where studies differed with regards to the age of acquisition a phoneme, the earliest age that the phoneme was reported in the phonetic or phonemic inventory is provided.

Error patterns. Although errors have been reported phoneme by phoneme (e.g., Smit, 1993), most studies report on patterns of errors. At its simplest, an *error pattern* describes a group of errors based on similar elements at the segmental, syllable, and word level. Error patterns may also be called "*phonological patterns*" or "*phonological processes.*" These terms can have a more theoretical orientation, as is the case for phonological processes within the framework of Natural Phonology (see Ingram, 1974; Grunwell 1981); but more recent research has tended towards a more neutral use of error patterns as a descriptive tool (e.g., James, 2001). Due to differences in theoretical orientation, the description of error patterns varies across studies. To simplify the comparison across studies in this chapter, the patterns have been grouped into three broad categories based on those proposed by Stoel-Gammon and Dunn (1985). Definitions and examples of error patterns are provided in in Chapter 2 and a summary is shown in Appendix 2.

Assimilation patterns describe error patterns that lead to changes in place, manner or voicing in the context of from the influence of a neighboring phoneme. This group of patterns includes labial, velar, or nasal assimilation; reduplication; prevocalic voicing; or final devoicing.

Substitution patterns describe error patterns that lead to changes in place, manner, or voicing of the target consonants. This group of patterns includes gliding, vowelization, stopping, depalatization, and velar fronting.

Syllable structure patterns describe changes to the syllable structure of the target word. This group of patterns includes syllable deletion, cluster reduction, consonant deletion, and epenthesis.

Within these three categories, I have grouped together error subtypes; for example, palatal fronting, alveolar fronting, and velar fronting have been grouped under the term "fronting." Once these subtypes of errors were formed, I used the data reported in each study to calculate a mean frequency of occurrence of the error pattern and the mean percent of children producing the error pattern across the studies. I have only listed error patterns when the percentages were above 5% for frequency of occurrence, or for percent of children using the pattern. These means are provided in the tables for each age range.

Phonological Development from the Age of Two to Nine Years

A common structure is used to summarize the results for each age group: Each section begins with a table that provides a summary of results for accuracy, inventory and error patterns. Next, a more detailed description of each of these facets is provided. Sidebars are used to summarize data that is relevant but only reported for one or two age groups. Children's ages are listed as years and months, separated by a semicolon, so that 2;11 refers to 2 years, 11 months.

Phonological Development at Two Years of Age

Two-year-olds were included in 22 of the studies reviewed for this chapter including those using longitudinal and cross sectional approaches [1-22, 31]. Three facets of the early development of the phonological system are reported here and are summarized in Table 6.2. Video file 6S1 contains an example of a 2;6 year old child producing words in a picture naming task (in this case the Goldman-Fristoe Test of Articulation-2).

Table 6.2. Summary of phonological development from 2;0 to 2;11 years of age

Facet	Measure	Result
Accuracy	Mean PCC (range across studies)	70% (52-76%)
	Mean PVC (range across studies)	91% (88-95%)
	Mean PPC	76%
Inventory	Phonemic Inventory (75% of children @ 2;0)	/m, n, ŋ, p, h/
	Phonemic Inventory (75% of children @ 2;11)	/m, n, ŋ, p, b, t, d, k, f, h, w, j/
	Phonotactic Inventory	CVC and CV together make up more than 60% of words
Error Patterns	Assimilation (greater than 5% frequency of occurrence)	Voicing Errors
	Substitution (greater than 5% frequency of occurrence)	Liquid deviations, stopping, deaffrication, fronting, gliding, velar deviation, depalatization, nasal and glide errors, vocalization, and vowel errors.
	Syllable Structure (greater than 5% frequency of occurrence)	Consonant cluster reduction, consonant deletion, and weak syllable deletion.

Access Video File 1 (Chapter 6)

6V1 Word productions of a girl, age 2;6.

Accuracy

Accuracy was studied using measures of percent consonants correct (PCC), percent vowels correct (PVC), and percent phonemes correct (PPC). Across the 5 studies that report on PCC among 2-year old children [8, 11, 16, 17, 19], the mean PCC reported was 70% with a range from a low of 52% to a high of 76%. In contrast, PVC was also reported in four studies [6, 11, 16, 17] in this age group and was considerably higher with a mean of 91 across these studies and a range of 88% to 95%. Overall PPC for this age group was only reported by one group of researchers [16, 17] who found that children have an average PPC of 76%. The results are quite consistent across studies, despite differences in the number of children included in each study, the variety of English spoken, and the type of speech sample used for the analysis.

Inventory

Consonants. Seven studies [8, 10, 11, 12, 15, 17] reported on the number and type of consonants produced by two year olds acquiring English. The type of consonants produced was reported in different ways across these studies. Only Prather et al. (1975) provided a phonemic inventory based on the consonants produced correctly by 75% or more of the children. The remaining studies provided a phonetic inventory by reporting consonants produced, accurately or otherwise, by 50% to 90% of children in the targeted age range. Phonetic and phonemic inventories were summarized in Table 6.3 below for children aged 2;0 and 2;11.

Children at 2;0 years of age produced an average of 12 consonants in initial position, 8 in final position, and only 5 of these consonants accurately (i.e., /m, n, ŋ, p, h/). By the end of their 2nd year, children produced 17 consonants in initial position, 13 in final position, and 12 consonants accurately. Children first began to produce glides and liquids in word initial position, but fricatives and affricates in word final position. Only two consonants are not attested to across these studies: /θ, tʃ/. Overall, children acquired a large number of consonants and made gains in accuracy of consonant production during their second year.

Consonant Clusters. Three studies [5, 10, 11] reported on consonant cluster inventories among children aged 2;0-2;11, but a greater number of studies reported on cluster reduction within an analysis of error patterns produced by children. The majority of children produced at least one instance of the following the clusters in word initial position: [pw, bw, kw, fw, tr, sp, st, sn, sl]; and in the following clusters in word final position: [nd, ts, ps, ntʃ, ŋk]. These results indicate that two-year-olds are producing a variety of consonant clusters; although they may not produce many consonant clusters accurately.

Vowels. Vowel inventories among two year olds were reported in two studies [2, 4]. Children produced a broad variety of vowels at this age: 75% of children produced /a, i, ɪ, ɛ, e, u, o, ʌ, ɔ [4]. Certain vowels, however, were produced more accurately than others at this age, for example /i, ɑ, e, æ/ had greater than 70% accuracy [2].

Phonotactic Inventory. At two years of age, children produced a variety of syllable shapes although monosyllabic words predominated, accounting for 80-85% of words [10,12]. For example at 2;0, more than 95% of children produced at least two words with the following shapes: CV and CVC; but less than 80% of children produce two words that were disyllabic (i.e., CVCV, or CVCVC) [8]. The occurrence of different syllable shapes did not change greatly between the ages of 2;0 and 2;11 [10]. Children produced CVC syllables (24-40% of word) and CV syllables (20% to 36%) most frequently, followed by VC syllables (8%), and finally V syllables (5%) [10, 12].

Table 6.3. Consonant inventory at 2;0-2;11 years of age

Age	Phonemic Inventory	/m/	/n/	/ŋ/	/p/	/b/	/t/	/d/	/k/	/ɑ/	/f/	/v/	/θ/	/ð/	/s/	/z/	/ʃ/	/ʒ/	/h/	/tʃ/	/d ʒ /	/ɹ/	/l/	/w/	/j/
2;0-2;6	Phonetic (word initial)	x	x		x	x	x	x	x	x	x	X			x				x					x	
	Phonetic (word final)	x	x		x		x		x						x	x			x						
	Phonemic (75% accuracy)	x	x	x	x														x						
2;6-2;11	Phonetic (word initial)	x	x		x	x	x	x	x	x	x				x				x			x	x	x	x
	Phonetic (word final)	x	x	x	x	x	x	x	x	x	x				x	x	x			x					
	Phonemic (75% accuracy)	x	x	x	x	x	x	x	x		x								x					x	x

Error Patterns

The production of phonological patterns were reported for two-year-olds in 11 studies [1, 7, 8, 9, 11, 13, 15, 17, 20, 21, 31]. As was noted above, error patterns were grouped into three broad categories to simplify the comparison across studies: assimilation patterns, substitution patterns and syllable structure patterns. An average frequency of occurrence of error patterns and percent of children producing each error pattern were calculated across the studies and are summarized in Table 6.4. Patterns that had a mean frequency of occurrence greater than 5% or that occur among more than 5% of children are reported here.

Table 6.4. Error patterns observed for children aged 2;0-2;11, reported by percentage frequency of occurrence across the group, and percent of children producing the pattern (n/a notes unavailable data)

Category of Error Pattern	Error Pattern Type	Percent Frequency of Occurrence	Percent of Children
Assimilation	Voicing error [17]	12	7
Substitution	Deaffrication [20]	20	27
	Depalatization [1]	11	43
	Fronting [1, 15, 17, 20, 21, 29, 31]	20	14
	Gliding [1, 15, 17, 20, 31]	43	60
	Liquid deviation [7, 11, 13]	48	n/a
	Nasal-Glide errors [7]	11	n/a
	Other [17]	21	20
	Stopping [1, 11, 13, 15, 17, 20, 31]	28	32
	Velar deviation [7,13]	22	n/a
	Vowelization [1,11,15]	13	21
	Vowel errors [1]	7	86
Syllable Structure	Cluster reduction [15, 31]	52	n/a
	Consonant deletion [11,15, 17, 31]	14	13
	Weak syllable deletion[17]	12	11

Assimilation Patterns. This group of error patterns included labial, alveolar, velar, or nasal assimilation; reduplication; prevocalic voicing; or final devoicing. The only pattern with a percent of occurrence that exceeded 5% was voicing errors with a frequency of occurrence of 12% and observed among 7% of children [17].

Substitution Patterns. This group of error patterns included gliding, vowelization, stopping, depalatization, velar fronting, and deaffrication. In addition, a subset of studies reported on the consonant class in error (e.g., liquid deviations, velar deviations). As can be seen in Table 3, children produced a broad range of error patterns both with regards to frequency of occurrence and number of children who produced each pattern. Two patterns had a frequency of occurrence greater than 40%: gliding and liquid deviations. Five patterns had a frequency of occurrence between 20% and 40%: deaffrication, fronting, stopping, velar deviation, and "other" patterns. In addition, three patterns had a frequency of occurrence between 5% and 20%: depalatization, nasal and glide errors, vowelization, and vowel errors.

Syllable Structure Patterns. Phonological patterns that change syllable structures were frequently observed among two-year-olds. At this age, consonant cluster reduction was the most common syllable structure pattern at 52%, followed by consonant deletion at 14% and weak syllable deletion at 12%.

Summary

Children at two years of age are rapidly building their phonological system by adding a number of consonants and vowels to their phonetic and phonemic inventories. Children tend to produce simple word-shapes and produce a number of error patterns.

Phonological Development at Three Years of Age

Fourteen studies reported on the phonological development of 6 three-year-olds, [11, 12, 18, 19, 20, 21, 22, 23, 24, 25, 26, 27, 30]. Most of these studies used a cross-sectional approach to describe phonological acquisition. A strength of this approach is that larger groups of children have been studied; however, unlike for two-year-olds, we have less information about an individual child's path of phonological development. A review of these studies will be presented measure-by-measure beginning with measures of accuracy, followed by inventory, and ending with descriptions of error patterns. Table 6.5 provides a summary of these measures. Video file 6S2 contains an example of a 3;1 year old child producing words in a picture naming task (in this case the Goldman-Fristoe Test of Articulation-2).

Table 6.5. Summary of phonological development from 3;0 to 3;11 years of age

Facet	Measure	Result
Accuracy	Mean PCC (range across studies)	73% (45 to 92)
	Mean PVC	97%
	Mean PPC	88%
Inventory	Phonemic Inventory (75% of children @ 3;6)	/m, n, ŋ, p, b, t, d, k, ɡ, f, v, s, ʃ, tʃ,ɹ, l, h, w, j/
	Phonemic Inventory (90% of children @ 3;0-3;11)	/m, n, ŋ, p, b, t, d, k, ɡ, f, v, s, z, h, w, j//
	Phonotactic Inventory	Monosyllabic words consist of 85% of words
Error Patterns	Assimilation (greater than 5% frequency of occurrence)	Alveolar and labial assimilation
	Substitution (greater than 5% frequency of occurrence)	Gliding, vowelization, stopping, deaffrication, fronting
	Syllable Structure (greater than 5% frequency of occurrence)	Weak syllable deletion, cluster reduction, consonant deletion

Access Video File 2 (Chapter 6)

6V2 Word productions of a girl age 3;1

Accuracy

Seven studies report on accuracy among three-year-olds [6, 11, 19, 22, 24, 27, 30]. The mean PCC increased to a mean of 73%, but with a broad range of 45% to 92% [11, 19, 24, 30]. The lowest PCC score was based on spontaneous speech of children aged 3;0 years. Vowel accuracy is considerably higher at 97% [6, 24]. The overall PPC also increased by the age of three years to 87.5% [24].

The Articulatory Competence Index (ACI) measures both PCC and the relative distortion of consonants is somewhat lower, ranging from 70% to 75% at this age [22]. The intelligibility index (II) measured by trained transcribers is 95.7% [27]. Measures of pMLU and PWP are higher, 4.7 and 83% respectively [30], representing an increase in the complexity and accuracy of targets that children are producing. Taken together, these measures indicate that three-year-olds have made important gains in their ability to accurately produce phonemes.

Inventory

Consonants. Five studies [11, 12, 23, 24, 26] have reported on the number and type of consonants produced by three-year-olds acquiring English. Four of these provide phonemic inventories, and one study [11] provides a phonetic inventory of the consonants produced, accurately or otherwise, by 60% children. By 3;11, 19 consonants are accurately produced by at least 75% of children.

The consonants produced accurately by 75% and 90% of children are listed in Table 6.6. Smit et al [26] reported on consonant accuracy by girls and boys separately. Girls tend to be more accurate overall, although boys acquired some consonants earlier than girls. For example, /n/ is produced accurately by 90% of boys at 3;0 but not until 3;6 by girls. Across the studies only three consonants were absent from the majority of children's inventories: /θ, ʒ, dʒ/.

Consonant Clusters. The production of clusters among 3-year-olds has been studied in a single study [11]. The type of consonant clusters produced twice by at least 60% of children was reported. In word initial position, these clusters include many labial stops or alveolars: /pw, bw, pl, st, sp/; in word final position, they produce these clusters mostly with alveolar stops: /nd, ts, nt, nz, st/.

These differences are likely explained by differences in phontactics of English: certain clusters predominate word initial position, while others are more common in word final.

Vowels. Vowels produced by 75% of children consisted of the following 12 vowels: /i, ɪ, e, ɛ, æ, a, u, ʊ, o, ɔ, ʌ, ɝ/ [4]. The majority of three-year-olds are producing monophthong vowels accurately.

Table 6.6. Consonant inventory at 3;0-3;11 years of age

Age	Phonemic Inventory	/m/	/n/	/ŋ/	/p/	/b/	/t/	/d/	/k/	/g/	/f/	/v/	/θ/	/ð/	/s/	/z/	/ʃ/	/ʒ/	/h/	/tʃ/	/dʒ/	/ɹ/	/l/	/w/	/j/
3;0	75% accuracy	x	x	x	x	x	x	x	x	x	x				x				x					x	x
3;6	75% accuracy	x	x	x	x	x	x	x	x	x	x	x			x		x		x	x		x	x	x	x
3;0-3;11	90% accuracy	x	x	x	x	x	x	x	x	x	x	x			x	x			x					x	x

Phonotactic Inventory. Approximately 85% of words produced by children are monosyllabic; Within monosyllabic words, children produce mostly of CVC words (53%), then CV words (26%), and the remaining words are V or VC [10].

Error Patterns

Error patterns were reported for three-year-old children in seven studies [1,11, 18, 20, 21, 24, 25]. As was done for the two-year-olds, the phonological patterns will be grouped to facilitate summarizing data across these studies. Patterns that have a mean frequency of occurrence greater than 5% and occur among more than 5% of children are reported here and summarized in Table 6.7.

Assimilation Patterns. This group of error patterns included labial, velar, or nasal assimilation; reduplication; prevocalic voicing; or final devoicing. Alveolar and labial assimilation were reported across these studies at a frequency of occurrence of 25% and 22% respectively [18].

Substitution Patterns. This group of error patterns includes gliding, vowelization, stopping, depalatization, velar fronting, and deaffrication. As can be seen in Table 7, children produced a range of these error patterns. Gliding had a frequency of occurrence at 34% and was the only substitution pattern that exceeded a frequency of occurrence of 20%. Four patterns had a frequency of occurrence that ranged from 5% to 20%: deaffrication, fronting, stopping, and vowelization. Higher rates of vowelization were reported for children acquiring Australian English[1], but since this was a feature of the speech of adult speakers of Australian English [1] it should not be considered clinically significant within this variety of English.

Syllable Structure Patterns. Children also produced phonological patterns that impact the syllable structure of words. Cluster reduction and weak syllable deletions both occurred at rates greater than 20%, and final consonant deletion occurred at a rate of 13%. Word length was affected by consonant deletion such that 42% of children deleted consonants in monosyllabic words, but 95% deleted consonants in disyllabic words [25]. Lower rates of consonant cluster reduction were observed as children approached their fourth birthday.

Table 6.7. Error patterns observed for children aged 3;0-3;11 reported by frequency of occurrence and percent of children producing the pattern (n/a notes unavailable data)

Category of Error Pattern	Error Pattern Type	Percent Frequency of Occurrence	Percent of Children
Assimilation	Assimilation: Alveolar [18]	25	n/a
	Assimilation: Labial [18]	22	n/a
Substitution	Deaffrication [20]	10	13
	Depalatization[1]	4	40
	Fronting [1, 18, 20, 21, 24]	13	12
	Gliding [1]	34	38
	Stopping [1, 11, 18, 20, 24]	11	25
	Vowelization [1,18]	18	34
	Vowel errors[1]	4	80
Syllable Structure	Cluster reduction [1, 11, 18, 20, 24, 25, 29]	27	78
	Consonant deletion [1, 18, 25,]	13	78
	Weak syllable deletion [18, 24]	31	24

Summary

By the end of their third year, children have expanded their phonetic inventory to 19 of 24 consonants, and their phonemic inventory includes 16 consonants for 90% of children. This increase in consonant inventory is reflected in an increase of PCC scores (i.e., above 85%). Consonant clusters are still somewhat problematic in both initial and final word position as indicated by the high rates of cluster reduction and the limited consonant cluster inventory reported. Among the most common error patterns, assimilation, gliding, and cluster reduction all exceed 20% frequency of occurrence.

Phonological Development at Four Years of Age

The ten studies describing phonological acquisition in four-year-old children were designed using a cross-sectional approach [6, 11, 18, 20, 21, 22, 23, 24, 26, 27]. A summary of the results is provided in Table 6.8. These studies are reviewed measure by measure beginning with accuracy and inventory, followed by descriptions of error patterns. Video file 6V3 contains an example of a 4;0 year old child producing words in a picture naming task (in this case the Goldman-Fristoe Test of Articulation-2).

Table 6.8. Summary of phonological development from 4;0 to 4;11 years of age

Facet	Measure	Result
Accuracy	Mean PCC	90%
	Mean PVC	99%
	Mean PPC	93%
Inventory	Phonemic Inventory (75% of children @ 4;0-4;11)	/m, n, ŋ, p, b, t, d, k, g, f, v, s, z, ʃ, ʒ, h, tʃ, dʒ, l, w/
	Phonemic Inventory (90% of children @ 4;0-4;11)	/m, n, ŋ, p, b, t, d, k, g, f, v, s, z, h, tʃ, dʒ, w, j/
	Phonotactic Inventory	Consonant deletion, cluster reduction, weak syllable deletion
Error Patterns	Assimilation (greater than 5% frequency of occurrence)	Labial assimilation
	Substitution (greater than 5% frequency of occurrence)	Vowelization, gliding, stopping, deaffrication, depalatization, fronting
	Syllable Structure (greater than 5% frequency of occurrence)	Weak syllable deletion, cluster reduction, consonant deletion

Access Video File 3 (Chapter 6)

6V3 Word productions of a boy age 4;0

Accuracy

Accuracy of phoneme production among four-year-olds was reported in five studies, [11, 27, 22, 24]. At this age, children had a PCC of 90% [24], a PVC of 99% [6, 11, 24], and a PPC of 93% [24]. The ACI was approximately 77% at 4;0-4;5 and rose to 80% at 4;6-4;11 [22]. The II was 97% [27] at this age.

Table 6.9. Consonant inventory at 4;0-4;11 years of age

Age	Phonemic Inventory	/m/	/n/	/ŋ/	/p/	/b/	/t/	/d/	/k/	/g/	/f/	/v/	/θ/	/ð/	/s/	/z/	/ʃ/	/ʒ/	/h/	/tʃ/	/dʒ/	/ɹ/	/l/	/w/	/j/
4;0-4;11	75% accuracy	x	x	x	x	x	x	x	x	x	x	x			x	x	x	x	x	x	x		x	x	x
4;0-4;11	90% accuracy	x	x	x	x	x	x	x	x	x	x	x			x	x			x	x	x			x	x

Inventory

Consonants. Three studies reported on the number and type of consonants produced among four-year-olds [23, 24, 26]. By 4;11, at least 75% of children produced 22 consonants accurately. The consonants produced accurately by 75% and 90% of children are listed in Table 6.9. Across these studies only two consonants were absent from the majority of children's inventories: /ɹ, θ/.

Consonant Clusters. Only two clusters, /tw, kw/, were accurately produced by 90% or more of children in this age range [26].

Error Patterns

Six studies reported on the phonological patterns produced by four-year-old children [1, 18, 20, 21, 24, 25]. The phonological patterns were grouped to facilitate summarizing data across these studies. Patterns had a mean frequency of occurrence greater than 5% and occur among more than 5% of children are reported here and summarized in Table 6.10.

Assimilation Patterns. This group of error patterns includes labial, velar, or nasal assimilation; reduplication; prevocalic voicing; or final devoicing. Only labial assimilation occurred at a frequency of occurrence that exceeded 5% with a rate of 14% [18].

Substitution Patterns. Four-year-old children used fewer substitution patterns in their productions, compared to younger children. Substitution patterns no longer exceeded 20%. Six patterns occurred at rates of 5% to 20%: gliding at 20%, vowelization at 18%, stopping at 10%, deaffrication at 8%, and depalatization and fronting at 5%. More than 5% of children produced the following patterns: deaffrication, depalatization, fronting, stopping, and vowelization.

Syllable Structure Patterns. Four-year-old children continued to produce error patterns that affect the structure of the word. They produced weak syllable deletion at a rate of 28%, cluster reduction at 11%, and consonant deletion at 10%. Children produced consonant deletion at lower rates in monosyllabic words (20%) than in di- or poly-syllabic words (89-96%) [25]. Although the frequency of occurrence was low for cluster reduction and consonant deletion, a high percentage of children produced these error patterns (61% and 76% respectively).

Table 6.10. Error patterns observed for children aged 4;0-4;11 reported by frequency of occurrence and percent of children producing the pattern (n/a notes unavailable data)

Category of Error Pattern	Error Pattern Type	Percent Frequency of Occurrence	Percent of Children
Assimilation	Assimilation: Labial[18]	14	n/a
Substitution	Deaffrication[20]	8	9
	Depalatization[1]	5	23
	Fronting[1, 20, 21, 24]	5	9
	Gliding[1, 18, 20, 24]	20	57
	Stopping[1, 20, 24]	10	19
	Vowelization[1, 18]	18	26
	Vowel errors[1]	4	100
Syllable Structure	Cluster reduction[18, 20, 24, 25]	10	61
	Consonant deletion[18, 25]	7	76
	Weak syllable deletion[18, 24]	16	5

Summary

By the age of 4 years, the phonemic inventory for 75% of children includes 22 of 24 consonants, and for 90% of children, it includes 18 to 24 of consonants. This increase in phonemic inventory is reflected in a PCC score of 90%. No error patterns exceed 20% frequency of occurrence, although many patterns still occur at rates greater than 5%.

Phonological Development from Five to Nine Years of Age

As in the studies of younger children, the six studies that report on five-year-olds were designed with a cross-sectional approach to describe the process of phonological acquisition1, [18, 23, 24, 25, 26]. Between the ages of 6 and 14 years of age, phonological development has been reported in 6 studies [20, 24, 25, 26, 27, 29]. The text will summarize the results tied to accuracy, inventory and error patterns and Table 6.11 provides an overview of these measures. Sound file 6S1 contains an example of a 6;1 year old child producing words in a picture naming task (in this case the Goldman-Fristoe Test of Articulation-2).

Table 6.11. Summary of phonological development from 5;0 to 9;11 years of age

	Measure	Result
Accuracy	Mean PCC at 5;0-7;0 (not reported above this age)	96% and greater
	Mean PVC at 5;0-7;0 (not reported above this age)	99%
	Mean PPC at 5;0-7;0 (not reported above this age)	97%
Inventory	Phonemic Inventory (75% of children @ 5;0-5;11)	/m, n, ŋ, p, b, t, d, k, ɡ, f, v, θ, ð, s, z, ʃ, ʒ, h, tʃ, dʒ, ɹ, l, w, j/
	Phonemic Inventory (90% of children @ 5;0-5;11; underlined attested to in 1 study but not the other)	/m, n, ŋ, p, b, t, d, k, ɡ, f, v, θ, ð, s, z, ʃ, ʒ, h, tʃ, dʒ, ɹ, l, w, j/
	Phonemic Inventory (90% of children @ 6;0-9;0)	/m, n, ŋ, p, b, t, d, k, ɡ, f, v, θ, ð, s, z, ʃ, ʒ, h, tʃ, dʒ, ɹ, l, w, j/
Error Patterns	Assimilation (greater than 5% frequency of occurrence)	*None*
	Substitution (greater than 5% frequency of occurrence)	Gliding at 5;0-5;11
	Syllable Structure (greater than 5% frequency of occurrence)	Cluster reduction from 5;0-6;11; weak syllable reduction at 5;0-5;11

Access Sound File 1 (Chapter 6)

6S1 Word productions of a girl, age 6;1

Accuracy

The accuracy of phoneme production among five-year-olds was reported in 3 studies [22, 24, 27]. Children had a PCC of 96% [24], a PVC of 99% [24], a PPC of 97% [24]. The ACI increased to 85% [27] and the II achieved was 98% [22]. By the ages of 7 and 8 years of age, II has reached a 99% [22].

Table 6.12. Consonant inventory at 5;0-9;0 years of age (phonemes marked with an asterisk (*) are attested in one of the two studies that cover this age range)

Age	Phonemic Inventory	/m/	/n/	/ŋ/	/p/	/b/	/t/	/d/	/k/	/g/	/f/	/v/	/θ/	/ð/	/s/	/z/	/ʃ/	/ʒ/	/h/	/tʃ/	/dʒ/	/ɹ/	/l/	/w/	/j/
5;0-5;11	75% accuracy	x	x	x	x	x	x	x	x	x	x	x	x	x	x	x	x	x	x	x	x	x	x	x	x
5;0-5;11	90% accuracy	x	x	*	x	x	x	x	x	x	x	x	x	x	*	*	*	*	x	*	x	*	x	x	x
6;0-9;0	90% accuracy	x	x	x	x	x	x	x	x	x	x	x	x	x	x	x	x	x	x	x	x	x	x	x	x

Inventory

Consonants. Three studies reported on the number and type of consonants produced among five-year-olds [23, 24, 26]. By 5;11 at least 75% of children accurately produced all of the consonants of English. According to Dodd et al.[24], 90% of children accurately produce all the consonants of English; however, according to Smit et al. [26], a number of consonants were not acquired by 90% of children. These consonants include /θ, s, z, ʃ, ʒ, tʃ, l/, and 90% of boys had not yet acquired the following additional consonants /f, v, θ, dʒ/. By the age of 6 to 9 years, 90% of children accurately produced all the consonants of English. These differences across studies are noted in Table 6.12.

Consonant Clusters. At five years of age, children produce a variety of consonant clusters and 90% of children accurately produce the following consonants: /pl, bl, kl, ɡl, fl/ [26].Between the ages of 6 to 9 years, 90% of children accurately produce the following consonant clusters: /sp, st, sk, sm, sn, sw, sl, skw, spl, stɹ, spɹ, skɹ, pɹ, bɹ, tɹ, dɹ, kɹ, ɡɹ, fɹ, θɹ/.

Error Patterns

Five studies have reported on’ phonological patterns produced by children age five to seven years [118, 20, 24, 25]. The phonological patterns will be grouped to facilitate summarizing data across these studies. Patterns that had a mean frequency of occurrence greater than 5% and occur among more than 5% of children are reported here and summarized in Table 6.13.

Assimilation Patterns. No assimilation patterns exceeded 5% frequency of occurrence or were produced by more than 5% of children for this age range.

Table 6.13. Error patterns observed for children aged 5;0-7;11 reported by frequency of occurrence and percent of children producing the pattern (n/a notes unavailable data)

		5;0-5 ;11		6;0-6;11		7;0-7;11	
Category of Error Pattern	Error Pattern Type	Percent Frequency of Occurrence	Percent of Children	Percent Frequency of Occurrence	Percent of Children	Percent Frequency of Occurrence	Percent of Children
Substitution	Fronting[1, 20, 24]	10	n/a	1.2	<1	<1	<1
	Gliding[1, 20, 24]	7	86	4	70	1	25
	Stopping[1, 24]	3	29	0.5	<1		
	Vowel errors[1]	2	86	1	70	2	88
Syllable Structure	Cluster reduction[1, 20, 24, 25]	4	56	7	92	0.4	50
	Consonant deletion[25]	2	70	2	66	2	61
	Weak syllable deletion[1, 18, 24]	7	n/a	n/a	n/a	n/a	n/a

Substitution Patterns. Fronting and gliding were the only substitution patterns that occurred at a rate above 5% within this age range. Three patterns were produced by more than 10% of children: gliding, stopping, and vowel errors, although these patterns had a low frequency of occurrence.

Syllable Structure Patterns. Only weak syllable deletions exceeded 5% frequency of occurrence. Consonant deletions were common in di- and poly-syllabic words (86% and 83% respectively [25]) and were produced by 15% [20] of children. Although the frequency of occurrence had decreased, the majority of children occasionally produced these error patterns.

Summary

Above the age of five years, children were fine-tuning their phonological system. By 5;11, 90% of children are producing between 19 and 24 consonants of English correctly. By 6 to 9 years, the final 5 consonants are accurately produced by 90% of children. The range of accurately produced consonant clusters become more diverse between the ages of 5 and 9 years. Error patterns have greatly decreased. Finally, children are also engaged in the fine-tuning of their prosodic system and this continues to the age of 13 years.

Overview of Phonological Development: One Facet at a Time

In addition to understanding what children can do at a given age, an overview of developmental trajectories with respect to accuracy, inventory, and error patterns provides important information towards a comprehensive perspective of development. To this end, a diachronic view of each of these three facets is presented here.

Accuracy

Measures of accuracy, specifically PCC, PVC, and PPC, were reported for children ranging from 2;0 to 7;0 years of age.

Figure 6.1 illustrates how these measures develop across this age range. The mean PVC scores across these studies showed that vowels are produced quite accurately from a young age. A majority of children, however, produced a few instances of vowel errors across the age range summarized above, as described in the Error Pattern section (e.g., Table 6.13 for vowel errors among 5;0 to 7;0 year olds). In contrast, the mean PCC began much lower at 70% and rose steadily through to the age of five years, followed by continued fine-tuning until the age of seven years. This increase in accuracy of consonant production was mirrored in the growing size of the phonemic inventory and the decrease in error patterns. PPC developed in parallel with these measures since it accounts for both consonant and vowel accuracy. Overall, even 2-year-old children were quite accurate in their vowel and consonant production and this accuracy continued to increase until the age of seven. Although children were variable in accuracy, the standard deviation reported across studies does rarely exceeded 15%. Thus, the majority of children, even during their second year, had accuracy rates for PCC that exceeded 65%.

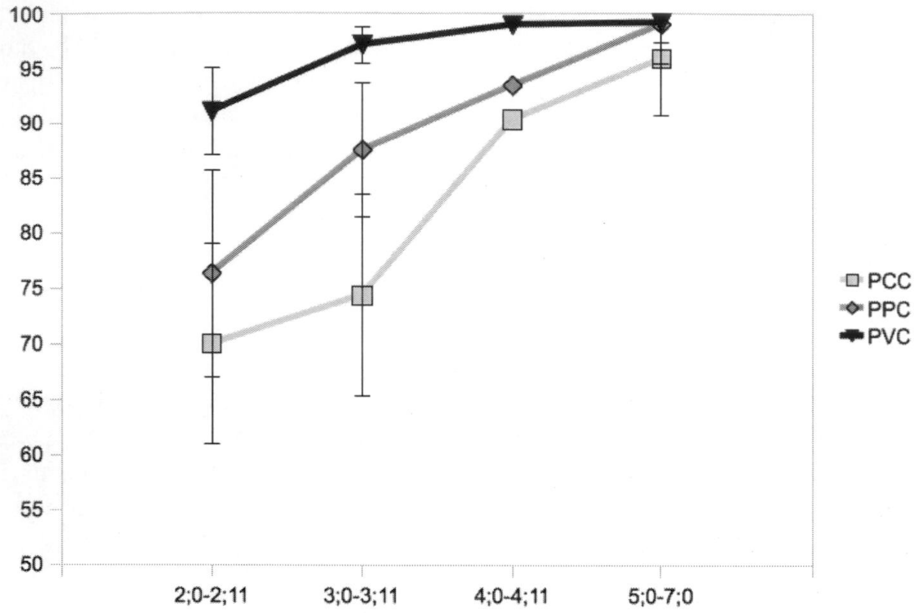

Figure 6.1. Measures of accuracy (PCC, PVC and PPC) across the targeted age range: means are represented by the points, and error bars represent +/- 1 standard deviation averaged across studies.

Inventory

As noted in the introduction, phonetic and phonemic inventories provide a more qualitative picture of children's phonological development.

Children build their phonemic inventory between the ages of two and six years. Table 6.14 summarizes phonetic and phonemic inventory for children aged 2 to 9 years of age. The majority of children produced a variety of consonants at a young age, but had difficulty using the correct consonant in the correct context. At two years of age, their phonetic inventory consisted of 18 of the 24 consonants of English, but only a subset of these consonants were present in their phonemic inventory. The majority of children had a large phonemic inventory for vowels, but only five types of consonants were accurately produced. By the end of their second year, 75% children added seven more consonants to their phonemic inventory. By the end of their third year, 90% children were producing these 13 consonants and an additional two consonants accurately. All but rhotic vowels were produced accurately by 75% of children by this age. By the age of five years, 90% of children were producing all but three consonants accurately according to one study [26], or all consonants accurately according to another study[12]. The last consonants to be added were /ʃ, ʒ, ɹ/, which were produced accurately by 90% of children between the ages of 6 and 9 years [26]. This summary of the development of phonemic inventory does not explore differences in order of acquisition reported for place of the consonant in the word, such as word initial, medial or final; or differences between boys and girls in the acquisition of consonants. The summary, however, provides a reference tool that should spur further investigation by the SLP when consonants and vowels are absent in the child's phonetic or phonemic inventory during an assessment.

Table 6.14. Phonetic and phonemic inventory for children across the targeted age range; blank cells denote accuracy below 75%; n/a notes unavailable data

	Phonetic Inventory	*Phonemic Inventory*					
Age	*2;0-2;11*	2;0-2;6	2;6-2;11	3;0-3;11	4;0-4;11	5;0-5;11	6;0-9;0
/m/	✓	75	75	90	90	90	90
/n/	✓	75	75	90	90	90	90
/ŋ/		75	75	90	90	90	90
/p/	✓	75	75	90	90	90	90
/b/	✓		75	90	90	90	90
/t/	✓		75	90	90	90	90
/d/	✓		75	90	90	90	90
/k/	✓		75	90	90	90	90
/g/	✓			90	90	90	90
/f/	✓		75	90	90	90	90
/v/	✓			90	90	90	90
/θ/						90	90
/ð/						90	90
/s/	✓			90	90	90	90
/z/				90	90	90	90
/ʃ/	✓			75	75	75*	90
/ʒ/					75	75*	90
/h/	✓	75	75	90	90	90	90
/ tʃ//	✓			75	90	90	90
/dʒ/					90	90	90
/ɹ/	✓			75		75*	90
/l/	✓			75		90	90
/w/	✓		75	90	90	90	90
/j/	✓		75	90	90	90	90
/ɑ, i, ɪ, ɛ, e, u, o ʌ, ɔ/		75	75	75	n/a	n/a	n/a
/æ, a, ʊ, ɝ/				75	n/a	n/a	n/a

Error Patterns

A range of studies on children age 2 to 7 years reported on three categories of error patterns: assimilation errors, substitution errors, and syllable structure errors. The measure of percent frequency of occurrence for these categories of error patterns age are presented in Figure 6.2 as a function of age. Among the three categories, assimilation error types were the least common; in contrast, substitution errors and syllable structure errors occurred frequently, particularly between the ages of 2 to 5 years of age. In general, the frequency of occurrence of the various error types diminished as children became older. Only two patterns, however, peaked at the age of three years then diminished (i.e., vowelization and weak syllable deletions).

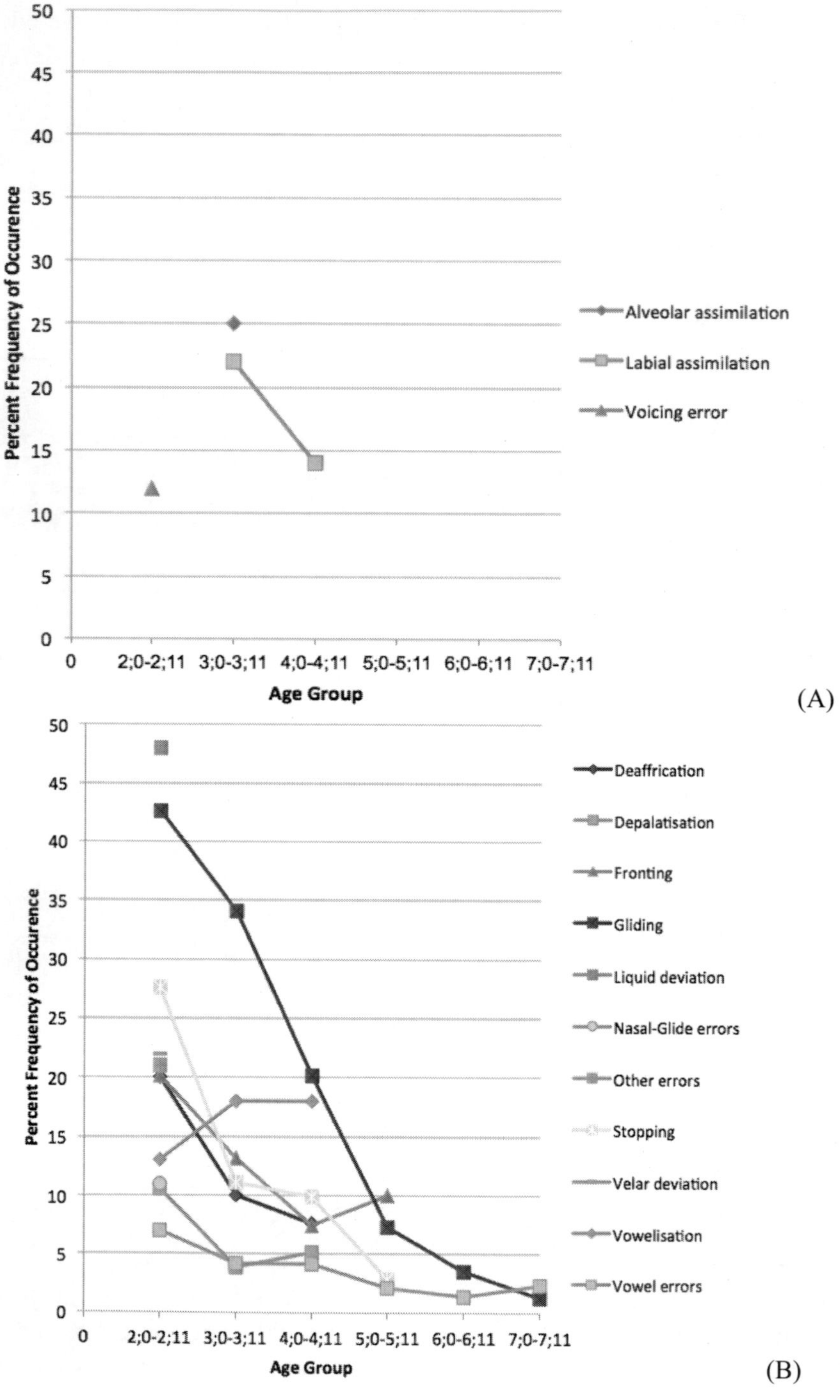

Figure 6.2. (Continued).

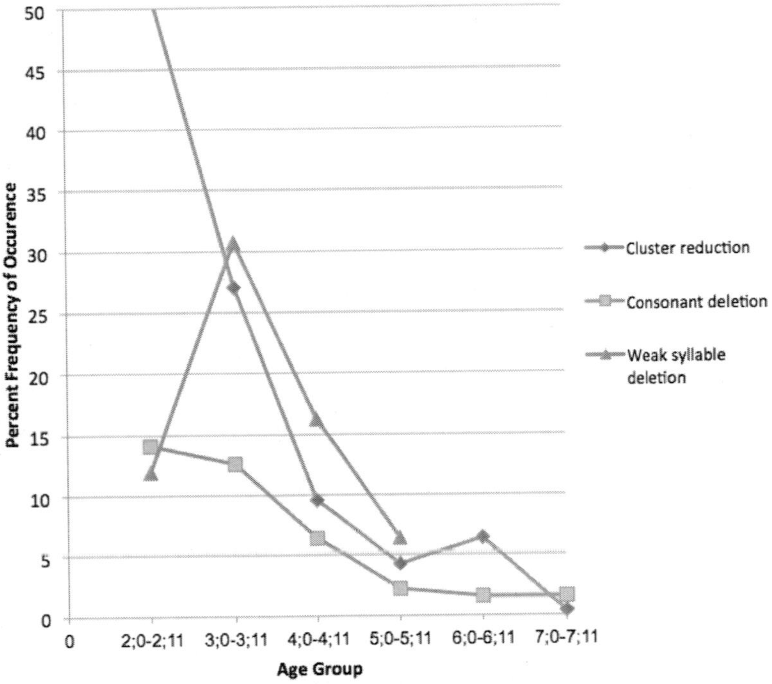

(C)

Figure 6.2. Percent Frequency of Occurrence of the three categories of error patterns across the targeted age range: (a) Assimilation Patterns; (2) Substitution Patterns; and (3) Syllable Structure Patterns.

In addition to generally decreasing in frequency of occurrence, fewer patterns were observed above the age of 4 years. Although patterns may be infrequent, the number of children in any given age group that produced a particular error patterns could be relatively high. For example, although cluster reduction had a frequency of occurrence of only 7% at 6 years of age, 92% of children produced this error. An understanding of phonological development is enriched by understanding the frequency of occurrence of each error pattern and the percent of children that produce these patterns.

Sidebar 6.1. Feature Production

Instead of looking at inventories, some researchers have reported on the development of feature contrasts. Children are thought to build their phonological system by establishing feature contrasts (Jakobson, 1968), thus the goal is to identify the features that children are contrasting and the order in which the feature contrasts are acquired. Stokes and colleagues [14] have reported on the percent of two-year-old children who contrast different features.

They found that 100% of children produced the consonantal, sonorant, coronal and voicing contrasts, that 75-95% of children produced the anterior, continuant and nasal contrasts, and that less than 50% of children produced a delayed release (i.e., affricates), lateral or strident contrasts.

Based on their research, Prather et al. [12] proposed the following order of feature acquisition (from earliest to latest): continuant, strident, diffuse, voice, nasal, grave.. To learn more about feature analyses and these terms, consult Prather et al. (1975).

Sidebar 6.2. Prosody

Beyond segmental accuracy, it is important to consider stress, intonation, and rate. As is noted in Chapter 7, few studies have described the prosody of preschool aged children, despite the important role it can play in word accuracy. Rate has been studied among three-year-old children from New Zealand and the United States of America [28].

This study showed that children from New Zealand speak a little faster than their American peers with a rate of syllables per minute of 208 for New Zealanders versus 182 for Americans. Regarding the length of utterances, the mean number of syllables per utterance was 4.7 for New Zealand and 4.5 for American children. Intonation has been studied among 5-year-old children [29]. Children were found to use the basic functions of intonation (e.g., chunking, affect, and focus). Children, however, have been found to have difficulty incorporating two words to correctly mark the stress of a compound word. For example, children have difficulty shifting the stress placement from the noun in "a black bird", to the first syllable in "a blackbird". Children at this age also have difficulty placing the phrase-level accent in non-final position for indicating a change in focus ("The CAT jumped on the hat").These abilities continue to improve through to the age of 13 years.

Connections

In this chapter, I have focused on typical development among monolingual children. Chapter 1 provides an overview of how theories of phonological acquisition have shaped how we study children. Chapter 2 provides a thorough description of the various measures used to describe children's speech, and a number of these measures are reported here. To understand how children are prepared for the rapid growth of their phonological system, you can turn to Chapter 3 to learn about the pre-linguistic stage and early words.

An overview of suprasegmental aspects of phonological development is provided in Chapter 7. Lastly, a series of Chapters in Section III of this volume provides details on phonological development across different languages and among bilingual children.

Concluding Remarks

The results of this analysis of 31 studies of English speaking children highlights the fast progress towards building their phonological systems made by typical children make between the ages of 2 and 9 years. During this age range, children acquire the main components of their phonological system: they quickly increase the number of phonemes in their inventory and these phonemes become more accurate by the age of four, leading to a drastic decrease in the frequency and type of error patterns around the same age. An understanding of typical phonological development is necessary for understanding speech sound disorders. An SLP needs to distinguish between typical development and disordered development in evaluation, and identify treatment goals that are realistic given the child's age and abilities. Although this chapter focused on phonological development at the segmental level based on what the child can produce, a multidimensional approach to phonological development includes an understanding of how children produce suprasegmental components of their phonological system (see Chapter 7 in this volume), how children perceive phonemes (e.g., Rvachew, Ohberg, Grawburt and Heyding, 2003), and how children acquire the sociolinguistic features of the language (e.g., Munson, Edwards and Beckman, 2005). Finally, phonological development does not occur independently of other components of language but likely interacts with other components such as lexical development (e.g., Stoel-Gammon, 2010).

Chapter Review Questions

1. Is an understanding of typical phonological development important to speech-language pathologists? Explain your answer.
2. What is the difference between a phonetic and a phonemic inventory?
3. What are the three categories of error patterns? Provide an example of error types for each category.

Suggestions for Further Reading

Cross-Sectional Study of Phonological Development

Smit, A. B., Hand, L., Freilinger, J. J., Bernthal, J. E., and Bird, A. (1990). The Iowa articulation norms project and its nebraska replication. *The Journal of Speech and Hearing Disorders*, *55*(4), 779-98.

Dodd, B., Holm, A., Hua, Z., and Crosbie, S. (2003). Phonological development: A normative study of British English-speaking children. *Clinical Linguistics and Phonetics*, *17*(8), 617-643.

Representations of Phonology

Munson, B., Edwards, J., and Beckman, M. E. (2005). Phonological knowledge in typical and atypical speech-sound development. *Topics in Language Disorders*, *25*(3), 190-206.

Interactions Between Phonology and Lexical System

Stoel-Gammon, C. (2010). The word complexity measure: Description and application to developmental phonology and disorders. *Clinical Linguistics and Phonetics*, *24*(4-5), 271-82.

Suggestions for Student Activities

Compare and contrast the acquisition of phonemes in English versus one of the languages described in the vignettes.

Answers to Chapter Review Questions

1. Is an understanding of typical phonological development important to speech-language pathologists? Explain your answer.

Understanding typical phonological development is important to SLPs. This understanding provides SLPs with better abilities to distinguish between typical and atypical development.

2. What is the difference between a phonetic and a phonemic inventory?

A phonetic inventory refers to a list of phonemes that a child can produce, even if the phoneme is not in the correct place or in the target word. A phonemic inventory refers to a list of phonemes that a child can produce that is in the correct place in the target and that matches the target word.

3. What are the three categories of error patterns? Provide an example of error types for each category.

Although error patterns can be sub-divided in many different ways, I have opted to use the following categories: error patterns describe touch assimilation (e.g., labial assimilation), others that describe substitutions (stopping), and patterns that describe changes to syllable structure (weak syllable deletion).

References

[1] Arlt, P. B., and Goodban, M. T. (1976). A comparative study of articulation acquisition as based on a study of 240 normals, aged three to six. *Language, Speech, and Hearing Services in Schools*, *7*(3), 173-180.

[2] Bland-Stewart, L. M. (2003). Phonetic inventories and phonological patterns of African American two-year-olds. *Communication Disorders Quarterly*, *24*(3), 109-120.

[3] Dodd, B., and McIntosh, B. (2010). Two-Year-Old phonology: Impact of input, motor and cognitive abilities on development. *Journal of Child Language*, *37*(5), 1027-1046.

[4] Dodd, B., Holm, A., Hua, Z., and Crosbie, S. (2003). Phonological development: A normative study of British English-speaking children. *Clinical Linguistics and Phonetics*, *17*(8), 617-643.

[5] Dyson, A. T. (1988). Phonetic inventories of 2-and 3-year-old children. *Journal of Speech and Hearing Disorders*, *53*(1), 89-93.

[6] Dyson, A. T., and Paden, E. P. (1983). Some phonological acquisition strategies used by two-year-olds. *Communication Disorders Quarterly*, *7*(1), 6-18.

[7] Flipsen, P. (2006). Measuring the intelligibility of conversational speech in children. *Clinical Linguistics and Phonetics*, *20*(4), 303-312.

[8] Grunwell, P. (1981). The development of phonology: A descriptive profile. *First Language*, *2*(6), 161.

[9] Haelsig, P. C., and Madison, C. L. (1986). A study of phonological processes exhibited by 3-, 4-, and 5-year-old children. *Language, Speech, and Hearing Services in Schools*, *17*(2), 107-114.

[10] Ingram, D. (1974). Phonological rules in young children. *Journal of Child Language*, *1*(01), 49-64.

[11] Ingram, D., and Ingram, K. D. (2001). A whole-word approach to phonological analysis and intervention. *Language, Speech, and Hearing Services in Schools*, *32*(4), 271.

[12] James, D. G. H. (2001). Use of phonological processes in Australian children ages 2 to 7; 11 years. *International Journal of Speech-Language Pathology*, *3*(2), 109-127.

[13] James, D. G., van Doorn, J., McLeod, S., and Esterman, A. (2008). Patterns of consonant deletion in typically developing children aged 3 to 7 years. *International Journal of Speech-Language Pathology*, *10*(3), 179-192.

[14] Kehoe, M., and Stoel-Gammon, C. (1997). Truncation patterns in English-speaking children's word productions. *Journal of Speech, Language, and Hearing Research*, *40*(3), 526-541.

[15] Kirk, C., and Demuth, K. (2005). Asymmetries in the acquisition of word-initial and word-final consonant clusters. *Journal of Child Language*, *32*(04), 709-734.

[16] Lowe, R. J., Knutson, P. J., and Monson, M. A. (1985). Incidence of fronting in preschool children. *Language, Speech, and Hearing Services in Schools*, *16*(2), 119-123.

[17] MacLeod, A.A.N., Laukys, K., Rvachew, S. (2011). Impact of bilingual language learning on whole-word complexity and segmental accuracy among children aged 18 and 36 months. *International Journal of Speech Language Pathology, 13*, 490-499.

[18] McIntosh, B., and Dodd, B. J. (2008). Two-Year-Olds' phonological acquisition: Normative data. *International Journal of Speech-Language Pathology*, *10*(6), 460-469.

[19] Otomo, K., and Stoel-Gammon, C. (1992). The acquisition of unrounded vowels in English. *Journal of Speech and Hearing Research*, *35*(3), 604-616.

[20] Pollock, K. E., and Berni, M. C. (2001). Transcription of vowels. *Topics in Language Disorders*, *21*(4), 22-40.

[21] Prather, E. M., Hedrick, D. L., and Kern, C. A. (1975). Articulation development in children aged two to four years. *Journal of Speech and Hearing Disorders*, *40*(2), 179-191.

[22] Preisser, D. A., Hodson, B. W., and Paden, E. P. (1988). Developmental phonology: 18-29 months. *Journal of Speech and Hearing Disorders*, *53*(2), 125-130.

[23] Robb, M. P., and Gillon, G. T. (2007). Speech rates of American English- and New Zealand English-speaking children. *Advances in Speech Language Pathology*, *9*(2), 173-180.

[24] Roberts, J. E., Burchinal, M., and Footo, M. M. (1990). Phonological process decline from 2 1/2 to 8 years. *Journal of Communication Disorders*, *23*(3), 205-217.

[25] Roulstone, S., Loader, S., Northstone, K., and Beveridge, M. (2002). The speech and language of children aged 25 months: Descriptive data from the avon longitudinal study of parents and children. *Early Child Development and Care*, *172*(3), 259-268.

[26] Rvachew, S., Ohberg, A., Grawburg, M., and Heyding, J. (2003). Phonological awareness and phonemic perception in 4-year-old children with delayed expressive phonology skills. *American Journal of Speech-Language Pathology*, *12*(4), 463.

[27] Schwarz, I. C., Burnham, D., and Bowey, J. A. (2006). Phoneme sensitivity and vocabulary size in 21/2-to 3-year-olds. In P. Warren and I. Watson (Eds.), Proceedings of the 11th Australian international conference on speech science and technology. (pp. 143-58). Auckland, New Zealand: University of Auckland.

[28] Selby, J. C., Robb, M. P., and Gilbert, H. R. (2000). Normal vowel articulations between 15 and 36 months of age. *Clinical Linguistics and Phonetics*, *14*(4), 255-265.

[29] Shriberg, L. D. (1993). Four new speech and prosody-voice measures for genetics research and other studies in developmental phonological disorders. *Journal of Speech and Hearing Research*, *36*(1), 105-140.

[30] Smit, A. B. (1993). Phonologic error distributions in the Iowa-Nebraska articulation norms project: Consonant singletons. *Journal of Speech and Hearing Research*, *36*(3), 533-47.

[31] Smit, A. B., Hand, L., Freilinger, J. J., Bernthal, J. E., and Bird, A. (1990). The Iowa articulation norms project and its Nebraska replication. *The Journal of Speech and Hearing Disorders*, *55*(4), 779-798.

[32] Stoel-Gammon, C. (1987). Phonological skills of 2-year-olds. *Language, Speech, and Hearing Services in the Schools*, *18*(4), 323-329.

[33] Stoel-Gammon, C. (2010). The word complexity measure: Description and application to developmental phonology and disorders. *Clinical Linguistics and Phonetics*, *24*(4-5), 271-82.

[34] Stoel-Gammon, C., and Dunn, C. (1985). Phonological development and disorders in children. Austin, TX: Pro-Ed.

[35] Stokes, S. F., Klee, T., Carson, C. P., and Carson, D. (2005). A phonemic implicational feature hierarchy of phonological contrasts for english-speaking children. *Journal of Speech, Language, and Hearing Research*, *48*(4), 817-833.

[36] Watson, M. M., and Scukanec, G. P. (1997). Profiling the phonological abilities of 2-year-olds: A longitudinal investigation. *Child Language Teaching and Therapy*, *13*(1), 3-14.

[37] Wells, B., Peppe, S., and Goulandris, N. (2004). Intonation development from five to thirteen. *Journal of Child Language*, *31*(04), 749-778.

[38] Wyllie-Smith, L., McLeod, S., and Ball, M. J. (2006). Typically developing and speech-impaired children's adherence to the sonority hypothesis. *Clinical Linguistics and Phonetics*, *20*(4), 271-291.

In: Comprehensive Perspectives …
Editors: Beate Peter and Andrea A. N. MacLeod

ISBN: 978-1-62257-041-6

Chapter 7

BEYOND SEGMENTS: HOW CHILDREN ACQUIRE PROSODY

Margaret Kehoe

INTRODUCTION

Most researchers working in the area of language acquisition are well aware of the important and crucial role that prosody plays in language development. Speech perception studies show that infants can discriminate different intonation contours and stress patterns from an early age. Their sensitivity to prosodic information allows them to distinguish different languages, isolate words, and organize the speech signal into grammatically relevant units. Speech production studies reveal that infants use consistent prosodic cues to express different pragmatic functions. Their sensitivity to prosodic information is evident in the fact that language-specific prosodic differences may appear in babbling and first words. Studies focusing on the development of prosodic phenomena, such as stress, timing and intonation, also indicate that children produce language-specific prosodic features very early in their words and phrases. More recently, prosodic assessment tools have been used to identify atypical prosody in clinical groups such as autism spectrum disorders, childhood apraxia of speech, and specific language impairment. One could assume that prosody has always occupied a central role in language acquisition research. However, the recognition of prosody as a key player in language acquisition is a relatively recent phenomenon that dates from the 1980s and 1990s. This period was associated with the development of linguistic theoretical frameworks (e.g., non-linear phonology, autosegmental phonology, metrical phonology, prosodic phonology) that offered a way to describe and explain prosodic structures, as well as the development of acoustic software that allowed for those acoustic correlate measurements associated with prosody to be easily accessible. Since this period, there has been an ever-increasing interest in the role of prosody in language development. The aim of this chapter is to provide an overview of prosodic development. The first part will be concerned with perceptual and productive aspects of early prosodic development, including different prosodic systems such as stress, timing, and intonation. Readers will be familiarized with different facets of prosody such as its acoustic correlates and cross-linguistic differences. The second part provides a description of atypical prosody and how it is affected in the presence of autism spectrum disorder, childhood apraxia of speech, and specific language impairments.

Sidebar 7.1. The Prosody Elephant

When defining prosody, we are reminded of the story of the blind men and the elephant. Each blind man felt different sections of the elephant (e.g., leg, tail, trunk) and came up with a different account of the "whole elephant." One man felt the leg and said the elephant was like a pillar; another man felt the tail and said the elephant was like a rope; yet another felt the trunk and said the elephant was like a tree branch, etc.

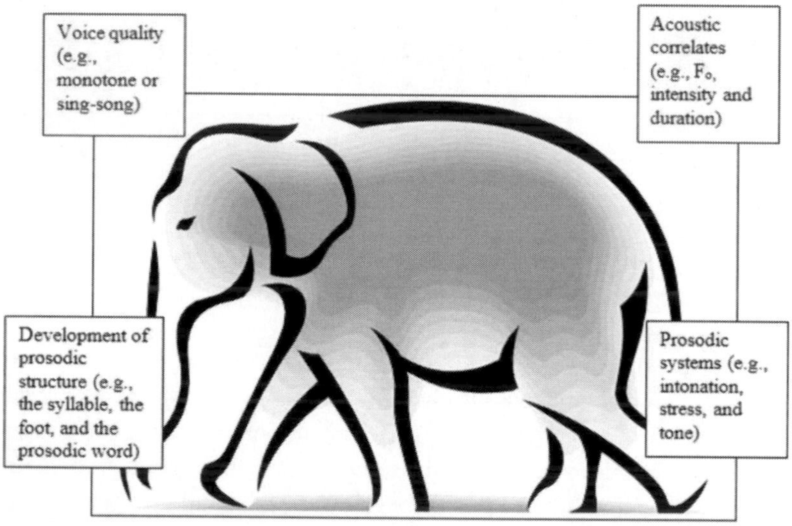

This simile is not original to prosody but has been used numerous times in the field of science. It has even been used in the field of speech and hearing sciences (e.g., the stuttering elephant; Johnson, 1958). It does seem to capture, however, the state of affairs in the discipline in which different components of prosody have been largely dealt with on an individual basis despite the fact that prosody is made up of multiple systems that interact.

Definition and Framework of Prosody

Providing a definition of prosody is not easy because it contains many different components and dimensions. Researchers working on prosody may focus on features of voice quality, that is, whether a voice sounds "sing-song" or "monotonous." Others may consider more traditional linguistic phenomena such as stress, timing, intonation, and tone. Yet another group may concentrate on the development of prosodic structures such as the syllable, the foot, the prosodic word and the phonological phrase. All of these above-mentioned aspects are concerned with prosody, because prosody refers to features of spoken language that involve more than a single consonant or vowel. It may refer to linguistic phenomena that apply across several segments, a word, or an entire utterance. The other term often used to refer to prosody is **suprasegmental**, which can be contrasted with the term **segmental**. (See Sidebar 7.1 for an illustration of these various perspectives on prosody.)

Prosody can be viewed on a continuum of functions and effects, ranging from non-linguistic at one end through paralinguistic to linguistic at the other end (Clark and Yallop, 1995), as shown in Figure 7.1. At the non-linguistic end are features of voice quality that reflect the nature of the speaker's larynx and vocal tract (e.g., size of the larynx and vocal tract, or the health of the larynx), or that reflect habitual characteristics such as a distinctive speech rhythm or intonation. These speech features are generally not considered to be under conscious control, but they enable us to identify a particular speaker or class of speaker. We refer to this function as **indexical** (Crystal, 1987). Mid-way along the continuum is the use of speech features to indicate the speaker's feelings and emotions. These features are generally under conscious control and they have an affective function. At the most linguistic end of the continuum are systems such as stress, timing, intonation, and tone. They may have two communicative functions: pragmatic and grammatical. Prosody may provide **focus** to highlight information in utterances as seen in the two different interpretations of the phrase "Mary drank a cup of coffee". For example, to emphasize who drank the coffee, we would say, "MARY drank a cup of coffee," or to emphasize what was drunk, we would say, "Mary drank a cup of COFFEE." Focus is associated with the notion of information structure and can be viewed as part of the pragmatic aspect of communication. Prosody may also demarcate the beginning and ends of syntactic phrases, distinguish whether an utterance is a question or a statement, or distinguish word-classes such as nouns and verbs (e.g., [ˈprɑʤɛkt] vs. [prəˈʤɛkt]). Thus, prosody may be used to provide grammatical information. In the current chapter, we will mainly focus on the linguistic end of the continuum.

The acoustic-phonetic correlates of prosody are variations in **fundamental frequency** (F_0) (perceived as pitch), amplitude or intensity (perceived as loudness), and duration (perceived as length). These correlates combine in different ways to convey different prosodic systems.

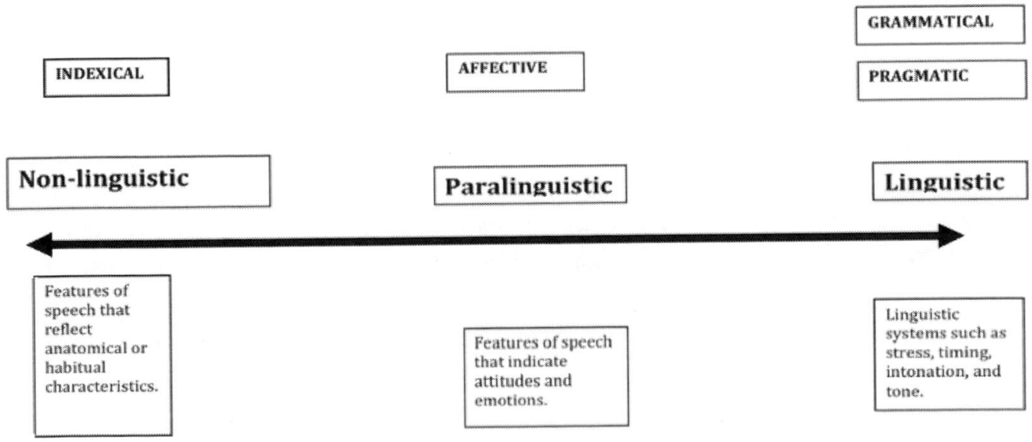

Figure 7.1. Functions and effects of prosody.

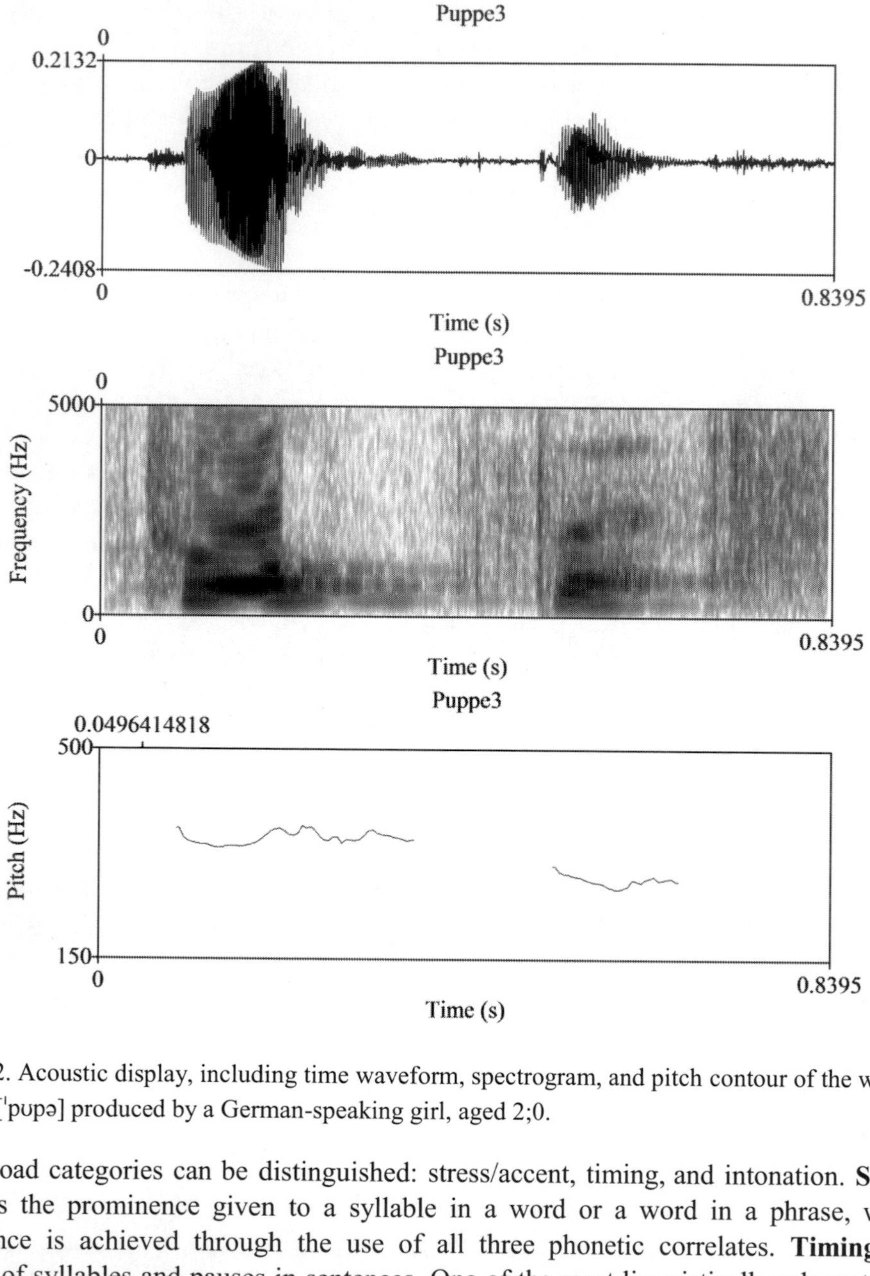

Figure 7.2. Acoustic display, including time waveform, spectrogram, and pitch contour of the word "*Puppe*" [ˈpʊpə] produced by a German-speaking girl, aged 2;0.

Three broad categories can be distinguished: stress/accent, timing, and intonation. **Stress** or **accent** is the prominence given to a syllable in a word or a word in a phrase, whereby prominence is achieved through the use of all three phonetic correlates. **Timing** is the duration of syllables and pauses in sentences. One of the most linguistically relevant aspects of timing is **phrase-final lengthening** which is the prolongation of the final syllable of a phrase or utterance. The overall pattern of timing and prominence effects contributes to our sense of the **rhythm of speech**. Finally, **intonation** is the patterning of pitch changes across words, whole phrases, and sentences.

The acoustic-phonetic correlates of prosody can be viewed easily using acoustic software equipment, such as PRAAT (Boersma and Weenink, 2005). Figure 7.2 shows an acoustic display of a German-speaking child saying the word "*Puppe*" ("doll").

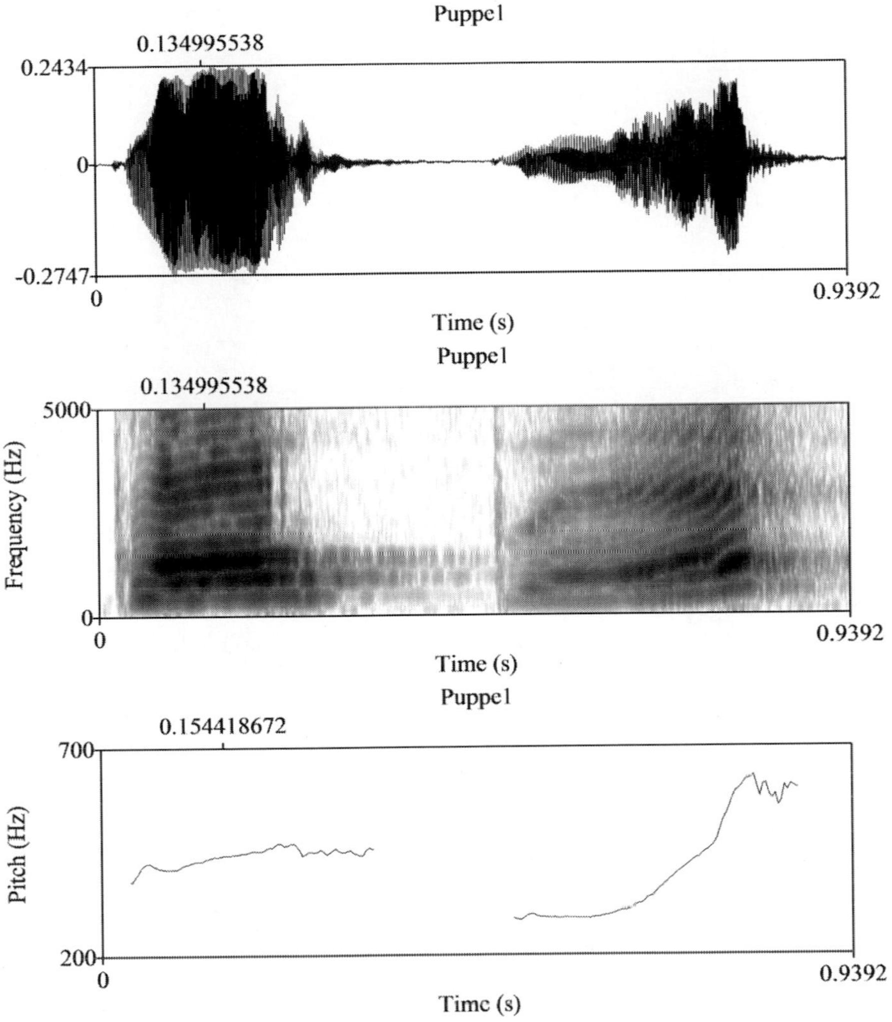

Figure 7.3. Acoustic display, including time waveform, spectrogram, and pitch contour of the word "*Puppe*" [ˈpʊpə] produced by a German-speaking girl, aged 2;0, with rising intonation.

Information from the time waveform (top diagram), the spectrogram (middle diagram) and the pitch contour (bottom diagram) help us to identify that the first syllable of the word is stressed. Figure 7.3 shows an acoustic display of the same German-speaking child saying "*Puppe*" ("doll") again. Information from the pitch contour display (bottom diagram) helps us to identify that the child is using rising intonation. More information about the acoustics of speech is described in Chapter 2.

The theory of prosodic phonology provides a way of representing different prosodic systems. Linguists have proposed a hierarchy of prosodic units that extends from **moras** at the bottom of the hierarchy to intonational phrases and utterances at the top of the hierarchy. Different versions of the prosodic hierarchy are available. The one shown in Figure 7.4 is an adaptation of Nespor and Vogel's (1986) conception of the prosodic hierarchy.

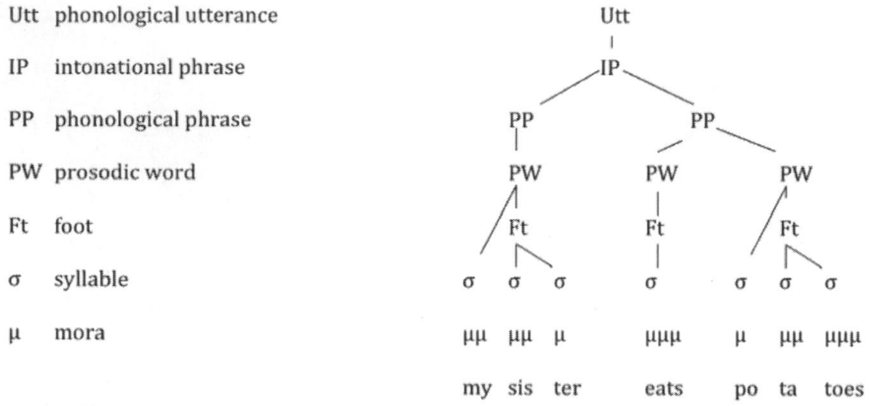

Figure 7.4. The prosodic hierarchy.

The higher-level units, such as the intonational phrase and the phonological phrase, are important in formalizing intonation and edge effects. The **foot** is important in capturing stress/accent and rhythm phenomena. At the bottom of the hierarchy are units such as the **syllable** and the mora. The mora is a unit of syllable weight that plays a role in stress assignment.

If we put together both the acoustic and the formal aspect of prosody, we arrive at a working definition of prosody, namely that it refers to acoustic patterns of fundamental frequency (F_0), duration, and amplitude that can best be accounted for by reference to higher-level structures of the prosodic hierarchy (adapted from Shattuck-Hufnagel and Turk, 1996).

Before we proceed to discussing prosodic development, there are some other important terminologies to be introduced. As mentioned above, the unit of stress analysis is the foot.There are two main types of feet: trochaic and iambic. A **trochee** or trochaic foot has the head (stressed or "strong") syllable on the left and the unstressed or "weak" syllable at the right, for instance as in the word "picture." An **iamb** or iambic foot has the head syllable on the right, for instance as in the word "guitar." These structures are shown in (1).

(1) Headedness of feet

At several times during the chapter, we will discuss rhythm types. Traditionally, languages have been classified into two main rhythm types: stress timed, such as English, German, and Dutch; and syllable-timed, such as Italian and French. A third rhythm type, mora-timed, is also posited, for instance for Japanese, where syllable durations depend on the number of moras in the syllables. Syllable-timed languages are thought to have syllables of equal length, which might sound like a machine gun, and stress timed languages are thought to have inter-stress intervals (or feet) of equal length while the individual syllables can vary in length, a pattern not unlike a Morse code (Abercrombie, 1967; Pike, 1945).

PROSODIC DEVELOPMENT

This section discusses important research that has been conducted in prosodic perception and production. Following an overview of the pre-linguistic and early linguistic period, three aspects of prosody that are relevant to English, stress, timing, and intonation are described.

Perception

Research in infant speech perception indicates that children are sensitive to prosodic information from an early age. Newborns and very young infants can discriminate words containing different stress and intonation contours, as well as discriminate phrases derived from different rhythmic groups. Older infants display sensitivity to prosodic cues at boundaries allowing them to segment sentences into clausal and phrasal constituents. They also show sensitivity to metrical patterns allowing them to isolate words. A summary of this research is provided below:

Discrimination Ability by Newborns and Young Infants

Several studies have found that very young infants, including newborns, can discriminate words containing different prosodic patterns. (See Chapter 3 for information on the prenatal development of the auditory system and the acoustic environment to which fetuses are exposed prior to birth.) Infants as young as two months can discriminate two syllables differing only in pitch contour (rising vs. falling) (Morse, 1972), or can detect differences between a monotone pitch contour and a rise-fall contour (Kuhl and Miller, 1975). Infants between one and four months can distinguish bisyllabic utterances differing only in stress patterns (e.g., [ˈbaba] vs. [baˈba]) (Jusczyk and Thompson, 1978; Spring and Dale, 1977). They can also detect change in each of the three prosodic parameters when isolated individually. For example, infants can discriminate two words in which the final vowels differ in duration (Eilers, Bull, Oller, and Lewis, 1984), amplitude (Bull, Eilers, and Oller, 1984) and F_0 (Bull, Eilers, and Oller, 1985). Nazzi, Floccia and Bertoncini (1998) also show that French newborns can discriminate lists of phonetically varied Japanese disyllabic words differing in pitch contour, indicating that they can extract consistent prosodic characteristics such as pitch despite phonetic variation.

Newborn infants can distinguish one language from another (Mehler, Jusczyk, Lambertz, Halsted, Bertoncini and Amiel-Tison, 1988). It has been hypothesized that rhythm type differences play the crucial role in this differentiation (see definition above and discussion of rhythm below). Infants can discriminate sentences drawn from different rhythmic groups, for example, from stress- versus syllable-timed languages (French-Russian, English-Italian, Mehler et al., 1988; English-Spanish, Moon, Cooper and Fifer, 1993) and from stress- versus mora-timed languages (English-Japanese, Nazzi, Bertoncini, and Mehler, 1998); they are unable to discriminate sentences drawn from the same rhythmic group (Dutch-English, Nazzi, et al., 1998).

Apart from discrimination abilities, infants show preferences for certain prosodic patterns. For example, they prefer their own ambient language to other languages (Mehler, Dupoux, Nazzi and Dehaene-Lambertz, 1996), and they prefer the exaggerated prosody of child-directed speech to the less intonated patterns of adult-directed speech (Fernald, 1985; Fernald and Kuhl, 1987; see Sidebar 7.2 Child Directed Speech).

Sidebar 7.2. Child-Directed Speech

Child-directed speech (CDS) or *"Motherese"* is a special style of speech used with infants and young children. CDS displays unique grammatical, lexical, and prosodic features. On the grammatical side, CDS consists of short, simple sentences containing frequent repetition, questions and imperatives. On the lexical side, CDS predominantly consists of words of one to two-syllables, diminutives, and frequent words of affection. On the prosodic side, CDS is characterized by higher pitch, wider pitch range, longer pauses, increased final-syllable-lengthening and a slower articulation rate than speech directed to adults (ADS) (Fernald and Simon, 1984; Fernald, Taeschner, Dunn, Papousek, de Boysson-Bardies and Fukui, 1989). Out of these prosodic features, high pitch and wide pitch range are the most important determinants of infants' preference for CDS. Fernald (1985) reports pitch ranges of 90 to 800 Hz for CDS in contrast to 90 to 300 Hz for ADS. The prosodic characteristics of CDS are found in all languages and in both mothers and fathers' speech, although different degrees have been reported (Fernald et al., 1989). For example, intonational modifications are more extreme in American English than in British English and in other languages such as French, German, Italian, and Japanese.

CDS may have a number of different functions, including expressing affection or attracting attention (Garnica, 1977; Fernald et al., 1989); however, it may also have an important linguistic function, namely, to help infants parse the syntactic structures of their native languages (see Sidebar 7.3 Prosodic Bootstrapping).

Clausal and Phrasal Segmentation

Prosody has been strongly implicated in recent theories of grammatical acquisition. According to the "prosodic bootstrapping hypothesis," infants use prosodic information in the speech signal to infer clausal and phrasal structure (Gleitman and Wanner, 1982; see Sidebar 7.3 Prosodic Bootstrapping). Clausal and, to a lesser extent, phrasal boundaries are marked by prosodic features such as heightened stress, changing intonational contours, pauses, and lengthening. Hirsh-Pasek, Kemler Nelson, Jusczyk, Wright Cassidy, Druss, and Kennedy (1987) found that infants between six and ten months orient significantly longer to more natural sounding speech samples which contain pauses coincident with clause boundaries than to samples containing pauses inserted unnaturally within clauses. Other studies have demonstrated sensitivity to the prosodic correlates of clauses as early as 4.5 months (Jusczyk, 1997).

Sidebar 7.3. The Prosodic Bootstrapping Hypothesis

According to the Prosodic Bootstrapping Hypothesis, acoustic cues in the speech stream provide infants with important cues to syntactic boundaries (Morgan and Newport, 1981; Gleitman and Wanner, 1982). The hypothesis presupposes three elements: 1. Acoustic properties cue syntactic boundaries; 2. Infants are sensitive to these properties; 3. Infants use these cues in processing the speech stream (Soderstrom, Seidl, Kemler Nelson, and Jusczyk, 2003). All of these elements have been confirmed in research studies. The acoustic properties most frequently associated with boundaries are phrase-final lengthening, pause duration, and changes in F_0. Young infants are sensitive to these acoustic properties, preferring passages with artificial pauses inserted at clause boundaries than at other places in the passage (Hirsh-Pasek et al., 1987). Infants also appear to use information coincident with phrasal and clausal units in the processing of speech (Nazzi, Kemler Nelson, Jusczyk, and Jusczyk, 2000; Soderstrom et al., 2003). Critics of this approach point out that there are prosody-syntax mismatches (Pinker, 1994; Fernald and McRoberts, 1996). In particular, phrases are less reliably cued by prosodic information than clauses (Gerken, Jusczyk, and Mandel, 1994), although certain studies reveal that infants use phrase-level prosodic cues in processing speech (Soderstrom et al., 2003).

The results discussed above indicate that infants are sensitive to the prosodic cues of syntactic boundaries; they do not show, however, that infants use these cues to structure incoming input. Researchers have shown that infants remember speech information better when it is packaged within a single prosodic unit versus presented as isolated words (Mandel, Jusczyk and Kemler Nelson, 1994). At 6 months, infants have been found to be able to use prosodic information associated with clausal units in their processing of fluent speech (Nazzi et al., 2000). Infants were better able to recognize a word sequence when it was part of a well-formed clause than when it constituted a non-unit made up of the last words of one clause and the beginning words of the next. Similar results have been observed with phrasal units. Soderstrom et al. (2003) found that infants aged 6 months were not only sensitive to phrasal level cues, but they were also able to deploy this sensitivity in the processing of fluent speech. Infants preferred passages containing a familiar phonological sequence when this sequence consisted of a well-formed phrasal unit, compared to when it corresponded to a syntactic non-unit. Previous studies had suggested that sensitivity to prosodic correlates of phrases occurs at about 9 months of age (Jusczyk, Hirsh-Pasek, Kemler Nelson, Kennedy, Woodward and Piwoz, 1992; Gerken et al., 1994) but Soderstrom et al.'s (2003) study suggests an earlier time line.

Word Segmentation

Not only does prosody contribute to children's knowledge of the major syntactic properties of a language, it is also implicated in children's ability to segment fluent speech into words. Studies reveal that children are sensitive to the predominant stress pattern of their language.

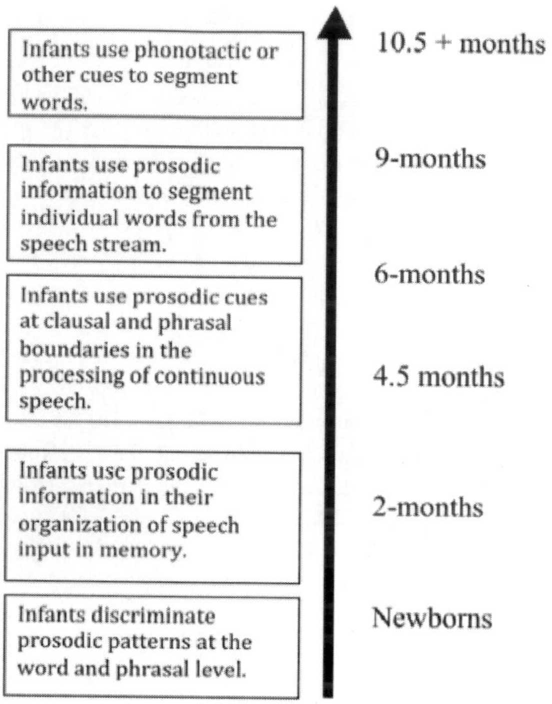

Figure 7.5. Timeline of infant perception of prosody.

Jusczyk, Cutler, and Redanz (1993) showed that 9-month-old infants display a preference for the trochaic stress pattern of English when presented with lists of trochaic and iambic disyllabic words. More recently, Höhle, Bijeljac-Babic, Herold, Weissenborn, and Nazzi (2009) found a preference for trochaic over iambic words in 6-month-old German-speaking children. They also found that 6-month-old French-speaking infants did not show a preference for either stress pattern. This result is consistent with the prosodic pattern of French, which is syllable-timed and which cannot be easily slotted into metrical distinctions such as trochaic and iambic.

Children's preferences for different metrical patterns seem to aid them in segmenting fluent speech into words. Jusczyk, Houston, and Newsome (1999) found that infants, aged 5 months, were able to segment trochaic but not iambic words from the fluent speech stream. The infants tended to segment iambic words at the beginning of the stressed syllable. Thus, the form "guitar is" was misperceived as the trochaic form "tar is." By 10.5 months, however, infants were able to segment words beginning with weak syllables suggesting that they were starting to acquire other cues (e.g., phonotactic) that mark the onset of words.

Findings on word segmentation from other languages suggest that segmentation abilities differ cross-linguistically as a function of the rhythm group. Nazzi, Iakimova, Bertoncini, Frédonie, and Alcantara (2006) propose that French infants use the syllable as the unit of prosodic segmentation. In a study of the word segmentation skills of 8-, 12-, and 16-month French infants, they observed no segmentation ability at 8 months, segmentation of final syllables at 12 months, and segmentation of disyllabic words at 16 months. A comparison of these results with findings from stress-timed languages reveals that prosodic segmentation (trochaic foot or syllable) occurs around 6.5 to 8 months and full word segmentation occurs later, at 10.5 months for the English infants and 16 months for the French infants. The later timeline in French may relate to a variety of cues at word boundaries that are still not yet well understood (Nazzi et al., 2006). A summary of an approximate time-line in infant speech perception of prosody is presented in Figure 7.5.

Production

Pre-Linguistic and Early Linguistic Period

This section focuses on the development of prosody during the pre-linguistic and early linguistic periods. Studies are grouped into three main areas: ambient language effects, differentiation according to pragmatic function, and the transitional phase between one- and two-word utterances. These studies are principally concerned with the development of prosody in general rather than with the development of individual prosodic phenomena such as stress, timing, and intonation, which will be addressed later in the chapter. This section focuses on production, but some brief references to comprehension will be made as well.

Ambient Language Effects

There is contradictory evidence for the presence of language-specific prosodic patterns in babbling. Engstrand, Williams, and Lacerda (2003) found that a group of expert listeners were unable to distinguish the babbles of 12- and 18-month-old English and Swedish children, supporting a series of earlier listening studies that have failed to find evidence for ambient language effects on babbling (Atkinson, MacWhinney, and Stoel, 1968; Olney and Scholnick, 1976; Thevenin, Eilers, Oller, and Lavoie, 1985). Those studies that have found ambient language effects point to the rhythmic and intonational properties of the target languages as playing the crucial role in differentiation (de Boysson-Bardies, Sagart, and Durand, 1984). These studies will be reviewed below.

Several studies employing acoustic analyses have revealed clear language-specific prosodic differences in infant babbling. Recent research even shows ambient language effects in newborn cries. For example, French newborns produce rising melody and intensity contours whereas German newborns most often produce falling contours, patterns that correspond to the prosodic contours perceived prenatally (Mampe, Friederici, Christophe and Wermke, 2009). Similar results have been obtained when examining the reduplicative babbling of French and English infants: perceptual judgments as well as acoustic analyses indicate a higher percentage of falling contours in the English infants' compared to the French infants' vocalizations (Whalen, Levitt, and Wang, 1991) and a higher percentage of longer final syllables in the French (54%) versus English infants' vocalizations (29%) (Levitt and Wang, 1991).

Despite the clear differences reported by Levitt, Whalen and colleagues, other researchers report rather modest ambient language effects at the onset of word use (see review by DePaolis, Vihman, and Kunnari, 2008). For example, Vihman and DePaolis (1998) did not find differences in the mean F_0 and vowel durations between French and English infants' vocalizations at the 4-word point (the first 30-minute session in which infants spontaneously produce four different words) (as reported by DePaolis et al., 2008). Similarly, DePaolis et al. (2008) found only isolated language-specific differences in the disyllabic (babbled) productions of English-, French-, Finnish-, and Welsh-speaking children at the same developmental stage. The most notable difference between languages was a reduced duration on the final syllables of Welsh and Finnish vocalizations. Finnish also distinguished itself from the other languages by having higher F_0 and intensity on the first syllable in the infant vocalizations and a greater number of perceived trochaic forms. Overall, these findings suggest that biological predispositions still predominate at the onset of word use, but that language-specific effects are emerging, particularly for those languages that are maximally distinctive (e.g., Finnish).

Whereas DePaolis et al. (2008) and Vihman and DePaolis (1998) observed minimal language-specific differences between French and English at the 4-word point, Vihman, DePaolis and Davis (1998) observed clear acoustic differences between the disyllabic (word and babble) productions of English- and French-speaking children at the 25-word point (the first 30 minute session in which infants spontaneously produce 25 different words). In both English and French, the second syllable of the disyllable was longer than the first syllable due to phrase final lengthening effects but more so in the case of French (mean duration ratio of 1:1.6) than English (mean duration ratio of 1:1.2). With respect to F_0 and amplitude, French children produced "more" of both on the second syllable whereas English children produced more of both on the first syllable, although with considerable variability. Similarly, Hallé, Boysson-Bardies, and Vihman (1991), comparing French and Japanese infants at the 25-word point, found that the French infants produced more rising contours than the Japanese infants. Thus, on the basis of acoustic studies, there is evidence that children display language-specific prosodic features in their early speech patterns, particularly after the onset of word production (i.e., the 25-word point and beyond).

Pragmatic Differentiation

How early do children use prosody to convey functional intention? In contrast to the contradictory findings with respect to ambient language effects, studies that have examined the relationship between infants' prosodic patterns and pragmatic intention tend to show consistent effects. These results have been demonstrated for cry vocalizations, babbling, and early words.

Studies of babies' cry vocalizations reveal that babies use intonation differently in different contexts. For example, D'Odorico (1984) observed that Italian-learning babies, aged 0;4 to 0;8, employed falling or level contours for discomfort cries, falling and rising contours for call cries, and mostly rising contours for requests. D'Odorico and Franco (1991) found that a variety of prosodic cues discriminated functional intentions up to the age of 0;8 or 0;9 among Italian infants. For example, rising contours distinguished "vocalizations during shared experiences" from "vocalizations during infant manipulation of a toy": functions requiring listener intervention led to higher pitch and more rising contours. After the age of 0;9, there did not appear to be any significant association between prosodic cues and context, suggesting a regression in prosodic development, a finding that has been reported by other researchers (see Sidebar 7.4 Regression in Prosodic Development).

Sidebar 7.4. Regression in Prosodic Development

Several researchers have noted a regression in infant's prosodic ability around the age of 0;10, lasting through the one-word period (D'Odorico and Franco, 1991; Levitt, 1993; Scollon, 1976). For example, Scollon (1976) reported a period of regression in his subject, Brenda, when she reverted to using a high percentage of level tones after having acquired falling tones. He posited that Brenda's prosodic regression was tied to her advances in segmental development. Levitt (1993) reported regression in children's development of phrase-final lengthening as they began to use their first words.

Snow and Balog (2002) posit two possible explanations for this regression: (1) a production-based explanation, in which children's focus on segmental complexity leads to a decline in prosodic complexity; or (2) a prosodic re-organization explanation, in which prosody moves from being biologically to being linguistically based. They hypothesize that up until the age of 0;9, pitch patterns reflect physiological or emotional tendencies, but after this period (0;9 to 2;0), the underlying basis is linguistic.

More recently, two studies by Papaeliou and colleagues, studying the vocalizations of English infants, aged 0;7 to 0;11, report consistent acoustic patterns according to whether vocalizations express emotion versus communicative functions, (Papaeliou, Minadakis, and Cavouras, 2002), or investigative (e.g., infant is holding or inspecting an object) versus communicative functions (e.g., infant is interacting with an adult, pointing or directing eye gaze to an adult) (Papaeliou and Trevarthen, 2006). They employed a pattern recognition system that classified infant vocalizations according to combinations of acoustic features. Vocalizations expressing emotion were characterized by longer duration, higher F_0, and lower overall intensity than vocalizations expressing communicative function, which in turn were characterized by shorter duration, higher F_0, and more variable F_0 than investigative vocalizations.

During the one-word period, several studies demonstrate that children use F_0 differently according to context or situation (Flax, Lahey, Harris, and Boothroyd, 1991; Furrow, 1984; Galligan, 1987; Halliday, 1975; Marcos, 1987). Halliday (1975) was one of the first to observe that his son, Nigel, used rising tones for all "pragmatic" utterances (those requiring a response) and falling tones for all "mathetic" utterances (those not requiring a response). Others have made similar observations. For example, Marcos (1987) found that French-speaking children, aged 1;2 to 1;10, used higher initial F_0 for repeated requests than for initial requests; high pitch and rising tones were more often associated with requests than with labeling. Similarly, Galligan (1987) found that her two subjects (aged 0;9 to 1;8) used more rises than falls in utterances directed towards their mother than in utterances directed towards others at the earliest period (around 1;3). She interpreted these patterns as being suggestive of a purposeful use of rising intonation to attract attention or gain a response, consistent with the pragmatic function of intonation. However, the functional distinction between pragmatic meaning and emotional level is difficult to make (Snow and Balog, 2002). When children are seeking a response, they may have greater strength of emotion than when not seeking a response (Marcos, 1987). Other studies show increasingly consistent associations between intonation and function with increased age and linguistic development (Furrow, 1984).

Transitional Phase between One- and Two-Word Utterances

In prosodic development, much discussion has been given to the transitional phase when children begin to combine two or more words. Two-word utterances of the transitional phase have been referred to as **Successive Single Word Utterances** (SSWU) (Bloom, 1973). Acoustic studies of transitional forms show that they differ from later, multi-word utterances in a number of ways. Successive single words may be characterized by unique intonational contours on each word, primary stress on each word, and significant pauses between words (Branigan, 1979; Fónagy, 1972). In contrast, two-word utterances typically have an integrated intonation contour, one syllable more stressed than the other, and no separation by a pause (Crystal, 1986b; Scollon, 1976).

Those authors who have studied this period of development emphasize the great deal of variability evident in the prosodic realization of children's early word combinations (Behrens and Gut, 2005; Branigan, 1979; Crystal, 1986b). Branigan and Stokes (1984) reported that utterances with and without pauses can coexist together for a period of time. Crystal (1986b) gives the example of the two-word combination "daddy eat" which he observed produced with 12 different prosodic realizations, involving different pause lengths, intonational contours, and stress patterns as seen in (2).

(2) Different prosodic realizations of the two word combination "daddy eat" (Crystal, 1986b, pp. 45-46) ("." indicates a short pause, "-" and "—" indicate pauses of increasing length; accents above vowels indicate falling and rising pitch contours; capitalization indicates stress; "/" indicates tone units or sense groups).

DÀDDY/ — ÈAT/	DÁDDY/ — ÈAT/
DÀDDY/ - ÈAT/	DÁDDY/ - ÈAT/
DÀDDY/ . ÈAT/	DÁDDY/ . ÈAT/
DÀDDY/ÈAT/	DÁDDY/ÈAT/
daddy ÈAT	DÁDDY eat/
DÀDDY eat	DÁDDY ÈAT/

Behrens and Gut (2005) report that syntactically different word combinations may be characterized by different prosodic patterns, which, in turn, may have different developmental trajectories. They studied four different word combinations (e.g., noun + noun repetitions, noun + particle combinations, noun + infinitive combinations, and determiner + noun combinations) in the speech of a German-speaking boy, aged 2;0 to 2;3. The noun + noun repetitions (e.g., "*Eichi Eichi*," "squirrel squirrel") functioned as a control condition, being analogous to SSWUs. These did not show any signs of increasing prosodic integration throughout the developmental period. The other three types of word combinations did undergo prosodic integration, but at different times and in different ways. Behrens and Gut (2005) underscore the difficulty of distinguishing SSWUs and two-word utterances purely on prosodic grounds. They also call for caution "when taking prosody as a diagnostic cue for syntactic development" (p. 22).

To summarize this section on early prosodic production:

- Acoustic studies indicate the presence of language-specific differences in prosody already during the babbling period, although the most consistent findings stem from the period in which children produce their first words.

- Children use different prosodic cues to indicate pragmatic (or emotional) intention from an early age.
- The transitional phase between one- and two-word utterances is marked by considerable variability such that children's early two-word utterances are not yet stable prosodic units.

The next sections of the chapter examine the development of different prosodic phenomena such as stress, timing, and intonation.

Stress

Stress refers to the increased prominence given to a syllable in a word or a word in a sentence. Thus, two types of stress can be distinguished: lexical (i.e., prominence given to a syllable in word) and phrasal (i.e., prominence given to a word in a sentence). Most attention in the literature has been given to the development of lexical stress, perhaps because much of the literature focuses on English, but there are isolated studies on the development of phrasal stress as well. When marking stress, children need to coordinate the phonetic features of stress (i.e., F_0, intensity, duration) to create prominence on one syllable. Several studies have also explored children's phonetic capacities to mark stress. This section first examines children's acquisition of the phonetic correlates associated with stress. It then goes on to examine children's acquisition of lexical stress, stress errors, phrasal and contrastive stress, and compound stress. Some discussion on children's sentence stress comprehension will be provided at the end of this section.

Acoustic Correlates of Stress

Children are already capable of producing multisyllabic vocalizations during babbling, in which one syllable is perceived as more prominent than the others. In a study of babbling by English infants 7 to 12 months of age, researchers found that the syllables perceived as stressed were characterized by increased values of all three correlates (F_0, intensity, duration) in 45% of disyllables, by increased values of two correlates in 40-45% of disyllables, and by a single correlate in 10% of disyllables (Davis, MacNeilage, Matyear, and Powell, 2000). Syllables perceived as evenly stressed were not characterized by any differences between acoustic parameters. When compared to adults, infants produced ratios of stressed to unstressed syllable values for F_0 and intensity that were virtually the same as adults'. Ratios for duration were different because adults displayed final syllable lengthening in contrast to infants who did not display a tendency to produce longer durations on final syllables. From this research, Davis et al. (2000) concluded that infants already control the acoustic correlates of stress in an adult-like manner in this pre-linguistic period. However, it must be remembered that no linguistic intent can be inferred from these vocalizations, simply that adult listeners agree that one syllable of the disyllable is stressed. Davis et al. (2000) posited that the task for children later in development is to link up their physiological capacity of producing perceptible stress to their lexical representations.

A number of studies have examined the acoustic correlates of stress in children's early word productions (Kehoe, Stoel-Gammon and Buder, 1995; Pollock, Brammer, and Hageman, 1993; Schwartz, Petinou, Goffman, Lazowski, and Cartusciello, 1996). All of them show that children develop adult-like use of the phonetic parameters of stress early on, albeit with considerable variability. In a study of imitated productions, Pollock et al. (1993) found that 3- and 4-year-old children use higher F_0, greater intensity, and longer duration to mark stressed syllables; however, 2-year-old children use a single cue, longer duration. In contrast, Kehoe et al. (1995) found that children as young as 1;6 mark differences between stressed and unstressed syllables in disyllabic words by all three parameters in spontaneous speech. This research suggests that children's control over phonetic parameters may emerge earlier in natural than imitated speech. An acoustic analysis of productions perceived to be incorrectly stressed revealed that the stressed syllable was often characterized by increased duration, but minimal F_0 and amplitude differences. In contrast, productions perceived to be correctly stressed were characterized by a coming together of all three phonetic parameters on the stressed syllable. Taken together, studies suggest that around 20-30% of two-year old children's multisyllabic productions may be ambiguous in terms of the acoustic marking of stress (Kehoe, 1995; Pollock et al., 1993).

One final question is whether children control one acoustic parameter earlier than another in stress acquisition and in prosodic acquisition in general. A tentative order has been proposed such that F_0 is controlled earlier than duration, which is controlled earlier than amplitude (Kehoe et al., 1995; Levitt, 1993; Prieto, Estrella, Thorson and Vanrell, 2011).

Stress Acquisition and Stress Errors

How do children acquire the stress pattern of their native language? Do children acquire stress on a word-by-word basis or by rule (Fikkert, 1994; Hochberg, 1988a, 1988b)? Children have heard most of the words that they will produce correctly stressed so they need only memorize the stress pattern of each individual word. Given that stress-rule learning is often complicated by large numbers of exceptional forms, memorization may be the easiest route for the learner to take. Several studies have examined children's stress production on exceptional stress forms. If children internalize a rule of stress, one should observe consistent and systematic stress errors when new words deviate from conventional stress.

One of the first researchers to study stress acquisition in detail and to situate it within modern linguistic theoretical frameworks (e.g., nonlinear and metrical phonology) was Fikkert (1994). In her study of the prosodic development of Dutch-speaking children, she observed greater numbers of stress errors in two-syllable words when the stressed syllable was the exception to the stress rule (i.e., word final in Dutch). This result confirmed Fikkert's (1994) thesis that metrical structure and rules were important in children's acquisition of stress. Several other studies have documented greater numbers of stress errors in irregular, compared to regular, stressed words and a strong tendency by children to regularize irregular patterns in various languages (Hochberg, 1988a, 1988b in Spanish, Kehoe (1997, 1998) in English, and Nouveau (1994) in Dutch). Examples of stress errors in English are provided in (3).

(3) Examples of stress errors in English in children aged 2;3 and 2;10 (from Kehoe, 1998; Kehoe and Stoel-Gammon, 1997):

(a) Two-syllable words with final stress

guitar	/gəˈtɑɹ/	[ˈgɪdə]	27f2
balloon	/bəˈlun/	[ˈbɑlu]	27f2
shampoo	/ʃæmˈpu/	[ˈʃɑpu]	27f6

(b) Three-syllable words with final stress

kangaroo	/ˌkæŋgəˈɹu/	[ˈtʰenʤəˌɹu]	34f2
chimpanzee	/ˌʧɪmpænˈzi/	[ˈʧɪbənˌdiː]	34f2

(c) Four-syllable words with initial stress

alligator	/ˈæləˌgeɾɚ/	[ˌæləˈgetɚ]	27m2
caterpillar	/ˈkæɾəˌpɪlɚ/	[ˌkæɾəˈpɪlɚ]	27m6

Thus, there seems to be evidence that children do not simply memorize stress patterns but use some sort of rule system (or set parameters). Nevertheless, there is a puzzling aspect to stress development, namely, that stress errors do not occur very often (Kehoe and Stoel-Gammon, 1997; Pollock et al., 1993; Prieto et al., 2011; Wijnen, Krikhaar, and Den Os, 1994).

Several investigators have observed that children may shift stress to an unstressed syllable for articulatory reasons (Klein, 1984; Hochberg, 1988a; Kehoe, 1997). For example, Hochberg (1988a) and Kehoe (1997) observed a shift of stress to syllables containing rhotacized vowels (see examples in (4)). To conclude, stress errors do seem to occur as the result of rule-based factors; however they tend to be infrequent and idiosyncratic (vary from child to child). Other factors, such as segmental focus or lack of mastery of the phonetic parameters of stress, may play a role in the perception of misplaced stress.

(4) Examples of stress errors associated with rhotacized vowels (adapted from Kehoe, 1997, p.404).

alligator	/ˈæləˌgeɾɚ/	[ˌælgəˈdɝ]	27m1
		[ˈæləˌgeˌtɝ]	27m2
helicopter	/ˈhɛləˌkɑptɚ/	[ˌhɛloˌkɑpˈtɝ]	27f1

Sound file 7S1 contains examples of English-speaking children's productions of multisyllabic words with correct and shifted stress. Sound files 7S2 and 7S3 illustrate correct lexical stress produced by two French-speaking children. Sound files 7S4 and 7S5 illustrate correct lexical stress produced by two German-speaking children. Sound file 7S6 illustrates correct lexical stress produced by a Spanish-speaking child.

Access Sound File 1 (Chapter 7)

7S1 English-speaking children, aged 2;10, producing "crocodile," "helicopter," and "kangaroo" with correct and shifted stress

Access Sound File 2 (Chapter 7)

7S2 French-speaking boy, aged 2;9, producing disyllabic words (“*cheval* ,“ “*fantôme*“)

Access Sound File 3 (Chapter 7)

7S3 French-speaking girl, aged 1;10, producing disyllabic words (“*biberon,*“ “*poisson,*“ “*tortue,*“ “*assiette*“)

Access Sound File 4 (Chapter 7)

7S4 German-speaking girl, aged 2;6, producing disyllabic words (“*Puppe*,” “*Sonne*,” “*Walde*”)

Access Sound File 5 (Chapter 7)

7S5 German-speaking boy, aged 2;6, producing disyllabic words (“*Hause*,” “*Henne*”)

Access Sound File 6 (Chapter 7)

7S6 Spanish-speaking boy, aged 2;6, producing disyllabic words (“*barco*,” “*bota*,” “*corto*,” “*gato*,” “*grande*,” “*malo*”)

Phrasal and Contrastive Stress

The few studies that have investigated children’s development of phrasal stress tend to show early productive competence, which includes awareness of semantic relationships in phrases and new information. Early research suggests that semantic relations even play a stronger role than syntactic categories and word position in determining which word is stressed in the phrase productions of children aged 1;9 to 2;5 years. Wieman (1976) observed that verb-locative constructions were characterized by stress on the locative element regardless of whether the locative was a noun ("play MUSEUM") or a preposition ("coming UP"), and regardless of whether it appeared in the first or second position ("HERE goes" or "goes HERE" for meaning "it goes here"). Exceptions to these patterns often arose because the child was marking new information. For example, Seth deviated from the typical pattern of stressing the noun in attributive phrases when introducing a word and then adding new information about it. Examples from Wieman (1976) are given in (5).

(5) Seth using stress to mark new information (Examples taken from Wieman, 1976, p.286)

Man. BLUE man.
Ball. NICE ball. ORANGE ball.
No sock. BLUE sock.

From the age of 2;9 to 4;6, children have been found to demonstrate a clear use of contrastive stress to signal new information when describing sequences of pictures or when responding to Yes-No questions (Baltaxc, 1984; Hornby and Hass, 1970). Contrastive stress is more prevalent when the contrasting element is in subject than when it is in the predicate position (either verb or object).

Compound Word versus Phrasal Stress

Another aspect of stress development is acquiring the distinction between a compound word and a phrase ("hotdog" vs. "hot dog"). A compound word receives stress on the first syllable whereas a phrase receives stress on the rightmost syllable, as shown in (6). Following Vogel and Raimy (2002), we display the difference between compound words and phrases according to grid convention, in which the grid mark at the highest level indicates primary stress. Examples of well-known compound nouns and their phrasal counterparts are given in (7).

(6) Compound vs. Phrasal Stress (Vogel and Raimy, 2002, p.228)

Compound	X		Phrase			X
Word	X	X	Word		X	X
Syllable	X	X	Syllable	X	X	X
	HOT	dog			hot	DOG

(7) Examples of compound nouns and noun phrases

Compound Noun	*Noun Phrase*
tightrope	tight rope
hotdog	hot dog
Big Bird (Sesame street character)	big bird
blackbird	black bird
White House (home of the president of the USA)	white house
greenhouse	green house

Two-year-old children can already produce compound words with the correct compound word stress pattern (Clark, Gelman, and Lane, 1985). Yet, detailed experimental studies reveal that the distinction between compound noun and phrasal stress is a later acquired phenomenon (Atkinson-King, 1973; Vogel and Raimy, 2002). Comprehension and production tests indicate that five-year-old children are unable to distinguish or produce compound or phrasal stress correctly, but by grade three, children's average performance is 78% on comprehension and more than half the children can make consistent distinctions in production (Atkinson-King, 1973; for similar results in comprehension see Vogel and Raimy, 2002). Children have also been found to display a strong preference for the compound interpretation for words they know, but a preference for the phrasal interpretation for words they don't know (Vogel and Raimy, 2002). Vogel and Raimy (2002) posited that the knowledge required to distinguish between compound and phrasal stress is abstract and requires access to higher level phonological constituents. This is why it takes longer to acquire than lexical stress does, which only requires access to lower level constituents such as the foot and prosodic word.

Comprehension versus Production Asymmetry in Phrasal and Sentence Stress

The production studies reviewed above revealed that children are capable of stressing new information in a phrase or sentence by the age range 2 to 4 years (Baltaxe, 1984; Hornby and Hass, 1970; Wieman, 1976). In contrast, comprehension studies indicate children have weaker abilities in using prosody for phrasal and sentence comprehension. It appears that only by the age of 6 years or later can children interpret stress and new information (Cutler and Swinney, 1987; Gualmini, Maciukaite, and Crain, 2003; Solan, 1980; see review by Grassman and Tomasello, 2010).

The asymmetry between production and comprehension in the acquisition of prosody is paradoxical since comprehension precedes production in most areas of language acquisition. Several authors have offered possible reasons for the asymmetrical findings, the most common one being differences in the nature of the experimental tasks (Grassman and Tomasello, 2010; Hendriks and Koster, 2010; Zhou, Su, Crain, Gao, and Zhan, 2011). Production studies have tended to use simpler tasks, such as picture description or question responses, in contrast to comprehension studies which have used more complex methodologies such as asking children about the meaning of sentences. Production studies have also been primarily concerned with the mapping between new information and stress, whereas comprehension studies have tended to go beyond this, examining the use of stress to disambiguate particular linguistic items (Chen, 2010).

More recently, studies using on-line methodologies (e.g., eye tracking) have revealed superior ability in sentence comprehension than has previously been indicated by off-line tasks (Chen, 2010; Grassman and Tomasello, 2010; Zhou et al., 2011). In sum, the proposed asymmetry between comprehension and the production of sentence prosody may be more apparent than real when experimental task differences are taken into account.

To summarize the section on stress:

- Children display adult-like use of the phonetic parameters of stress from an early age, although up to 20-30% of their early multisyllabic productions may be unreliable in terms of stress placement. Pitch appears to be the phonetic parameter mastered the earliest.

- Analyses of children's stress errors indicate that children internalize rules of stress, although, in general, stress misplacement errors are infrequent. The perception of misplaced stress may also arise from segmental factors.
- Children display awareness of semantic relations and new information in their early use of phrasal stress.
- The distinction between compound and phrasal stress appears to be a later-acquired phenomenon.
- There appears to be a production versus comprehension asymmetry in children's acquisition of phrasal and sentence stress. Children acquire the productive aspects of contrastive stress earlier than their understanding of them. Some of this disparity may relate to methodological differences between production versus comprehension studies.

Timing

Timing refers to the temporal aspects of prosody. It plays a major role in our perception of speech rhythm and is implicated in the marking of boundary phenomena such as phrase final lengthening. This section considers studies on rhythm and phrase final lengthening in young children's speech.

Rhythm

Rhythm is an area of prosody that is very difficult to quantify. Most definitions of rhythm refer to two phenomena: accentuation and timing, with the primary emphasis given to timing in recent acoustic measurement procedures. Discussions of rhythm also refer to a dichotomy of rhythm types. As mentioned above, some languages (e.g., English, German) are said to have a temporal organization based on stress, the so-called stress-timed languages, whereas other languages (e.g., French, Italian, and Spanish) have a temporal organization based on syllables, the so-called syllable-timed languages (Dauer, 1983, 1987; Pike, 1945; Roach, 1982). In a stress-timed language, the intervals between stressed syllables are thought to be roughly of equal length, whereas in a syllable-timed language, the syllables are roughly of equal length. Numerous studies have measured the length of inter-stress intervals and the lengths of syllables in a variety of the world's languages, yet none has confirmed the notion of isochronous units (equal time intervals). Nevertheless, time intervals and temporal organization are essential to the concept of rhythm and have been taken up in more recent acoustic quantifications that involve the measurement of vowel and consonant durations (Low, Grabe and Nolan, 2001; Ramus, Nespor and Mehler, 1999).

Two main approaches to the measurement of rhythm have been developed which involve segmenting an utterance into a succession of vocalic and consonantal intervals. An interval refers to either one vowel or to one consonant, or to a sequence of vowels and consonants, regardless of whether they belong to the same syllable or not.

In Ramus et al.'s (1999) approach, the duration of vocalic and consonantal intervals is submitted to three calculations:

- the percent of vocalic intervals within the sentence (%V),
- the standard deviation of the duration of vowel intervals (ΔV),
- the standard deviation of the duration of consonantal intervals (ΔC),

whereby %V and ΔC have been found to be the most robust predictors of rhythm types. In Low et al.'s (2001) approach, differences in the duration between successive pairs of intervals are measured using a metric called the Pairwise Variability Index (PVI). The main insight of both of these procedures is that when the duration of successive intervals is relatively similar, low standard deviations and low variability indices will be computed. This is the case in syllable-timed languages that tend to have syllables of similar length. They will also have high %V scores due to the absence of vowel reduction and stress-related effects. When the duration of successive intervals is highly variable, high standard deviations and high variability indices should be computed. This is the case in stress-timed languages that have syllables of different lengths due to the effects of stress, vowel reduction, and syllable structure.

Several different studies have applied these measures, in particular the PVI, to the productions of children acquiring languages traditionally considered stress- and syllable-timed (English, French and German in Grabe, Gut, Post and Watson,1999a, Grabe, Post, and Watson, 1999b; English and Spanish in Bunta and Ingram, 2007; Spanish and German in Kehoe and Lleó, 2005; Kehoe, Lleó, and Rakow, 2011; English and Cantonese in Mok, 2011). Collectively, these findings show that cross-linguistic differences in rhythmic patterns are evident in the speech of three- to four-year old children. These cross-linguistic results are consistent with the rhythmic patterns of the ambient languages and with the distinction of stress versus syllable timed. Another important finding of these studies is that the syllable-timed pattern appears to be linguistically less **marked** from a developmental point of view than the stress-timed pattern.

Overall, findings are consistent with a bias towards syllable timing in the speech of young children. Here, we are reminded of earlier statements on rhythmic development made three decades ago by Allen and Hawkins (1979, 1980). Their definition of rhythm encompassed two main areas: syllable weight and accentuation. They noted that it was the syllable weight that posed the most problems at the early stages: two-year old children use far fewer reduced syllables and more uniform syllable structure than adults, giving the impression that all syllables are equally heavy. Learning phrase rhythm, in their view, involved learning to reduce heavy syllables with full vowels.

Measuring rhythm based on consonant and vowel durations has shown considerable promise in distinguishing languages traditionally classified as stress or syllable timed (Grabe and Low, 2002; Low et al., 2001; Ramus et al., 1999) and in distinguishing cross-linguistic prosodic patterns in early child speech (Bunta and Ingram, 2007; Grabe et al., 1999a, 1999b; Kehoe and Lleó, 2005; Kehoe et al, 2011; Mok, 2011). Nevertheless, several authors have recently criticized current acoustic measurement techniques, noting, in particular, their over reliance on vowel and consonant duration and their failure to take into account prominence or other physical properties (Kohler, 2009; Nolan and Asu, 2009). Thus, the task of defining and quantifying rhythm remains an ongoing enterprise.

Phrase Final Lengthening

Phrase final lengthening (PFL) is a timing feature associated with syntactic boundaries. It refers to the process by which the last syllable of a phrase is lengthened (Oller, 1973). The corresponding feature with respect to pitch is the declination of F_0 at the end of phrase and clause boundaries. This section discusses PFL; the next section discusses the use of intonation to mark boundaries.

There has been much discussion in the literature concerning the origin and function of PFL. Some consider it to be a physiological tendency, closely linked to intonation (Lyberg, 1979). Others consider it a learned grammatical effect which helps the listener to segment syntactic units (Klatt, 1975). Studies on the acquisition of PFL and intonation should help to tease out these competing theories. According to the first view, referred to as the F_0 dependent model (Lindblom, 1978), final syllables are lengthened in order to accommodate the F_0 contour, thus, implying a close association between intonation and PFL in development. According to the second view, intonation and PFL are learned at different times (Snow, 1994). Studies that have examined the acquisition of PFL present conflicting findings. Some find it present in pre-linguistic speech (e.g., Robb and Saxman, 1990); others find it develops later (e.g., Davis et al., 2000; Oller and Smith, 1977).

One of the most definitive studies of PFL is that of Snow (1994) who investigated PFL and intonation in nine children at the one-word stage of linguistic development (aged 1;0 to 1;8). Snow (1994) reported a U-shaped acquisition pattern, in which the final lengthening contrast declined to a minimum point, half way through the testing period and then re-established itself later. The re-emergence of PFL was most closely time-locked to the beginning of combinatorial speech. Snow (1994) argued that the earlier presence of PFL was possibly due to biological factors (see *Sidebar 4 Regression in Prosodic Development)*. The later reappearance of PFL suggests that it is an acquired phenomenon closely associated with the development of syntax. The discontinuity in PFL occurred in the absence of a change in intonation development, indicating that PFL is not an epiphenomenon of tone production.

Cross-linguistic differences in the development of PFL have been reported. Whereas PFL is associated with the appearance of combinatorial speech in English (Oller and Smith, 1977; Snow, 1994), it appears earlier in French possibly due to the fact that the stress pattern is simpler and it is also phrase-final (Konopczynsky, 1990). D'Odorico and Carubbi (2003) found that Italian-speaking children, aged 1:3 to 2;4, followed a similar developmental pattern to English speaking children. However, they also lengthened the stress bearing non-final syllable as well as the final syllable, consistent with the prosodic characteristics of Italian, in which stressed syllables are long. D'Odorico and Carubbi's (2003) results were in accordance with Snow (1994); they found that children control intonation and PFL independently; however, they still observed that PFL was partially influenced by different intonation models.

To summarize the section on timing:

- Recent acoustic measures of rhythm show that three- to four-year old children display cross-linguistic differences in rhythmic variability consistent with the distinction stress versus syllable timing.
- Several sources of evidence suggest that syllable-timed rhythm is less marked than stress-timed.
- Phrase-final lengthening appears to be a learned phenomenon associated with the development of combinatorial speech. It is acquired independently of intonation.

Intonation

Intonation involves the patterning of pitch changes in utterances. Some important questions that have been asked in intonation research are how early do children acquire adult-like intonation and whether intonation is more closely tied to lexical versus grammatical development. Many researchers claim that children acquire intonation before they produce their first words. Others claim that children acquire intonation later in development. Certain authors observe that growth in intonation coincides with the appearance of two-word combinations, at around 18-months (Snow, 2006). Other authors argue that intonation production is more closely related to lexical knowledge (Chen and Fikkert, 2007; Prieto et al., 2011). The general consensus is that children do not control intonation before they produce their first words (Snow and Balog, 2002). Rather, they control certain aspects of intonation by the time they have amassed a certain number of words. There still remains some debate as to whether this occurs before of after the onset of combinatorial speech (Prieto et al., 2011; Snow and Balog, 2002).

Intonation serves several different functions (e.g., affective, pragmatic, and grammatical). It is also characterized by several different formal features relating to the direction and complexity of the pitch contour as well as to the magnitude of pitch change. Thus, any review of intonation development should consider its functional as well as its formal aspects. By the former, we mean: how early do children use intonation to convey affective, pragmatic, and grammatical intention? By the latter, we mean: how early do children produce intonation that resembles adult-like intonation in terms of the direction, complexity, and magnitude of pitch contour? There are two main linguistic frameworks for the measurement of intonation. One is the nuclear tone approach, which represents intonation in terms of contours such as fall and rise (Cruttenden, 1997). The other is the autosegmental metrical approach, which represents intonation in terms of level pitch targets and high-low tone melodies (Pierrehumbert, 1980). The autosegmental metrical approach has only recently been applied to children's speech; however, advocates claim that it provides a more fine-grained tool to analyze pitch contours than the traditional dichotomy of fall versus rise.

Functional Development of Intonation

Children's use of pitch contours to signal meaning was already discussed above in the section on pragmatic differentiation. This review showed that infants use distinct pitch contours in different contexts from early on, suggesting that the functional aspects of intonation are acquired very early. Nevertheless, some researchers question whether early intonation signals pragmatic intent or simply an emotional level (Snow and Balog, 2002). The distinction is often difficult to make. The current section focuses on children's acquisition of the grammatical use of intonation. A clear illustration of children's grammatical use of intonation is the marking of utterance-final position by a falling tone. The classical approach of assessing children's use of falling intonation is to compare the width of pitch change in accented final and accented non-final syllables. Snow refers to this method of assessing children's intonation as the contrast criterion. Using this approach, he and other researchers have observed that children around 1;6 years and older produce utterance-final syllables with lower F_0 than non-final syllables, thus, suggesting that they can control the boundary marking function of intonation (Branigan, 1979; Fónagy, 1972; Snow, 1994). One-year-old children, however, do not produce a wider pitch contrast in final than in non-final syllables, indicating that they have not yet acquired the grammatical use of intonation (Snow, 2004).

Formal Development of Intonation

Important formal features of intonation are: direction (whether rising or falling), complexity of contour (i.e., whether a fall or rise is preceded by a pitch change in the opposite direction), and degree of accent change (Snow and Balog, 2002). Over three decades ago, Crystal (1986b) proposed a tentative order of tonal development in English, which included contrasts involving direction and range, as shown in (8).

(8) Stage 1: falling tones
Stage 2: falling vs. level tones
Stage 3: falling vs. high rising tones
Stage 4: falling vs. high falling tones
Stage 5: rising vs. high rising tones
Stage 6: falling vs. high rising-falling tones
Stage 7: rising vs. falling-rising tones
Stage 8: Later contrasts, e.g., high vs. low rising-falling tones

These stages (referred to as tonal contrasts by Crystal, 1986b) were based on his own work as well as findings by Halliday (1975) and Menn (1976). Verification of this order of tonal contrasts in a large scale study appears to be lacking; however, different studies support certain aspects of this order such as the fact that falling tones are acquired before rising tones and that simple (unidirectional) contours are acquired before complex (bidirectional) ones. Snow (1995) observed a great deal of variability in children's acquisition of complexity between the ages of 1;6 and 2;0, suggesting that children vary considerably in the later stages of tonal contrast.

In studying accent range, Snow (1995, 2004) uses the term magnitude criterion to refer to whether the width of the pitch change of the nuclear tone in child speech is comparable to that of an adult speaker. In fact, many studies report a high proportion of level contours in infant speech suggesting that children's production of accent range is not adult-like (Snow and Balog, 2002). For example, Marcos (1987) found that more than half the numbers of utterances in her study of French-speaking infants, aged 1;2 to 1;10, were level contours. Snow (2002, 2004) observed that one-year-old infants produce monosyllabic falling tones with a narrower accent range than four-year-olds, indicating that they have not acquired intonation based on the magnitude criterion. In contrast, four-year-olds, when imitating declarative sentences with falling intonation, produce an accent range that is comparable to that of adults. In between these age groups, there is some evidence that children aged 1;6 are able to produce accent ranges that approach those of preschool-aged children (see discussion in Snow and Balog, 2002).

Are Falling Contours Less Marked than Rising Contours?

Many studies on children's early intonation have observed a predominance of falling over rising contours (Behrens and Gut, 2005; Chen and Fikkert, 2007; Chen and Kent, 2009; Kent and Murray, 1982; Snow, 2006). A physiological explanation has been proposed to explain the preponderance of falling over rising tones since a falling contour corresponds to the natural decline of subglottal pressure at the end of an utterance (Lieberman, 1986). Nevertheless, language experience can alter this natural tendency; cross-linguistic studies show that language-specific intonation patterns, including rising tones, may be evident in babbling and first words (Hallé et al., 1991; Whalen et al., 1991). Despite these cross-linguistic trends, there is some evidence that falling contours are acquired earlier than rising contours (Snow, 2002), are less variable than rising tones (Snow and Stoel-Gammon, 1994), are substituted for rising contours (Lleó, Rakow, and Kehoe, 2004), and are by far the most frequent contours of children at the two-word stage (Behrens and Gut, 2005). Prieto et al. (2011) question the "**unmarked**" status of falling tones. They point out that this notion stems from an over-reliance on the holistic/contour approach in which intonation has only been classified into two possible patterns. More recent work in intonation shows that children are capable of producing more complex melodies than rising and falling contours from an early age. Furthermore, falling contours are the predominant pattern in many of the languages studied in developmental intonation research and, therefore, it is not surprising that they appear to be produced first.

Later Intonation Development

Most studies on intonation development focus on the preschool years, but there are some indications that intonation continues to develop after the age of five years (Cruttenden, 1974; see Sidebar 7.5: Late Intonation). Wells, Peppé and Goulandris (2004) administered a battery of prosodic tasks, which tapped the production and comprehension of different aspects of intonation, to children aged 5 to 13 years. They found that, in general, the productive aspects of intonation were acquired by 5 years, but that certain aspects of intonation comprehension continued to develop through to the age of 10 years and beyond. This finding is reminiscent of the asymmetry between production and comprehension discussed earlier in the case of contrastive stress (see Cutler and Swinney, 1987). Findings on the comprehension tasks correlated with the results of receptive and expressive language tests, suggesting that intonation comprehension develops hand in hand with grammatical development.

Sidebar 7.5. Late Intonation

Cruttenden (1974) tested children's use of intonation to predict the results of a football match. For example, children heard a radio or TV announcer producing the phrase *"Liverpool, three/ Everton..."* and they were required to determine whether the score was going to be a draw, a win, or a loss for the home team. On the basis of intonation, the outcome of the game is predictable. The first team and its score (e.g., Liverpool three) are produced with a rising pitch contour. The second team and its score (e.g., Everton…) is characterized by a falling pitch contour for a draw; by a lower tone for a home win; and by a higher tone and increased emphasis for a home loss. A schematic representation of the pitch contours is shown below (adapted from Crystal, 1986a, pp. 235-236).

Cruttenden (1974) played recordings of typical announcer intonation to a group of 28 boys, aged 7 to 10 years. He found that most of the children, even those who were football fanatics, were unable to perform this task. Most of the 10-year-olds hadn't reached the competence levels of adults, and only one of the 28 children scored all items correct.

To summarize the section on intonation:

- Children as young as 1;6 years produce a wider accent range in final than in non-final syllables, suggesting that they control the boundary-marking function of intonation. This is an illustration of the grammatical use of intonation. Children's use of intonation to signal other functions (pragmatic, affective) appears to be acquired very early (see Section on Pragmatic Differentiation).

- There is some debate as to whether intonation development is more closely associated with lexical or grammatical development. The main generalization appears to be that children display an "intonation burst" after they can produce a certain number of words.
- Children somewhere between the ages of 1;6 and 4;0 years are capable of producing accent ranges that approximate adult values.
- Many (but not all) sources of evidence suggest that falling contours are acquired before rising contours.
- Intonation development, particularly comprehension of intonation, continues to develop after the pre-school years.

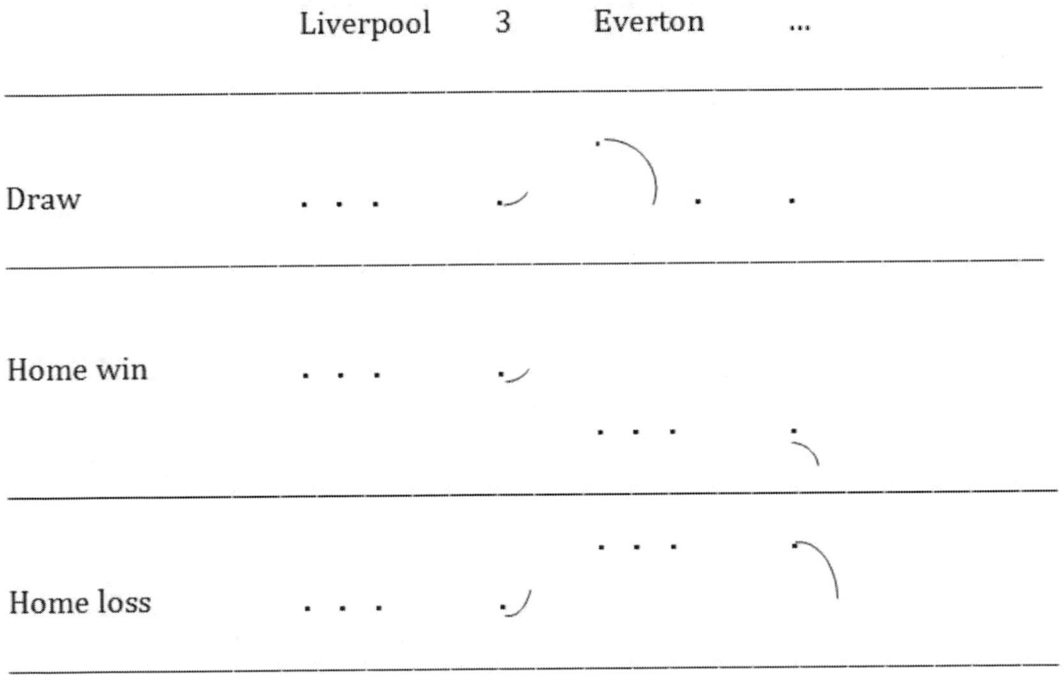

Atypical Prosody

Atypical prosody is associated with certain clinical populations such as autism spectrum disorder (ASD), childhood apraxia of speech (CAS), and specific language impairment (SLI). A brief summary of prosodic differences follows.

Sidebar 7.6. Atypical Prosody in a Normally Developing Child

Some normally developing children may display unusual prosodic patterns at certain times in development. In Kehoe and Stoel-Gammon's (1997) study of English-speaking children's multisyllabic productions, one child (28m2), aged 2;4, appeared to operate with an iambic template as shown in the examples below:

picture	/ˈpɪktʃɚ/	[pɪkˈtʃɝ]
apple	/ˈæpl/	[æˈboʊː]
banana	/bəˈnænə/	[næˈnɑː]
helicopter	/ˈhɛləˌkɑptɚ/	[kæˈtʰɝ]

Possible foot structure for 28m2:

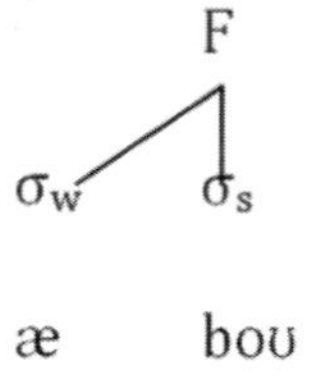

Many of his productions of three- and four-syllable words involved reduplications of stressed syllables and epenthesis in what appeared to be an attempt to produce two stressed feet. The pattern that resulted was (WS) (S) or (WS) (WS) as shown in the examples below.

dinosaur	/ˈdaɪnəˌsɔr/	[haɪˈnɪs ˈhɔː]
elephant	/ˈɛləfɪnt/	[aˈfɪt ˈhɪt]
octopus	/ˈɑktəpʊs/	[aˈbʌtəˌpʊs]

Sound file 7S7 illustrates examples of 28m2's unusual prosodic patterns.

Access Sound File 7 (Chapter 7)

7S7 English-speaking child, aged 2;4, producing multisyllabic words ("alligator," "elephant," "potato," " avocado," "helicopter," "dinosaur," "octopus," "telephone") with several examples of unusual prosodic patterns.

Autism Spectrum Disorder

The speech of individuals with ASD has been described as monotone, sing-song, robotic, stilted, or dull, suggesting they have atypical expressive prosody.

In McCann and Peppé's (2003) review of studies on prosody and autism between the years 1980 to 2002, the most consistent finding in these studies was that individuals with ASD display difficulty with the realization and placement of contrastive stress; however, the authors noted that many of the studies suffered from methodological weaknesses and had contradictory findings. For example, one study indicated that intonation production posed difficulty for children with ASD (Fosnot and Jun, 1999); another did not (Baltaxe and Simmons, 1985).

More recent studies that have tested both perception and production of prosody, and have assessed across different prosodic functions, tend to show that those prosodic areas particularly affected in autism relate to affective and pragmatic functions and those that are less affected are those relating to grammar (e.g., Chevallier, Noveck, Happé and Wilson, 2009; Peppé, McCann, Gibbon, O'Hare, and Rutherford, 2007).

Childhood Apraxia of Speech (CAS)

Atypical prosody was listed as one of the specific features unique to CAS in a position statement issued by the American Speech-Language-Hearing Association in 2007 (http://www.asha.org/docs/html/PS2007-0027html). In particular, an inappropriate use of lexical or phrasal stress appears to be frequent in this clinical group. Shriberg, Aram, and Kwiatkowski (1997c) pooled the results of three studies (Shriberg et al., 1997a,b,c) comparing the segmental and prosodic abilities of children with speech disorders and children suspected of CAS. Approximately half of the children with CAS displayed inappropriate phrasal stress, whereas only 10% of the speech disordered group did. Shriberg et al. (1997c) argue that the presence of inappropriate stress appears to be a diagnostic marker for a subtype of CAS. They dismiss suggestions that it is a compensatory strategy used by children to enhance intelligibility since they did not find inappropriate stress to be more prevalent in older versus younger subjects or in long complex phrases versus short simple phrases. If inappropriate stress was a compensatory pattern, one would expect to see it more developed in older subjects and used more frequently for more complex linguistic material. This was not the case. Shriberg et al. (1997c) argue that the prosodic difficulties of CAS stem from a phonological representational deficit rather than a motor speech one. Sound file 7S8 is an example of conversational speech recorded from an 11-year-old boy with a history of severe CAS, and sound file 7S9 was recorded from his identical twin brother, also with a history of severe CAS. What do you notice about lexical stress, intonation, and rate?

Access Sound File 8 (Chapter 7)

7S8 Conversational speech of a boy, age 11, with a history of severe childhood apraxia of speech.

Access Sound File 9 (Chapter 7)

7S9 Conversational speech of the identical twin brother of the boy in 7S9, also with a history of severe childhood apraxia of speech.

Specific Language Impairment (SLI)

Numerous studies have examined the prosodic abilities of children with SLI; some studies find evidence for disordered prosody and some find less evidence. For example, children with SLI have been found to have difficulty using and processing prosodic cues in acquiring the formal properties of a language (Weinert, 1992). In the area of expressive prosody, several studies report increased percentages of weak syllable omissions among the SLI population in comparison to younger, normally developing language-age matched children (Bortolini and Leonard, 2000; Owen, Dromi, and Leonard, 2001). This suggests that phonology is a vulnerable area for SLI children. Certain studies also show a correlation between the percentage of weak syllable omissions in words and the percentage of grammatical morphemes in sentences (Bortolini and Leonard, 2000). While it is acknowledged that phonological/prosodic limitations may explain some of the morphological errors of SLI children, most authors concede that the phonological and morphological deficits of SLI are separate to some degree (Bortolini and Leonard, 2000; Owen et al., 2001).

Apart from deficits in syllable-based phonological processes, prosody does not appear to be a core impairment of children with SLI. Snow (2001) did not find any differences between SLI children and an age-matched control group in an intonation imitation task. This was despite the fact that the SLI group had significantly lower segmental phonological abilities as determined by the percentage of consonants correct. Snow (2001) concluded that segmental and prosodic levels of phonology are disassociated in SLI children.

Other studies have found isolated differences between SLI children and age-matched controls on certain subtests of the Profiling Elements of Prosodic Systems-Children test (PEPS-C, Peppé and McCann, 2003), but no differences have been found between SLI children and language-matched controls (Wells and Peppé, 2003; Marshall, Harcourt-Brown, Ramus, and van der Lely, 2009). In general, children with SLI do not display difficulty discriminating and imitating prosodic forms, but they display weaknesses in those receptive prosodic tasks that interact with the grammatical and pragmatic functions of prosody. This is consistent with the results reported for children with ASD. In other words, children with ASD or SLI do not have difficulty with the formal but rather with the functional aspects of prosody, namely with those tasks in which prosody interacts with linguistic function. In the case of autistic children, it was observed principally with affective and pragmatic functions and in SLI children, with pragmatic and grammatical functions.

To summarize the section on atypical prosody:

- Atypical prosody may be associated with certain clinical groups (ASD, CAS, SLI).
- Autistic children may experience difficulty in prosodic areas related to affective and pragmatic functions.
- Children suspected of having CAS may display inappropriate use of lexical and phrasal stress.
- Children with SLI display certain prosodic difficulties such as increased weak-syllable deletions, and difficulty interpreting grammatical and pragmatic functions in receptive prosodic tasks. Prosody does not appear to be a core impairment of SLI, however.

Connections

Tools for evaluating prosody are described in Chapter 2. Chapter 18, on motor impairment, describes the speech characteristics of childhood apraxia, which was introduced here, in greater detail. Chapter 19 contains additional information about speech characteristics observed in children with autism spectrum disorder. Chapter 20 describes how to assess a child's speech abilities from a clinical perspective.

Concluding Remarks

The aim of this chapter was to provide a comprehensive review of the development of prosody. The first part of the chapter considered perceptual and productive aspects of early prosodic development, as well as individual prosodic systems such as stress, timing, and intonation. The second part of this chapter focused on disordered prosody in several developmental disabilities.

It is clear that a single chapter cannot do justice to the enormous literature base on prosodic development that has amounted in recent years. In particular, we have been unable to cover certain topics such as the phonological aspects of prosodic development or the interface of prosody with semantic, pragmatic and grammatical development. We have also been unable to dwell sufficiently on rapidly growing areas such as the perception of prosody, sentence comprehension, and the development of tone. The fact that the field of prosodic acquisition is expanding is a strong indication of its relevance to key questions in language acquisition such as how children process the incoming speech stream and acquire the grammatical units of the language. This chapter should serve as a comprehensive base for a further exploration of the field of prosodic acquisition.

Chapter Review Questions

1. What are the four main functions of prosody?
2. Cite some of the remarkable speech perception abilities of neonates with respect to prosody.
3. Are there ambient language effects on prosody in infant babbling?
4. Identify possible reasons for misplaced stress in two-year-olds' productions of multisyllabic words.
5. What is the main insight from recent acoustic measurement procedures of rhythm?
6. What are some of the formal aspects of intonation that children need to acquire?
7. Select a clinical group (e.g., ASD, CAS, SLI) and describe some of the prosodic difficulties that may be associated with this group.

Suggestions for Future Reading

Bernhardt, B. and Stemberger, J. (1998). *Handbook of phonological development*. San Diego: Academic Press

Crystal, D. (1986). Prosodic development. In P. Fletcher and M. Garman (Eds.), *Language acquisition: Studies in first language development. Second Edition*. Cambridge, England: Cambridge University Press, pp. 33-48.

Fikkert, P. (1994). *On the acquisition of prosodic structure*. Dordrecht: ICG Printing (HIL Dissertations).

Snow, D. and Balog, H. (2002). Do children produce the melody before the words? A review of developmental intonation research. Lingua, 112, 1025-1058.

Vihman, M. (1996). *Phonological development. The origins of language in the child.* Cambridge, Massachusetts: Blackwell Publishers.

Suggestions for Student Activities

1. As the early section of this chapter emphasized, finding a definition of prosody is not easy. On the basis of what you know about prosody, can you develop your own definition of prosody?
2. Open Sound File 7S1 in an acoustic software program and compare the acoustic parameters of stress in the correctly and incorrectly produced words.
3. Listen to Sound Files 7S2 through 7S6, which consist of disyllabic productions by German-, Spanish-, and French-speaking children. Analyze the acoustic correlates of stress using an acoustic software program such as PRAAT. Do you observe any systematic differences between languages?
4. Import sound files 7S8 and 7S9 into an acoustic software program and observe the following characteristics: durations of stressed and unstressed syllables, average F_0, and intonational contours. Interpret your observations in light of the fact that the two speakers, 11-year-old twin brothers, both had a history of severe CAS.

ANSWERS TO CHAPTER REVIEW QUESTIONS

1. What are the four main functions of prosody?

The four main functions of prosody are:

a) *Indexical_*– Prosody enables us to identify a particular speaker or class of speaker
b) *Affective* – Prosody may indicate a speaker's feelings and emotions
c) *Pragmatic* – Prosody provides focus or highlights information in utterances. (Other examples of pragmatic functions are discussed in the section Pragmatic Differentiation)
d) *Grammatical_*– Prosody may have many grammatical uses. It may demarcate the beginning and ends of syntactic phrases, distinguish whether an utterance is a question or a statement, and distinguish word-classes such as nouns and verbs.

2. Cite some of the remarkable speech perception abilities of neonates with respect to prosody.

Newborns and very young infants can discriminate words containing different stress and intonation contours. For example they can discriminate disyllables differing in stress pattern (ˈbaba vs. baˈba) (Jusczyk and Thompson, 1978; Spring and Dale, 1977), and they can discriminate syllables containing rising vs. falling intonation (Morse, 1972). In addition, they can discriminate intonation differences in the presence of phonetic variations (Nazzi, Floccia and Bertoncini, 1998). Researchers have also shown that newborns can distinguish languages derived from different rhythmic groups (Mehler, Jusczyk, Lambertz, Halsted, Bertoncini and Amiel-Tison, 1988). They also show preferences for certain prosodic patterns: They prefer their own ambient language to other languages (Mehler, Dupoux, Nazzi and Dehaene-Lambertz, 1996) and the exaggerated prosody of child-directed speech to the less intonated patterns of adult-directed speech (Fernald, 1985; Fernald and Kuhl, 1987).

3. Are there ambient language effects on prosody in infant babbling?

There is contradictory evidence for the presence of language-specific prosodic patterns in babbling. Several studies, in which expert listeners have been required to distinguish the babbles of children from different languages, have failed to find evidence for ambient language effects on babbling (Atkinson, MacWhinney, and Stoel, 1968; Engstrand, Williams, and Lacerda, 2003; Olney and Scholnick, 1976; Thevenin, Eilers, Oller, and Lavoie, 1985). Nevertheless, certain studies employing acoustic analyses have revealed clear language-specific prosodic differences in infant babbling. For example, Whalen and colleagues, when comparing the babbles of English- and French-speaking children, found a higher percentage of falling contours in the English infants' compared to the French infants' vocalizations (Whalen, Levitt, and Wang, 1991) and a higher percentage of longer final syllables in the French versus English infants' vocalizations (Levitt and Wang, 1991). The clearest evidence for ambient language effects in prosody, however, is reported after the onset of word production (i.e., the 25-word point and beyond) (Vihman, DePaolis and Davis, 1998).

4. Identify possible reasons for misplaced stress in two-year-olds' productions of multisyllabic words.

Possible reasons for misplaced stress in two-year-olds' word productions include incorrect rule usage (e.g., failure to apply the stress rule), lack of mastery of the phonetic parameters of stress, and segmental focus (shift of stress to a syllable for articulatory reasons).

5. What is the main insight from recent acoustic measurement procedures of rhythm?

In acoustic measurement procedures, such as the ones designed by Ramus, Nespor, and Mehler (1999) and Low, Grabe, and Nolan (2001), speech is segmented into vocalic and consonantal intervals. In Ramus et al.'s (1999) measure, the percent of vocalic intervals within the sentence (%V) as well as the standard deviation of vocalic and consonantal intervals is determined. In Low et al.'s (2001) measure, an index called the Pairwise Variability Index is computed, which calculates differences in duration between successive pairs of intervals. The main insight of both of these procedures is that when the duration of successive intervals is relatively similar, low standard deviations and low variability indices will be computed. This is the case in syllable-timed languages that tend to have syllables of similar length. They will also have high %V scores due to the absence of vowel reduction and stress-related effects. When the duration of successive intervals is highly variable, high standard deviations and high variability indices will be computed. This is the case in stress-timed languages that have syllables of different lengths due to the effects of stress, vowel reduction, and syllable structure. Thus, the rhythm indices distinguish stress vs. syllable timed languages.

6. What are some of the formal aspects of intonation that children need to acquire?

Formal features of intonation that children need to acquire are direction of contour (whether rising or falling), complexity of contour (i.e., whether a fall or rise is preceded by a pitch change in the opposite direction), and degree of accent change (i.e., width of the pitch change) (Snow and Balog, 2002).

7. Select a clinical group (e.g., ASD, CAS, SLI) and describe some of the prosodic difficulties that may be associated with this group.

ASD

Earlier studies report difficulty with the realization and placement of contrastive stress (McCann and Peppé, 2003). More recent studies report prosodic difficulties relating to affective and pragmatic functions and few difficulties relating to the grammatical function (e.g., Chevallier, Noveck, Happé and Wilson, 2009; Peppé, McCann, Gibbon, O'Hare, and Rutherford, 2007).

CAS

Atypical prosody was listed as one of the specific features unique to CAS in a position statement issued by the American Speech-Language-Hearing Association in 2007 (http://www.asha.org/docs/html/PS2007-0027html). In particular, inappropriate use of lexical or phrasal stress appears to be frequent in this group (Shriberg, Aram, and Kwiatkowski, 1997).

SLI

Prosody does not appear to be a core impairment of children with SLI. Nevertheless, several studies have identified prosodic difficulties in SLI children. They include:

a. Difficulty using and processing prosodic cues in acquiring the formal properties of a language (Weinert, 1992);
b. Increased percentages of weak syllable omissions in comparison to younger, normally developing language-age matched children (Bortolini and Leonard, 2000; Owen, Dromi, and Leonard, 2001);
c. Some difficulties in receptive prosodic tasks that interact with the grammatical and pragmatic functions of prosody (Wells and Peppé, 2003; Marshall, Harcourt-Brown, Ramus, and van der Lely, 2009).

REFERENCES

Abercrombie, D. (1967). Elements of general phonetics. Edinburgh: University Press.

Allen, G. and Hawkins, S. (1979). Trochaic rhythm in children's speech. In H. Holien and P. Hollien (Eds.), Current issues in the phonetic sciences. Amsterdam: *John Benjamin,* pp. 927-933.

Allen, G. and Hawkins, S. (1980). Phonological rhythm: Definition and development. In G. Yeni-Komshian, J. Kavanagh, and C. Ferguson (Eds.), Child Phonology: Volume 1. Production. New York: Academic Press, pp. 227-256.

Atkinson-King, K. (1973). Children's acquisition of phonological stress contrasts. Unpublished doctoral dissertation, University of California, Los Angeles.

Atkinson, K., MacWhinney, B. and Stoel, C. (1968). An experiment on the recognition of babbling. Language Behavior Research Laboratory Working Paper. University of California, Berkeley, 14.

Baltaxe, C. (1984). Use of contrastive stress in normal, aphasic, and autistic children. *Journal of Speech and Hearing Research,* 27, 97-105.

Baltaxe, C. A. and Simmons, J. Q. (1985), Prosodic development in normal and autistic children. In E. Schopler and G. B. Mesibov (Eds), Communication Problems in Autism. New York: *Plenum,* pp. 95–125.

Behrens, H. and Gut, U. (2005). The relationship between prosodic and syntactic organization in early multiword speech. Journal of Child Language, 32, 1-34.

Bloom, L. (1973). One word at a time. The Hague: Mouton.

Boersma, P., and Weenink, D. (2005). Praat: doing phonetics by computer (Version 4.3.01) [Computer program]. Retrieved from http://www.praat.org/.

Bortolini, U. and Leonard, L. (2000). Phonology and children with specific language impairment: Status of structural constraints in two languages. *Journal of Communication Disorders,* 33, 131-150.

Bunta, F., and Ingram, D. (2007). The acquisition of speech rhythm by bilingual Spanish- and English-speaking 4- and 5-year-old children. *Journal of Speech, Language, and Hearing,* 50, 999-1014.

de Boysson-Bardies, B., Sagart, L., and Durand, C. (1984). Discernible differences in the babbling of infants according to target language. *Journal of Child Language,* 11, 1-15.

Branigan, G. (1979). Some reasons why successive single word utterances are not. *Journal of Child Language,* 6, 411-421.

Branigan, G. and Stokes, W. (1984). An integrated account of utterance variability in early language development. In C. Thew and C. Johnson (Eds.), Proceedings of the Second International Congress for the Study of Child Language. Vol. 2. Lanham, Md: University Press of America, pp. 73-88.

Bull, D., Eilers, E. and Oller, D. (1984). Infants' discrimination of intensity variation in multisyllabic contexts. *Journal of the Acoustical Society of America,* 76, 1-13.

Bull, D., Eilers, E. and Oller, D. (1985). Infants' discrimination of final syllable fundamental frequency in multisyllabic stimuli. *Journal of the Acoustical Society of America,* 77, 289-295.

Chen, A. (2010). Is there really an asymmetry in the acquisition of the focus-to-accentuation mapping? *Lingua,* 120, 1926-1939.

Chen, A. and Fikkert, P. (2007). Intonation of early two-word utterances in Dutch. In J. Trouvain and W. Barry (Eds.), Proceedings of the XVIth International Congress of Phonetic Sciences. Dudweiler: *Pirrot GmbH,* pp. 315-320.

Chen, L-M. and Kent, R. (2009). Development of prosodic patterns in Mandarin-learning infants. *Journal of Child Language,* 36, 73-84.

Chevallier, C., Noveck, I., Happé, F., and Wilson, D. (2009). From acoustics to grammar: Perceiving and interpreting grammatical prosody in adolescents with Asperger Syndrome. *Research in Autism Spectrum Disorders,* 3(2), 502-516.

Clark, E., Gelman, S., and Lane, N. M. (1985). Compound nouns and category structure in young children. *Child Development,* 56, 84-94.

Clark, J. and Yallop, C. (1995). An Introduction to phonetics and phonology. Second Edition. Oxford: Blackwell.

Cruttenden, A. (1974). An experiment involving comprehension of intonation in children from 7 to 10. *Journal of Child Language,* 1, 221-231.

Cruttenden, A. (1997). Intonation. Second Edition. Cambridge University Press: Cambridge.

Crystal, D. (1986a). Listen to your child. Harmondsworth: Penguin.

Crystal, D. (1986b). Prosodic development. In P. Fletcher and M. Garman (Eds.), Language acquisition: Studies in first language development. Second Edition. Cambridge, England: Cambridge University Press, pp. 174-19.

Crystal, D. (1987). The Cambridge encyclopedia of language. Cambridge: Cambridge University Press.

Cutler, A. and Swinney, D. (1987). Prosody and the development of comprehension. *Journal of Child Language,* 14, 145-16.

Dauer, R. (1983). Stress-timing and syllable-timing reanalyzed. *Journal of Phonetics,* 11, 51-62.

Dauer, R. (1987). Phonetic and phonological components of language rhythm. Proceedings of the 11th International Congress of Phonetic Sciences, Talinn, Estonia, pp. 447-450.

Davis, B., MacNeilage, P., Matyear, C., and Powell, J. (2000). Prosodic correlates of stress in babbling: An acoustical study. *Child Development,* 71, 1258-1270.

DePaolis, R., Vihman, M., and Kunnari, S. (2008). Prosody in production at the onset of word use: A cross-linguistic study. *Journal of Phonetics,* 36, 406-422.

D'Odorico, L. (1984). Non-segmental features of prelinguistic communication: an analysis of some types of infant cry and non-cry vocalizations. *Journal of Child Language,* 11, 17-2.

D'Odorico, L. and Carubbi, S. (2003). Prosodic characteristics of early multi-word utterances in Italian children. *First Language,* 23, 97- 116.

D'Odorico, L. and Franco, F. (1991). Selective production of vocalization types in different communication contexts. *Journal of Child Language,* 18, 475-499.

Eilers, E., Bull, D., Oller, D., and Lewis, D. (1984). The discrimination of vowel duration by infants. *Journal of the Acoustical Society of America,* 75, 213-218.

Engstrand, O., Williams, K., and Lacerda, F. (2003). Does babbling sound native? Listeners' responses to vocalizations produced by Swedish- and American 12- and 18-month-olds. *Phonetica,* 60, 17-44.

Fernald, A. (1985). Four-month-old infants prefer to listen to motherese. *Infant Behavior and Development,* 8, 181-195.

Fernald, A. and Kuhl, P. (1987). Acoustic determinants of infant preference for motherese speech. *Infant Behavior and Development,* 10, 279-293.

Fernald, A. and McRoberts, G. (1996). Prosodic bootstrapping: A critical analysis of the argument and the evidence. In J. Morgan and K. Demuth (Eds.), From signal to syntax: Bootstrapping from speech to grammar in early acquisition. Hillsdale, NJ: Erlbaum, pp. 365-388.

Fernald, A. and Simon, T. (1984). Expanded intonation contours in mothers' speech to newborns. *Developmental Psychology,* 20, 104-113.

Fernald, A., Taeschner, T., Dunn, J., Papousek, M., de Boysson-Bardies, B. and Fukui, I. (1989). A cross-language study of prosodic modifications in mothers' and fathers' speech to preverbal infants. *Journal of Child Language,* 16, 477-501.

Fikkert, P. (1994). On the acquisition of prosodic structure. Dordrecht: ICG Printing (HIL Dissertations).

Flax, J., Lahey, M., Harris, K., and Boothroyd, A. (1991). Relations between prosodic variables and communicative functions. *Journal of Child Language,* 18, 3-19.

Fónagy, I. (1972). A propos de la genèse de la phrase enfantine. Lingua, 30, 31-71.

Fosnot, S. M. and Jun, S. (1999), Prosodic characteristics in children with stuttering or autism during reading and imitation. *Proceedings of the 14th International Congress of Phonetic Sciences,* pp. 1925–1928.

Furrow, D. (1984). Young children's use of prosody. *Journal of Child Language,* 11, 203-213.

Galligan, R. (1987). Intonation with single words: purposive and grammatical use. *Journal of Child Language,* 14, 1-21.

Garnica, O. (1977). Some prosodic and paralinguistic features of speech to young children. In C. Snow and C. Ferguson (Eds.), Talking to children. Language input and acquisition. Cambridge, England: Cambridge University Press, pp. 63-88.

Gerken, L., Jusczyk, P., and Mandel, D. (1994). When prosody fails to cue syntactic structure: Nine month olds' sensitivity to phonological versus syntactic phrases. *Cognition,* 51, 237-265.

Gleitman, L. and Wanner, E. (1982). Language acquisition: The state of the state of the art. In E. Wanner and L. Gleitman (Eds.), Language acquisition: The state of the art. Cambridge, England: Cambridge University Press, pp. 3-48.

Grabe, E. and Low, E. (2002). Durational variability in speech and the rhythm class hypothesis. Papers in Laboratory Phonology Cambridge: Cambridge University Press, pp. 515-546.

Grabe, E., Gut, U., Post, B., and Watson, I. (1999a). The acquisition of rhythm in English, French, and German. In I. Barrière, G. Morgan, S. Chiat and B. Woll (Eds.), Current research in language and communication: Proceedings of the child language seminar. London: *City University,* pp. 157-163.

Grabe, E., Post, B., and Watson, I. (1999b). The acquisition of rhythm in English and French. *Proceedings of the Intonational Congress of Phonetic Sciences,* 2, 1201-1204.

Grassman, S. and Tomasello, M. (2010). Prosodic stress on a word directs 24-month-olds' attention to a contextually new referent. *Journal of Pragmatics,* 42, 3098-3105.

Gualmini, A., Maciukaite, S., Crain, S. (2003). Children's insensitivity to contrastive stress in sentences with ONLY. Proceedings of the 25th Penn Linguistics Colloquium, pp. 87-110.

Hallé, P., Boysson-Bardies, B., and Vihman, M. (1991). Beginnings of prosodic organization: Intonation and duration patterns of disyllables produced by Japanese and French infants. *Language and Speech,* 34, 299-318.

Halliday, M. (1975). Learning how to mean: Explorations in the development of language. London: Edward Arnold.

Hendriks, P. and Koster, C. (2010). Production/comprehension asymmetries in language acquisition. *Lingua,* 120, 1887-189.

Hirsh-Pasek, K., Kemler Nelson, D., Jusczyk, p., Wright Cassidy, K., Druss, B., and Kennedy, L. (1987). Clauses are perceptual units for young infants. *Cognition,* 26, 269-286.

Hochberg, J. (1988a). First steps in the acquisition of Spanish stress. *Journal of Child Language,* 15, 273-292.

Hochberg, J. (1988b). Learning Spanish stress: Developmental and theoretical perspectives. *Language,* 64, 675-68.

Höhle, B., Bijeljac-Babic, R., Herold, B., Weissenborn, J., and Nazzi, T. (2009). Language specific prosodic preferences during the first half year of life: Evidence from German and French infants. *Infant Behavior and Development,* 32, 262-274.

Hornby, P. and Hass, W. (1970). Use of contrastive stress by preschool children. *Journal of Speech and Hearing Research,* 13, 395-399.

Johnson, W. (1958). Introduction: The six men and the stuttering. In J. Eisenson (Ed.,), Stuttering: A symposium. New York: Harper and Row, pp. 123-166.

Jusczyk, P. (1997). The discovery of spoken language. Cambridge, MA: MIT Press.

Jusczyk, P., Cutler A., and Redanz, N. (1993). Preference for the predominant stress patterns of English words. *Child Development,* 64, 675-68.

Jusczyk, P., Hirsh-Pasek, K., Kemler Nelson, D., Kennedy, L., Woodward A., and Piwoz, J. (1992). Perception of acoustic correlates of major phrase units by young infants. *Cognitive Psychology,* 24, 252-293.

Jusczyk, P., Houston, D., and Newsome, M. (1999). The beginnings of word segmentation in English-learning infants. *Cognitive Psychology,* 39, 159-20.

Jusczyk, P. and Thompson, E. (1978). Perception of a phonetic contrast in multisyllabic utterances by 2-month-old infants. *Perception and Psychophysics,* 23, 105-109.

Kehoe, M. (1995). An investigation of rhythmic processes in English-speaking children's word productions. Unpublished doctoral dissertation, University of Washington, Seattle, Washington.

Kehoe, M. (1997). Stress error patterns in English-speaking children's word productions. *Clinical Linguistics and Phonetics,* 11, 389-409.

Kehoe, M. (1998). Support for metrical stress theory in stress acquisition. *Clinical Linguistics and Phonetics,* 12, 1-23.

Kehoe, M., and Lleó, C. (2005). The emergence of language specific rhythm in German-Spanish bilingual children. Arbeiten zur Mehrsprachigkeit: Working Papers in Multilingualism 58. Hamburg: SFB 538.

Kehoe, M., Lleó, C., and Rakow, M. (2011). Speech rhythm in the pronunciation of German and Spanish monolingual and German-Spanish bilingual 3-year-olds. *Linguistische Berichte,* 227, 323-352.

Kehoe, M., and Stoel-Gammon, C. (1997). The acquisition of prosodic structure: An investigation of current accounts of children's prosodic development. *Language*, 73(1), 113-144.

Kehoe, M., Stoel-Gammon, C., and Buder, E. (1995). Acoustic correlates of stress in young children's speech. *Journal of Speech and Hearing Research,* 38, 338-350.

Kent, R. and Murray, A. (1982). Acoustic features of infant vocalic utterances at 3, 6, and 9 months. *Journal of the Acoustical Society of America,* 72, 353-365.

Klatt, D. (1975). Vowel lengthening is syntactically determined in a connected discourse. *Journal of Phonetics,* 3, 129-140.

Klein, H. (1984). Learning to stress: A case study. *Journal of Child Language,* 11, 375-390.

Kohler, K. (2009). Rhythm in speech and language. A new research paradigm. *Phonetica,*66, 29-45.

Konopczynski, G. (1990). Le Language emergent: caractéristiques rythmiques. Hamburg: Helmut Buske Verlag.

Kuhl, P. and Miller, J. (1975). Speech perception in early infancy: Discrimination of speech sound categories. *Journal of the Acoustical Society of America,* 58, S56(A).

Levitt, A. (1993). The acquisition of prosody: Evidence from French- and English-learning infants. *Haskins Laboratories Status Report on Speech Research, SR*-113, 41-50.

Levitt, A. and Wang, Q. (1991). Evidence for language-specific rhythmic influences in the reduplicative babbling of French- and English-learning infants. *Language and Speech,* 34, 235-249.

Lieberman, P. (1986). The acquisition of intonation by infants: Physiology and neural control. In C. Johns-Lewis (Ed.). Intonation and discourse. London: *Croom Helm,* pp. 239-25.

Lindblom, B. (1978). Final lengthening in speech and music. In E. Garding, G. Bruce, and R. Bannert (Eds.), Nordic prosody: Papers from a symposium. Department of Linguistics, Lund University, Sweden, pp. 86-101.

Lleó, L., Rakow, M. and Kehoe, M. (2004). Acquisition of language-specific pitch accent by Spanish and German monolingual and bilingual children. In T. Face (Ed.), Laboratory approaches to Spanish phonology. Berlin: Mouton de Gruyter.

Low, E., Grabe, E., and Nolan, F. (2001). Quantitative characteristics of speech rhythm: Syllable-timing in Singapore English. *Language and Speech,* 43, 377-401.

Lyberg, B. (1979). Final lengthening – partly a consequence of restrictions on the speed of fundamental frequency change? *Journal of Phonetics,* 7, 187-196.

Mampe, B., Friederici, A., Christophe, A., and Wermke, K. (2009). Newborns' cry melody is shaped by their native language. *Current Biology,* 19, 1994-199.

Mandel, D., Jusczyk., and Kemler Nelson, D. (1994). Does sentential prosody help infants organize and remember speech information? *Cognition,* 29, 143-178.

Marcos, H. (1987). Communicative functions of pitch range and pitch direction in infants. *Journal of Child Language,* 14, 255-268.

Marshall, C., Harcourt-Brown, S. Ramus, F. and van der Lely, H. (2009). The link between prosody and language skills in children with specific language impairment (SLI) and/or dyslexia. *International Journal of Language and Communication Disorders,* 44(4), 466-488.

McCann, J. and Peppé, S. (2003). Prosody in autism spectrum disorders: A critical review. *International Journal of Language and Communication Disorders,* 38, 325-350.

Mehler, J., Dupoux, E., Nazzi, T., and Dehaene-Lambertz, G. (1996). Coping with linguistic diversity: the infants' viewpoint. In J. Morgan and K. Demuth (Eds.), From signal to syntax: Bootstrapping from speech to grammar in early acquisition. Hillsdale, New Jersey: *Lawrence Erlbaum Associates,* pp. 101-116.

Mehler, J., Jusczyk, P., Lambertz, G., Halsted, N., Bertoncini, J., and Amiel-Tison, C. (1988). A precursor of language acquisition in young infants. *Cognition,* 29, 143-178.

Menn, L. (1976). Pattern, control, and contrast in beginning speech: A case study in the development of word-form and function. Unpublished Ph.D thesis, University of Illinois, Urbana-Champaign.

Mok, P. (2011). The acquisition of speech rhythm by three-year-old bilingual and monolingual children: Cantonese and English. Bilingualism: *Language and Cognition,* 14, 458-472.

Moon, C., Cooper, R., and Fifer, W. (1993). Two-day-olds prefer their native language. *Infant Behavior and Development,* 16, 495-500.

Morgan, J. and Newport, E. (1981). The role of constituent structure in the induction of an artificial language. *Journal of Verbal Learning and Verbal Behavior,* 20, 67-85.

Morse, P. (1972). The discrimination of speech and nonspeech stimuli in early infancy. *Journal of Experimental Child Psychology,* 13, 477-492.

Nazzi, T., Bertoncini, J., and Mehler, J. (1998). Language discrimination by newborns: Toward an understanding of the role of rhythm. Journal of Experimental Psychology: *Human Perception and Performance,* 24(3), 756-766.

Nazzi, T., Floccia, C., and Bertoncini, J. (1998). Discrimination of pitch contours by neonates. *Infant Behavior and Development,* 21 (4), 779-784.

Nazzi, T., Iakimova, I., Bertoncini, J., Frédonie, S., and Alcantara, C. (2006). Early segmentation of fluent speech by infants acquiring French: Emerging evidence for crosslinguistic differences. *Journal of Memory and Language,* 54, 283-299.

Nazzi, T., Kemler Nelson, D., Jusczyk, P., and Jusczyk, A. (2000). Six month olds' detection of clauses embedded in continuous speech: Effects of prosodic well-formedness. *Infancy,* 1, 123-14.

Nespor, M. and Vogel, I. (1986). Prosodic phonology. Dordrecht: Foris.

Nolan, F. and Asu, E. (2009). The pairwise variability index and coexisting rhythms in language. *Phonetica,* 66, 64-7.

Nouveau, D. (1994). Language acquisition, metrical theory, and optimality. A study of Dutch word stress. Utrecht, the Netherlands: OTS Dissertation Series.

Oller, D. (1973). The effect of position in utterance on speech segment duration in English. *Journal of the Acoustical Society of America,* 54, 1235-123.

Oller, D. and Smith, B. (1977). The effect of final-syllable position on vowel duration in infant babbling. *Journal of the Acoustical Society of America,* 62, 994-99.

Olney, R. and Scholnick, E. (1976). Adult judgments of age and linguistic differences in infant vocalizations. *Journal of Child Language,* 3, 145-155.

Owen, A. J., Dromi, E., and Leonard, L. B. (2001). The phonology-morphology interface in the speech of Hebrew-speaking children with specific language impairment. *Journal of Communication Disorders,* 34, 323-33.

Papaeliou, C., Minadakis, G., and Cavouras, D. (2002). Acoustic patterns of infant vocalizations expressing emotions and communicative functions. *Journal of Speech, Language, and Hearing Research,* 45, 311-31.

Papaeliou, C. and Trevarthen, C. (2006). Prelinguistic pitch patterns expressing 'communication' and 'apprehension'. *Journal of Child Language,* 33, 163-178.

Peppé , S., and McCann, J. (2003). Assessing intonation and prosody in children with atypical language development: The PEPS-C test and the revised version. *Clinical Linguistics and Phonetics,* 17, 345–354.

Peppé , S., McCann, J., Gibbon, F., O'Hare, A., and Rutherford, M. (2007). Receptive and expressive prosodic ability in children with high-functioning autism. *Journal of Speech, Language, and Hearing Research,* 50, 1015–1028.

Pierrehumbert, J. (1980). The phonology and phonetics of English intonation. PhD dissertation, MIT.

Pike, K. (1945). The intonation of American English. Ann Arbor, MI: University of Michigan Press.

Pinker, S. (1994). Language learnability and language development. Cambridge, MA: Harvard University Press.

Pollock, K., Brammer, D., and Hagerman, C. (1993). An acoustic analysis of young children's productions of word stress. *Journal of Phonetics,* 21, 183-203.

Prieto, P., Estrella, A., Thorson, J., and Vanrell, M. (2011). Is prosodic development correlated with grammatical development? Evidence from emerging intonation in Catalan and Spanish. *Journal of Child Language* Available on CJO 2011 DOI:10.1017/S030500091100002X.

Ramus, F., Nespor, M., and Mehler, J. (1999). Correlates of linguistic rhythm in the speech signal. *Cognition,* 73, 265-292.

Roach, P. (1982). On the distinction between "stress-timed" and "syllable-timed" languages. In D. Crystal (Ed.), Linguistic controversies, London: *Edward Arnold,* pp. 73-79.

Robb, M. and Saxman, J. (1990). Syllable durations of preword and early word vocalizations. *Journal of Speech and Hearing Research,* 33, 583-593.

Schwartz, R., Petinou, K., Goffman, L., Lazowski, G. and Cartusciello, C. (1996). Young children's production of syllable stress: An acoustic analysis. *Journal of the Acoustic Society of America,* 99, 3192-3200.

Scollon, R. (1976). Conversations with a one year old: A case study of the developmental foundation of syntax. Honolulu: The University Press of Hawaii.

Shattuck-Hufnagel, S. and Turk, A. (1996). A prosody tutorial for investigators of auditory sentence processing. *Journal of Psycholinguistic Research,* 25(2), 193-24.

Shriberg, L. D., Aram, D. M., and Kwiatkowski, J. (1997a). Developmental apraxia of speech: I. Descriptive perspectives. *Journal of Speech, Language, and Hearing Research,* 40, 273–285.

Shriberg, L. D., Aram, D. M., and Kwiatkowski, J. (1997b). Developmental apraxia of speech: II. Toward a diagnostic marker. *Journal of Speech, Language, and Hearing Research,* 40, 286–312.

Shriberg, L. D., Aram, D. M., and Kwiatkowski, J. (1997c). Developmental apraxia of speech: III. A subtype marked by inappropriate stress. *Journal of Speech, Language, and Hearing Research,* 40, 313-33.

Snow, D. (1994). Phrase-final syllable lengthening and intonation in early child speech. *Journal of Speech and Hearing Research,* 37 (4), 831-840.

Snow, D. (1995). Formal regularity of the falling tone in children's early meaningful speech. *Journal of Phonetics,* 23, 387-405.

Snow, D. (2001). Imitation of intonation contours by children with normal and disordered language development. *Clinical Linguistics and Phonetics,* 15(7), 567- 584.

Snow, D. (2002). Intonation in the monosyllabic utterances of 1-year-olds. *Infant Behavior and Development,* 24, 393-40.

Snow, D. (2004). Falling intonation in the one- and two-syllable utterances of infants and preschoolers. *Journal of Phonetics,* 32, 373-393.

Snow, D. (2006). Regression and reorganization of intonation between 6 and 23 months. *Child Development,* 77, 281-296.

Snow, D. and Balog, H. (2002). Do children produce the melody before the words? A review of developmental intonation research. *Lingua,* 112, 1025-1058.

Snow, D. and Stoel-Gammon, C. (1994). Intonation and final lengthening in early child language. In M. Yavas (Ed.), First and second language phonology. San Diego, CA: Singular Publishing Group, pp. 81-105.

Soderstrom, M., Seidl, A., Kemler Nelson, D., and Jusczyk, P. (2003). The prosodic bootstrapping of phrases: Evidence from prelinguistic infants. *Journal of Memory and Language,* 49, 249-26.

Solan, L. (1980). Contrastive stress and children's interpretation of pronouns. *Journal of Speech and Hearing Research,* 23, 688-698.

Spring, D. and Dale, P. (1977). The discrimination of linguistic stress in early infancy. *Journal of Speech and Hearing Research,* 20, 224-231.

Thevenin, D., Eilers, R., Oller, D., and Lavoie, L. (1985). Where's the drift in babbling drift. A cross-linguistic study. *Applied Psycholinguistics,* 6, 3-15.

Vihman, M. and DePaolis, R. (1998). Perception and production in early vocal development: Evidence from the acquisition of accent. In M. Gruber, D. Higgins, K. Olson, and T. Wysocki (Eds.), Chicago Linguistic Society, 34, Part 2: Papers from the Panels. Chicago, IL: Chicago Linguistic Society, pp. 373-386.

Vihman, M., DePaolis, R., and Davis, B. (1998). Is there a "trochaic bias" in early word learning? Evidence from infant production in English and French. *Child Development,* 69, 935-949.

Vogel, I. and Raimy, E. (2002). The acquisition of compound vs. phrasal stress: The role of prosodic constituents. *Journal of Child Language,* 29, 225-250.

Weinert, S. (1992). Deficits in acquiring language structure: The importance of using prosodic cues. *Applied Cognitive Psychology,* 6, 545–571.

Wells, B. and Peppé , S., (2003). Intonation abilities of children with speech and language impairments. *Journal of Speech, Language and Hearing Research,* 46, 5–20.

Wells, B., Peppé, S. and Goulandris, N. (2004). Intonation development from five to thirteen. *Journal of Child Language,* 31, 749-778.

Whalen, D., Levitt, A., and Wang, Q. (1991). Intonational differences between the reduplicative babbling of French- and English-learning infants. *Journal of Child Language,* 18, 501-516.

Wieman, L. (1976). Stress patterns of early child language. *Journal of Child Language,* 3, 283-286.

Wijnen, F., Krikhaar, E., and Den Os, E. (1994). The (non)realization of unstressed elements in children's utterances: Evidence for a rhythmic constraint. *Journal of Child Language,* 21, 59-83.

Zhou, P., Su, Y., Crain, S., Gao, L. Q., and Zhan, L. K. (2011). Children's use of phonological information in ambiguity resolution: A view from Mandarin Chinese. *Journal of Child Language Available on CJO* 2011 DOI: 10.1017/S0305000911000249.

In: Comprehensive Perspectives …
Editors: Beate Peter and Andrea A. N. MacLeod
ISBN: 978-1-62257-041-6

Chapter 8

ACQUISITION OF A PHONOLOGICAL SYSTEM IN ADULTHOOD

Amber Franklin

INTRODUCTION

The reasons for learning a second language as an adult are many. High school and university students in North America often take foreign language classes to fulfill educational requirements. Some adults learn a second language to facilitate and enrich the experience of traveling abroad or to become more competitive in the job market. Immigrants may learn a second language in order to better integrate into the host country. The recent US Census data indicate that over 55 million people over the age of 5 years speak a language other than English at home. This number accounts for 19.7% of the U.S. population. Of this number, 55.9% report speaking English "very well" while 19.8% and 16.3% report speaking English "well" and "not well" respectively (FILES: U.S. Census 2010).

Learning a new language in adulthood presents challenges that are less likely to be encountered by children who are exposed to two languages early in life (see Chapters 13 and 14 for a review of childhood bilingualism). This observation is particularly true with respect to learning the phonological system of a new language. Although some research indicates that it is possible for adults to acquire a new phonological system with native-like proficiency (Moyer 1999, Abu-Raiba and Kehat 2004, Munro and Mann, 2005), native-like phonological acquisition of a new language in **adult language learners** is generally the exception to the rule (Flege, Munro, and McKay, 1995). Consequently, the average adult learner of a new language will speak that language with a discernable foreign accent.

This chapter presents some of the theoretical frameworks that help explain why adult second language learners are more likely to speak with a foreign accent. This will be followed by an exploration of the different dimensions used to characterize pronunciation proficiency in non-native speakers and the variables that affect foreign accent. Finally, we will explore accent modification in clinical practice and some of the sociolinguistic considerations for non-native speakers of English. Although the following discussion can apply to adults learning any new language, this chapter will focus primarily on adult learners of English.

Additionally, the term **target language (TL)** will be used rather than second language because the concepts discussed in this chapter can apply to any new language being learned, regardless of how many languages the individual has acquired or learned previously. Note that a speaker's **native language (NL)** is sometimes referred to as L1 and a subsequent language, as L2.

LEARNING A NEW TARGET LANGUAGE AS AN ADULT

Age of Learning and Pronunciation Proficiency

The terms language *learning* and language *acquisition* are sometimes used in the literature in distinct ways. In the strict sense, language acquisition occurs when an individual eventually understands and speaks a language without the benefit of explicit instruction.

Thus, the process by which most people learn their first language is through language acquisition. Some adults acquire a TL when they are immersed in the TL community and develop proficiency over time primarily through exposure and language use. In the strict sense, language learning occurs when an individual receives explicit instruction to help them speak and understand a language. Many adults are explicitly taught a TL through classes, instructional books, and audio material. For the purposes of this chapter a strict distinction between language learning and language acquisition will not be established since many adults develop proficiency in a TL through a combination of processes.

Studies have demonstrated that a relationship exists between the age an individual learns a TL and the extent to which the TL pronunciations approximate those of monolingual speakers (Abu-Raiba and Kehat, 2004; Flege, Munro, and MacKay, 1995; Munro and Mann, 2005; Tsukada, Birdsong, Bialystock, Mack, Sung and Flege, 2005; Yeni-Komshian, Flege, and Liu, 2000). The general consensus is that "earlier is better," especially when it comes to learning the phonological features of a TL. The **critical period hypothesis (CPH)** was first proposed by Lenneberg in 1967 to account for the observation that adults experience greater difficulty acquiring native command of a TL than do children. The CPH maintains that changes in neuroplasticity during puberty make it much more difficult for individuals beyond that age to attain complete mastery of a new language. Since then, other researchers (Patkowski, 1990; Scovel, 1969) have conducted studies supporting the existence of an age-related critical period.

However, some reports have identified a small number of individuals who are capable of achieving native-like pronunciation proficiency despite have been exposed to the TL later in childhood (MacLeod and Stoel-Gammon, 2010) and even well after puberty (Abu-Rabia and Kehat, 2004; Moyer, 1999, 2004; Munro and Mann, 2005). A study of native Korean ESL speakers arriving in the U.S. investigated NL and TL pronunciation proficiency as a function of **age of arrival (AOA)** (Yeni-Komshian, Flege and Liu, 2000). English and Korean sentences that were spoken by the Korean participants were rated for pronunciation proficiency and degree of accent. The results indicated that AOA accounted for 73% of the variance in English pronunciation ratings. However, the findings did not indicate a precipitous drop in pronunciation proficiency after puberty. Instead, there was a sigmoidal relationship between AOA and English pronunciation proficiency. A sigmoidal relationship can be illustrated as an s-shaped curve. This curve indicates that during young AOAs pronunciation proficiency is relatively high and does not change much with increasing age. As the AOA increases past early childhood, there is a sharp decrease in pronunciation proficiency with increasing age resulting in a steep slope. This is followed by a leveling off at older AOAs where proficiency is relatively low and stable. An additional finding that conflicts with the claims of the CPH is that improved pronunciation proficiency in English sometimes came at the expense of native-like pronunciation in Korean. This and similar studies (Munro and Mann, 2005) have led researchers to reinvestigate the CPH as a "hard and fast" predictor of success in second language learning.

Besides the critical period hypothesis, four alternative hypotheses have been proposed to help explain the relationship between the age one learns a new language and the degree of perceived foreign accent (Munro and Mann, 2005). One alternative is the **sensitive period model** (Oyama, 1976) that broadened the chronological window within which native-like proficiency of a TL was possible. A model of constant ability suggests that all speakers retain the ability to achieve native accents in a newly learned language regardless of age (Moyer, 1999). By contrast, a model of linear decline proposes a gradual decline in the ability to acquire native-like pronunciation proficiency throughout the entire lifespan (Flege, Munro, and McKay, 1995). Finally, Flege and Fletcher (1992) propose a sigmoid model of TL acquisition which is categorized by three distinct phases: (1) the first phase is brief and predicts near native TL pronunciation proficiency at early ages; (2) phase two is characterized by an s-curve slope wherein high variability exists in TL pronunciation proficiency as a function of age; (3) the final phase predicts TL acquisition that is far from native at later ages of exposure.

Flege's Speech Learning Model (SLM)

The **Speech Learning Model (SLM)** (Flege, 1995) provides an explanation for the presence of foreign accents in second language learners. The SLM states that with increasing age there exists a reduced likelihood that the speaker will establish new phonetic categories for second language sounds that do not already exist in the NL. This phenomenon results in a foreign accent that is, in part, a function of the phonological disparity between the speaker's NL and the new TL. In this way, the SLM accounts for the observation that pronunciation proficiency in a TL decreases with age of learning. However, this model also posits that the same processes underlying NL acquisition can be applied to TL learning (Mack, 2003). As such, this decrease in pronunciation proficiency with increased age of learning is gradual rather than precipitous because the phonetic systems of adults remain malleable throughout their lifetime.

Flege proposes two mechanisms that affect speech perception and, consequently, production in the TL: **category assimilation** and **category dissimilation** (Yeni-Komshian, Flege, and Liu, 2000). Category assimilation occurs when a speaker has difficulty forming a new category for a TL sound because a very similar sound exists in the speaker's native phonetic system. Because this similar NL phoneme is not identical to the TL phoneme in question, the learner assimilates the TL phoneme into the existing NL phonetic category. As such, the NL phoneme morphs to accommodate the similar TL sound and the learner perceives the two phonemes as equivalent; this is also called equivalence classification. As a result, neither the NL nor the TL phoneme is produced with native-like precision.

Category dissimilation occurs when the learner does indeed form a new phonetic category for the TL speech sound. Category dissimilation is most likely to occur in children who are learning the TL at a relatively young age. As a result of the new and accurate production of the TL sound, the learner attempts to maximize the phonetic contrast among the different phonemes in phonetic space. This may cause some adjustments in the characteristics of the phonemes in the NL and TL. Therefore both category assimilation and dissimilation may affect a bilingual speaker's production of phonetic segments in his or her NL or TL. However, category assimilation is more likely to be observed in adults learning a new language than in children.

Category assimilation and category dissimilation represent but two of the seven hypotheses proposed by Flege under the SLM. The other five hypotheses are as follows: (1) An allophonic perceptual relationship exists between phonetic segments in the NL and the TL. (2) New phonemic categories are formed in the TL when an individual can differentiate between a TL phoneme and its most similar NL phoneme. (3) An individual can more readily distinguish between a TL phoneme and the closest NL phoneme when the phonetic distance between those two phonemes increases. (4) An individual's ability to distinguish between NL and similar TL phonemes decreases with age. (5) An individual's production of a TL phoneme will be reflective of that phoneme's long-term memory representation.

Quantifying Second Language Pronunciation Proficiency

Flege's SLM explains why particular phonemes may be difficult for speakers of a new TL language to pronounce accurately. Production accuracy at the segmental level (consonants and vowels) is indeed one way to quantify second language pronunciation proficiency. In fact, a variety of accent modification assessment programs require the clinician to conduct an analysis of segmental accuracy (Compton, 1983; Pennington and Richards, 1986; Sikorski, 2005). For this type of analysis, the adult English language learner is required to read a list of words that have been selected to represent a variety of vowel and consonants in a variety of word positions. Segmental accuracy is best analyzed using phonetic transcription which requires specialized training (Pollock and Berni, 2001). Phonetic transcription provides valuable information regarding the phonemes that are being substituted for the English targets. Specific knowledge of the substitution, addition or elimination patterns can allow the clinician to provide appropriate specialized instruction during accent modification training.

In addition to segmental accuracy, global pronunciation proficiency can be assessed using a number of different concepts (Derwing and Munro, 2005; Derwing et. al, 2004; Derwing and Munro, 1997). Among them are **intelligibility**, **comprehensibility**, **accentedness**, and **fluency**. Intelligibility refers to the extent to which a naïve listener actually understands an utterance and it is generally measured through orthographic transcription of utterances spoken by the non-native speaker. The percentage of words correctly identified by the naïve listener constitutes the outcome measure of intelligibility. Comprehensibility can be defined as a listener's perception of how difficult it is to understand a speaker or the degree of effort one must exert when listening to a speaker. Comprehensibility may sound very similar to intelligibility. However, it is important to keep in mind that while two speakers may be equally intelligible, a listener may have to devote more effort when listening to one speaker over the other. The speaker to whom a listener must devote more effort is said to speak with lower comprehensibility. Accentedness refers to a listener's perception of how different a speaker's accent is from that of the TL community. Finally, fluency can be defined as how smooth and free-flowing an individual's speech is. Comprehensibility, accentedness and fluency are often subjectively measured using a scalar judgment task that ranges from 1 to 9. The higher the number on the scale, the less comprehensible, more strongly accented or less fluent an individual's speech is.

These dimensions of global proficiency, while different, are not completely independent measures. For example, one study investigating the relationship between accent, intelligibility and comprehensibility noted that accent ratings were often more severe than comprehensibility ratings for the same group of speakers.

Additionally, comprehensibility ratings were often more severe than intelligibility scores. Therefore it is possible for a heavily accented speaker to also be fairly intelligible (Derwing, Rossiter, Munro, and Thompson, 2004; Munro and Derwing, 1995). A different study indicated that fluency ratings are significantly correlated with comprehensibility ratings but not highly correlated with accentedness ratings. Additionally, accent judgments appear to be based primarily on segmental and suprasegmental features such as consonant and vowel accuracy and intonation contours. By contrast, fluency and comprehensibility measures are affected primarily by prosodic or temporal features such as speaking rate, pause time, false starts and the presence of fillers. The aforementioned findings indicate the importance of using a variety of measures when quantifying pronunciation proficiency in non-native speakers.

Many non-native speakers of English take **oral proficiency** exams to qualify for jobs that place a high demand on verbal communication. Government agency employees or international students who intend to work as teaching assistants and instructors in universities and colleges are often expected to take the Oral Proficiency Interview (OPI) or the Speaking Proficiency English Assessment Kit (SPEAK) test. The OPI was developed by the American Council on the Teaching of Foreign Languages (ACTFL) and is conducted over the phone or in-person by a trained ACTFL tester. The results of the OPI categorize the oral proficiency of non-native speakers on a scale ranging from Novice to Superior. The SPEAK test was developed by the Test of English as a Foreign Language (TOEFL) program. Like the OPI, the SPEAK test assesses oral language proficiency as it relates to fluency, grammar, and comprehensibility in addition to pronunciation. Both tests require the speaker to answer general open-ended questions, and engage in conversational role-play. Additionally, the SPEAK test includes some picture description tasks.

Studies have demonstrated that a speaker's performance on oral proficiency tests depends not only on the speaker's command of the language, but also on the examiner's familiarity with the test-taker's accent. Examiners sometimes assign higher scores to test takers who have accents that are familiar to the examiner (Carey, Mannell and Dunn, 2010). Another variable that can affect test results is the type of accent exhibited by the speaker. One study compared the differential results on the SPEAK test between speakers from Asian and European language backgrounds (Kim, 2001). The results indicated that some scales of the SPEAK test assessed proficiency more effectively than other scales depending on the speaker's NL. For example, the "Grammar" scale more effectively discriminated among European NL speakers than the "Pronunciation" scale. Conversely, the "Pronunciation" scale more effectively discriminated among Asian NL speakers than the "Grammar" scale. These two studies suggest a need for more research to investigate and improve the reliability and validity of oral proficiency exams.

Motivation as a Variable Affecting Accentedness

As stated earlier, accentedness refers to how different a speaker's accent is from that of the TL community. Several variables have been found to affect the strength of accent in adult learners of a new TL. The primary biological variables are the age at which one learns a second language the difference between the speaker's NL phonetic inventory and the phonetic inventory of the TL. Another variable that has been demonstrated to affect pronunciation proficiency is motivation.

Motivation as it relates to second language learning can be subdivided into two branches, instrumental motivation and integrative motivation (Flege, Munro and MacKay, 1995). Instrumental motivation is based on a desire to achieve native-like proficiency in a TL in order to attain particular goals related to economic and career advancement. Integrative motivation refers to a desire to achieve native-like proficiency in a second language for cultural or social reasons (Gass and Selinker, 2001). Instrumental and integrative motivation are also termed extrinsic and intrinsic motivation, respectively (Smit and Dalton, 2000). In one study of English speakers learning German as a second language, the variable that correlated most highly with achieving native-like pronunciation proficiency in German was professional motivation (Moyer, 2004).

Motivation can also be viewed as a concept comprising a number of different subcomponents that intersect. These subcomponents include learner related, classroom related and subject related variables (Smit and Dalton, 2000). Smit and Dalton included intrinstic and extrinsic motivation as well as a learner's attitude toward the TL community and accent under the umbrella of subject related variables. Classroom related variables included class goals, teaching styles, feedback and learning strategies. Finally learner related variables included language use and anxiety, self-perception of TL accent and self-efficacy. While motivation is an important factor in second language learning in general, this study suggested that the motivation underlying pronunciation learning in adults is different from the motivation underlying language learning in general.

Other variables that have been demonstrated to affect accentedness include the frequency of spoken interactions in the TL, the length of residence in the country/community in which the TL is natively spoken and the number of years of formal instruction in the TL. For a more in-depth discussion of some of these variables, refer to the text by Moyer (2004).

Accent Modification in Clinical Practice

The Role of the Speech-Language Pathologist

In a paper reviewing research related to the critical period, Scovel stated, "Despite the fact that foreign accents emerge early in adulthood and, with rare exception remain indelible after puberty, adult learners can, should and do improve their pronunciation and intelligibility in a second language" (Scovel, 2000, pp17). **Accent modification** is a growing area of practice for speech-language pathologists (SLPs) and English as a Second Language (ESL) teachers in a variety of clinical, vocational and educational settings (Sikorski, 2005). Accent modification clients are generally adults since children who learn a TL are more likely to achieve near-native pronunciation proficiency. The aim of accent modification is to change pronunciation and improve speech intelligibility by targeting pronunciation and prosodic differences between the speaker's NL and the TL. The terms accent reduction and accent elimination have also been used by service providers to describe this same process; however, accent *modification* is a more accurate term since clients are simply learning to modify their current accent in favor of an accent that more closely approximates that of the native speakers of the TL. Ultimately, there is no stereotypically pure form of a TL. Speech patterns among native speakers of any language vary considerably because of regional, ethnic and social dialects. So the idea that one can learn to speak a stereotypically pure form of a language is misleading. For this reason, the ultimate goal of accent modification should be improved intelligibility.

It is important to realize that individuals who speak with a foreign accent are not exhibiting a speech disorder but a speech *difference* (ASHA Joint Subcommittee of the Executive Board on English Language Proficiency, 1998). The SLP is traditionally seen as a provider of health care services. Therefore, when providing accent modification services to non-native speakers, clinicians risk sending the message that an accent is a speech disorder in need of remediation (Muller, Ball and Guendouzi 2000). Consequently, when working with adult learners of a new language clinicians should be careful to avoid terminology that is frequently used when referencing individuals with speech or language disorders. For example, individuals seeking accent modification services should be referred to as *clients* rather than patients and the service they receive should be called pronunciation or accent *training* or *instruction* rather than therapy.

Clinicians must address a number of pedagogical issues surrounding accent modification. Among these are: (1) the types of speech sample elicitation strategies to use during assessment, (2) the features of pronunciation to be addressed during training, and (3) the type, duration and intensity of training methods that will provide the most effective results (Burgess and Spencer, 2000; Moyer, 2004). There is currently no standard approach to guide clinicians in providing accent modification services as non-native speakers vary in terms of speech patterns they exhibit and their response to particular types of instruction (Macdonald, Yule and Powers, 1994; Munro, 1993). Consequently, accent modification programs should be designed and implemented in a way that is tailored to individual clients' needs (Derwing and Munro, 2005).

Speech Sample Elicitation

Before an individual can participate in an accent modification program, his or her speech must be analyzed for sound patterns and differences that will be targeted during service delivery. Clinicians have several speech elicitation options to consider: (1) written single words, (2) written sentences, (3) written paragraphs, (4) spontaneous conversation and (5) picture description tasks. The first three options have the advantage of allowing the clinician to pre-select the specific phonemes, syllable structures, and prosodic patterns attempted by the speaker. Spontaneous conversation and picture description tasks provide a more naturalistic speech sample. Different types of speech samples have been shown to result in different foreign accent ratings for the same speaker. In a study investigating the age of immersion as a predictor of foreign accent, Munro and Mann (2005) collected four different types of speech samples (single words, sentences, paragraphs, and picture narration) from Mandarin ESL speakers. Native speakers of English rated each type of sample for degree of accentedness. The results indicated that the paragraphs were often assigned the most foreign accent rating followed by sentences and single words. However, the spontaneous picture description task was assigned ratings that were more native than the paragraphs. These findings suggest that accent ratings based on single words tend to overestimate a speaker's pronunciation proficiency. Ratings based on spontaneous speech samples may also minimize a speaker's foreign accent because the speaker is able to avoid difficult articulatory patterns by selectively choosing the words they use. The type of speech sample elicited has also been shown to affect ratings of fluency in non-native speakers (Derwing et al., 2004). When speech samples produced during a picture description task, a monologue task, and a dialogue task were compared and rated for fluency, the picture description task received the lowest fluency ratings. Of the three spontaneous speech tasks, the picture description task did not provide the speaker with as much freedom in terms of vocabulary choice, syntactic structure and content thus resulting in the lower fluency rating. A thorough speech pattern analysis should include a variety of speech elicitation strategies in order to get the most complete view of the nature of a client's accent. Lists of single words have the advantage of allowing a variety of phonemes to be examined in a number of different word positions. Spontaneous speech samples provide the best reflection of naturalistic speech and give the most accurate account of a client's speech rate, rhythm, and prosodic patterns. Written paragraphs have the benefit of allowing the clinician to pre-select specific words while still providing a continuous speech sample. However, written sentences and paragraphs should be used with caution because reading errors, pauses, and hesitations may give a false impression of high accentedness and low fluency (Munro and Derwing, 1994). It is therefore important to familiarize non-native speakers with the words and grammatical structures in sentences and passages used to elicit speech samples.

Target Selection

The SLP must also pay careful consideration to target selection during pronunciation instruction. Pronunciation instructors may choose to target non-native speech at the suprasegmental level by focusing on intonation and stress patterns, and at the segmental level by focusing on consonants and vowels (Burgess and Spencer, 2000; Pennington and Richards, 1986). Targeting the segmental, rather than suprasegmental aspects of speech yields different results after pronunciation training. One study revealed that clients who received intensive training in consonant and vowel production alone received better accent ratings during a sentence reading task than clients who exclusively received suprasegmental training targeting intonation, rhythm and speaking rate (Derwing, Munro, and Weibe, 1998). However, only the clients who received suprasegmental training demonstrated improved comprehensibility and fluency ratings on a picture description task. Suprasegmental instruction appears to equip the speakers with the ability to be more fluent and comprehensible in spontaneous speech while segmental instruction enables the speaker to make specific corrections if a communication breakdown has occurred. Therefore a comprehensive approach to accent modification should address both individual speech sounds as well as more global aspects of pronunciation such as intonation, rhythm, stress patterns and speech rate (Ferrier, Reid and Chenausky, 1999). One potentially important aspect of target selection related to individual speech sounds is the concept of functional load. Functional load refers to the effect that a particular type of error has on the intelligibility of TL speech. For example, the substitution of /t/ for / θ/ ("ting" instead of "thing") may be less detrimental to intelligibility than the substitution of /b/ for /p/ ("bit" for "pit") (Derwing andMunro, 2005).

Therefore, clinicians should consider targeting errors in speech segments that carry the greatest functional load. In the speech signal, vowels are generally more salient than consonants and are the primary carriers of prosody and intonation (Mehler, Dupoux, Nazzi and Dehaene-Lambertz, 1996). Variability in TL vowel production is a noticeable component of foreign-accented speech (Sikorski, 2005) and errors in vowel production contribute greatly to decreased speech intelligibility (Nazzi, 2005). Finally, the relatively high density of the English vowel system compared to other languages (Maddieson, 1997) suggests that ESL speakers may encounter English vowels that pose some pronunciation difficulties for them. As such, clinicians should pay particular attention to improving the production of English vowels as part of a comprehensive accent modification program (Sikorski, 2005, Wang and Munro, 2004). Ultimately, determining the relative functional load of individual segments is not an exact science. However, Brown (1991) identified several factors that contribute to the functional load of phonemes including the position of the phoneme within a word, the number and frequency of minimal pairs produced by a phoneme substitution and the perceived social stigma associated with the substitution pattern. A 2006 investigation by Munro and Derwing demonstrated that errors affecting phonemes with high functional load resulted in stronger TL accentedness scores and lower TL comprehensibility scores than errors with low functional load. While this study provides preliminary evidence that functional load does impact perceived accent and comprehensibility, functional load is only one of a number of factors that clinicians should consider when choosing appropriate targets for pronunciation instruction.

Sociolinguistic and Sociocultural Considerations

Accent and Identity

When we consider factors that shape our sense of identity, we often think of biological and physiological variables such as race, ethnicity, gender and age. We may also consider social variables such as religious or philosophical beliefs, level of education, NL, social status and place of birth or place of residence. In addition to the aforementioned variables, adults who are learning a new language and who may eventually become fully bilingual often find themselves negotiating bilingual and bicultural identities (Kanno, 2003). The process and extent of identity reorganization may differ depending on whether the non-native speaker plans to immigrate permanently to a new country or reside there only temporarily.

In a paper titled "Never Quite a Native speaker: Accent and Identity in the L2 – and the L1," Marx (2002), a native speaker of English, describes a process of identity formation that mirrored a shift in accent as she learned German while living in Germany for over three years. Marx discovered that as she gained greater proficiency in her German accent, there was a simultaneous conformity to German culture in the form of appearance and social behavior that marked a shift in her cultural identity.

Additionally, improvement in German proficiency was accompanied by decreased proficiency in English. This process of language loss became evident when Marx spoke English with German intonation patterns. Loss of L1 is a natural process experienced by language learners who are completely immersed in the TL environment. Marx's German-accented English persisted for some time after she moved back to Canada and this necessitated another shift in identity relative to her native culture. In recounting her experience, Marx suggests that as more adults live or study abroad for set periods of time, temporary internal and cultural identity shifts related to language learning and foreign accent will become more common.

The way a non-native speaker perceives his or her own degree of accentedness and communicative competence also shapes the speaker's sense of identity and belonging in a new cultural context. In a recent study, Gluszek and Dovidio (2010) asked English speaking adults from a variety of language backgrounds to rate the strength of their own accent, complete a scale assessing perceived stigmatization, and answer a questionnaire related to communication problems and the speakers' sense of belonging in the U.S. context. The results indicated that non-native speakers who rated their accents as being relatively strong also indicated that they were more heavily stigmatized in society by native speakers of English. The results of this study also indicated that speakers with Asian and Latino accents had a greater sense of perceived societal stigmatization than speakers with European accents. Additionally, individuals who spoke with foreign accents experienced a lower sense of belonging in the U.S. than native speakers of English. One very interesting finding related to this study is that native speakers of English sometimes perceived non-native speakers as having more problems communicating than the non-native speakers report. One potential consequence of this incorrect assumption is that native speakers of English may avoid communicating with non-native speakers because they assume that communication is too uncomfortable for the non-native speaker. As a result, opportunities for intercultural communication are missed.

Accent Discrimination and Language Rights

Non-native speakers of English sometimes face accent discrimination in a variety of contexts (Munro, 2003). Although accent discrimination can be difficult to prove, there is legal protection of **language rights** for non-native speakers. Title VII of the Civil Rights Act of 1964 protects individuals in the U.S. from any discrimination based on national origin (Nguyen, 1993).

Additionally, the Equal Opportunities Employment Commission declared that speech accent is related to national origin and thereby falls under the purview of Title VII. While employers are not required to hire anyone whose communication materially interferes with satisfactory job performance, they are also required to show impartiality with respect to different types of accents. In other words, employers have to be careful not to show a preference for French accents over Japanese accents.

Speech Samples

To illustrate various aspects of non-native productions of English, two sets of speech samples were recorded. The first set. 8S1 through 8S6, consists of sentences read by non-native speakers with a variety of language backgrounds. The second set, 8S7 through 8S22, were recorded from four native speakers of Indonesian, Mandarin, German, and French, respectively.

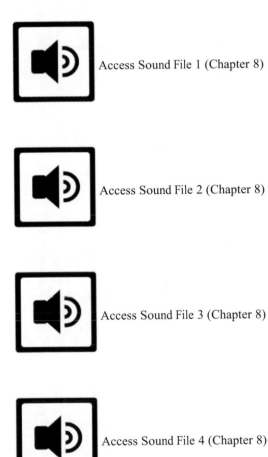

Access Sound File 1 (Chapter 8)

8S1 Sample 1.

Access Sound File 2 (Chapter 8)

8S2 Sample 2.

Access Sound File 3 (Chapter 8)

8S3 Sample 3.

Access Sound File 4 (Chapter 8)

8S4 Sample 4.

Access Sound File 5 (Chapter 8)

8S5 Sample 5.

Access Sound File 6 (Chapter 8)

8S6 Sample 6.

Access Sound File 7 (Chapter 8)

8S7 Native speaker of Indonesian: Summary of experience with English.

Access Sound File 8 (Chapter 8)

8S8 Native speaker of Indonesian: Rainbow Passage.

Access Sound File 9 (Chapter 8)

8S9 Native speaker of Indonesian: Stella Passage.

Access Sound File 10 (Chapter 8)

8S10 Native speaker of Indonesian: Rainbow narrative in Indonesian.

Access Sound File 11 (Chapter 8)

8S11 Native speaker of Mandarin: Summary of experience with English.

Access Sound File 12 (Chapter 8)

8S12 Native speaker of Mandarin: Rainbow Passage.

Access Sound File 13 (Chapter 8)

8S13 Native speaker of Mandarin: Stella Passage.

Access Sound File 14 (Chapter 8)

8S14 Native speaker of Mandarin: Rainbow narrative in Mandarin.

Access Sound File 15 (Chapter 8)

8S15 Native speaker of German: Summary of experience with English.

Access Sound File 16 (Chapter 8)

8S116 Native speaker of German: Rainbow Passage.

Access Sound File 17 (Chapter 8)

8S17 Native speaker of German: Stella Passage.

Access Sound File 18 (Chapter 8)

8S18 Native speaker of German: Rainbow narrative in German.

Access Sound File 19 (Chapter 8)

8S19 Native speaker of French: Summary of experience with English.

Access Sound File 20 (Chapter 8)

8S20 Native speaker of French: Rainbow Passage.

Access Sound File 21 (Chapter 8)

8S21 Native speaker of French: Stella Passage.

Access Sound File 22 (Chapter 8)

8S22 Native speaker of French: Rainbow narrative in French.

Each speaker provided a personal narrative about his or her experience with English, a reading of the Rainbow Passage, a reading of the Stella passage, and a few comments about rainbows spoken in the speaker's native language.

CONNECTIONS

This chapter discusses how the phonological system of English is acquired at an age when the first phonological system has long been established. Chapter 9 reviews how children speaking languages other than English go about establishing their phonological systems.

Chapters 13 and 14 focus on aspects of bilingual speech acquisition in children who are exposed to two or more languages either simultaneously or sequentially.

CONCLUDING REMARKS

Learning a new language and phonological system can be a challenging and rewarding experience. While it is well established that phonological acquisition of a new language is easier when one is exposed to that language as a young child, research also demonstrates that adults are capable of learning a new phonological systems. Research on adult target language learning has helped drive the development of theoretical frameworks and models of second language learning. The factors that affect pronunciation accuracy when learning a new language are varied.

However, high motivation related to professional development or societal acculturations are strong predictors of native-like accent ratings when adults learn a new language. As the population and linguistic landscape of North America becomes increasingly diverse, Speech Language Pathologists are more likely to encounter non-native speakers seeking accent modification to help improve their English intelligibility and accent. While foreign-accented speech is a communication difference rather than a disorder, it is important for clinicians to provide these services with the same professional standards applied to other speech and language services.

Finally, as with any culturally and linguistically diverse community, clinicians should take the time to understand how the client's cultural and linguistic identity affects his or her communication goals in a variety of contexts.

CHAPTER REVIEW QUESTIONS

1. Define the following global measures of pronunciation proficiency: accentedness, comprehensibility, intelligibility, and fluency. Are these measures completely independent of one another? Explain your answer.
2. Why is accent *modification* a more appropriate term to use rather than accent *reduction* or accent *elimination*?
3. Describe three different types of speech sample elicitation strategies used to assess non-native speech. What is an advantage of each type?

SUGGESTIONS FOR FURTHER READING

Derwing, T. M. and Munro, M. J. (2005). Second language accent and pronunciation teaching: a research-based approach. *Language Learning,* 58(3), 479-502.

Gluzek, A. and Dovidio, J.F. (2010). Speaking with a non-native accent: Perceptions of bias communication difficulties and belonging in the United States. *Journal of Language and Social Psychology*, 29 (2), 224-234.

Moyer, A. (2004). *Age, accent, and experience in second language acquisition: An integrated approach to critical period inquiry*. Clevedon: Multilingual Matters.

SUGGESTIONS FOR STUDENT ACTIVITIES

Activity 1.

Interview a non-native speaker of English. Try to find someone who speaks English with a noticeable foreign accent.

Ask your interviewee the following questions related to her/his demographic background and sociocultural experiences as a non-native speaker of English:

1) What is your native language?
2) How old were you when you first started learning English and where were you living?
3) Describe how you were taught English. Was your teacher a native speaker or non-native speaker of English?
4) What was your motivation for learning English?
5) How long have you been living in an English speaking country (U.S., Canada, England etc.)?
6) In what situations or with whom do you feel *most* confident speaking English?
7) In what situations or with whom do you feel *least* confident speaking English?
8) Do native speakers of English ever have difficulty understanding you? Give examples of specific situations if possible.
9) If you are not understood by others, do you use any strategies to express yourself more clearly? Explain.
10) From your perspective, do native speakers of English view your accent in a positive way or in a negative way? Explain.
11) Do you feel that you have been discriminated against or treated poorly because of your accent? If possible please give an example.
12) How do YOU view your accent?
13) Are there particular sounds (consonants or vowels) or words that you know you have a difficult time pronouncing correctly in English?
14) Have you ever received specialized training to change your accent? Is accent modification a service that you would consider receiving? Why or why not?

Group discussion: Bring your interview responses to class with you and share your responses with other members of a group. Are there any common themes or patterns apparent in the responses? For example, do the non-native speakers feel uncomfortable speaking English in similar contexts? Are speakers from European language backgrounds less likely to feel discriminated against than speakers from Asian language backgrounds? Consider other differences and similarities in the interview responses.

Activity 2.

The table below provides demographic information for the speakers featured in speech samples 8S1 through 8S6 that were recorded for this chapter. Each speaker is reading a sentence from the Sentence Intelligibility Test. Without looking at the target sentences, listen to each sample and transcribe what you hear orthographically. Then compare your orthographic transcription with the target sentences provided in the table at the end of this chapter. For each sample, calculate intelligibility using the following formula (number of words correctly transcribed/ number of target words) x 100%. Use the rating scales below to rate each speaker's comprehensibility and accentedness. Compare your results with others in a group. How similar or different are your results from those of other group members? What do you think accounts for the differences?

		Comprehensibility Rating	Accentedness Rating	Percent Intelligibility
Sample 1 Spanish Peru	Female age 33 AOL 23 YSE 10			
Sample 2 Spanish Peru	Male age 42 AOL 40 YSE 2			
Sample 3 Korean	Female age 29 AOL 13 YSE 3			
Sample 4 Korean	Male age 32 AOL 13 YSE 12			
Sample 5 Japanese	Female age 39 AOL 13 YSE 0.25			
Sample 6 Japanese	Male age 35 AOL 12 YSE 21			

AOL: Age of learning YSE: Years speaking English.

*AOL refers to the age the speaker first began learning English. This may have taken place in school in the speaker's native country or when the speaker first moved to the United States. AOL generally corresponds to the age when the speaker was first exposed to English vocabulary and grammar but he or she may not have begun speaking English in conversation at that time. YSE refers to the number of years the speaker has been speaking English for work or in social settings. This may have begun in the speaker's native country but usually begins when the speaker first moves to an English speaking country.

Comprehensibility – the listener's perception of the degree of difficulty encountered when trying to understand an utterance

1	2	3	4	5	6	7
extremely easy	easy	very little work	some attention required	a lot of attention required	difficult	extremely difficult

Accentedness – a listener's perception of how different a speaker's accent is from that of native speakers

1 no accent	2 barely notice-able accent	3 very mild accent	4 mild accent	5 moderate accent	6 heavy accent	7 extremely strong accent

Orthographic transcription of sentences for speech samples

	Sentence	Number of target words
Sample 1	My mother nursed me in the wings and in dressing rooms	11
Sample 2	I was worried about what I was going to say to him	12
Sample 3	When her son graduated from college with honors she beamed with pride	12
Sample 4	As long as one can admire and love, then one is young forever	13
Sample 5	It is unrealistic to expect any human personality to remain frozen for two decades.	14
Sample 6	After what seemed like hours of waiting, the taxi finally showed up	12

Sidebar 8.1 Other Ingredients in Acquiring a Target Language as an Adult

The phonetic and phonologic repertoire of a TL is only one of many components to be acquired by adult learners. Other components include the vocabulary, morphology, syntax, and even the written form of the language. An example of a person who expertly mastered all aspects except the phonetic and phonological systems of English is Henry Kissinger, who, despite having lived in the United States for most of his long adult life, never quite lost his German accent. Is the phonology different? Why would an adult acquiring a TL experience greater difficulty achieving native-like proficiency in phonology compared to grammar and vocabulary? The critical period has been more closely tied to phonology than to other areas of language such as morphology, syntax and pragmatics. However, in an article published in 2000 entitled "A critical review of the critical period research," Scovel stated the following: "Despite the fact that foreign accents emerge in early adulthood and, with rare exception, remain indelible after puberty, adult learners can, should and do improve their pronunciation and intelligibility in a second language." (Scovel, 2000 page 17).

Activity 3.

In the sound files 8S7 through 8S22,

a. Attempt to construct a NL phoneme inventory from the comments about rainbows in the speaker's native language.
b. Observe any suprasegmental features in the NL language
c. List any distortions, substitutions, insertions, and omissions you detect in the TL productions
d. List any suprasegmental differences in the TL productions
e. Finally, describe any patterns of NL-to-TL transfer, assimilations, or dissimilations in the segmental and suprasegmental TL productions.

ANSWERS TO CHAPTER REVIEW QUESTIONS

1. Define the following global measures of pronunciation proficiency: accentedness, comprehensibility, intelligibility, and fluency. Why would it be important for a clinician to gather ratings on several of these measures when assessing pronunciation proficiency?

Accentedness is the extent to which a nonnative speaker's pronunciation patterns differ from that of the target language community.

Comprehensibility is a listener's perception of how difficult it is to understand a speaker or the degree of effort one must exert when listening to a speaker. Intelligibility is the extent to which a naïve listener understands an utterance and fluency is how smooth and free-flowing an individual's speech is.

Clinicians should gather ratings on more than one of these measures because it is possible for a speaker with a heavy accent to be fully intelligible and have good comprehensibility. A client may improve in comprehensibility and intelligibility as a result of pronunciation instruction even if he or she retains a noticeable accent.

2. Why is accent *modification* a more appropriate term to use rather than accent *reduction* or accent *elimination*?

Accent modification is a more appropriate term than accent reduction or elimination because it acknowledges that everybody speaks with an accent. In seeking pronunciation training, a nonnative speaker is simply trying to modify his or her accent toward that of the target language community. The terms accent reduction and accent elimination suggest that one can speak without an accent at all.

3. Describe three different types of speech sample elicitation strategies used to assess non-native speech. What is an advantage of each type?

Non-native speech patterns can be assessed using single words, paragraphs or through spontaneous conversation.

Written single words and paragraphs can allow the clinician to pre-select the specific phonemes, syllable structures, and prosodic patterns attempted by the speaker. However, spontaneous conversation provides a more naturalistic speech sample.

REFERENCES

American Speech-Language-Hearing Association Joint Subcommittee of the Executive Board of English Language Proficiency. (1998). Students and professionals who speak English with accents and non-standard dialects: Issues and recommendations. Position statement and technical report. *ASHA,* 40 (suppl 18), 28-41.

Abu-Rabia, S. and Kehat, S. (2004). The critical period for second language pronunciation: Is there such a thing? Ten case studies of late starters who attained a native-like Hebrew accent. *Educational Psychology,* 24 (1), 77-98.

Brown, A. (1991). Functional load and the teaching of pronunciation. In Brown, A. (Ed.), Teaching English pronunciation: A book of readings, (pp. 221-224). London: Routeledge.

Burgess, J. and Spencer, S. (2000). Phonology and pronunciation in integrated language teaching and teacher education. *System,* 28, 191-215.

Carey, M.D., Mannell, R.H. and Dunn, P.K. (2010). Does a rater's familiarity with a candidate's pronunciation affect the rating in oral proficiency interviews? *Language Testing*, 28 (2), 201-219.

Compton, A.J. (1983). Phonological assessment of foreign accent. San Francisco: Carousel House.

Derwing, T. M. and Munro, M. (1997). Accent, intelligibility, and comprehensibility. Evidence from four L1s. *Studies in Second Language Acquisition,* 19 (1), 1-16.

Derwing, T. M. and Munro, M. J. (2005). Second language accent and pronunciation teaching: a research-based approach. *Language Learning,* 58(3), 479-502.

Derwing, T. M. and Munro, M. J. (2006). The functional load principle in ESL pronunciation instruction: An exploratory study. *System, 24,* 520-531.

Derwing, T.M., Rossiter, M.J., Munro, M.J., and Thompson, R.I. (2004). Second language fluency: Judgments on different tasks. *Language Learning*, 54 (4), 655-679.

Derwing, T., Munro, M.J., and Weibe, G. (1998). Evidence in favor of a broad framework for pronunciation instruction. *Language Learning,* 48 (3), 393-410.

FILES: 2007 American Community Survey United States/prepared by the U.S. Census Bureau, 2010.

Ferrier, L.J., Reid, L.N., and Chenausky, K. (1999). Computer-assisted accent modification: A report on practice effects. *Topics in Language Disorders,* 19 (4), 35-48.

Flege, J. (1995). Second language speech learning: Theory, findings, and problems. In W. Strange (ed.), Speech perception and linguistic experience: Issues in cross-language research, pp. 233-277. Timonium, MD: York Press.

Flege, J.E. and Fletcher, K.L. (1992). Talker and listener effects on the perception of degree of foreign accent. *Journal of the Acoustical Society of America,* 91, 370-389.

Flege, J. E., Munro, M. J. and MacKay, I. R. A. (1995). Factors affecting strength of perceived foreign accent in a second language. *Journal of the Acoustical Society of America,* 97 (5), 3125-3134.

Gass, S.M. and Selinker, L. (2001). *Second Language Acquisition: An introductory course.* Mahwah, NJ: Lawrence Erlbaum Associates.

Gluzek, A. and Dovidio, J.F. (2010). Speaking with a non-native accent: Perceptions of bias communication difficulties and belonging in the United States. *Journal of Language and Social Psychology,* 29 (2), 224-234.

Kanno, Y. (2003). Negotiating Bilingual and Bicultural Identities. Japanese Returnees Betwixt Two Worlds. Mahwah, NJ: Lawrence Earlbaum Associates.

Kim, Mikjung. (2001). Detecting DIF across the different language groups in a speaking test. *Language Testing,* 18(1), 89-114.

Lenneberg, E. H. (1967). Biological foundations of language. New York: Wiley.

Macdonald, D., Yule, G. and Powers, M. (1994). Attempts to improve English L2 pronunciation: The variable effects of different types of instruction. *Language Learning,* 44 (1), 75-100.

Mack, M. (2003). The phonetic systems of bilinguals. In M. T. Banich and M. Mack (eds.), Mind, brain, and language: Multidisciplinary perspectives, (pp. 309-349). Mahwah, NJ: Lawrence Earlbaum Associates.

MacLeod, A. and Stoel-Gammon, C. (2010). What is the impact of age of second language acquisition on the production of consonants and vowels among childhood bilinguals? *The International Journal of Bilingualism, 14(4),* 400-421.

Maddieson, I. (1997). Phonetic universals. In W. J. Hardcastle and J. Laver (eds.), *The Handbook of Phonetic Sciences,* pp. 619-639. Cambridge: Blackwell Publishers Inc.

Marx, N. (2002). Never quite a native speaker: Accent and identity in the L2 – and the L1. Canadian Modern Language Review, 59 (2), 264-281.

Mehler, J., Dupoux, E., Nazzi, T. and Dehane-Lambertz, g. (1996). Coping with linguistic diversity: The infant's viewpoint. In J. L. Morgan and K. Demuth (eds.), Signal to Syntax, pp. 101-116. Mahwah,NJ: Lawrence Erlbaum Associates.

Moyer, A. (1999). Ultimate attainment in L2 phonology. *Studies in Second Language Acquisition,* 21, 81-108.

Moyer. A. (2004). Age, accent, and experience in second language acquisition: An integrated approach to critical period inquiry. Clevedon: Multilingual Matters.

Muller, N., Ball, M. J., and Guendouzi, J. (2000). Accent reduction programmes: Not a role for speech-language pathologists? *Advances in Speech-Language Pathology,* 2(2), 119-154.

Munro, M. J. (1993). Productions of English vowels by native speakers of Arabic: Acoustic measurements and accentedness ratings. *Language and Speech,* 36 (1), 39-66.

Munro, M.J. (2003). A primer on accent discrimination in the Canadian context. *TESL Canada Journal,* 20 (2), 38-51.

Munro, M.J. and Derwing, T.M. (1994). Evaluations of foreign accent in extemporaneous and read material. *Language Testing,* 11, 253-266.

Munro, M. J. and Mann, V. (2005). Age of immersion as a predictor of foreign accent. *Applied Psycholinguistics,* 26, 311-341.

Nazzi, T. (2005). Use of phonetic specificity during the acquisition of new words: differences between consonants and vowels. *Cognition,* 98, 13-30.

Nguyen, B. (1993). Accent discrimination and the Test of Spoken English: A call for an objective assessment of the comprehensibility of nonnative speakers. *California Law Review,* 81(5), 1325-1337.

Oyama, S. (1976). A sensitive period of the acquisition of a nonnative phonological system. *Journal of Psycholinguistics Research,* 5, 261-283.

Patkowski, M.S. (1990). Ace and accent in a second language: A reply to James Emil Flege. *Applied Linguistics,* 11 (1), 73-89.

Pennington, M. C. and Richards, J. C. (1986). Pronunciation revisited. *TESOL Quarterly,* 20 (2), 207-225.

Pollock, K.E. and Berni, M.C. (2001). Transcription of vowels. *Topics in Language Disorders,* 21 (4), 22-40.

Smit, U. and Dalton, C. (2000). Motivational patterns in advanced EFL pronunciation learners. *IRAL,* 38, 229-246.

Scovel, T. (1969). Foreign accents, language acquisition, and cerebral dominance. *Language Learning,* 19, 245-253.

Scovel, T. (2000). A critical review of the critical period research. *Annual Review of Applied Linguistics,* 20, 213-223.

Sikorski, L. D. (2005). Regional accents: A rationale for intervening and competencies required. *Seminars in Speech and Language,* 26 (2), 118-125.

Tsukada, K., Birdsong, D., Bialystock, E., Mack, M., Sung, H. and Flege, J. (2005). A developmental study of English vowel production and perception by native Korean adults and children. *Journal of Phonetics,* 33, 263-290.

Wang, X. and Munro, M. J. (2004). Computer-based training for learning English vowel contrasts. *System,* 32, 539-552.

Yeni-Komshian, G. H., Flege, J. E. and Liu, S. (2000). Pronunciation proficiency in the first and second languages of Korean-English bilinguals. *Bilingualism: Language and Cognition,* 3 (2), 131-149.

III. Beyond English: Children Acquiring Other Languages or Multiple Languages

In: Comprehensive Perspectives …
Editors: Beate Peter and Andrea A. N. MacLeod
ISBN: 978-1-62257-041-6

Chapter 9

Cross-Linguistic Trends in the Acquisition of Speech Sounds

Krisztina Zajdó

Introduction

Starting at the end of the 19th century, parental diary studies documenting speech acquisition mostly in monolingual English-speaking children served as primary sources of information on children's speech development. Interest in the search for *universal trends* in speech acquisition processes across languages was ignited by the work of Russian linguist Roman Jakobson (1896-1982). As a structural linguist, Jakobson had a strong interest in the development of new techniques to map out sound systems in various languages. As described in Chapter 1, structural linguistics is an approach to studying language that focuses on underlying structures and levels such as sentences, phrases, lexical components, and speech sounds, where the speech sounds of a language are systematically organized in language-specific ways. While exploring regularities in the sound systems of languages, Jakobson noticed that the laws of sound systems also guide the order of speech sound acquisition in children. This chapter retraces the history of cross-linguistic research regarding the acquisition of phonologic systems and shows how speech sound development follows certain universal trends across many different languages.

The Laws of Irreversible Solidarity

Jakobson (1941/1968) gathered the available data from the then-nascent field of phonological theory coupled with child speech data based on anecdotal evidence of children acquiring speech in various language communities. As a linguist, he attempted to identify common trends in sound systems across languages. Jakobson proposed the laws of *irreversible solidarity* to account for the sound system structures associated with diverse languages. This term refers to the observation that the presence of certain sound classes (e.g., front vowels) presupposes the availability of others (e.g., back vowels) in the sound repertory of languages. Similarly, Jakobson noted that languages with fricatives also have stops in their consonant inventory. He argued that the existence of fricatives in a language presupposes the presence of stops in that language. *Implicational hierarchy* is a more contemporary term used to describe the idea that if one element is present, certain others will be present as well. Jakobson also observed that languages with back consonants in their consonant inventory typically also have front consonants. Jakobson concluded that some phonological features (or sound classes) can be considered "more basic" than others, indicated by their widespread presence in the languages of the world. He proposed that phonological features (or sound classes) that are documented in a smaller number of languages mandate the presence of other features (or sound classes) that are observed more frequently in sound systems cross-linguistically. The term *markedness* refers to the less basic elements or features. In this terminology, a marked sound or feature is the less basic one, whereas the unmarked sound or feature is the more basic or common one.

Jakobson theorized that the presence or absence of phonological features also dictate a universal order of speech sound acquisition in children. When studying sound systems in various languages, he observed the presence or absence of phonological features in various languages. Relying mostly on anecdotal evidence gathered from child speech descriptions, Jakobson suggested that speech sound acquisition in children begins with "more basic" (unmarked) followed by "less basic" (marked) features in speech sounds. Thus, unmarked features that are more commonly observed cross-linguistically emerge in children's speech earlier than marked ones that have been documented less frequently in various languages.

Jakobson's work, which in essence constitutes the first attempt at formulating a theory of speech acquisition, has been criticized by many since its publication, most frequently due to its incompleteness. However, even today, theories of speech sound acquisition build on and stem from many of Jakobson's observations to explain certain trends in the acquisition of speech sounds cross-linguistically. In the following sections, we will review several (but not all) of the claims put forward by Jakobson pertaining to the order of the acquisition of phonemic contrasts.

THEORETICAL FRAMEWORK

In his often-cited work, Jakobson (1941/1968) proposed that children acquire speech by establishing and learning to produce maximal contrasts such as the difference between a consonant and a vowel. A maximally closed bilabial stop followed by a low vowel would constitute an example of maximal contrast.

According to Jakobson, the law of maximal contrast determines a universal order of speech sound acquisition. Speech acquisition begins with Step 1, the production of low vowels (such as the wide /ɑ/) and consonants produced with most closure (e.g., bilabials such as /b/). When sequenced, these sounds constitute a consonant-vowel (CV) structured syllable. Subsequently, the child continues with Step 2, contrasting nasal with oral stops. Thus, it is proposed that nasal sounds as a class are acquired in opposition to orals sounds. The next step of learning to contrast sounds involves contrasting labials with non-labials (e.g., dentals). Overall, Step 3 is interpreted as the earlier acquisition of front (as opposed to less fronted or back) consonants. The next step of development, Step 4, involves creating a contrast between low and high vowels. Thus, low vowels would be acquired before high ones. The trend to contrast speech sounds continues with Step 5, opposing front and back vowels, or with the acquisition of high and mid vowels. The order of emerging speech sound classes reflects the proposed order of acquisition. Thus, Jakobson proposed a universal order of speech sound acquisition that is determined by the law of contrast. Children learn to speak through developing a concept of contrasting speech sounds and acquiring the production of *binary oppositions* while developing speech skills.

However, Jakobson also pointed out that the child is not fully able to distinguish between certain phonemes that are somewhat similar from the child's perspective. In some cases, children substitute members of a sound class with a sound from a different sound category. Examples of substitution include confusing and substituting /m/ for /n/, or substituting the stops /t/ or /d/ for labials such as /b/. Overall, while many children make speech sound errors, Jakobson hypothesized that child speech is characterized by learning an increasing number of sound contrasts in a pre-determined order.

Cross-Linguistic Studies of Speech Sound Acquisition

Jakobson's theory was based on data from more than a dozen languages. Large-scale follow-up studies of speech sound development in various languages were not available in the 1930s. Since then, there has been much progress in mapping out speech phenomena in children speaking English (see Chapters 4 through 7 that focus on pre-speech through to the development of speech sounds and intonation). However, only a very limited amount of progress in child speech research focusing on languages other than English has been achieved.

Research focused on the acquisition of speech sounds and sound systems in monolingual children cross-linguistically has only started to take momentum during the last twenty years. Recently, an increase in the number of studies documenting speech sound acquisition in various languages has been witnessed. Data gathered to document the acquisition of speech segments has been slowly becoming available during recent years from English-speaking communities where one or more of the non-standard varieties of English are spoken. Additionally, results of a limited amount of child speech research from non-English-speaking countries have become accessible.

Different languages are characterized by various system properties including different consonant and vowel inventories, different frequency distribution of speech sounds, various syllable types, and different stress and intonation systems used. Children learning various languages proceed through the acquisition process via different pathways. Formulating theories of speech and language acquisition requires a most detailed understanding of the mechanisms at work during the acquisition process in many language communities. As a result of gaining insight into processes of speech sound acquisition in many diverse languages in addition to English, various pieces of knowledge pertaining to the acquisition of speech sounds previously considered evident may be replaced with new information. It is reasonable to speculate that progress in the acquisition of speech sounds in English may not only reflect universal features of learning to speak, but rather mirrors both universal and language-specific steps in speech sound acquisition.

LIMITATIONS OF RESEARCH ON THE ACQUISITION OF SPEECH SOUNDS CROSS-LINGUISTICALLY

Constructing theories of speech sound acquisition requires the availability of child speech data from various languages resulting from studies that yield comparable results. Up until now, cross-linguistic studies applying identical or very similar methodology have been rare, leading to concerns regarding comparability of study results. Studies differ greatly in many aspects, including: variations in study design (e.g. cross-sectional or follow-up study), sample size (e.g. case study vs. group study), subject selection criteria (selection and elimination of potential participants from the study), speech elicitation strategies (e.g. speech produced during picture naming vs. spontaneous conversation), and recording techniques (e.g. the specifics of recording attributes and the recording tools used). Importantly, studies focusing on speech sound acquisition apply diverse working definitions for basic concepts. Interpretation of study results requires a thorough understanding of all working definitions used in the study, such as, for example, how the authors used the term "accuracy", what constituted "stable" or "variable" production or how the criteria for the label "acquired sounds" were determined.

Due to important differences in how child speech studies have been conducted throughout the world, caution is required when interpreting the results. It is important to recognize the limits on the amount and types of currently available data. However, making observations of speech acquisition processes is still a viable option in spite of the different methods used in individual research studies. Various questions generated by examining the data are supposed to guide future research and thus bring us closer to a fuller understanding of cross-linguistic trends in speech acquisition as a complex human behavior.

Despite the fact that the methodology used in cross-linguistic studies varies to a great extent, examining child speech data from diverse languages is a worthwhile process in as much as it highlights interesting child speech phenomena that may not be observable from studies focusing on speech acquisition data from individual languages.

To provide a picture of the wide variety of results on child speech studies from diverse languages, three short reviews of the phonological acquisition of French, Brazilian Portuguese, and Korean are provided in Chapters 10, 11, 12.

UNIVERSAL STEPS IN VOWEL ACQUISITION PROPOSED BY JAKOBSON

Despite many limitations of the currently available research results, the data has been examined and statements about common trends in speech sound acquisition proposed by Jakobson (1941/1968) found full or partial support. Pertaining to vowels in speech development, Jakobson proposed that 1) children learn to differentiate vowels and consonants early in development (Step 1 of speech acquisition); 2) children learn to contrast low and high vowels at a certain stage during speech development (Step 4); and that 3) the final stage of speech sound development (Step 5) is learning to contrast front and back or high and mid vowels.

Universal Trends in Vowel Acquisition Signaled by Cross-Linguistic Studies

As stated earlier, many researchers have attempted to evaluate Jakobson's proposals about developmental steps in speech sound acquisition. As for the acquisition of vowels, support for Step 1 of the acquisition process comes from one of the earliest occurring pre-speech phenomena in infants, the stage of canonical babbling. During this stage, consonant-like and vowel-like sounds are sequenced in vocalizations. The most frequently occurring production patterns documented in babbling include CV, VC, or CVCV sequences (Oller, 1980), clearly indicating the exploration of contrasts in these sound categories both within the same syllable and across syllable boundaries. CV structured syllables have been reported to be the most commonly occurring syllable type cross-linguistically (e.g., Blevins, 1995; Clements, 1990), serving as a reminder of these early explorations of contrasts in vocalization segments.

Support for Steps 4 and 5 can also be found. Data from canonical babbling production of children reared in various language environments including communities speaking French, Romanian, Dutch, Tunisian Arabic and Turkish indicates that mid and low front and central vowels are most frequently produced by infants at this stage of pre-speech development (Kern and Davis, 2009). Similar findings have been reported by others from various other language communities (for a review, see Locke, 1983; for American English, see Stoel-Gammon and Herrington, 1990). With the exception of Tunisian Arabic, infants examined in the study of Kern and Davis produced mid vowels most frequently, followed by low vowels. High vowels were the least frequently produced in sound class in all languages examined. Thus, the data lends some support for Jakobson's claim that contrasts between low or mid and high vowels appear later during development, since there are less opportunities for acquiring the contrast between a low frequency vowel class and other vowels.

Additionally, results from Kern and Davis (2009) also show that the occurrence of back vowels is significantly less frequent than the production of central and front vowels in canonical babbling. Again, it is reasonable to speculate that learning to contrast front and back vowels is a later occurring step in speech-like behavior in children, due to the low frequency of back vowels that hinders acquisition of this vowel class and those that serve as contrasts. Later occurrence and lower frequency of back vowel production in canonical babbling is likely to lead to later acquisition of the contrast between them and other classes of vowels.

As noted in Chapters 4 and 5, previous research has already shown a certain amount of phonetic continuity between babbling and speech (for American English, see Stoel-Gammon and Cooper, 1984; for reviews, see Oller, 1980; and Kern, Davis and Zink, 2009). Thus results indicate that learning to produce vocalizations during babbling benefits children's later occurring speech behavior cross-linguistically.

Cross-Linguistic Vowel Acquisition Data: Observations from Several Languages

Many publications on speech development contain statements about the early acquisition of vowels. Table 1 contains cross-linguistic data on the proportions of vowels produced "correctly" by children in various age groups from various studies done all over the world. For the purposes of this analysis, data from languages that are typologically distinct were selected. Languages examined include Greek, Sesotho, American English, Hungarian, Cantonese, Puthongua and Finnish. With the exception of Sesotho, these studies examined relatively large groups of children; the numbers of participants varied between 34 and 1600. These languages differ with respect to their linguistic roots (Greek and American English have Indo-European roots, Hungarian and Finnish are Uralic languages, Puthongua and Cantonese belong to the Sino-Tibetan language family, and Sesotho is a Bantu language from the Niger-Congo language family). Importantly, the above-mentioned seven languages are characterized by different vowel inventories: Greek has 5, Sesotho has 9, and Hungarian has 14 monophthong vowels in their vowel inventory. The vowel system of American English includes 18 or 19 monophthongs and 3 or 4 diphthongs (see Pollock and Berni, 2003). Cantonese has 8 monophtongs (with 3 allophones) and 11 diphthongs, bringing the size of its vowel inventory to 19 + 3 vowels. Puthongua has 9 monophthongs, 9 diphthongs and 4 triphthongs. The most sizeable vowel inventory examined here is the Finnish one which includes 26 vowels: 8 monophthongs and 18 diphthongs. Languages with different vowel inventory size allow for the examination of the impact of vowel inventory size on the speed of acquisition in children. Working definitions of "correct production" vary among these studies.

The majority of studies report a speech sound to be correctly produced if 90% of children in a given age group produce the speech sound in a way that is perceived to be a correct production by one or more native speakers. However, these studies differ in speech elicitation techniques (e.g. picture naming, vs. spontaneous conversation), the position of the sound within words examined (e.g. only speech sounds in word initial or word medial contexts are examined), the effects of the surrounding consonants on vowel production, as well as recording attributes. Although cross-linguistic studies often differ in the methodology used, it is important to keep in mind that the lack of consistency in data gathering and analysis techniques limits the validity of conclusions drawn from results.The claim that vowels are acquired early (earlier than consonants) appears to be only partially supported by cross-linguistic data. Table 9.1 shows results about the percentage of vowels correctly produced by monolingual typically developing children acquiring seven languages. Among the languages listed, some are characterized by a lower number of vowels while others have a more sizeable vowel inventory. Languages are listed in an order from the lowest to the highest number of vowels in their inventory. Results from early speech (1;6-2;0 [years;months]) from two languages, General American English and Putonghua (Modern Standard Chinese) indicate the percentage correct values for vowels at or above 80%. As Table 9.2 shows, consonants produced by typically developing children in a relatively comparable age range (1;3-2;0) speaking Turkish, Putonghua and German are characterized by lower levels of accuracy. While correct production is associated with vowels earlier during development than with consonants, examining the data allows for some interesting observations.

Table 9.1. Percentage of vowels correct (PVC) in children speaking seven languages

Greek Papadopoulou 2000		Sesotho Demuth 2007		Hungarian Zajdó 2002		American English Pollock and Berni 2003		Cantonese So and Dodd 1995		Putonghua Zhu and Dodd 2000		Finnish Pietarinen 1987	
Size of vowel inventory (+ allophones)													
5 monophthongs		9 monophthongs		14 monophthongs		21/23= 18/19 monophthongs + 3/4 diphthongs*		22= 8 (3 allophones) + 11 diphthongs		22 = 9 monophthongs + 9 diphthongs + 4 triphthongs		26= 8 monophthongs + 18 diphthongs	
n = 34		n = 4		n = 80		n = 165		n = 272		n = 129		n = 1600	
Age	PVC	Age	PVC	Age	PVC	Age	PVC	Age	PVC	Age	PVC	Age	PVC
						1;6-1;11	82.00			*1;6-2;0*	80.00		
		2;0	75.00	*2;0*	85.20	*2;0-2;5*	92.00	*2;0-2;5*	98.80	*2;1-2;6*	82.40		
		2;6	80.00	*2;6*	90.10	*2;6-2;11*	94.00	*2;6-2;11*	99.20	*2;7-3;0*	83.60		
		3;0	90.00	*3;0*	90.40	*3;0-3;5*	97.00	*3;0-3;5*	99.70	*3;1-3;6*	87.90		
				3;6	96.80	*3;6-3;11*	97.00	*3;6-3;11*	99.70	*3;7-4;0*	90.80		
4;0	90% of all children have acquired all vowels	*4;0*	100.00	*4;0*	95.10	*4;0-4;5*	98.00	*4;0-4;5*	99.60	*4;1-4;6*	89.10		
						4;6-4;11	99.00	*4;6-4;11*	99.60				
						5;0-5;5	99.00	*5;0-5;5*	99.80			*5;0*	98.60
						5;6-5;11	99.00	*5;6-5;11*	100.0				
						6;0-6;5	98.00						
						6;6-6;11	99.00						

* In American English, the number of monophthongs increases to 19 if we count the /ɔ/ vowel; the number of diphthongs increases to 4 if we count /ju/ as a diphthong (Smit, 2007).

Table 9.2. Percentage of consonants correct (PCC) in seven languages

Cantonese So and Dodd 1995		Turkish Topbaş and Yavaş 2006				Putonghua Zhu 2007		German Fox and Dodd 1999		Hungarian Nagy 1980		Jordanian Arabic Amayreh and Dyson 1998		Sesotho Demuth 2007	
Size of consonant inventory (+ allophones)															
19		20				22		24		25 (7)		28 (6)		39 (2) or 65 (2)*	
n = 272		n = 665				n = 129		n = 178		n = 7602		n = 180		n = 4	
Age	PCC	Age	**	PCC	SD	Age	PCC	Age	PCC	Age	PCC	Age	PCC	Age	PCC
		1;3-2;0	M	41.10	13.21										
			F	44.27	11.80	*1;6-2;0*	63.90	*1;6-1;11*	73.95						
			A	42.80	12.42										
2;0-2;5	85.60	*2;1-3;0*	M	68.50	12.76	*2;1-2;6*	74.40	*2;0-2;5*	78.81			*2;0-2;4*	52.00	*2;0*	75.00
			F	74.00	8.77										
			A	71.42	11.05										
2;6-2;11	91.70					*2;7-3;0*	81.00	*2;6-2;11*	87.41			*2;6-2;10*	62.00	*2;6*	80.00
3;0-3;5	95.80	*3;1-4;0*	M	94.88	4.29	*3;1-3;6*	86.40	*3;0-3;5*	90.99	*3;0*	82.10	*3;0-3;4*	75.00	*3;0*	90.00
			F	94.78	4.87										
3;6-3;11	96.40		A	94.85	4.44	*3;7-4;0*	89.50	*3;6-3;11*	94.25			*3;6-3;10*	75.00		
4;0-4;5	98.10	*4;1-5;0*	M	98.72	2.26	*4;1-4;6*	92.20	*4;0-4;5*	95.14	*4;0*	90.80	*4;0-4;4*	81.00	*4;0*	100.00
			F	97.78	2.53										
4;6-4;11	97.80		A	98.19	2.44			*4;6-4;11*	96.20			*4;6-4;10*	78.00		

* In Sesotho, the number of consonants in the inventory increases to 65 (2) if we count labialized consonants as contrastive phonemes.

** M=Male, F=Female, A=All.

Cantonese So and Dodd 1995		Turkish Topbaş and Yavaş 2006				Putonghua Zhu 2007		German Fox and Dodd 1999		Hungarian Nagy 1980		Jordanian Arabic Amayreh and Dyson 1998		Sesotho Demuth 2007	
Size of consonant inventory (+ allophones)															
19		20				22		24		25 (7)		28 (6)		39 (2) or 65 (2)*	
n = 272		n = 665				n = 129		n = 178		n = 7602		n = 180		4	
Age	PCC	Age	**	PCC	SD	Age	PCC	Age	PCC	Age	PCC	Age	PCC	Age	PCC
5;0-5;5	99.50	*5;1-6;0*	M	97.54	3.21			*5;0-5;5*	97.43	*5;0*	93.20	*5;0-5;4*	86.00		
			F	98.33	2.39										
5;6-5;11	99.20		A	97.92	2.85			*5;6-5;11*	98.08			*5;6-5;10*	84.00		
		6;1-7;0	M	98.52	2.53					*6;0*	96.20	*6;0-6;10*	90.00		
			F	98.80	2.18										
			A	98.66	2.35										
		7;1-8;0	M	99.56	1.31					*7;0*	99.70				
			F	99.22	1.76										
			A	99.42	1.51										
		8;0 <	M	99.40	1.13					*8;0*	99.90				
			F	99.54	1.37										
			A	99.47	1.25										

* In Sesotho, the number of consonants in the inventory increases to 65 (2) if we count labialized consonants as contrastive phonemes.

** M=Male, F=Female, A=All.

Table 9.3. Age of acquisition of consonants in ten languages (in years;months)

Target consonant	**Jordanian Arabic** 1 Amayreh & Dyson (1998)	**Jordanian Arabic** 2 Amayreh (2003)	**Jordanian Arabic** 3 Hamdan & Amayreh (2007)	**Cantonese** 1 Tse (1982)	**Cantonese** 2 (Cheung (1990)	**Cantonese** 3 Tse (1991)	**Cantonese** 4 So & Dodd (1995)	**Putonghua** 75% group crit* (Zhu & Dodd, 2000)	**Putonghua** 90% group crit (Zhu & Dodd, 2000)	**German** 75% crit (Fox & Dodd, 1999)	**German** (Fox & Dodd, 1999)	**Greek** 75% criterion (PAL, 1995)	**Greek** (Papadopoulou, 2000)	**Hungarian** (Nagy, 1980)	**Japanese** 1 (Sakauchi, 1967)	**Japanese** 2 (Takagi and Yashuda, 1967)	**Japanese** 3 (Noda et al., 1969)	**Japanese** 4 (Nakanishi et al., 1972)	**Korean** (Kim & Pae, 2005)	**Maltese** 75% criterion (Grech, 1998)	**Thai** 80% criterion (Boonyathitisuk, 1982 and Dardarananda, 1993)	
	180	60	100	3	155	1	272	129		178		300	34	7602	134	133	446	1689	220	21	1032	number of participants
	2;0- 6;4	6;6-8;4	avg. 6;4	1;7-2;8	2;1-6;0	1;2-3;0	1;2-5;11	1;6- 4;6		1;6- 5;11		2;6- 6;0	3;7- 4;6	3;0- 8;0	2;10- 4;8	3;6- 6;0	2;0- 6;6	4;0- 6;11	2;6- 6;5	2;0- 3;6	3;0- 8;0	age range
	28 (6)			19				22		24		20 (11)		25 (7)	15 (9)				19 (1)	22	21	Inventory size: Phonemic consonants (+ allophones)
p				1;7	2;1	1;3	2;0	2;6	3;0	1;6 -1;11	1;6-1;11	2;6-3;0	3;7-4;0	<3;0	2;10-3;3	3;0-3;5	3;6-3;11	4;0-4;5	early 3	2;0	2;8-3;0	plosives
p*																			late 2			
p^h				2;5	3;1	1;11	3;6	2;6	4;0										late 2		3;1-3;6	
? p																					>7;0	
b	3;0	nd****	nd							1;6-1;11	2;0-2;5	2;6-3;0	3;7-4;0	4;0	2;10-3;3	5;0-5;5	3;0-3;5	4;0-4;5		2;0	2;8-3;0	
t	2;6	nd	nd	2;0	2;1	1;6	2;0	2;0	2;0	1;6-1;11	2;6-2;11	2;6-3;0	3;7-4;0	<3;0	2;10-3;3	3;0-3;5	3;0-3;5	4;0-4;5	early 3	2;0	3;1-3;6	
t*																			late 2			
t^h				2;5	3;1	1;11	3;6	2;0	3;0										early 3		3;1-3;6	
? t																					>7;0	

Target consonant	**Jordanian Arabic** 1 Amayreh & Dyson (1998)	**Jordanian Arabic** 2 Amayreh (2003)	**Jordanian Arabic** 3 Hamdan & Amayreh (2007)	**Cantonese** 1 Tse (1982)	**Cantonese** 2 (Cheung (1990)	**Cantonese** 3 Tse (1991)	**Cantonese** 4 So & Dodd (1995)	**Putonghua** 75% group crit* (Zhu & Dodd, 2000)	**Putonghua** 90% group crit (Zhu & Dodd, 2000)	**German** 75% crit (Fox & Dodd, 1999)	**German** (Fox & Dodd, 1999)	**Greek** 75% criterion (PAL, 1995)	**Greek** (Papadopoulou, 2000)	**Hungarian** (Nagy, 1980)	**Japanese** 1 (Sakauchi, 1967)	**Japanese** 2 (Takagi and Yashuda, 1967)	**Japanese** 3 (Noda et al., 1969)	**Japanese** 4 (Nakanishi et al., 1972)	**Korean** (Kim & Pae, 2005)	**Maltese** 75% criterion (Grech, 1998)	**Thai** 80% criterion (Boonyathitisuk, 1982 and Dardarananda, 1993)	
t̲	6;4	8;4	≤6;4																			
d	3;0	nd	nd							1;6-1;11	1;6-1;11	3;0-3;6	3;7-4;0	<3;0	2;10-3;3	3;0-3;5	4;6-4;11	4;0-4;5		2;0		
d̲	>6;4	7;4	6;4																			
ç								2;6	3;0	3;0-3;5	4;0-4;5	3;0-3;6	4;1-4;6	4;0-5;0	>4;8	4;0-4;5	4;0-4;5	4;0-4;5				
k	2;6	nd	nd	2;0	3;7	1;8	3;0	2;6	3;6	2;6-2;11	2;6-2;11	2;6-3;0	3;7-4;0	3;0	2;10-3;3	4;0-4;5	3;6-3;11	4;0-4;5	early 4	2;0	2;8-3;0	
k*																			early 3			
kʰ				>2;8	4;1	>3;0	3;6	2;6	3;6										early 4		2;1-2;6 3;7-4;0*** >7;0	
ʔ k																						
kʷ				>2;8	3;7	>3;0	3;9															
kʷʰ				>2;8	3;7	>3;0	4;9															
g										2;6-2;11	3;0-3;5	2;6-3;0	3;7-4;0	3;0-4;0	2;10-3;3	3;0-3;5	3;6-3;11	4;0-4;5		3;0		
ⁿg												nd	>4;6									
q	>6;4	7;4	6;4																			
ʔ	<2;0	<6;6	<6;4							n d.	n.d									2;0	2;1-2;6	
m	<2;0	nd	nd	2;0	2;1	1;8	2;6	2;0	2;0	1,6-1;11	1;6-1;11	2;6-3;0	3;7-4;0	3;0	2;10-3;3	3;0-3;5	3;0-3;5	4;0-4;5	early 3	2;0	2;1-2;6	nasals
n				2;0	2;7	1;11	2;0	2;0	2;6	1,6-1;11	2;0-2;5	3;0-3;6	3;7-4;0	3;0	3;4-3;8	3;6-3;11	4;0-4;5	4;0-4;5	late 3	2;0	2;1-2;6	
ɲ												2;6-3;0	3;7-4;0	3;0-4;0	nd	nd	nd	nd				
ŋ				1;7	3;1	2;10	2;6			2;6-2;11	2;6-2;11	nd	nd	nd	nd	nd	nd	nd	early 4		3;7-4;0	

Table 9.3. (Continued)

Target consonant	**Jordanian Arabic** 1 Amayreh & Dyson (1998)	**Jordanian Arabic** 2 Amayreh (2003)	**Jordanian Arabic** 3 Hamdan & Amayreh (2007)	**Cantonese** 1 Tse (1982)	**Cantonese** 2 (Cheung (1990)	**Cantonese** 3 Tse (1991)	**Cantonese** 4 So & Dodd (1995)	**Putonghua** 75% group crit* (Zhu & Dodd, 2000)	**Putonghua** 90% group crit (Zhu & Dodd, 2000)	**German** 75% crit (Fox & Dodd, 1999)	**German** (Fox & Dodd, 1999)	**Greek** 75% criterion (PAL, 1995)	**Greek** (Papadopoulou, 2000)	**Hungarian** (Nagy, 1980)	**Japanese** 1 (Sakauchi, 1967)	**Japanese** 2 (Takagi and Yashuda, 1967)	**Japanese** 3 (Noda et al., 1969)	**Japanese** 4 (Nakanishi et al., 1972)	**Korean** (Kim & Pae, 2005)	**Maltese** 75% criterion (Grech, 1998)	**Thai** 80% criterion (Boonyathitisuk, 1982 and Dardarananda, 1993)	
r	5;6	nd	nd											5;0-6;0							>7;0	trills
ʁ	6;0	nd	nd							2;6-2;11	3;0-3;5											
ɾ												nd	nd		>4;8	>6;6	4;0-4;5	4;0-4;5	nd			tap/flap
ɸ															2;10-3;3	3;6-3;11	4;0-4;5	4;0-4;5				fricatives
f	2;6	nd	nd	2;3	3;1	>3;0	4;0	3;0	3;0	2;6-2;11	2;6-2;11	3;6-4;0	3;7-4;0	<3;0						2;5	4;1-4;6	
v										2;0-2;5	2;6-2;11	3;0-3;6	3;7-4;0	3;0-4;0						3;0		
θ	>6;4	>8;4	>6;4									4;0-4;6	>4;6									
δ	>6;4	>8;4	>6;4									4;0-4;6	4;1-4;6									
δ̲	>6;4	>8;4	>6;4																			
s	5;0	nd	nd	2;3	5;7	>3;0	4;0	4;6	4;6	2;0-2;5	2;6-2;11	3;6-4;0	>4;6	5;0	>4;8	>6;6	5;0-5;5	5;0-5;5	>late 6	2;5	5;1-5;6	
s*																			>late 6			
s̲	>6;4	nd	nd																			
z	>6;4	nd	≤6;4							2;0-2;5	2;6-2;11	3;6-4;0	>4;6	5;0-6;0	>4;8	5;6-5;11	5;6-5;11	5;6-5;11		3;6		
ʂ								4;6	>4;6													
ʃ	5;0	nd	nd							3;6-3;11	4;6-4;11			5;0						2;5 - 3;6		

Target consonant	**Jordanian Arabic** 1 Amayreh & Dyson (1998)	**Jordanian Arabic** 2 Amayreh (2003)	**Jordanian Arabic** 3 Hamdan & Amayreh (2007)	**Cantonese** 1 Tse (1982)	**Cantonese** 2 (Cheung (1990)	**Cantonese** 3 Tse (1991)	**Cantonese** 4 So & Dodd (1995)	**Putonghua** 75% group crit* (Zhu & Dodd, 2000)	**Putonghua** 90% group crit (Zhu & Dodd, 2000)	**German** 75% crit (Fox & Dodd, 1999)	**German** (Fox & Dodd, 1999)	**Greek** 75% criterion (PAL, 1995)	**Greek** (Papadopoulou, 2000)	**Hungarian** (Nagy, 1980)	**Japanese** 1 (Sakauchi, 1967)	**Japanese** 2 (Takagi and Yashuda, 1967)	**Japanese** 3 (Noda et al., 1969)	**Japanese** 4 (Nakanishi et al., 1972)	**Korean** (Kim & Pae, 2005)	**Maltese** 75% criterion (Grech, 1998)	**Thai** 80% criterion (Boonyathitisuk, 1982 and Dardarananda, 1993)	
ʒ														5;0-6;0								
ɕ								2;6	3;0						4;4-4;8	>6;6	5;6-5;11	4;6-4;11				
ʝ												3;0-3;6	3;7-4;0									
x								2;0	3;0	2;6-2;11	2;6-2;11	3;0-3;6	3;7-4;0	n.d.								
χ	4;6	nd	nd																			
h	5;0	nd	nd	1;7	2;7	1;3	3;0			2;0-2;5	2;6-2;11			<3;0	2;10-3;3	4;0-4;5	4;0-4;5	4;0-4;5	late 2**	2;0	2;1-2;6	
ħ	2;6	nd	nd																			
ʕ	>6;4	7;4	≤6;4																			
pf										2;6-2;11	3;0-3;5											affricates
ts				2;0	4;1	2;10	4;0	>4;6	>4;6	3;0-3;5	4;0-4;5	4;6-5;0	4;1-4;6	5;0	>4;8	>6;6	5;6-5;11	5;0-5;5				
tʂ								>4;6	>4;6													
tsʰ				1;7	4;1	2;7	4;6	>4;6	>4;6													
tʂʰ								>4;6	>4;6													
tɕ								2;6	4;6										late 3		3;1-3;6	
tɕ*																			early 3			
tɕʰ								2;6	4;6										early 3		>7;0	

Table 9.3. (Continued)

Target consonant	**Jordanian Arabic** 1 Amayreh & Dyson (1998)	**Jordanian Arabic** 2 Amayreh (2003)	**Jordanian Arabic** 3 Hamdan & Amayreh (2007)	**Cantonese** 1 Tse (1982)	**Cantonese** 2 (Cheung (1990)	**Cantonese** 3 Tse (1991)	**Cantonese** 4 So & Dodd (1995)	**Putonghua** 75% group crit* (Zhu & Dodd, 2000)	**Putonghua** 90% group crit (Zhu & Dodd, 2000)	**German** 75% crit (Fox & Dodd, 1999)	**German** (Fox & Dodd, 1999)	**Greek** 75% criterion (PAL, 1995)	**Greek** (Papadopoulou, 2000)	**Hungarian** (Nagy, 1980)	**Japanese** 1 (Sakauchi, 1967)	**Japanese** 2 (Takagi and Yashuda, 1967)	**Japanese** 3 (Noda et al., 1969)	**Japanese** 4 (Nakanishi et al., 1972)	**Korean** (Kim & Pae, 2005)	**Maltese** 75% criterion (Grech, 1998)	**Thai** 80% criterion (Boonyathitisuk, 1982 and Dardarananda, 1993)	
cɕ															2;10-3;3	3;0-3;5	3;0-3;5	4;0-4;5				
tʃ														4;0-5;0						3;0		
cç														4;0-5;0								
ɟz															3;4-3;8	3;0-3;5	3;6-3;11	4;0-4;5				
dʒ	>6;4	>8;4	>6;4											nd						3;6		
ɟj														4;0								
w	<2;0	nd	nd	2;5	2;7	1;3	2;6								3;4-3;8	3;0-3;5	4;6-4;11	4;0-4;5		2;0	2;8-3;0	approximants
l	3;6	nd	nd	2;3	2;7	2;9	3;6	4;6	4;6	2;6-2;11	2;6-2;11	3;6-4;0	3;7-4;0	3;0-4;0					early 5	2;0	3;1-3;6	
ɹ								4;6	4;6											2;5		
j	6;0	6;6	≤6:4	1;7	2;1	1;3	2;0			2;6-2;11	3;0-3;5			3;0-4;0	2;10-3;3	3;0-3;5	3;0-3;5	4;0-4;5		2;0	2;1-2;6 3;1-3;6	
ʎ												4;0-4;6	4;1-4;6									

* Crit in this table stands for criterion. For example, "75% group crit" means that the author reports the age (in years;months) at which 75% of a group of children produced the observed sound correctly. Unless otherwise noted, authors report 90% correct levels, either indicating an age of acquisition when a child produced 90% of the examined sound correctly, or at which 90% of a group of children produced the sound correctly.

** It is not known whether pharyngeal or glottal /h/ (see Kim and Pae, 2007).

*** This sound is not commonly used in everyday speech (Lorwatanapongsa & Maroonroge, 2007).

**** nd: no data was provided about the acquisition of this sound.

First, the majority of studies examining vowel production in boys vs. girls did not document substantial differences between vowel accuracy results in the two genders. Thus, the data is reported for all children. Second, it is interesting to examine the potential effects of vowel inventory size on vowel accuracy. Greek has only 5 monophthong vowels in its inventory, but at the age of 4;0 years, only 90% of children have acquired all of them (Papadopoulou, 2000). In Sesotho, a Bantu language spoken in South Africa, the 9 monophthongs in the vowel inventory are produced correctly by children 100% of the time at 4;0 years (Demuth, 2007). Hungarian has 14 monophthong vowels, and children acquiring Hungarian produce the vowels correctly 95.1% of the time at 4;0 years (Zajdó, 2002; Zajdó and Stoel-Gammon, 2003; Zajdó, 2007). Acquisition data from Cantonese, a language with 22 vowels in its inventory, shows that correctly produced vowels account for 99.6% of the data between 4;0-4;5 (So and Dodd, 1995).

Data from Putonghua reflects an equally high number (89.10%) of correct vowels between 4;1-4;6, even though this language community uses 9 monophthongs, 9 diphthongs and 4 triphtongs in its vowel inventory (Zhu and Dodd, 2000). It appears that the size of the vowel inventory may not have a substantial effect on vowel accuracy in children.

Data from General American English (Pollock and Berni, 2003), Cantonese (So and Dodd, 1995), and Finnish (Pietarinen, 1987) reflects vowel errors in children even at the age of 5;0 years. Thus, the production of some vowels poses a challenge for some children speaking various languages even at that age. In Cantonese, both systematic and non-systematic vowel errors are reported for the age range 2;0-5;5, including the reduction of triphthongs and diphthongs and vowel errors co-occurring with consonant deletion (So and Dodd, 1995). Further, in General American English, vowel errors are reported for the age group 6;6-6;11 (Pollock and Berni, 2003).

In this study, errors in non-rhotic vowel production varied from 0-4% in children between 3;0 and 6;9 years. In General American English, many vowel errors are associated with rhotic vowel production in children between 3;0-8;0 years (Templin, 1957).

Nagy (1980) examined the production of the front vowels in children acquiring Hungarian. Vowel errors included substituting the front rounded vowels /y/ and /y:/ in the age group 7;11-8;0. Phonological studies of speech impaired children also show that triphthongs and diphthongs, rhotic vowels and rounded vowels, especially front rounded vowels are often produced erroneously, indicating the potentially more challenging production patterns needed to generate these speech sounds.

Taken together, this data suggests that, while vowel production in general is characterized by relatively high levels of accuracy early in development, the production of certain vowels takes many years for typically developing children to reach adult-like accuracy levels. In the light of cross-linguistic investigations of child speech, vowel acquisition appears to be a more challenging process for many children than previously thought.

Theories of speech sound acquisition and clinical intervention for vowel-disordered children will benefit greatly from advanced research on the acquisition of vowels across languages.

Universal Steps in Consonant Acquisition Proposed by Jakobson

As mentioned above, Jakobson (1941/1968) proposed several ideas about developmental steps in the acquisition of speech sound inventory in his early work. Specifically, Jakobson suggested that children learn to produce maximally closed consonants (e.g., bilabial stops) as part of the earliest step in speech sound acquisition (Step 1). The next phase of speech sound production is proposed to be the acquisition of nasals vs. oral stop contrasts (Step 2). A subsequent step in consonant production is the exploration of contrast between labials and non-labials (e.g., dentals; Step 3).

Universal Trends in Consonant Acquisition Signaled by Cross-Linguistic Studies

Cross-linguistic studies lend some support for Jakobson's claims on consonant acquisition. Table 9.2 shows consonant accuracy data from seven languages, including Cantonese, Turkish, Putonghua, German, Hungarian, Jordanian Arabic and Sesotho.

These languages differ in their linguistic roots and the size and composition of their consonant inventory. Turkish is a representative of Turkic languages, which is proposed by some to belong to the Altaic language family. Similarly to English, German belongs to the Germanic branch of the Indo-European language family. Jordanian Arabic is a Semitic language. Consonant inventory size in these languages varies greatly: Cantonese has 19, Turkish has 20, Puthoghua has 22, German has 24, Hungarian has 25, Jordanian Arabic has 28, and Sesotho has 39, if we do not count the allophones present. Interestingly, the consonant inventory size for Sesotho increases greatly, from 39 to 65, if we count labialized consonants as constrastive phonemes.

Thus, by making observations about consonant production in these languages, trends in acquisition in relation to consonant inventory size may become apparent.

Table 9.3 shows consonant acquisition data from ten languages including Jordanian Arabic (Amayreh and Dyson, 1998), Cantonese (Cheung, 1990; So and Dodd, 1995; Tse, S.M. 1982; Tse, A.C.Y. 1991), Putonghua (Zhu and Dodd, 2000), German (Fox and Dodd, 1999), Greek (PAL, 1995; Papadopoulou, 2000), Hungarian (Nagy, 1980), Japanese (Nakanishi et al., 1972; Noda et al., 1969; Sakauchi, 1967; Takagi and Yashuda, 1967), which belongs to the Japonic language family, Korean (Kim and Pae, 2005), Maltese (Grech, 1998), which is considered either a language isolate or related to the Altaic languages, and Thai (Boonyathitisuk, 1982; Dardaranandra, 1993), which belongs to the Tai-Kadai language family. The age designators in years;months indicate age of mastery, where the standards for mastery differed among the studies. With the exception of two studies reporting on the acquisition of consonants in Cantonese (Tse, S.M. 1982; Tse, A.C.Y. 1991), results are reported from sizeable groups of children; the numbers of participants vary from 21 to 7602.

While the majority of these studies applied a cross-sectional study design rather than a longitudinal one examining the development of speech in children during longer periods of time, the data still allows for making some basic observations. Jakobson's claim that "closed consonants" (e.g. bilabial stops) are acquired early appear to be supported by that data from many (but not all) languages. In languages that include stops differentiated by voicing, voiceless bilabial stops are reported to be acquired earlier than their voiced cognates, indicating the challenging nature of producing vocal fold vibrations while building up pressure in the oral cavity and releasing closure of the lips.

It is to be noted that consonant production with additional markers such as aspiration and affrication, labialization of a consonant, labialization of a consonant coupled with aspiration, the insertion of a glottal stop before the plosive, or producing emphatic consonants (e.g., in Jordanian Arabic) that are characterized by a secondary pharyngeal articulation requiring the tongue to be pulled backwards in the direction of the pharyngeal region (Hamdan and Amayreh, 2007) appear to delay the acquisition of consonant varieties examined cross-linguistically. In phonology, these speech sounds are considered marked, due to their low frequency in the speech sound inventories examined across languages.

Sidebar 9.1 So, what if some of your consonants are not accurate, anyway?

The term *lisp* is used as an everyday term by the general public to indicate the non-conventional quality of a group of speech sounds, mostly sibilants. It is also used as a specific term by SLPs to indicate the perceived quality resulting from non-conventional articulation characteristics of certain speech sounds. Nowadays, English-speaking SLPs consider this speech phenomenon a treatment target.

It is important to recognize that people throughout history have evaluated lisping and other speech impediments in various ways, depending on the historical context and cultural environment that served as background.

For example, in Ancient Greece, Alcibiades (circa 450 BC – 404 BC), the famous Athenian statesman, orator and general who was a disciple of Socrates downright flaunted his lisping, and people of high standing thought it made his speech lovely and peculiar. Writings of Plutarch indicate that Alcibiades' son even imitated his father's speech production patterns. While lisping was considered erroneous speech production, Alcibiades was not working on remediation (Rose, 2003).

The proposed order of acquiring early on the opposition of nasal versus oral bilabial stops is only partially supported by the data. Data from several languages examined signal the acquisition of nasals earlier, either before 2;5 (e.g., for German /m/ and /n/; Fox and Dodd, 1999) or between 2;0-3;0 years of age (e.g., Jordanian Arabic, see Amayreh and Dyson, 1998). In several languages, similar ages of acquisition are reported (see 3 out of 4 studies on Japanese, such as Nakanishi et al., 1972; Sakauchi, 1967; Takagi and Yashuda, 1967), Greek (PAL, 1995; Papadopoulou, 2000) and Korean (Kim and Pae, 2005, 2007). Studies of speech acquisition in Cantonese (Cheung, 1990; So and Dodd, 1995; Tse, A.C.Y. 1991; Tse, S.M. 1982) and Hungarian (Nagy, 1980) indicate the appearance of higher levels of accuracy in nasal production relatively later than that of the oral bilabial stops. Overall, no clear order of acquisition can be determined on the basis of the data examined.

As for contrasting labials with non-labials (e.g., dentals) during speech acquisition, the data from the ten languages examined generally support Jakobson's that the more frontal consonants are acquired earlier than those produced posteriorally cross-linguistically. However, certain exceptions are noted. For example, data from Putonghua (Zhu and Dodd, 2000) shows that front consonants were acquired at about the same age as back consonants. In several languages including Cantonese (e.g., Tse, S.M. 1982), German (Fox and Dodd, 1999), Japanese (e.g., Sakauchi, 1967), Maltese (Grech, 1998), and Thai (Boonyathitisuk, 1982; Dardarananda, 1993), glottal fricatives are acquired earlier than consonants produced in a more anterior positioning of the articulators. So many exceptions make one rethink the position of /h/ within the consonant systems examined across languages.

Cross-Linguistic Consonant Acquisition Data: General Observations from Several Languages

Compared to vowels, consonants are typically produced with lower levels of accuracy early in development. As mentioned previously in this volume, accuracy is a rather difficult term to define (see insert). "One person's voice disorder is another person's phoneme" – cautioned Ladefoged (1983, p. 351), referring to the challenge of declaring a speech sound accurate. Nevertheless, many studies report lower levels of accuracy for consonants as opposed to vowels so it is reasonable to speculate that the production of consonants is indeed more challenging than that of vowels.

Table 2 shows data from seven languages about percentage of correctly produced (accurate) consonants in typically developing children. Caution has to be exercised when interpreting the results due to important differences in research methodology. Data for the individual languages is ordered by consonant size inventory, from the lowest consonant inventory size examined to the highest one. In general, 90% accuracy levels of consonants are observed in children at different ages. In Cantonese, children produce consonants accurately 90% of the time relatively early, between 2;6-2;11 years (So and Dodd, 1995). Sesotho children are reported to reach the same level of consonant accuracy sometime between 2;0 and 3;0 years (Demuth, 2007). German-speaking children reach the 90% accuracy level in consonant production between the ages of 3;0-3;5 (Fox and Dodd, 1999). Children acquiring Putonghua reach the 90% accuracy level somewhere between the ages of 4;1-4;6 years (Zhu, 2007). In contrast, children acquiring Jordanian Arabic produce correct consonants 90% of the time much later, between the ages of 6;0 and 6;10 (Amayreh and Dyson, 1998). It is indeed true that Jordanian Arabic has a relatively sizeable consonant inventory with 28 consonants and 6 allophones. However, a closer examination of the data does not reveal a clear connection between consonant inventory size and the age of reaching higher levels of consonant accuracy.

An interesting observation can be made about increases in consonant accuracy levels between the ages of 7;0 and 8;0 years based on results from two large cohort studies of children acquiring Hungarian and Turkish. Results gathered from several hundred children reflect a slight increase pertaining to consonant accuracy in Hungarian-speaking children during this period (Nagy, 1980). Data from Turkish-speaking children also shows a slight increase in the production of well-formed consonants between these ages (Topbaş and Yavaş, 2006). Thus, consonant errors are still detectable in 8-year-old children acquiring Hungarian and Turkish.

Other universal trends observable from the data shown in Table 3 include the relatively earlier acquisition of voiceless consonants compared to their voiced cognates in languages where both classes of sounds are included in the consonant inventory. In general, the acquisition of stops precedes that of fricatives. Across several languages examined, apical trills are acquired relatively late. Affricates are characterized by high levels of accuracy only later in development (with the exception of Cantonese, see data in Table 3 by Tse, A.C.Y. 1991; Tse, S.M. 1982). Overall, approximants are generally acquired prior to 4;0 years in several languages, but the voiced palatal approximant /j/ in Jordanian Arabic (Amayreh and Dyson, 1998; Amayreh, 2003; Hamdan and Amayreh, 2007) and the Korean voiced alveolar approximant /l/ (Kim and Pae, 2005) appear to be exceptions to this regularity.

Even less is known about the acquisition of consonant clusters in different languages. Typically, the correct production of consonant clusters has been shown to present a challenge for young children. Often, it is the "more challenging" (and, according to some theories based on Jakobson's view, later acquired) consonant that gets deleted from a sequence of consonants, such as the word "crocodile" is pronounced as /kokodaɪl/ instead of /kɹokodaɪl/. However, some children choose a different path and articulate the sound sequence /ɹokodaɪl/ instead. Detailed studies including cross-linguistic comparisons of the production of consonant clusters in diverse languages are needed to shed more light on processes guiding their acquisition (see also Chapter 7 for prosodic explanations of consonant deletion in consonant clusters).

Universal Trends in the Occurrence and Elimination of Phonological Processes

In the previous sections, we have reviewed data on the acquisition of individual speech sounds. The limitations of this review are due to the limited amount of results generated so far along with differences in research methodology. When trying to identify common trends in phonological processes and their elimination, the reader is faced with the availability of even less data on speech error patterns in child speech in various language communities. A wide range of studies on English (e.g., Bowen, 1998; Grunwell, 1997, and Galea in Chapter 11 of this volume on Brazilian Portuguese) report the presence of phonological processes in early child speech, including syllable reduction or deletion, final consonant deletion, word-final devoicing, consonant harmony (assimilation), fronting, cluster reduction, gliding of liquids, etc. Some studies report approximate age periods by which these processes are observed to be eliminated from the speech of typically developing children, presumably due to maturation of the speech mechanisms or the emergence of more sophisticated phonemic representations.

To date, no detailed study of phonological processes and their elimination based on cross-linguistic data is available. Detailed analyses of these processes and their elimination will have to be carried out by building on the results of research from various languages to account for their presence and absence and to evaluate their usefulness for speech and language assessment and remediation across languages.

Connections

In this chapter, general patterns of acquisition of vowels and consonants across many languages were described. In particular, predictions based on a structural linguistics framework were evaluated in light of evidence from many languages. More information about structural linguistics is found in Chapter 1 of this volume.

Specific information about the acquisition of the English phonological system is found in the chapters in Section II of this volume. How monolingual children acquire the phonological systems of French, Brazilian Portuguese, and Korean is described in Chapters 10 through 12, respectively. Chapters 13 and 14 focus on aspects of multilingual speech acquisition.

Concluding Remarks

In this chapter, predictions about patterns in the acquisition of phonological sound systems across many languages were evaluated based on evidence from multiple studies. Questions about vowel and consonant acquisition were considered separately. While trends indicated that vowels are mastered earlier than consonants, full mastery of the entire inventory did not occur until school age in both categories.

Language-specific (unique) patterns in sound acquisition can only be determined through detailed studies of both typically developing and speech disordered children at different ages. Currently, the paucity of data on non-English languages does not allow for constructing detailed accounts of speech sound acquisition cross-linguistically. Results suggest that age of acquisition for a speech sound can differ wildly across languages in some cases. For example, the typical age of acquisition for the (across languages perceptually rather similar speech sound) /l/ may differ by three years in Maltese vs. Korean. That is, age of acquisition for a speech sound appears to be language specific.

From the perspective of universal versus language-specific trends in the order of speech sound acquisition, much remains to be explored. In terms of vowel production, studies of *acoustic phonetics* documenting vowel system structure in children are needed since perceptual studies of speech acquisition often leave important aspects of vowel production hidden (see van der Stelt et al., 2005; Zajdó et al., 2011).

The effects of vowel duration and consonantal context (see, for example, Buder and Stoel-Gammon, 2002; Zajdó and Stoel-Gammon, 2002), stress patterns and tones on vowel accuracy remain under-explored in diverse language communities. The potential impact of syllable and word position on vowel accuracy and production patterns will need to be documented in detail across languages. The effects of language-specific phoneme frequency on vowel acquisition have not been examined in detail cross-linguistically.

With respect to the acquisition of language-specific trends in consonant production, much remains to be mapped out. Acoustic studies documenting in detail developmental phases in consonant production will help with drawing well-established conclusions about universal and language-specific patterns in consonant acquisition. In addition, cross-linguistic studies will have to explore developmental steps during the acquisition of consonant clusters. The work started by Jakobson has to continue in order to understand fully the complexities of speech and its acquisition as a uniquely human activity.

CHAPTER REVIEW QUESTIONS

1. How did child phonology benefit from cross-linguistic observations of sound systems in various languages?
2. What are the major steps of speech sound acquisition in children according to Jakobson's theory?
3. List at least 5 universal and 5 language-specific acquisition patterns from cross-linguistic data examined in this chapter.

SUGGESTIONS FOR FURTHER READING

S. McLeod (Ed., 2007), *The International Guide to Speech Acquisition.* Clifton Park,NY: Thomson Delmar Learning.

Zhu Hua and B. Dodd (Eds., 2006), *Phonological development and disorders in children: A multilingual perspective.* Clevedon, UK: Multilingual Matters Ltd.

SUGGESTIONS FOR STUDENT ACTIVITIES

1. Identify at least 10 universal trends in speech sound acquisition reflected by the data in Tables 1, 2, and 3.
2. Find vowel and consonant acquisition data from an additional 3 languages. Evaluate whether the data supports or refutes certain universal trends in the order of speech sound acquisition proposed by Jakobson.
3. Carry out a small case study of a child acquiring English. Record the child's speech once a month during a period of at least 3 months. Compare and contrast the results of vowel and consonant accuracy levels to data provided in Tables 1, 2, and 3.

ANSWERS TO CHAPTER REVIEW QUESTIONS

1. How did child phonology benefit from cross-linguistic observations of sound systems in various languages?

Child phonology benefited greatly from cross-linguistic observations since these studies allowed for identifying phonological trends that are present in many languages. Jakobson proposed a universal order of speech sound acquisition. While the data available today does not support the existence of a fully universal acquisition order, it is true that some trends in speech sound acquisition are identifiable in several (but not all) languages, others are observed in the vast majority of language communities. Information about frequently occurring phonological trends in vowel and consonant acquisition and the appearance and elimination of phonological processes provide insight into normative processes in speech acquisition on a language-by-language basis. Comparing the properties of typically developing speech in several languages calls attention to the hard-to-grasp concept of which sounds or sound sequences may be considered “easy” or “more difficult” (earlier vs. later acquired) in one vs. another language as well as cross-linguistically. Knowledge of normative data from several languages also has clinical implications in as much as it guides speech evaluations and therapy in special populations, including bilingual, multilingual or adopted (e.g. second language learner) children.

2. What are the major steps of speech sound acquisition according to Jakobson’s theory?

According to Jakobson, speech sounds are learned by children through the production of binary oppositions, in the following order of steps:

Step 1. Contrasting low vowels vs. consonants produced with the most closure
Step 2. Contrasting nasals vs. oral stops
Step 3. Contrasting labials vs. non-labials (e.g. dentals)
Step 4. Contrasting low vs. high vowels
Step 5. Contrasting front vs. back vowels, or high vs. mid vowels

3. List at least 5 universal and 5 language-specific acquisition patterns from cross-linguistic data examined in this chapter.

Examples of universal trends in speech sound acquisition:

1. Typically, vowels are acquired earlier than consonants.
2. Typically, back vowels are acquired earlier than front ones.
3. Typically, front rounded vowels are acquired latest.
4. Typically, stops are acquired earlier than fricatives.
5. Typically, bilabial nasals are acquired somewhat earlier than alveolar nasals.

Examples of language-specific trends in speech sound acquisition:

1. In Jordanian Arabic, the voiced palatal approximant is acquired quite late, between 6 to 7 years, compared to the other languages observed, where it is acquired several years earlier.
2. In Hungarian, the voiced palatal affricate is acquired earlier than its voiceless counterpart. In this language, as well as cross-linguistically, the acquisition of voiceless as opposed to voiced counterparts in a sound pair is typically achieved earlier but the case mentioned is an exception.
3. In Greek (and, according to some studies, in Japanese), the acquisition of the typically early acquired voiceless bilabial plosive sound is rather late in comparison to many other languages.
4. The voiced bilabial plosive is typically acquired later than the voiceless alveolar plosive, but German appears to be an exception, since /b/ in this language community is acquired earlier than /t/.

5. In Maltese, the typically challenging voiced alveolar lateral approximant is acquired by 2;0, making it the only language community among those examined where this sound is acquired rather early, among the first sounds produced correctly.

References

Amayreh, M.M. (2003). Completion of the consonant inventory of Arabic. *Journal of Speech, Language and Hearing Research,* 46, 517-529.

Amayreh, M.M., Dyson, A.T. (1998). The acquisition of Arabic consonants. *Journal of Speech, Language, and Hearing Research,* 41, 642-653.

Blevins, J. (1995). The syllable in phonological theory. In J. Goldsmith (Ed.), *The handbook of phonological theory* (pp. 206-244). Cambridge, Massachusetts: Basil Blackwell.

Boonyathitisuk, P. (1982). Articulatory characteristics of kindergarten children aged three to four years eleven months in Bangkok. Unpublished Master's thesis, Mahidol University, Bangkok, Thailand.

Bowen, C. (1998). Developmental phonological disorders. A *practical guide for families and teachers. Melbourne: ACER Press.*

Buder, E.H., Stoel-Gammon, C. (2002). American and Swedish children's acquisition of vowel duration: Effects of vowel identity and final stop voicing. *Journal of the Acoustic Society of America,* 111(4), 1854-1864.

Cheung, P. (1990*). The acquisition of Cantonese phonology in Hong Kong: A cross-sectional study.* Unpublished final year B.Sc. project, University College London.

Clements, G. (1990). The role of the sonority cycle in core syllabification. In J. Kingston and M. Beckman (Eds.), Pa*pers in laboratory phonology I: Between the grammar and physics of speech* (pp. 283-333). Cambridge: Cambridge University Press.

Dardarananda, R. (1993*). The Life and Work of Professor Dardarananda: Collection of Articles from Ramathibodi Hospital.* Division of Communicative Disorders, Mahidol University, Bangkok, Thailand.

Demuth, K. (2007). Sesotho speech acquisition. In S. McLeod (Ed.), *The International Guide to Speech Acquisition* (pp. 528-538). Clifton Park, NY: Thomson Delmar Learning.

Fox, A.V., Dodd, B.J. (1999). Der Erwerb des phonologischen Systems in der deutschen Sprache. *Sprache – Stimme – Gehör,* 23, 183-191.

Grunwell, P. (1997). Natural phonology. In M. Ball and R. Kent (Eds.), *The New Phonologies: Developments in clinical linguistics.* San Diego: Singular Publishing Group, Inc.

Grech, H. (1998). Phonological development of normal Maltese speaking children. Unpublished PhD dissertation, University of Manchester, UK.

Hamdan, J. M., Amayreh, M.M. (2007). Consonant profile of Arabic-speaking school-age children in Jordan. *Folia Phoniatrica et Logopaedica,* 59, 55-64.

Jakobson, R. (1941/1968). Kindersprache, Aphasie und allgemeine Lautgesetzte. Child Language, aphasia and phonological universals. The Hague: Mouton.

Kern, S., Davis, B. (2009). Emergent complexity in early vocal acquisition: Cross-linguistic comparisons of canonical babbling. In F. Pellegrino, E. Marsico, I. Chitoran and C.

Coupé (Eds.), *Approaches to phonological complexity* (pp. 353-375). Berlin: Mouton de Gruyter.

Kern, S., Davis, B., Zink, I. (2009). From babbling to first words in four languages: Common trends across languages and individual differences. In D'Errico, F., and J-M. Hombert (Eds.), *Becoming eloquent: Advances in the emergence of language, human cognition, and modern cultures* (pp. 205-234). Amsterdam: John Benjamins.

Kim, M., Pae, S. (2005). The percentage of consonant correct and the ages of consonantal acquisition for [the] "Korean Test of Articlation for Children" [in Korean]. *Korean Journal of Speech Sciences,* 12 (2), 139-152.

Kim, M., Pae, S. (2007). Korean speech acquisition. In S. McLeod (Ed.), *The International Guide to Speech Acquisition* (pp. 472-482). Clifton Park, NY: Thomson Delmar Learning.

Ladefoged, P. (1983). The linguistic use of different phonation types. D. Bless and J. Abbs (Eds.), Vocal fold physiology: Contemporary research and clinical issues (pp. 351–60). San Diego: College Hill Press.

Locke, J.L. (1983). Phonological acquisition and change. New York, NY: Academic Press.

Lorwatanapongsa, P., Maroonroge, S. (2007). Thai speech acquisition. In S. McLeod (Ed.), *The International Guide to Speech Acquisition* (pp. 554-565). Clifton Park, NY: Thomson Delmar Learning.

Nagy, J. (1980). Öt-hat éves gyermekeink iskolakészültsége [Preparedness for school of our five-six years old children]. Budapest: Akadémiai Kiadó.

Nakanishi, Y., Owada, K., Fujita, N. (1972). K_onkensa to sono kekka ni kansuru k_satsu. *Tokyo Gakugei Daigaku Tokushu Kyoiku Shisetsu Hokoku,* 1, 1-19.

Noda, M., Iwamura, Y., Naito, K., Asukai, K. (1969). Y_ji no k_onn_ryoku no hattatsu ni kansuru kenky_. *Nihon S_g_ Aiiku Kenky_sho Kiy_,* 4, 153-170.

Oller, D.K. (1980). The emergence of the sounds of speech in infancy. In G. Yeni-Komshian, J.F. Kavanagh, and C.A. Ferguson (Eds.), *Child Phonology: Vol. 1. Production* (pp.93-112). New York: Academic Press.

PAL (Panhellenic Association of Logopedics). (1995). Assessment of phonetic and phonological development. Athens, Greece: PAL.

Papadopoulou, K. (2000). Phonological acquisition of Modern Greek. Unpublished BSc Honors dissertation, University of Newcastle upon Tyne, UK.

Pietarinen, A. (1987). Vantaalaisten v. 1980 syntyneiden lasten viisivuosisseulalla mitatut kielelliset häiriöt ja niiden yhteydet kehityksen muihin osatekijöihin. Unpublished Master's thesis, University of Helsinki (Finland), Department of Phonetics.

Pollock, K.E., Berni, M.C. (2003). Incidence of non-rhotic vowel errors in children: Data from the Memphis Vowel Project. *Clinical Linguistics and Phonetics,* 17, 393-401.

Rose, M.L. (2003). The staff of Oedipus: Transforming disability in ancient Greece. Ann Arbor, MI: The University of Michigan Press.

Sakauchi, T. (1967). Kodomo no k_on n_ryoku nit suite. *Gengo Sh_gai Kenky_,* 68, 13-26.

Smit, A.B. (2007). General American English speech acquisition. In S. McLeod (Ed.), *The International Guide to Speech Acquisition* (pp. 128-147). Clifton Park, NY: Thomson Delmar Learning.

So, L.K.H., Dodd, B. (1995). The acquisition of phonology by Cantonese-speaking children. *Journal of Child Language,* 22, 473-495.

Stoel-Gammon, C., and Cooper, J. (1984). Patterns of early lexical and phonological development. *Journal of Child Language,* 11, 247-271.

Stoel-Gammon, C., and Herrington, P. (1990). Vowel systems of normally developing and phonologically disordered children. *Clinical Linguistics and Phonetics,* 4, 145 – 160.

Takagi, S., Yasuda, A. (1967). Seij_y_ji no k_onn_ryoku. *Sh_ni Hoken Igaku,* 25, 23-28.

Templin, M.C. (1957). Certain language skills in children (Monograph Series No. 26). Minneapolis, MN: University of Minnesota, The Institute of Child Welfare.

Topbaş, S., Yavaş, M. (2006). Phonological acquisition and disorders in Turkish. In Zhu Hua and B. Dodd (Eds.), Phonological development and disorders in children: A multilingual perspective (pp. 233-261). Clevedon, UK: Multilingual Matters Ltd.

Tse, A.C.Y. (1991). The acquisition process of Cantonese phonology: A case study. Unpublished M. Phil. thesis, University of Hong Kong.

Tse, S.M. (1982). The acquisition of Cantonese phonology. Unpublished PhD thesis, University of British Columbia, Canada.

van der Stelt, J.M., Zajdó, K., Wempe, T.G. (2005). Investigating the acoustic vowel space in two-year-old children: Results for Dutch and Hungarian. *Speech Communication,* 47, 143-159.

Zajdó. K. (2002). The acquisition of vowels in Hungarian-speaking children aged two to four years: A cross-sectional study. Unpublished doctoral dissertation, University of Washington (Seattle), USA.

Zajdó. K. (2007). Hungarian speech acquisition. In S. McLeod (Ed.), *The International Guide to Speech Acquisition* (pp. 412-436). Clifton Park, NY: Thomson Delmar Learning.

Zajdó, K., and Stoel-Gammon, C. (2002). The acquisition of rhyme-internal timing in American English versus Swedish: Similarities and differences in speech development. In R. Rapp (Ed.), Sprachwissenshaft auf dem Weg in das Dritte Jahrtausend: Akten des 34. Linguistischen Kolloquiums, Germersheim, 1999 / Linguistics on the way into the third Millennium: Proceedings of the 34th Linguistics Colloquium, Germersheim, 1999 (vol. 1., pp. 845-853). Frankfurt: Peter Lang.

Zajdó, K., Stoel-Gammon, C. (2003). The acquisition of vowels in Hungarian: Developmental data. In M.J. Solé, D. Rescasens and J. Romero (Eds.), Proceedings of the 15th International Congress of Phonetic Sciences, Barcelona, 3-9 August, 2003 (vol. 3., pp. 2229-2232). Barcelona: Universitat Autònoma de Barcelona.

Zajdó, K., Wempe, T.G., van der Stelt, J.M., Pols, L.C.W. (2011). The acquisition of Hungarian high front unrounded short vs. long vowels. In W-S.V. Lee and Y.Y.E. Zee (Eds.), Proceedings of the 17th International Congress of Phonetic Sciences, Hong Kong, 17-21 August, 2011 (pp. 2252-2255). Hong Kong: Department of Chinese, Translation and Linguistics at the City University of Hong Kong.

Zhu, H. (2007). Putonghua (Modern Standard Chinese) speech acquisition. In Zhu H., Dodd, B. (Eds.), Phonological development and disorders in children: A multilingual perspective (pp. 516-527). Clevedon, UK: Multilingual Matters Ltd.

Zhu, H., Dodd, B. (2000). The phonological acquisition of Putonghua (Modern Standard Chinese). *Journal of Child Language,* 27 (1), 3-42.

In: Comprehensive Perspectives ...
Editors: Beate Peter and Andrea A. N. MacLeod

ISBN: 978-1-62257-041-6

Chapter 10

ACQUIRING FRENCH

Andrea A. N. MacLeod

INTRODUCTION

This brief chapter on phonological development of French speaking-children begins with an overview of French speakers in the world and a description of the phonetics and phonology of French. The phonological development of French-speaking children is described from babbling to the age of five years and compared to the development of children acquiring English. The chapter ends with an appraisal of research needs in the area of speech sound disorders in French-speaking children.

FRENCH SPEAKERS IN THE WORLD

French is spoken in a number of countries around the world by more than 220 million speakers as a first language (Yannick, 2010). For example, it is spoken in Europe (France, Belgium, Switzerland), North America (Canada, Haiti), and Africa (Algeria, Rwanda, Congo). As with English or Spanish, there are various dialects of French, each with distinct phonologies, vocabularies, and grammars. An example of phonological differences include the allophones of /t, d/ in French spoken in the province of Québec, Canada: /t, d/ become affricated before high front vowels (eg., "*tu*" ("you") is produced [tsy]). An example of grammatical differences includes the use of double clitics in Québecois French: "*tu veux tu?*" ("you, do you want?"). To hear an example of French spoken by an adult from France and an adult from Canada, listen to the sound file below (10S1). An awareness of dialect differences is important to consider when working with young children: SLPs must distinguish between language delays or disorders and language differences.

Access Sound File 1 (Chapter 10)

10S1 Speech sample based on the first two sentences of a standard text used by the Projet Phonologie du français contemporain: (http://www.projet-pfc.net/index.php) by two speakers of French: one from France and the second from Canada.

Phonetics and Phonology of French

Despite the various dialects, there are many general characteristics of French phonetics and phonology. The phonological inventory of consonants and vowels for French is illustrated in Figures 10.1 and 10.2, respectively. French has a relatively large phonetic inventory consisting of 20 consonants and 16 monophthong vowels.

English and French share many consonants with only three that would be new to speakers of English, the voiced velar fricative /ʁ/ (e.g., *"rose"* ("rose") /ʁoz/), the palatal nasal /ɲ/ (e.g., *"agneau"* ("young sheep") /aɲo/), and the labial-palatal glide /ɥ/ (e.g., *"huit"* ("eight") /ɥit/). As for the vowels, there are several new vowels that would be unfamiliar to an English speaker since French contrasts vowels based not only on their height and tongue advancement, but also on lip rounding of front vowels (eg., "*vie*" ("life") /vi/ vs. "*vue*" ("*view*") /vy/) and nasality (eg., "*ta*" ("your") /ta/ vs. "*temps*" ("time") /tɑ̃/).

The syllable structure of French begins with single vowel as the minimal syllable shape: for example words such as "*eau*" ("water") /o/, "*eux*" ("them") /ø/. Syllables can be quite complex allowing for up to three consonants in the onset or coda of the syllable, and up to four consonants in word medial positions. These large consonant clusters, however, are limited in composition to /s/ + obstruent + liquid + glide. This results in words such as "*froid*" ("cold") /fʁwa/ (obstruent + liquid + glide) or "*instruit*" ("educated") /□̃strɥi/ (s + obstruent + liquid + glide). In children's vocabulary, there is a tendency for early words in French to be longer than those of English. If we compare the words found in the MacArthur-Bates Communication Development Inventory, two thirds of words typically attempted by young French children have more than one syllable whereas two thirds of words attempted by English children have one syllable.

The phonotactics of French include four key phenomena: *liaison, enchainement, elision,* and the "*loi de position*" (Rose and Wauquier, 2007; Tranel, 1995; Tranel, 2000). These phenomena lead to the addition of consonants, the deletion of consonants, or changes in syllabification. They also interact with the morphology of French. For example, *liason* describes the process where word final consonants that appear in the orthography but are not pronounced become the onset of the following word if the word begins with a vowel. For example, *"les"* ("the") /lɛ/ + *"ânnes"* ("donkeys") /ɑn/ is pronounced /lɛ.zɑn/. *Enchainement* is a similar process where word final consonants that are pronounced can become the onset for the following word if it begins with a vowel. For example, "*jeune arbre*" ("young tree") is pronounced /ʒœ.naʁ.bʁə/.

	Bilabial	Labiodental	Dental	Alveolar	Postalveolar	Palatal	Velar	Uvular
Plosive	p b			t d			k g	
Nasal	m			n		ɲ		
Trill								
Tap or Flap								
Fricative		f v		s z	ʃ ʒ			ʁ
Approximant	w[1]					j ɥ[2]		
Lateral approximant				l				

[1]/w/ produced with a restriction at the bilabial and velar places of articluation
[2]/ɥ/ produced with a restriction at the bilabial and palatal places of articulation

Figure 10.1. IPA chart of French consonants.

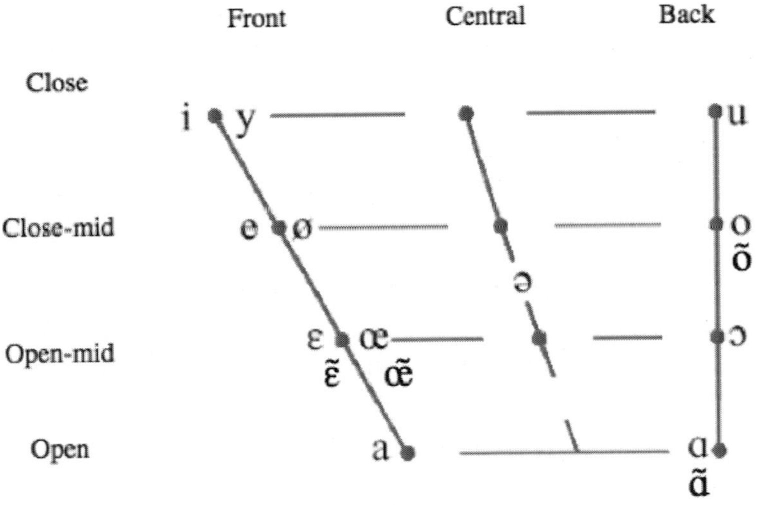

Figure 10.2. IPA chart of French vowels.

The process of *elision* describes the deletion of a vowel in the clitics when the clitic appears before vowel-initial words, a process that is reflected in the orthography: "*le*" + "*arbre*" ("the" + "tree") is written "*l'arbre*" and pronounced [laʁ.bʁə]. The *loi de position* is a process that favors the appearance of lax vowels in closed syllables and tense vowels in open syllables. As a result, it is difficult to find minimal pairs for certain vowels since they rarely appear in the same context, for example /e/ and /ɛ/: "*thé*" ("tea") /te/ but "*tête*", ("head") /tɛt/.

The prosody of French is quite different from English. Whereas the multisyllabic words in English tend to bear the stress on the first syllable (Cutler and Carter, 1987), French multisyllabic words tend to carry stress on the last syllable.

Phonological Development in French

Our knowledge of phonological development in French is based on longitudinal case studies (e.g., dos Santos, 2007; Rose, 2000), diary studies (Demuth and Johnson, 2003), small group studies (e.g., Hilaire-Debove and Kehoe, 2004, Kern and Davis, 2009; Vinter, 2001; Whalen, Levitt and Wang, 1991), and a large group study (MacLeod, Sutton, Trudeau and Thordardottir, 2011). Together, these studies capture development from infancy to 5 years of age.

Three cross-linguistic studies have described the babbling stage of infants acquiring French. French infants have been found to produce more rising intonation than English infants (Whalen, Levitt and Wang, 1991), similar to the prosodic pattern of French multisyllabic words. In a cross-linguistic study of the babbling of 20 infants from French, English, Cantonese, and Arabic language environments, infants from each language environment were found to produce vowels that were similar to those produced by adults of the same language (De Boysson-Bardies, Halle, Sagart and Durant, 1989). For example, French infants produced more diffuse vowel formants than the Cantonese and Arabic infants, in other words their vowels were more distinct from one another than the vowels of Cantonese or Arabic infants. One explanation is based on the differences in vowel inventory between these languages: French has a relatively large vowel inventory, whereas Cantonese and Arabic have smaller vowel inventories.

A more recent cross-linguistic study reporting on Turkish, French, Romanian, Dutch, and Tunisian Arabic children observed that the French infants produced more nasals, more labial consonants, and more variegated babbling than the infants from the other languages (Kern and Davis, 2009). Taken together, these studies support the notion that even during the babbling period children have begun to tune into the language spoken around them and produce speech sounds more characteristic of this language.

Three studies have investigated how French children acquire aspects of their phonology at the first word stage. At approximately 2 years of age, the spontaneous speech of French toddlers has been found to include more monosyllabic words than bisyllabic words (Vinter, 2001)—despite the observation that the inventory of early words consists of only 1/3 monosyllabic words. Common error patterns at the age of two were syllable simplification, substitutions, and assimilations (Vinter, 2001). Word-final consonants were also studied and found to be produced more frequently in monosyllabic words than in bisyllabic words (Hilaire-Debove and Kehoe, 2004). Interestingly, the error pattern differed based on the length of the word: children tended to produce substitutions in monosyllabic words and omissions in bisyllabic words (Hilaire-Debove and Kehoe, 2004). Children have been found to produce word initial clusters more frequently in word-initial position than in word-final position (Demuth and Kehoe, 2006).

In a large group study, 156 children between the ages of 20 and 53 months participated in a picture-naming task (MacLeod et al., 2011). Forty different words were elicited that contained the phonemes of French in word-initial, medial and final position. An *independent analysis* was conducted by exploring the consonant inventory regardless of their accuracy. This analysis revealed that even before their second birthday (i.e., at 20 to 23 months of age), children produced a broad range of consonants consisting of /p, b, t, d, k, m, n, f, s, j/. By the age of 41 months, these children were able to produce all sounds in French – although not necessarily in the correct target form. Two main *relational analyses* were conducted: consonant mastery and percent consonant correct. Consonant mastery was found to begin slowly with only /t, m, n, z/ mastered (i.e., correctly produced by 90% of the children) before the age of 36 months. The period of greatest change occurred between 36 and 53 months during which children mastered the following phonemes: /p, b, d, k, g, ɲ, f, v, ʁ, l, w, ɥ/. Finally, four phonemes were not mastered by the age of 53 months: /s, ʒ, ʃ, j/). Percent consonants correct followed a similar trend; percent consonant correct began at 57% at 20-23 months and increased to 88% by 36-41 months, and reached 95% at 48-53 months. As with English-speaking children, children produced consonants less accurately when they appeared in consonant clusters (MacLeod et al., 2011). Two main differences can be detected between the acquisitions of consonant by French speaking children compared to English speaking children (based on Smit et al., 1990). First, the mastery of the lateral, /l/, and rhotic, /ʁ/, in French occurs at a much younger age than in studies of English. In French, these phonemes are mastered by 90% of children by the age of 53 months, but in English /l/ and /ɹ/ mastery extends to the age of 7 and 8 years, respectively (Smit et al., 1990). Second, the mastery of voiced consonants is a little slower in French, occurring by 53 months for 90% of children, whereas it has occurred by 36 months for /b/, 42 months for /d/ and 48 months for /g/ by English speaking children (Smit et al., 1990). Despite these differences, English and French both show a similar and drawn-out pattern of fricative consonant acquisition that extends past 53 months in French and into school-aged years in English.

Speech Sound Disorders in French

Research on phonological development among French speakers has been increasing gradually over the past decade. Although we expect that phonological disorders have a similar frequency of occurrence in French than in English, we have no published reports on speech sound disorders in French.

Connections

The second section of this book described typical phonological development among monolingual English speakers. As can be seen from this chapter, some aspects of phonological development are common to both English and French, while others appear to be language specific. Chapter 9 provides a description of cross-linguistic trends and a theoretical framework for understanding these trends. The chapters on Brazilian Portuguese and Korean provide other perspectives on phonological development across languages. Lastly, Chapters 13 and 14 focus on the acquisition of speech sounds in two or more languages.

Concluding Remarks

Although French is spoken by a large number of individuals around the world, an understanding of the phonological development of this language has only begun to be explored. Many aspects need to be addressed before we have a full understanding of typical phonological development in French, including the developmental trajectory of consonant clusters, the influence of phonotactics, and phonological development past the age of four-and-a-half. In addition, speech sound disorders have yet to be described and studied in depth. SLPs working with French-speaking children have used their clinical judgment and descriptions based on the literature about English-speaking children to identify and treat children with speech sound disorders.

Future research will surely explore these issues and provide an evidence base to support the work of French SLPs.

Chapter Review Questions

1. Identify three key features the phonetic and phonological system of French.
2. What differences have been observed between English and French phonological development?

Suggestions for Further Reading

MacLeod, A.A.N., Sutton, A., Trudeau, N., and Thordardottir, E. (2011). The acquisition of consonants in Québécois French: A cross-sectional study of pre-school aged children. *International Journal of Speech-Language Pathology, 13*(2), 93-109.

Kern, S. and Davis, B. (2009). Emergent Complexity in Early Vocal Acquisition: Cross-linguistic Comparisons of Canonical Babbling. In I. Chitoran, F. Pellegrino and E. Marsico (eds.), *Approaches to Phonological Complexity, 353-375*. Berlin: Mouton de Gruyter.

Suggestions for Student Activities

1. Compare the inventory consonant and vowel inventories of English and French. Identify similarities and differences between these two inventories. Given what you know about phonological development in English and French (1) what overlapping sounds are acquired earlier? later? and (2) what different sounds are acquired earlier? later?

Answers to Chapter Review Questions

1. Identify three key features the phonetic and phonological system of French.

A large vowel and consonant inventory, syllable structure that can be quite complex with up to three consonants in a cluster, and four phonotactic phenomena, three that govern sound sequences at word boundaries and one that governs vowels in closed and open syllables.

2. What differences have been observed between English and French phonological development?

Two main differences can be detected between the acquisitions of consonant by French speaking children compared to English speaking children (based on Smit et al., 1990). First, the mastery of the rhotic and lateral in French occurs at a much younger age than in studies of English. Second, the mastery of voiced consonants is a little slower in French.

REFERENCES

Cutler, A., and Carter, D.M. (1987). The predominance of strong initial syllables in the English vocabulary. *Computer, Speech and Language*, 2, 133-142.

De Boysson-Bardies, B., Halle, P., Sagart, L. and Durant, C. (1989). A crosslinguistic investigation of vowel formants in babbling. *Journal of Child Language,* 16, 1-17.

Demuth, K., and Johnson, M. (2003). Truncation to subminimal words in early French. *Canadian Journal of Linguistics*, 48(3/4), 211-242.

Demuth, K. and Kehoe, M. (2006). The acquisition of word-final clusters in French. *Catalan Journal of Linguistics,* 5, 59-81.

Dos Santos, C. (2007). Développement phonologique en français langue maternelle: Une étude de cas. Unpublished doctoral thesis.

Hilaire-Debove, G. and Kehoe, M. (2004). Acquisition des consonnes finales (codas) chez les enfants francophones des universaux aux spécificités de la langue maternlle. In Actes de la 25ème Journée d'Études sur la Parole. Fez: Moracco, pp. 265-268.

Kern, S. and Davis, B. (2009). Emergent Complexity in Early Vocal Acquisition: Cross-linguistic Comparisons of Canonical Babbling. In I. Chitoran, F. Pellegrino and E. Marsico (eds.), Approaches to Phonological Complexity, 353-375. Berlin: Mouton de Gruyter.

MacLeod, A.A.N., Sutton, A., Trudeau, N., and Thordardottir, E. (2011). The acquisition of consonants in Québécois French: A cross-sectional study of pre-school aged children. *International Journal of Speech-Language Pathology, 13*(2), 93-109.

Martin, P. (2002). Vowel system of Quebec French. From acoustics to phonology. *La Linguistique,* 38, 71-88.

Mehler, J., Lambertz, G., Jusczyk, P., and Amiel-Tison, C. (1986). Discrimination of the mother tongue by newborn infants. *C R Acad Sci III,* 303(15), 637-640.

Rose, Y. (2000). Headedness and prosodic licensing in L1 acquisition of phonology. Unpublished doctoral thesis.

Rose, Y. and Wauquier-Gravelines, S. (2007). French speech acquisition. In S. McLeod, ed., *The International Guide to Speech Acquisition*, New York: Thomson Delmar Learning, 364-384.

Smit, A.B., Hand, L., Freilinger, J.J., Bernthal, J.E. and Bird, A. (1990). The Iowa articulation norms project and its Nebraska replication. *Journal of Speech and Hearing Disorders,* 55, 779-798.

Tranel, B. (1995). Current issues in French phonology: liaison and position theories. In J. A. Goldsmith (ed.), *The Handbook of Phonological Theory.* Cambridge: Blackwell, 798-816.

Tranel, B. (2000). Aspects de la phonologie du français et la théorie de l'optimalité. *Langue Française,* 126, 39-72.

Vinter, S. (2001). Habiletés phonologiques chez l'enfant de deux ans. *Glossa,* 77, 4-19.

Whalen, D.H., Levitt, A.G., and Wang, Q.I. (1991). Intonational differences between the reduplicative babbling of French- and English-learning infants. *Journal of Child Language,* 18, 501-516.

Yannic, A. (2010). Rapport du sécrétaire général de la francophonie. Paris: Burlet Graphics.

In: Comprehensive Perspectives …
Editors: Beate Peter and Andrea A. N. MacLeod ISBN: 978-1-62257-041-6

Chapter 11

ACQUIRING BRAZILIAN PORTUGUESE

Daniela Evaristo dos Santos Galea

INTRODUCTION

The purpose of this chapter is to present a brief description of phonological development in Brazilian Portuguese-speaking children, mainly from São Paulo, a city in the southeastern region of the country.

The first part of the chapter reviews the phoneme inventory of Brazilian Portuguese relative to syllabic and word position. The second part summarizes the findings of research about the phonological development in Portuguese-speaking typically developing children. Two types of analysis are shown: age of acquisition of each phoneme and the age of elimination of various phonological processes. In general, this chapter focuses more on consonants than on vowels.

PORTUGUESE SPEAKERS AROUND THE WORLD

Portuguese is a Romance language spoken in Europe (Portugal), South America (Brazil), Africa (Mozambique, Angola, Cape Verde, Guiné-Bissau, and São Tomé e Príncipe), and Asia (Macau, East Timor, and Goa).

It is the sixth-most spoken language in the world. The Portuguese alphabet has 26 letters and five diacritics to denote stress, vowel height, contraction, nasalization, and other sound changes (these are: acute accent, grave accent, circumflex accent, tilde, and cedilla). In some parts of Brazil, /t/ and /d/ have the affricate allophones [tʃ] and [dʒ], respectively, before /i/ and /ĩ/. Other characteristics of Brazilian Portuguese phonology are described in the next part of this chapter.

THE PHONOLOGY OF BRAZILIAN PORTUGUESE

The classification of Brazilian Portuguese consonants proposed by Bechara (1988) lists the following categories and subcategories: occlusives (i.e., stops and nasals) and constrictives (i.e., fricatives, laterals, flaps and trills). Brazilian Portuguese has six stops, the bilabials /p/ and /b/, the prealveolars /t/ and /d/ and the velars /k/ and /g/. Fricatives are divided into labiodentals /f/ and /v/, alveolars /s/ and /z/ and palatals /ʃ/ and /ʒ/. As shown, each voiceless sound has its voiced counterpart. Other classes of consonants include only voiced segments. The bilabial /m/, dental /n/ and palatal /ɲ/ are all voiced nasals. Other voiced consonants include the alveolar lateral approximant /l/ and the palatal lateral approximant /ʎ/ as well as the alveolar flap /ɾ/, all three of which are considered liquids. The status of the velar /ʁ/ is debated; some authors consider it as a trill (Cunha, 1980; Bechara, 1988; Câmara Júnior, 2001), others propose that it is a liquid (Hernandorena and Lamprecht, 1997; Mezzomo and Ribas, 2004). Some researchers argue that this speech sound should be considered the voiceless velar fricative /x/ (Silva, 1999; Wertzner et al., 2001).

Brazilian Portuguese has seven oral vowels, /a, e, ɪ, o, u, ɛ, ɔ/, and five nasal vowels, /ã, ẽ, ɪ̃, õ, ũ/ (Silva, 1999; Cunha, 1980). In addition, there are several oral diphthongs and triphthongs.

The majority of Portuguese words are polysyllabic. Syllables consist of vowels (V) and consonants (C). Vowels serve as the nucleus of the syllable and thus they are compulsory elements. However, consonants are optional (Silva, 1999). Consonants can appear in either pre-vocalic or post-vocalic position. Syllables including a post-vocalic element are closed syllables. Syllables without a post-vocalic element are open (or "free") syllables (Bechara, 1988). In Portuguese, free syllables are predominant (Câmara Júnior, 2001). The most frequently occurring syllable type is the CV syllable (Teixeira and Davis, 2002; Matzenauer, 2004).

In polysyllabic words, consonants can appear as a syllable onset word initially, word medially, and in coda positions word medially or word finally. Additionally, consonants can serve as the second pre-vocalic consonant word initially or medially (Câmara Júnior, 1975; Silva, 1999; Matzenauer, 2004). Whereas 16 consonants can appear as a syllable onset word initially, 19 consonants can appear as syllable onsets inside the word (Silva, 1999).

Regarding the coda, only the following consonants can be placed in this position: /S, R, l, n/, and some restrictions apply to these consonants. Note that the capital letters /S, R/ denote archiphonemes, which are sounds that can be realized in a wide variety of ways depending on factors such as regional dialect. The actual realizations of archiphonemes may exceed those variants typically described as allophones of a phoneme; for example, a given archiphoneme can have voiced and voiceless realizations. Regarding the regional dialects of Brazilian Portuguese, /R/ is more velarized in Rio de Janeiro than in São Paulo and the /S/ is pronounced /s/ in São Paulo and / ʃ / in Rio de Janeiro. The /l/ in the final syllable tends to be subjected to a vowelization process, so that some distinct minimal pairs (e.g., "*mal*" – "bad" – adverb, noun, "evil" or "badly," vs. "*mau*" – "bad" - adjective) are produced identically in São Paulo (Câmara Júnior, 2001, Silva, 1999). However, in the south of Brazil, the /l/ appears as a final consonant as there is some obstruction of the air in the oral cavity as the tongue moves in the direction of the upper teeth.Word finally, the consonant /n/ nasalizes the preceding vowel. Since some authors (e.g., Câmara Júnior, 2001) suggest that nasal vowels constitute a junction of the vowel with the /n/, some descriptions of Portuguese list only the seven oral vowels in the phonological system.

In Portuguese, the most common combinations of clusters include a sequence of two segments, an obstruent followed by a liquid sound. The first segment can be /p, b, t, d, k, g, v, f/, and the second segment must be a liquid, /ɾ/ or /l/. However, not all combinations between these segments are allowed. For example, there is neither a /vɾ/ in the beginning of a word nor /dl/ or /vl/ in any word position. The use of /tl/ is restricted to some words (Silva, 1999; Ribas, 2004). Many clusters such as /gn, mn, pn, pt, tm/ appear only infrequently (Cunha, 1980; Bechara, 1988).

Typical Phonological Development

Research on phonological development in typically developing children is well established. Areas of study include not only phonemic inventories and phonological processes but also factors related to syllabic structure and metrical phonology. Understanding typical phonological development in a specific language is very important because this knowledge guides the assessment of delay or disorder, and influences treatment decisions in phonological intervention. Knowing the typical path of development in a specific language can lead to earlier diagnosis. In addition, children who have delays or disorders may also present with difficulties in phonological awareness skills and consequently, problems during the acquisition of reading and writing. The research on typical phonological development of Brazilian Portuguese has focused on children from the South and Southeast regions of Brazil.

The Acquisition of Individual Speech Sounds

The nasals /m/ and /n/ are acquired rather early in Brazilian Portuguese, between 1;6 and 1;8 years (Freitas, 2004). The palatal nasal /ɲ/ was found to be acquired later, after 1;7 years. Hernandorena (1999) studied the production of the palatal nasal /ɲ/ in 130 children from 2;0 to 4;1 years. Results showed that /ɲ/ is acquired by age 2;0, although the nasal is still substituted or omitted by children with low frequency.

Fricatives were found to be acquired between 3;0 and 4;0 years, with the exception of the /ʒ/ in final and initial syllables (Wertzner and Carvalho, 2000). In a later study examining the speech of children between 2;1 to 5;6 years, Wertzner et al. (2002) found that /f, v, s, z/ were acquired earlier than /ʃ, ʒ/. In this age group, substitutions were more frequent than omissions. The results of Oliveira's (2003) study with children between 1;0 to 3;9 years showed that the voiceless alveolar fricative /f/ is acquired by children aged 1;9, and its voiced counterpart, /v/ emerges earlier at 1;8 years.

The voiceless post-alveolar fricative /ʃ/ is acquired at 2;10 years and /ʒ/ at 2;6 years. Children substitute /s/ and /z/ for /ʃ/ and /ʒ/, respectively. Oliveira (2004) concluded that the voiceless alveolar fricative /s/ is acquired by 2;6 whereas its voiced counterpart /z/ is acquired by 2;0 years. Several studies showed that voiced fricatives appear in child speech before their unvoiced counterparts (Oliveira, 2003). In contrast, some studies show a different order of acquisition (e.g. Matzenauer, 2003).

Table 11.1 Phonemes and clusters in two groups (2;1 to 2;6 years and 2;7 to 3;0 years) as elicited in a picture naming task

Age Group	Position	Not Acquired	In Acquisition	Customary Production	Acquired
Group I (2;1 through 2;6)	Initial	pr, bl, br, s, x, S	v	t.	p, b, k, g, d, f, m
	Medial	ʎ	s, z	l, ʃ	p, b, d
	Final	ɾ, x	s, z, ʒ	t, d, l	p, k, ʃ, m, n, ŋ
Group 2 (2;7 through 3;0)	Initial	pr, br, R	s, x, S	v, g	p, b, t, d, k, f, l, m
	Medial		ʎ, z	s, ʃ	p, b, d, l
	Final	vr, ʎ, R	s, z, ɾ, ʒ	ʃ, x	p, d, t, k, g, f, l, m, n, ŋ

Legend: Not acquired = produced by fewer than 25% of the children; In acquisition = produced by 25% up to 50% of the children; Customary production = produced by 50% up to 75% of the children; Acquired = produced by 75% or more of the children.

As for the acquisition of the voiceless velar fricative, Hernadorena and Lamprecht (1997) and Mezzomo and Ribas (2004) reported that /x/ is acquired between age 3;4 and 3;5 years in the South of Brazil. Wertzner et al. (2001) and Galea (2003) reported that this sound is acquired by age 3;0 years.

Hernadorena and Lamprecht (1997) studied 310 children from the South of Brazil between 2;0 and 7;1 years examining their liquid sounds. Results showed that in word initial position the voiced alveolar lateral /l/ is acquired between 2;8 and 2;9 years. Word medially, the same sound is acquired later, between 3;0 and 3;1 years. Mezzomo and Ribas (2004) reported that the /l/ is acquired before the other liquids, being acquired word initially at 2;6. However, in syllable onset position inside the word it is only acquired later, at 3;0 years.

The palatal lateral /ʎ/ and the flap /ɾ/, that appear only in syllable onsets within words, are acquired between 4;0 and 4;1 years and between 4;2 and 4;3 years, respectively (Hernadorena and Lamprecht, 1997). Hernandorena (1999) studied the palatal lateral /ʎ/ in 130 children from 2;0 to 4;1 years. Results showed that /ʎ/ is acquired between 2;6 and 2;7 years. However, the palatal lateral is still deleted or substituted by children until 4;0 to 4;1 years. Common errors in the production of both phonemes include omission or gliding. Another study (Mezzomo and Ribas, 2004) showed that the simple flap /ɾ/ is acquired at 4;2 years. Substituting this sound by /l/ and gliding have been shown to be the most frequent errors for this speech sound. The authors showed that the /ʎ/ is acquired at 3;6 years.

Wertzner (1994) studied children from 3;0 to 7;0 years and noted that the archiphoneme /S/ is acquired by 3;0 years.

However, the archiphoneme /R/ is acquired later, at 4;6 years in final syllable position and at 6;0 years in initial syllable position. Mezzomo (2004) stated that /S/ is acquired in word final codas at 2;6 years, and in word-medial codas at 3;0 years. According to this author, the /R/ in syllable codas is already acquired at 3;10 years.

Pertaining to consonant clusters in Brazilian Portuguese child speech, Wertzner (1994) reported that clusters with the /ɾ/ as the second segment were acquired between 3;7 and 5;0 years. Clusters with an /l/ as the second segment were acquired between 4;7 to 5;0 years. In the speech of children in South Brazil (Ribas 2003, 2004), these clusters appear at 1;8 years, showing speech errors until their complete acquisition at 5;2 years.

Galea (2008) studied all consonants of Portuguese and their phase of acquisition among 88 children age 2;1 to 3;0 years who were acquiring Portuguese Brazilian in a monolingual context. Data were analyzed separately for 41 children age 2;0 to 2;6 (Group I) and 47 children age 2;6 to 3;0 (Group II). They were all typical developing children.

The data were collected using three types of tasks: imitation and naming tasks (both using a standard tests; see Wertzner, 2000) and a spontaneous speech task. Results showed that children had similar performances in imitation and spontaneous speech, thus only the naming task will be considered in this chapter. Table 1 shows the acquisition of the phonemes for this naming task.

This study used a method of classification of acquisition of phonemes that is based on the percentage of children in each group who accurately produced a certain segment or cluster. If from 75% to 100% of children had acquired the target, it was considered "acquired"; from 50% to 74.99% of children that had acquired the target, it was considered in "customary production," from 25% to 49.99%, it was considered "in acquisition," and between 0% to 24.99%, "not acquired." The targets were analyzed in initial, medial and final position only if at least half of the children had accurately produced the target.

The stops /p, b, k/ were fully acquired in all syllable positions tested, but /d/ was acquired in all syllables with the exception of the final position for the children aged 2;0 to 2;6. The stop /t/ was in customary production by the children aged 2;0 to 2;6, and was acquired by the children aged 2;7-3;0. The stop /ɡ/ was acquired in initial position for the children 2;0-2;6 but was in customary production for the children aged 2;7-3;0; it was acquired in the final position for children aged 2;7-3;0. Nasals were all acquired by both age groups.

The fricative /f/ was analyzed in initial syllable of both groups and was acquired in that position. In final position, it was only analyzed for the children 2;0-2;6 and was also acquired. The fricative /v/ was in acquisition for the children 2;0-2;6 and in customary production for the children 2;7-3;0. The fricative /s/ was still not acquired in initial position for the children 2;0-2;6. In other positions, it was in acquisition for both age groups, with the exception of the medial position for the older group where it was in customary production. The fricative /z/ was in acquisition across all positions. The fricative /ʃ/ was acquired in the final position for the children 2;0-2;6; however, it was in customary production in the medial position for the children 2;0-2;6, and in the medial and final positions for the children 2;7-3;0. The voiced fricative /ʒ/ was in acquisition for both groups in the only position tested, the final position. The velar /x/ was analyzed in initial and final syllables and was found to be not acquired among the younger children but was in acquisition in initial position and in customary production in final position for the older children.

The flap /ɾ/ was not acquired for the children aged 2;0-2;6 but was in acquisition for children aged 2;7-3;0. In medial position, the same pattern was observed for /ʎ/. It was not acquired for the children aged 2;0-2;6 but was in acquisition for children aged 2;7-3;0. In final position, the /ʎ/ was analyzed only for the older children and was found to be not acquired. The /l/ was in customary production for the children aged 2;0-2;6 and acquired for the children aged 2;7-3;0.

The archiphoneme /S/ was analyzed in initial syllable position. In the younger group, it was not acquired and for the older children it was in acquisition. On the other hand, the archiphoneme /R/ was not acquired by either groups. As can be seen in Table 11.1, all clusters were considered not acquired.

PHONOLOGICAL PROCESSES

In the south of Brazil, Yavaş (1988) studied the phonological processes and the age of their elimination in typically developing children between 2;4 to 4;6 years. Results show that cluster reduction is still present in children at 4;6 years. Devoicing is still detectable in children at 4;6 years. Fronting and final liquid deletion has been documented in children at 4;0 years. Unstressed syllable deletion, final fricative deletion, gliding, and liquid substitution are still characteristics of child speech at 3;6 years. Intervocalic liquid deletion and backing are still in use in 3;0 year-old children. Liquid onset deletion, stopping, and assimilation have been found to be present in 2;6 year-old children, whereas reduplication and pre-vocalic voicing are used until 2;6 years.

In a longitudinal study of twelve children between 2;9 to 5;5 years, Lamprecht (1991,1993) showed that only eight phonological processes appear in the speech of children from the south of Brazil. These processes include cluster simplification, non-lateral liquid deletion in coda position inside the word, fricative devoicing in coda within the word, liquid substitution, palatal fronting, devoicing, backing of fricative and metathesis. Results of a research study carried out in the city of Santa Maria, also in the south of Brazil (Cigana et al., 1995), showed that the most frequently used phonological processes in kindergarten children included cluster reduction and final liquid deletion in the coda of a syllable inside the word.

Moving from the south to the southeast region of Brazil, several differences have been documented in the order of phonological acquisition in children. The differences identified may stem from differences in the pronunciation of regional dialects and the variable research methods used in these studies, among other important factors.

Galea et al. (1999) observed five phonological processes in children from São Paulo: assimilation, syllable deletion, stopping, and devoicing of stops and fricatives in children from 2;1 to 3;0 years. Children used these processes with a frequency of less than 25% of all cases. A decrease was detectable in the use of these processes with increasing age. Galea et al. (2001) analyzed syllable deletion in 15 children between 2;1 to 2;6 years and 20 children between 2;7 to 3;0 years. Results revealed that younger children use this phonological process more frequently than older ones. However, the process was documented to be used only with low frequency. Also in São Paulo, Wertzner et al. (2001) observed the presence of velar simplification (omission or substitution of the /x/) in children of the same age range.

The authors concluded that, up to age 3;0 years, velar simplification is a productive phonological process, although an increase in the correct production and a decrease of omissions and substitutions with increasing age was documented. Wertzner (1998) noted the process of liquid simplification to be the most frequent substitution pattern in children from 3;1 to 5;6 years. Results showed omissions and substituting the glide /j/ for all liquids.Although the results of many studies were mentioned above, this chapter primarily focuses on reviewing the findings of two studies: Wertzner (1992, 1994) and Galea (2003). These research studies documented phonological processes in monolingual Brazilian Portuguese-speaking children that are frequently used for assessment and treatment in this population.The first study examined children between 3;0 to 7;0 years (Examples 4 to 10) whereas the second study explored the speech characteristics of children between 2;1 to 3;0 years (Examples 1 to 3 and 11 to 13). Phonological processes and the age of their elimination by typical phonological developing children are listed in Table 11.2.

Table 11.2. Description of phonological processes in children acquiring Brazilian Portuguese

Phonological Process	Example	Age of Elimination (years; months)
1. Syllable omission	/'patʊ/ - [pa] – "duck"	2;6
2. Assimilation (a feature of a phoneme influences another phoneme)	/ma'kakʊ/ - [ka'kakʊ] – "monkey"	2;6
3. Stopping of fricatives (stops are substituted for fricatives)	/'sapʊ/ - ['tapʊ] – "frog" /'vaka/ - ['baka] – "cow"	2;6
4. Backing to velar (a velar, /k/ or /g/, is substituted for an alveolar, /t/ or /d/)	/sa'patʊ/ - [sa'pakʊ] – "shoe" /'dosɪ/ - ['gosɪ] – "sweet"	3;0
5. Backing to palatal (palatals /ʃ/ or /ʒ/ are substituted for alveolars /s/ or /z/)	/'sapʊ/ - ['ʃapʊ] - "frog" /'zebɾa/ - ['ʒebɾa] - "zebra"	4;6
6. Velar fronting (alvelar stops, /t/ or /d/, are substituted for velars /k/ or /g/)	/'kaɾʊ/ - ['taɾʊ] – "expensive" /'gaRfʊ/ - ['daRfʊ] –"fork"	3;6
7. Palatal fronting (alveolars /s/ or /z/ are substituted for a palatals /ʃ/ or /ʒ/)	/'ʃavɪ/ - ['savɪ] – "key" /'ʒelʊ/ - ['zelʊ] – "ice"	4;6
8. Liquid simplification (a liquid is omitted, replaced by another liquid, or semivocalized)	/'kaɾa/ - ['kala] – "face" /'bolʊ/ - ['bojʊ] – "cake" /pa'ɾedɪ/ - [pa'edɪ] – "wall"	4;6
9. Coda consonant simplification (a coda of a syllable, either /S/ or /R/ is omitted or replaced)	/'baɾkʊ/ - ['bajkʊ] – "boat" /'pasta/ - ['pata] - "paste"	7;0
10. Cluster reduction or simplification (the second consonant of a cluster, a liquid, is omitted or substituted)	/'pɾatʊ/ - ['patʊ] – "plate" /'klubɪ/ - [kɾubɪ] – "club"	7;0
11. Stop voicing (an unvoiced stop is replaced by its voiced counterpart)	/'patʊ/ - ['batʊ] – "duck" /'kaɾa/ - ['gaɾa] – "face" /tia/ - [dia] – "aunt"	Prior to 2;0

Table 11.2. (Continued)

Phonological Process	Example	Age of Elimination (years; months)
12. Fricative voicing (an unvoiced fricative is replaced by its voiced conterpart)	/'faka/ - ['vaka] – "knife" /'sapʊ/ - ['zapʊ] – "frog" /ʃa/ - [ʒa] – "tea"	Prior to 2;0
13. Stop devoicing (a voiced stop is replaced by its unvoiced counterpart)	/'bala/ - ['pala] – "candy" /'gaRfʊ/ - ['karfʊ] – "fork " /dia/ - [tia] – "day"	2;6
14. Fricative devoicing (a voiced fricative is replaced by its unvoiced counterpart)	/'vaka/ – ['faka] - "knife" /'zebɾa/ – ['sebɾa] - "zebra" /ʒa/ – [ʃa] - "now"	2;6
15. Velar simplification (/x/ is omitted or replaced)	/'xua/ – ['ua] - "street"	3;0

The second study was conducted with 88 children from 2;1 through 3;0 years divided into two groups (Group I: 41 children from 2;1 through 2;6 years and Group II: 47 children from 2;7 through 3;0 years) in the same region of the city of São Paulo (Galea, 2003). Children were similar in their socioeconomic background.

Some phonological processes were used more frequently by the older group. Other processes were identified with higher frequency in the younger group. Overall, results showed the gradual acquisition of Brazilian Portuguese phonology. Cluster simplification, final consonant simplification, and velar simplification were the most frequently occurring phonological processes used by both groups. Fricative devoicing was used frequently in the younger group, but this process had almost completely disappeared in the older children. However, although fricative devoicing was not present in all children, those who used this process applied it in more than 25% of the cases. These results indicate a gradual acquisition of phonology and call attention to the substantial degree of individual variability during the acquisition process of phonology.

Children aged 2;0-2;6 presented the following processes from the most to the least frequently used: cluster simplification, velar simplification, final consonant simplification, liquid simplification, palatal fronting, fricative devoicing, backing to palatal, stopping, stop devoicing, velar fronting, syllable deletion, assimilation, backing to velar, stop voicing and fricative voicing. Older children (i.e., aged 2;7-3;0) presented the following processes from the most to the least frequently used: cluster simplification, final consonant simplification, velar simplification, liquid simplification, palatal fronting, backing to palatal, stopping, fricative devoicing, velar fronting, fricative devoicing, syllable reduction, assimilation, backing to velar, fricative voicing and stop voicing.

Connections

This chapter is one of three chapters describing the acquisition of languages other than English. Chapter 10 focuses on French and Chapter 12, on Korean. Chapter 9 outlines some common trends in cross-linguistic acquisition processes.

Concluding Remarks

This chapter reviewed the phonological acquisition in Brazilian Portuguese. It is important to acknowledge the impact of dialectal diversity in Brazil before trying to compare the results of studies based on child speech data gathered from various geographical regions of the country. Results of child speech studies examining phonological acquisition in Brazilian Portuguese are often similar.

However, several findings differ from each other substantially. Overall, results show that children acquire Brazilian Portuguese phonology by about 7;0 years of age. The last phonological processes to be eliminated are processes involving more complex syllables like CCV and CVC syllables, and those that contain liquids.

Chapter Review Questions

1. What are the first and last sounds to be acquired in Brazilian Portuguese?
2. What are the last phonological processes to disappear in the productions of children?
3. What are the most frequently observed phonological processes in children during acquisition?

Suggestions for Further Reading

Silva, T. C. (2007). Fonética e Fonologia do Português - Roteiro de Estudos e Guia de Exercícios. 9. ed. São Paulo: Editora Contexto.

Suggestions for Student Activities

1. Compare the acquisition of consonants in Brazilian Portuguese to that in English, using the information in Chapter 6 (toddlers and preschoolers). What similarities and differences do you see?
2. Compare the phonological processes in Brazilian Portuguese to those commonly seen in English-acquiring children. What similarities and differences to you see?
3. Consult Chapter 9 for some general trends in the acquisition of phonemes. How closely does Brazilian Portuguese fit these trends?

Answers to Chapter Review Questions

1. What are the first and last sounds to be acquired in Brazilian Portuguese?

The earliest sounds to be acquired are the stops and nasals. The last sounds to be acquired include the archiphoneme /R/ and the consonant clusters, which are composed of a stop followed by a liquid.

2. What are the last phonological processes to disappear in the productions of children?

The processes containing liquids and with more complexed syllable structure as coda consonant simplification and cluster omission or simplification (Wertzner, 1992).

3. What are the most frequently observed phonological processes in children during acquisition?

Some of the oldest children whose productions were analyzed for phonological processes were Kindergarden children in the south of Brazil (Cigana et al., 1995). The most frequently observed processes included cluster reduction and final liquid deletion in midword coda positions. In children age 3;1 to 5;6, Wertzner (1998) observed liquid simplification (omissions or substitutions) as the most commonly used phonological process. In the south of Brazil, Yavaş (1988) cluster reduction and devoicing in children at age 4;6.

References

Bechara, E. (1988). Moderna gramática portuguesa (32nd ed.). São Paulo: Companhia Editora Nacional.

Câmara Júnior, J. M. (1975). História e estrutura da língua portuguesa. Rio de Janeiro: Padrao.

Câmara Júnior, J. M. (2001). Estrutura da língua portuguesa (34th ed.). Petrópolis: Editora Vozes.

Cigana, L. B., Cechella, C., Mota, H. B. E Chiari, B. M. (1995). Perfil do desenvolvimento fonológico de crianças de creches da rede municipal de Santa Maria, Rio Grande do Sul, na faixa etária de 4:0 a 6:2 anos. *Pró-Fono Revista de Atualização Científica, 7* (2), 15-20.

Cunha, C. (1980). Gramática do português contemporâneo, de acordo com a nomenclatura gramatical brasileira (8th ed.). Rio de Janeiro: Padrão.

Freitas G. C. M. (2004). Sobre a Aquisição das Plosivas e Nasais. In: LAMPRECHT, R.R. Aquisição Fonológica do Português: perfil de desenvolvimento e subisídios para a terapia. Porto Alegre: Artmed, chap 4.

Galea, D. E. S.(2003). Análise do sistema fonológico em crianças de 2;1 a 3;0 anos de idade. São Paulo. Dissertação (Mestrado em Semiótica e Lingüística Geral) - Faculdade de Filosofia Letras e Ciências Humanas Universidade de São Paulo.

Galea, D. E. S. (2008). Percurso da Aquisição dos Encontros Consonantais, Fonemas e Estruturas Silábicas em Crianças de 2:1 a 3:0 Anos de Idade. São Paulo. Dissertação (Doutorado em Semiótica e Lingüística Geral) - Faculdade de Filosofia Letras e Ciências Humanas Universidade de São Paulo.

Galea D. E. S., Almeida, R. C. ,Wertzner, H. F. (1999). Uso dos Processos Fonológicos de Ensurdecimento de Plosivas e Fricativas, Plosivação de Fricativas, Harmonia Consonantal e Redução de Sílaba em Crianças de 2;1 a 3;0 anos de idade. In: Congresso Internacional de Fonoaudiologia, 6; Encontro Ibero-Americano de Fonoaudiologia., 3., 1999, São Paulo. *Anais*... São Paulo: [s.n.], 51 – complimentary volume.

Galea, D. E. S.; Wertzner, H. F. (2005). Análise das Consoantes Líquidas no desenvolvimento fonológico típico. In: Congresso Brasileiro de Fonoaudiologia, 13, Santos. *Anais*... São Paulo: [s. n.].

Galea, D. E. S., Wertzner, H. F. And Almeida, R. C. (2001). Ocorrência e Análise Métrica do Processo Fonológico de Redução de Sílaba. In: Congresso Brasileiro de Fonoaudiologia, 9, Guarapari. Anais... São Paulo: [s.n.], 403.

Hernandorena, C. L. M. (1999). Aquisição da Fonologia e implicações teóricas: um estudo sobre as soantes palatais. In: Lamprecht, R. R. Aquisição da Linguagem – questões e análises. Porto Alegre: *EDIPUCRS*, 81-94.

Hernandorena, C. L. M., Lamprecht, R. R. (1997). A aquisição das consoantes líquidas do português. *Letras de Hoje,32* (4), 7-22.

Lamprecht, R. R. (1991). A teoria da fonologia natural nas pesquisas sobre a aquisição da fonologia. *ABRALIN, 12*, 129-133.

Lamprecht, R. R. (1993). A aquisição da fonologia do português na faixa etária dos 2;9-5;5. *Letras de Hoje, 28* (2), 99-106.

Matzenauer, C. L. B. (2003). A aquisição das fricativas coronais com base em restrições. *Letras de Hoje*, *38* (2), 123-135.

Matzenauer, C. L. B. (2004). Bases para o entendimento da aquisição fonológica. In: Lamprecht, R.R. Aquisição Fonológica do Português: perfil de desenvolvimento e subisídios para a terapia. Porto Alegre: Artmed, chap 2.

Mezzomo, C. L. (2004). Sobre a aquisição da coda. In: Lamprecht, R. R. Aquisição Fonológica do Português: perfil de desenvolvimento e subisídios para a terapia. Porto Alegre: Artmed, chap 8.

Mezzomo, C. L.; Ribas, L. P. (2004). Sobre a aquisição das líquidas. In: Lamprecht, R.R. Aquisição Fonológica do Português: perfil de desenvolvimento e subisídios para a terapia. Porto Alegre: Artmed, chap 6.

Oliveira, C. C. (2003). Perfil da aquisição das fricativas /f/, /v/, ʃ/ e /ʒ do português brasileiro: um estudo quantitativo. *Letras de Hoje*, 38. (2), 97-110.

Oliveira, C. C. (2004). Sobre a aquisição das fricativas. In: Lamprecht, R.R. Aquisição Fonológica do Português: perfil de desenvolvimento e subisídios para a terapia. Porto Alegre: Artmed, chap 5.

Ribas, L. (2003). Onset complexo: características da aquisição. *Letras de Hoje*, 38 (2), 23-31.

Ribas, L. (2004). Sobre a aquisição do onset complexo. In: Lamprecht, R.R. Aquisição Fonológica do Português: perfil de desenvolvimento e subisídios para a terapia. Porto Alegre: Artmed, chap 9.

Silva, T. C. (1999). Fonética e Fonologia do português – roteiro de estudos e guia de exercícios (2nd ed.) São Paulo: Contexto.

Teixeira, E. R., Davis, B. L. (2002). Early Sound patterns in the speech of two Brazilian Portuguese speakers. *Language and Speech, 45* (2), 179-204.

Wertzner, H. F. (1992). Articulação: Aquisição do Sistema Fonológico dos três aos Sete Anos. Tese (Doutorado – Departamento de Lingüística) - Faculdade de Filosofia, Letras e Ciências Humanas da Universidade de São Paulo, São Paulo.

Wertzner, H. F. (1994). Aquisição da articulação: um estudo em crianças de três a sete anos. *Estudos de Psicologia*, 11 (1,2), 11-21.

Wertzner, H. F. (1998). Typical Substitutions of the Liquids Phonemes in the Phonological Acquisition of Brazilian Children. Proceedings of Speech Pathology Australia National Conference, School of Speech and Hearing Sciences, and Curtin Printing Services, Curtin University of Technology, 175-180.

Wertzner, H. F. Fonologia. (2000). In: Andrade, C. R. F.; Befi-Lopes, D. M.; Fernandes, F. D. M.; Wertzner, H. F. ABFW; teste de linguagem infantil nas áreas de fonologia, vocabulário, fluência e pragmática. Carapicuíba: Pró-Fono, chap 1.

Wertzner, H. F., Carvalho, I. A. M. (2000). Ocorrências de "erros" nos fonemas fricativos durante o processo de aquisição do sistema fonológico. *Jornal Brasileiro de Fonoaudiologi, 2* (2), 67-74.

Wertzner, H. F., Galea, D.E.S., Almeida, R.C. (2001). Uso do processo fonológico de simplificação de velar em crianças de 2;1 a 3;0 anos de idade. *Jornal Brasileiro de Fonoaudiologia, 8*,233-238.

Wertzner, H. F., Galea, D. E. S., Teruya, N. M. (2002). Acquisition of the Fricative Phonemes in Brazilian Children. *The ASHA Leader. American Speech- Language- Hearing Association, 7* (15), 158.

Yavas, M. (1988). Padrões de aquisição da fonologia do português. *Letras de Hoje*, *23*, 7-30.

In: Comprehensive Perspectives …
Editors: Beate Peter and Andrea A. N. MacLeod
ISBN: 978-1-62257-041-6

Chapter 12

ACQUIRING KOREAN

Minjung Kim

INTRODUCTION

This chapter provides an introduction to the sound patterns of standard Korean and an overview of how Korean children acquire their native phonology. Age and order of acquisition of Korean speech sounds are described. In addition, information about phonological error patterns is provided.

KOREAN SPEAKERS IN THE WORLD

Korean is the official language of both South and North Korea and is spoken by about 78 million Korean speakers worldwide. The major countries outside the Korean peninsula with a sizable Korean population are China, USA, Japan, and the former Soviet Union. The Korean language belongs to Altaic languages, is agglutinative in its morphology, and has the order of Subject-Object-Verb in its syntax. Korean vocabulary consists of native words (35%), Sino-Korean words (60%) and loan words (5%), and has the indigenous phonetic writing system called *Hangul* (Sohn, 1999).

THE SOUND PATTERNS OF KOREAN

Vowels

Korean vowels can be categorized as high, mid, and low vowels by tongue height, front and back vowels by tongue advancement, and unrounded and rounded vowels by lip rounding.

Table 12.1. Korean vowels

	Front	Back	
	Unround	Round	Unround
High	i	u	ɯ
Mid	ɛ	o	ʌ
Low			ɑ

In terms of the number of Korean vowels, there is discrepancy across studies and it ranges from seven to ten monophthongs (Shin, Cha, and Kiear, in press). The ten vowels of the Korean language include three unrounded front vowels, /i, e, ɛ/, two rounded front vowels, /y, ø/, three unrounded back vowels, / ɨ, ə, a/, and two rounded back vowels, /u, o/ (Sohn, 1999). Shin and Cha (2003), however, argued that two vowels, /e/ and /ɛ/, are no longer contrastive perceptually and acoustically, and /y/ and /ø/ are pronounced as diphthongs by contemporary standard speakers.

Based on this observation, they suggested that a seven-vowel system might be most appropriate to reflect the spoken language of Korea. Table 12.1 displays the seven-vowel system of Korean (Shin, Cha, and Kiear, in press).

With respect to Korean diphthongs, three semivowels or glides (/j, w, ɰ/) are combined with other vowels to create ten diphthongs (/jɛ, jɑ, ju, jʌ, jo, wi, wɛ, wɑ, wʌ, ɰi/). The phonotactics of Korean suggest that these are diphthongs and not glide + vowel sequences such as we would find in English (e.g., "you" /ju/).

Consonants

There are 19 consonants in Korean. Table 12.2 provides the classification of Korean consonants according to the place and manner of articulation.

Table 12.2. Korean consonants

		Labial	Alveolar	Alveolo-palatal	Velar	Glottal
Stops (Plosives)	Tense	p*	t*		k*	
	Aspirated	p^h	t^h		k^h	
	Lax	p	t		k	
Affricates	Tense			tɕ*		
	Aspirated			$tɕ^h$		
	Lax			tɕ		
Fricatives	Lax		s			h
	Tense		s*			
Nasals		m	n		ŋ	
Liquid (Lateral approximant)			l			

Note: The different laryngeal types have been termed differently in the literature; "tense-aspirated-lax" or "fortis-aspirated-lenis." In this chapter, the terms "lax-tense-aspirated" are used.

Korean obstruents (i.e., stops, fricatives, and affricates) have an unusual system in terms of variations in laryngeal types. While most languages use a voicing contrast to distinguish among obstruents produced at the same place of articulation, Korean obstruents are characterized by a three-way contrast among stops and affricates (i.e., tense, aspirated, and lax) and a two-way fricative contrast (i.e., tense and lax).

All these obstruents are voiceless phrase-initially, and word-initially in words produced in isolation. In word-final position, the distinctions among the different laryngeal types of Korean obstruents are neutralized; Korean stops are produced as lax stops, and Korean alveolo-palatal affricates and Korean alveolar fricatives are neutralized to a lax stop /t/ (Kim, 1979; Kim and Jongman, 1996; Sohn, 1999).

The three types of Korean stops are produced at the three places of articulation: labial, alveolar, and velar. In phrase initial position, including single word productions, tense stops are described as unaspirated and laryngealized, aspirated stops as strongly aspirated, and lax stops as slightly aspirated and breathy (Cho, Jun, and Ladefoged, 2002). While tense and aspirated stops are always voiceless regardless of the phonetic context, lax stops become voiced in word- or phrase- medial position (Jun, 1995; Kim, 1965; Shin, 1997).

Whereas most language have stop consonants categorized by voicing and aspiration that are described using voice onset time (VOT), the three types of Korean word-initial stops can be distinguished by three acoustic-phonetic properties: VOT, fundamental frequency (f_0) of the following vowel, and voice quality at the onset of the following vowel (Cho *et al.*, 2002; Kim *et al.*, 2002). In general, mean VOT values are shortest for tense stops, intermediate for lax stops, and longest for aspirated stops, and VOT values markedly differentiate between tense stops and aspirated stops. However, VOT ranges often overlap (Han and Weitzman, 1970; Hardcastle, 1973; C.-W. Kim, 1965). A supplementary acoustic feature that serves to distinguish Korean stops is fundamental frequency (f_0) of the following vowel. The f_0 at the onset of the vowels following lax stops is generally lower than the following tense or aspirated stops (e.g., Ahn, 1999; Cho *et al.*, 2002; Hardcastle, 1973; Kim *et al.*, 2002). As for the voice quality of the following vowel, the voice onset after a lax stop has a breathy quality, and the voice onset after a tense stop has a creaky (or pressed) quality. The difference in amplitude between the first and second harmonics (*H*1-*H*2) at the onset of voicing is greater for lax stops and aspirated stops relative to tense stops in Korean (Cho *et al.*, 2002). The similar acoustic features across different laryngeal types are applied to Korean alveolo-palatal affricates.

As for Korean alveolar fricatives (i.e., /s, s*/), acoustic studies report that the lax /s/ is produced with frication followed by aspiration whereas the tense /s*/ has frication followed by glottalization at the onset of the following vowel. The frication duration of the tense /s*/ is longer than that of the lax /s/ word initially (Cho *et al.*, 2002; Shin, Cha, and Kiear, in press). Kagaya (1974) categorized the Korean fricative /s/ as aspirated because of the presence of aspiration and laryngeal gestures similar to other aspirated consonants through the fiberscopic study. However, the absence of aspiration and the presence of voicing in the production of the /s/ in intervocalic position supports the view that this sound may be lax rather than aspirated (Cho *et al.*, 2002; Shin, Cha, and Kiear, in press).

The remaining Korean consonants are /m, n, ŋ, l/. All consonants except for the nasal /ŋ/ occur in word-initial position, although /l/ is restricted to occur only in loan words; however, only seven consonants (i.e., /p, t, k, m, m, ŋ, l/) can occur in syllable-final position. The phonetic syllable structure of Korean is formed as (C)(G)V(C), and consonant clusters do not occur within the same syllable. Consonant clusters may occur across syllables in word-medial position. For example, the word "*kamja,*" meaning "potato," is pronounced as /kɑm-tɕɑ/ with a two-consonant sequence word-medially.

SPEECH SOUND DEVELOPMENT OF KOREAN

Age and Order of Phoneme Acquisition

Compared to acquisition studies of English, there are fewer studies investigating the acquisition of Korean. Most studies reported phonological patterns in Korean children through the perceptual analysis based on phonetic transcription (Kim and Pae, 2005; Kim, 1992, 1996; Y.-T. Kim and Shin, 1992; Pae, 1994; Um, 1994). These studies revealed that Korean stops are acquired earlier than other Korean consonants, as predicted by Jakobson's universal theory.

There are a few large-scale normative studies of the acquisition of Korean obstruents. Um (1994) analyzed Korean consonants produced by 150 typically developing Korean children aged 3, 4, and 5 years. She reported that all three different types of stops and affricates were produced correctly by over 90% of the children at each age level, while correct production of fricatives occurred in approximately 50% of the children at age 3, and 60% at ages 4 and 5. With a criterion of 75% children who correctly produced the target phoneme, all the initial and final consonants except for /l, s, s*/ were acquired by age 3. The initial /l/ was acquired by age 5, but /s, s*/ were not acquired by age 5.

More recently, Kim and Pae (2005) provided normative data on phonemic development of 220 Korean children aged 2;6 to 6;5, speaking the Seoul dialect. They analyzed the production accuracy of Korean consonants and age of acquisition of consonants in syllable-initial (SI) and syllable-final (SF) positions. Table 12.3 summarizes the findings from Kim and Pae (2005).

The results revealed similar patterns of development of Korean consonants compared to those found in other normative studies. In general, Korean children acquired stops and nasals first, followed by affricates, and then fricatives. While all Korean stops and affricates except for /k^h/ were acquired by 75% of children at age 4;0, Korean alveolar fricatives were not acquired by age 6;5. With respect to the acquisition of phonemes in different word position, all seven consonants except for /l/, which can occur syllable-finally, were acquired earlier in syllable-initial position than in syllable-final position. As for /l/, syllable-final /l/ was mastered at age 3;6 but syllable-initial /l/ was not acquired until 5;6.

Kim and Stoel-Gamon (2010) investigated phoneme development in children aged 2;6, 3;0, 3;6, and 4;0. This study focused on the age and order of acquisition of Korean word-initial obstruents with particular interest in the order of acquisition of different laryngeal types.

In this study, they examined *age of emergence* and *age of mastery* for word-initial obstruents. *Age of emergence* was defined as the age at which 75% of the children produced at least one correct production of the target phoneme. For *age of mastery*, two criteria of 75% and 90% of children who produced target phonemes with at least 75% accuracy were utilized.

Table 12.3. Developmental patterns of Korean consonants by syllable-initial and syllable final position (Kim and Pae, 2005)

Age	Consonants customarily produced Syllable-initial (SI)	Consonants customarily produced Syllable-final (SF)	Consonants acquired SI	Consonants acquired SF	Consonants mastered SI	Consonants mastered SF
2;6	t^h, t, k*, k^h, k, tɕ*, $tɕ^h$, m, n	p, t, k, m, n, ŋ, l	p*, p^h, p, t*, h			
3;0					p*, t*	
3;6	tɕ, l		t, k, tɕ*, $tɕ^h$	p, m	p^h, p, k*, t^h, m, n, h	t, l
4;0	s		tɕ	n		p
4;6			k^h	k, ŋ	t, k, tɕ*, $tɕ^h$, tɕ	m, n
5;0	s*				k^h	k, ŋ
5;6			l			
6;0					l	
6;5						

Note: A phoneme is "customarily produced," "acquired," and "mastered" when produced correctly by 50%, 75%, and 90% of children, respectively.

The results showed that all tense stops were acquired by 90% of children at age 2;6. Aspirated stops and lax stops emerged in most children at age 3;0 but lax stops were not acquired until age 4;0 whereas aspirated stops were mastered at age 3;6. The three types of affricates emerged in all children at age 3;6 and were acquired by over 75% of children at the same age. The Korean fricatives /s/ and /s*/, on the other hand, emerged at age 3;6 and 4;0, respectively, but were not mastered by age 4;0.

With respect to the order of acquisition of different laryngeal types, Korean stops were acquired in the order of tense, aspirated, and lax. This finding was consistent with that of Kim and Pae's (2005) study except for /k^h/. They attributed the late acquisition of /k^h/, relative to other stops and affricates, to the fact that the test word had a diphthong, which might have made the target phoneme hard to produce. While Kim and Pae (2005) also reported later acquisition of the lax category in the acquisition of Korean affricates, the pattern was not as clear as for stops in Kim and Stoel-Gamon's (2010) study, in which the relatively small number of tokens were assessed to examine the acquisition process for affricates.

Kim and Stoel-Gamon's (2009) acoustic study of Korean word-initial stops proposed that the late acquisition of lax stops may be related to their phonetic and phonological characteristics. Korean lax stops are perceptually less salient with weaker articulation, and context-sensitive by being slightly aspirated in utterance-initial position but being voiced intervocalically. In addition, lax stops are realized with low f_0 of the following vowel when the laryngeal state for voiceless stops typically leads to high f_0. This means that the production of lax stops will be articulatorily more complex than that of tense or aspirated stops because it may require an additional laryngeal adjustment for lowering f_0 (Löfqvist *et al.*, 1989). Although supralaryngeal articulation differs in the production of stops versus affricates, the laryngeal settings for stops and affricates are similar and lax affricates are also produced with low f_0.

As for Korean fricatives, on the other hand, a lax fricative appears to be acquired earlier than a tense counterpart given the customary production of the lax fricative at age 4;0 versus the tense one at age 5;0 (Kim and Pae, 2005). Kim and Stoel-Gamon (2010) interpreted the earlier development of the lax category in Korean fricatives based on the acoustic and articulatory properties that are common between /s/ and aspirated obstruents in word-initial position. Korean children's frequent substitution of / t^{h}/ or / tɕ^{h}/ for /s/ also supports this view. In contrast, later acquisition of the tense /s*/ than the lax /s/ can be explained by increased articulatory complexity. The /s*/ is produced with longer frication that is often followed by glottalization at the onset of the following vowel. It is also suggested that /s*/ is realized with a relatively smaller cavity in front of the constriction, and possibly greater velocity of airflow in the front cavity (Cho *et al.*, 2002).

With regard to acquisition of Korean vowels, all the vowels are acquired before age 3 except for some diphthongs. Diphthongs such as /wɛ, wɑ/ are acquired by age 5 (Um, 1994).

Phonological Error Patterns

In the development of Korean consonants, children demonstrate some errors that conform to Jakobson's universal theory while others appear to be language-specific (Kim, 2006; Kim and Pae, 2000; Kim and Shin, 1992; Kim and Stoel-Gammon, 2010). For example, substitutions of stops for affricates or fricatives frequently occurred in productions of young Korean children as in children acquiring other languages; however, substitution of a tense stop for a lax or an aspirated stop (i.e., tensing) is specific to Korean. In addition, the fronting of velar stops to alveolar stops is less common than in other languages since velar stops are acquired as early as alveolar stops in Korean (Kim and Shin, 1992; Um, 1994).

Kim (2006) investigated productions of 220 Korean children aged 2;6 to 6;5 to propose a preliminary norm of the phonological error patterns for the Korean-Test of Articulation for Children (K-TAC). She reported phonological processes that occurred more than three times in more than 10% of late 2-year-olds. She categorized the phonological processes by whole-word process and segment-change process as proposed in Bankson and Bernthal (2004). As whole-word processes, reduplication (e.g., /sɑt^{h}ɑŋ/ → [t^{h}ɑŋ t^{h}ɑŋ], "candy") or consonant harmony (e.g., /nɑmu/ → [mamu], "tree"), word-final consonant deletion (e.g., /tɕ^{h}ɛk/ → [tɕ^{h}ɛ], "book"), and intersyllabic cluster simplification (e.g., /oks*usu/ → [os*usu], "corn") were reported.

As for segment-change process, tensing or deaspiration (e.g., /p^{h}odo/ → [p*ot*o], "grape"), velar fronting (e.g., /kʌbuki/ → [dʌbudi], "turtle"), nasalization or stopping of liquid (e.g., /kolɛ/ → [konɛ] or [kodɛ], "whale"), liquid simplification (e.g., /kolɛ/ → [kojɛ], "whale"), affrication (e.g., /s*ɑl/ → [tɕ*ɑl], "rice"), palatalization (e.g., /p^{h}odo/ → [p^{h}od^{j}o], "grape"), stopping of fricative or affricate (/tɕɑdoŋtɕ^{h}ɑ/ → [tɑdoŋt^{h}ɑ]), and interdentalization of fricative (e.g., /sɑt^{h}ɑŋ/ → [s̪ɑt^{h}ɑŋ]) were included. Among these phonological processes, reduplication/consonant harmony, word-final consonant deletion, nasalization/stopping of liquids, velar fronting, tensing, and deaspiration were suppressed by age 3. By age 4, intersyllabic cluster simplification, liquid simplification, affrication, and palatalization disappeared. Stopping of fricatives or affricates, on the other hand, persisted until the age of 5.

Kim and Stoel-Gammon (2010) have provided in-depth descriptions on error patterns across different laryngeal types in Korean obstruents. They reported that aspirated stops were produced as either tense or lax stops before age 3;6, and lax stops were produced as either tense or aspirated stops in younger age groups but only as aspirated stops in 3;6 and 4;0 year-old children. In the case of affricates, substitutions of stops were predominant with a tendency toward preserving the original laryngeal type.

This substitution error (i.e., stopping) decreased substantially after age 3;6. With regard to Korean alveolar fricatives, substitutions of [t^h] or [$tɕ^h$] for /s/ were most common. The substitution of [t^h] (i.e., stopping) for /s/ was more common in younger age groups whereas the substitution of [$tɕ^h$] (i.e., affrication) for /s/ occurred more frequently in older children. The similar developmental pattern was found for the target /s*/ which was replaced by [t*] or [tɕ*].

Connections

This chapter is one of three chapters describing the acquisition of languages other than English.

Chapter 10 focuses on French and Chapter 12, on Brazilian Portuguese. Chapter 9 outlines some common trends in cross-linguistic acquisition processes. For an overview of phonological processes in English, see Appendix 2.

Concluding Remarks

Korean has an unusual sound system in terms of variations in laryngeal types. The three-way word-initial Korean stops and affricates are acquired by the age of 4.

The two-way Korean alveolar fricatives, however, are not acquired until after age 6;5. Further research in older children is required to understand the age of acquisition for Korean fricatives. With regard to sound errors, both language-universal and language-specific error patterns were present.

Chapter Review Questions

1. Which speech sound classes are acquired earliest in Korean?
2. Name at least 5 phonological processes (error patterns) that occur in child speech in Korean.
3. How do different stops differ in Korean and why?

Suggestions for Further Reading

Kim, M. and Stoel-Gammon, C. (2011). Phonological development of word-initial Korean obstruents in young Korean children. *Journal of Child Language*, 38(2), 316-340.

Suggestions for Student Activities

Find a Korean speaker and listen to his/her plosives. Can you reliably identify all types of Korean plosives? If you cannot find a native speaker of Korean, try to find Korean speech data on the internet.

Answers to Chapter Review Questions

1. Which speech sound classes are acquired earliest in Korean?

Stops and nasals.

2. Name at least 5 phonological processes (error patterns) that occur in child speech in Korean.

Consonant harmony, word-final consonant deletion, intersyllabic cluster simplification, tensing, deaspiration, velar fronting, liquid simplification, stopping, etc.

3. How do different stops differ in Korean?

Korean stops have a three-way contrast (i.e., tense, aspirated, and lax). All these types of stops are phonetically all voiceless in phrase-initially, and word-initially in words produced in isolation. Tense stops are realized as unaspirated and laryngealized, aspirated stops as strongly aspirated, and lax stops as slightly aspirated and breathy. While tense and aspirated stops are always voiceless regardless of the phonetic context, lax stops become voiced in word- or phrase- medial position.

References

Ahn, H. (1999). Post-release phonatory processes in English and Korean: Acoustic correlates and implications for Korean phonology. PhD dissertation, University of Texas at Austin.

Bankson, N. W. and Bernthal, J. E., (2004). Phonological assessment procedure. In J. E. Bernthal and N. W. Bankson (Eds.), Articulation and phonological disorders (5th ed.). Boston, MA: Allyn and Bacon.

Cho, T., Jun, S.-A., and Ladefoged, P. (2002). Acoustic and aerodynamic correlates of Korean stops and fricatives. *Journal of Phonetics,* 30(2), 193-228.

Han, M. S., and Weitzman, R. S. (1970). Acoustic features of Korean /P,T,K/, /p,t,k/ and /p^h,t^h,k^h/. *Phonetica,* 22(2), 112-128.

Hardcastle, W. J. (1973). Some observations of the tense-lax distinction in initial stops in Korean. *Journal of Phonetics,* 1, 263-271.

Jakobson, R. (1968). Child language, aphasia, and phonological universals. The Hague: Mouton.

Jun, S.-A. (1995). Asymmetrical prosodic effects on the laryngeal gesture in Korean. In B. Connell and A. Arvaniti (Eds.), Phonology and phonetic evidence: papers in laboratory phonology IV (pp. 235-253). Cambridge, U.K.: Cambridge University Press.

Kagaya, R. (1974). A fiberscopic and acoustic study of the Korean stops, affricates and fricatives. *Journal of Phonetics,* 2, 161-180.

Kim, C.-W. (1965). On the autonomy of the tensity feature in stop classification (with special reference to Korean stops). Word, 21, 339-359.

Kim , C.-W. (1979). Neutralization in Korean revisited. *Studies in the Linguistic Sciences,* 9, 147-155.

Kim, M. and Stoel Gammon, C. (2011). Phonological development of word-initial Korean obstruents in young Korean children. *Journal of Child Language,* 38(2), 316-340.

Kim, M. and Stoel-Gammon, C. (2009). The acquisition of Korean word-initial stops. *Journal of the Acoustical Society of America,* 125(6), 3950-3961.

Kim, M.-J. (2006). The phonological error patterns of preschool children in the Korean-test of articulation for children. *Korean Journal of Communication Disorders,* 11, 17–31.

Kim, M. -J., and Pae, S. (2005). The study on the percentage of consonants correct and the ages of consonantal acquisition for 'Korean-test of articulation for children (K-TAC)'. *Korean Journal of Speech Science,* 12, 139–149.

Kim, M.-R., Beddor, P. S., and Horrocks, J. (2002). The contribution of consonantal and vocalic information to the perception of Korean initial stops. *Journal of Phonetics,* 30(1), 77-100.

Kim, H. S., and Jongman, A. (1996). Acoustic and perceptual evidence for complete neutralization of manner of articulation in Korean. *Journal of Phonetics,* 24(3), 295-312.

Kim, Y.-T. (1992). Study on developmental phonological processes of 2-6 year-old children in Seoul and Kyunggi regions. *Malsori,* 21, 3-24.

Kim, Y.-T. (1996). Study on articulation accuracy of preschool Korean children through picture consonant articulation test. *Korean Journal of Communication Disorders,* 1, 7-33.

Kim, Y.-T., and Shin, M.-J. (1992). The phonological processes of Korean children (II): focused on substitution. *Korean Journal of Speech and Hearing Disorders,* 2(1), 29-51.

Löfqvist, A., Baer, T., McGarr, N. S., and Story, R. S. (1989). The cricothyroid muscle in voicing control. *Journal of the Acoustical Society of America,* 85(3), 1314-1321.

Pae, S. (1994). Development of normal speech sounds (I): children aged 1;4-3;11. In Korean Speech Pathology Association (Ed.), Treatment of children's articulation disorder. Seoul: Kunja press.

Shin, J. (1997). Consonantal production and coarticulation in Korean. PhD dissertation, University of London, London.

Shin, J. and Cha, J.(2003). The sound system of Korean. Seoul: Hankookmunhwasa.

Shin, J., Cha, J., and Kiear, J. (in press). The sounds of Korean. Cambridge: Cambridge University Press.

Sohn, H. (1999). *The Korean language.* Cambridge: Cambridge University Press.

Um, J.-H. (1994). Development of normal speech sounds (II): children aged 3, 4, and 5 years. In Korean Speech Pathology Association (Ed.), Treatment of children's articulation disorder. Seoul: Kunja press.

In: Comprehensive Perspectives …
Editors: Beate Peter and Andrea A. N. MacLeod
ISBN: 978-1-62257-041-6

Chapter 13

UNDERSTANDING BILINGUAL PHONOLOGICAL DEVELOPMENT

Andrea A. N. MacLeod

INTRODUCTION

Although bilinguals make up the majority of the world's population (Grosjean, 1982), bilingual language abilities are targeted in a relatively small body of research that is often relegated to the sidelines of academic debates. Despite demographic changes within North America and around the world, the focus of research and clinical SLP training has been on monolingual speakers. The study of bilingual populations is important for societal and theoretical reasons. The societal motivation is based on the premise that research should reflect the population in which the research takes place. For the same reasons it is important to study participants with diverse ethnic and socio-economic status, it is also important to study participants with varied language backgrounds. Around the world, monolingual speakers are not the norm; instead, bilingual and multilingual language abilities are prevalent. Approximately one-half to two-thirds of the world's population speak more than one language. Estimates of the number of bilingual speakers vary due to differences in the definition of "bilingual". One strategy is to estimate the prevalence of bilingualism by looking at the number of languages that exist (approximately 6000) compared with the number of countries (approximately 200) (Richard, 1999).

In addition to the societal motivation to studying bilinguals, theoretical motivation for the study of bilinguals is based on the need to evaluate current theories of language production and perception in this population. Bilingual speakers provide a unique window into speech production and speech perception since some adult second-language learners have been found to achieve near-native mastery of vocabulary and grammar; however, these same individuals typically fall short of native-like speech pronunciation (Moyer, 1999). In contrast, native-like speech production in a second language has been observed in adults who learned two languages during childhood and who have continued to speak those languages into adulthood (Flege, 1988; MacLeod and Stoel-Gammon, 2009; MacLeod, Stoel-Gammon and Wassink, 2009; Munro, Flege, and MacKay, 1996). The goal of this chapter is to provide an introduction to bilingual development starting with definitions of the term "bilingual," followed by a summary of theoretical frameworks used to study this population, the effect of age on bilingual language learning, and a summary of research on bilingual speech sound development among typically developing children and children with speech sound disorders. In this chapter, I will present research on children who are acquiring two languages – either both languages from a very young age, or a second language learned upon beginning school. In Chapter 14, the authors provide a specific example of bilingual phonological development among children who have learned their second language in kindergarten; Chapter 8 addresses how adults acquire the phonology of a second language.

DEFINING "BILINGUAL"

Bilingualism can be conceptualized on two main levels: *societal bilingualism* or *individual bilingualism* (Fishman, 1980). Societal bilingualism refers to a community, region, or country that supports two languages. This may be on an official level, such as in Canada, resulting in the use of both languages by the government, in law, in education, and in public media. Societal bilingualism may be less official, such as in California, where a number of private services are available in languages other than English, and where some government documents are available in languages other than English. Although societal bilingualism refers to the co-existence of two languages within one society, individuals within this society are not necessarily bilingual. Research on societal bilingualism tends to focus on questions of language preservation, language interaction, and the impact of language policies on the society. In contrast, individual bilingualism refers to the presence of two languages within an individual. Kohnert and Bates (2002) defined bilingual language proficiency as knowledge and performance skills in each of the two languages, as well as control of the dual-language system. In other words, a bilingual can speak in either of her languages and can alternate between the two languages to translate, *code-switch,* or process mixed-language input. The description of a bilingual individual must take into consideration a variety of factors that relate to the ease with which both languages are used by the individual while speaking, reading, writing, and listening. The factors that contribute to this ease include the age when the languages were learned, the linguistic relationships between the languages being acquired, the social contexts of language acquisition, and the social status of the languages (Birdsong, 2006; Flege, 1988; Kohnert and Bates, 2002). When studying the phonology of bilingual speakers, it is important to identify the social contexts of language use and the amount of exposure to each language because these factors affect the degree of bilingual proficiency that can be attained. Language proficiency may be nearly equal in both languages in the case of a balanced bilingual, or one of the languages may be better mastered than the other resulting in language dominance. Mastery may also differ depending on the language task such as speaking, writing, or reading. As circumstances change across one's lifetime, the mastery of each language may also vary. For example, a person may move to a monolingual community as an adult, and have few daily opportunities to use one of their languages; or a person may have few opportunities to write in one of their languages despite speaking the language daily; or a person may move to a new linguistic environment for educational purposes and acquire a technical vocabulary in that language that was not acquired in the language of origin. Finally, the opportunity to use each language may differ from person to person depending on which language is used at home, in the workplace, in school, in the community, with friends, or in religion. Although there are several ways to define the term bilingual, in this chapter I will use the term "bilingual" to refer to individuals who are proficient in two languages. Some bilinguals may be exposed to two languages from birth (i.e., *simultaneous bilinguals*); other bilinguals may have been exposed to two languages sequentially (i.e., *sequential bilinguals*), thus they have a first and a second language. An individual's "second language" (L2) is the language that the individual was exposed to after 3 or 4 years of age; an individual's "first language(s)" (L1) is the language that the individual was exposed to prior to this age. Lastly, some individuals acquire more than two languages and the term "multilinguals" is commonly used to refer to them.

Theoretical Frameworks for Understanding Bilingual Development

Research on bilingual language development has been motivated by two main hypotheses: the Unitary System Hypothesis (Volterra and Taeschner, 1978), and, more recently, the Dual Systems Hypothesis (Paradis and Genesee, 1996). These hypotheses focus on the degree to which bilinguals' have separate language systems and are described in greater detail below (see also Figure 13.1).

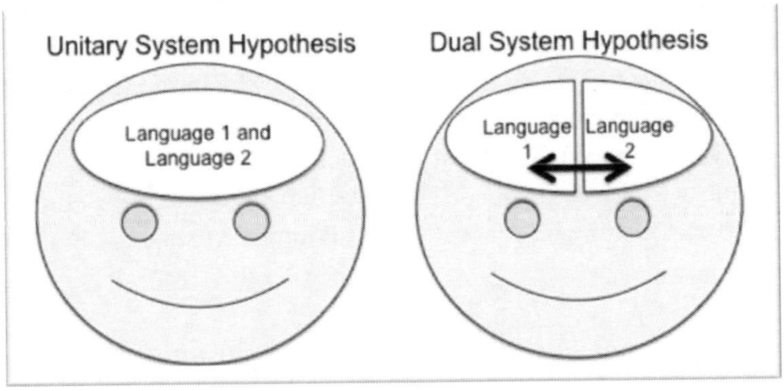

Figure 13.1. Conceptualization of the Unitary System Hypothesis and the Dual System Hypothesis.

Unitary System Hypothesis

The Unitary System Hypothesis proposed that bilingual children begin with a single linguistic system that becomes differentiated through experience with two languages (Volterra and Taeschner, 1978). According to this hypothesis, a bilingual toddler would have a single lexical system that included words of both languages but rarely translation equivalents. In other words, a bilingual child would not learn a word in each language for the same thing (e.g., in French "*chien*" and in English "dog" both refer to the canine household pet) but instead would learn words in each language for different things (e.g., French word for cat ,"*chat,*" but English word for dog). With time, children recognize two different lexicons although they may continue to apply a single syntactic structure. As a result, a bilingual child begins learning translation equivalents, but applies a single syntax: for example, "dog brown" and "*chien brun*", where the child uses the same noun-adjective order for both languages (in this case the French order). Finally, children develop separate, language-specific linguistic systems. This hypothesis motivated a number of studies across different language domains, but, as we will see, it has not been upheld.

Dual System Hypothesis

In the mid 1990s, researchers presented the *Dual System Hypothesis* that proposes that children's linguistic systems are differentiated at an early age (Paradis and Genesee, 1996). Following this hypothesis, two types of bilingual language development can occur: either the two languages develop independently and resemble monolingual development in each language, or the two languages interact resulting in differences when compared to monolingual development (Paradis and Genesee, 1996). This systematic influence of the grammar of one language on the grammar of the other during acquisition could lead to three different effects in bilingual speech and language development: *acceleration* in the acquisition of a structure when this structure occurs in the two languages; *deceleration* in the acquisition of a structure when it is not shared by the two languages; and *transfer* of a structure from one language to the other language (Paradis and Genesee, 1996). For example, acceleration may explain the earlier acquisition of a phoneme in one language than would be expected among monolingual children. Deceleration may explain the slower acquisition of a phoneme in one language. Finally, transfer effects can explain errors that are atypical in monolingual development but which can be explained by the influence of one language on the other. Phonological development provides an exciting area of study to test the Dual Systems Hypothesis because it is possible to identify language-specific structures (e.g., phonemes and prosody) during the very early stages of linguistic development. In contrast, one must wait until children are older to study language differentiation in syntax and morphology.

Three Main Approaches in Studying Bilingual Phonological Abilities

Researchers have investigated bilingual phonetic and phonological abilities among children and adults using three approaches: (1) the *monolingual comparison approach;* (2) the *shared-separate approach;* and (3) the *age-effect approach* (Mack, 2003). The monolingual comparison approach, which analyzes bilingual speech systems in reference to monolinguals, investigates the extent to which bilingual speakers are two speakers in one body (Mack, 2003). The shared-separate approach, which analyzes bilingual speech systems in reference to themselves, investigates the extent of the independence or dependence of the bilingual speaker's phonological systems (Mack, 2003). The age-effect approach, which analyzes productions of bilingual speakers who differ in terms of age of acquisition/learning of the L2, investigates the effect of different ages of acquisition on the development of two phonological systems (Mack, 2003). The research resulting from these three approaches has begun to clarify the patterns of bilingual phonological systems in both children and adults. However, these approaches have yet to be unified within a theoretical model that can account for both the phonological abilities of adult second language learners and the phonological abilities of children acquiring two languages.

AGE AND EXPOSURE IN BILINGUAL DEVELOPMENT

Learning a language is a complicated and lengthy process that requires learning a new pragmatic system, vocabulary, syntax, morphology, phonology, and phonetics. As noted above, bilingual language proficiency varies due to factors such as age of acquisition, the environment of language learning, and the current environment of language use (Watson, 1991; Flege, Yeni-Komshian, and Liu, 1999; Moyer, 1999). We will focus on the age of acquisition and exposure to each language since these factors are have been the topic of a number of studies and thus we have a better understanding of how they influence bilingual speech and language development in preschool aged children.

Age of Language Learning

Age of language learning is a key factor in bilingual proficiency. We know that a *critical period* exists for learning one's first language and that this period extends from birth to approximately three or four years of age. Until the age of three or four, children seem to learn language "automatically." Studies of speech perception demonstrate that infants from birth to 8 months of age can perceive subtle contrasts between speech sounds, even if the sounds are not part of their language environment (Werker and Lalonde, 1988); then by 10 to 12 months, children begin to focus on the phonemic distinctions in their ambient language while losing their ability to discriminate between some foreign speech sounds (Kuhl, 2000; Werker and Lalonde, 1988). Finally, data from children adopted internationally before the age of two indicate that children can learn a new language and approach monolingual norms after approximately one year following adoption (Glennen and Masters, 2002). Children adopted at older ages also make quick gains but they take longer to achieve abilities that are comparable to their monolingual peers (Glennen, 2007). Although bilingual language learning benefits from early exposure to two languages, older children and adults can also become bilingual.

Simultaneous bilingual development refers to a situation where the child is exposed to two languages from a very young age. In simultaneous bilingual language learning, the language input can come from various sources. Some children grow up in a home where the parents speak different languages, other children hear and speak one language at home but another in daycare, and still others may spend time with grandparents or other relatives that expose them to their second language. In each of these scenarios, the quantity of language exposure can vary day to day (for example, weekends are spent mostly with parents resulting in more exposure to Chinese, but weekdays are spent mostly in daycare resulting in more exposure to English), but also during longer periods due to changes in child-care, divorce, relocation, and even the influence of other family members.

In sequential bilingual language learning, the child has begun the process of acquiring her first language when exposure to the second language occurs. The introduction to a second language often occurs in daycare or school, as is the case for the children described in

Chapter 14. In some contexts, families may be able to choose the language of schooling but in many cases the language of schooling is imposed. Children learning a second language use learning mechanisms similar to those used in first language learning, but also have access to structures learned in the first language (MacWhinney, 2005). As a result, sequential bilinguals often produce "errors" that can be explained by the transfer of a linguistic structure in one's first language to the language being learned. Transferring structures from one's first language to the second has advantages in the early stages of second language communication, but as they become embedded in one's second language system they can lead to accented speech (Flege and Davidian, 1984). A *sensitive period* for bilingual language learning extends to adolescence (Birdsong, 2006). During this period, children can learn a second language easier and more accurately than an adult (Birdsong and Molis, 2001; Flege, 1988; Johnson and Newport, 1989). In many countries, formal second language teaching begins during this age range. Although learning a second language as an adolescent or adult is possible, it is more effortful and the process is more conscious (Flege, 1988). As many of you who have studied a foreign language in school may have done, adult learners often memorize vocabulary lists, complete innumerable worksheets to practice new morphological forms or syntactic structures, and perhaps have practiced producing the new consonants or vowels of this language. Vocabulary, syntax and morphology appear to be easier to master than pronunciation (Moyer, 1999); however, most people who learned their second language after the age of twelve speak with an accent in their second language. Chapter 8 provides an in-depth description of the acquisition of a phonological system in adulthood.

Language Exposure

Direct language exposure is crucial to bilingual language development – thus watching the television or hearing others speak a language is not sufficient for acquiring the language (Pearson, Fernández, Lewedeg and Oller, 1997). In their study of lexical development among Spanish-English bilingual children, Pearson and her colleagues (2007) reported on three key findings: (1) a relationship was found between amount of exposure to each language and vocabulary size; (2) even low exposure to each language resulted in word learning, and (3) children who were exposed to one of their languages less than 20% of the time were less likely to produce utterances in that language willingly or spontaneously. It is important to keep in mind that ongoing language exposure may change and vary across time (Pearson et al., 1997). Research has shown that language status in the community and broader society, and attitudes about bilingual language learning play an important role in bilingual language development: children become bilingual when they have regular opportunities to interact in both of their languages (Pearson, 2007).

Bilingual Speech Sound Development

Bilingual speech sound development refers to the learning of two phonemic inventories, learning the acoustic and articulatory values for each phoneme, and learning the phonotactics and prosody of each language. Research on adult bilingual speech proficiency has focused on two main levels of analysis: the segmental level (i.e., production of consonants and vowels) and the sentence level (i.e., production of segmental and prosodic elements) (Birdsong, 2007). According to some, the segmental level is the most challenging test of L2 pronunciation accuracy and is a necessary condition for being perceived as a native-speaker of a language (Birdsong, 2007). At the sentence level, one can study the phonotactics and prosody of speech but it can be difficult to exclude the effects that go beyond the phonology on a speaker's productions such as syntax and vocabulary. Research on phonological development among bilingual children has focused on the segmental level of analysis.

Typical Bilingual Phonological Development

As was noted in early chapters on monolingual speech sound development, an uncontested generalization about speech sound production during preschool years is that *children are variable*. This variability can be observed both within the same child, but also across children. In this respect, bilingual children are no different than their monolingual peers. In addition to individual variability, the study of bilingual children is complicated by differences across a number of variables including, but not limited to, age of acquisition, exposure to each language, and the pair of languages compared. As a result, studies of bilingual children have yielded mixed findings with regards to the degree of *interaction* between bilingual children's language and evidence has been found for acceleration, deceleration and transfer. The following paragraphs summarize research on typical bilingual phonological development from the early word period to the end of the preschool years. A summary of this research is also presented in Table 13.1. The description of bilingual phonological development during the early word period has focused mainly on case studies of bilingual children that track development across a period of months, and even years. Although each study reports on a small number of children, the languages targeted are varied including English, French, German, Hebrew, Hungarian, Norwegian, Portuguese, and Spanish. One study of a Spanish-English bilingual child from the ages of 1;1 to 3;9 identified four stages of consonant acquisition starting with pre-systematic variation, the formation of a single system, the separation into two language-specific systems, and ending with the production of adult-targets with some transfer (Schnitzer and Krasinski, 1994). In contrast, another longitudinal study of a Spanish-English bilingual child from 1;6 to 4;6 identified consistent separation of the two languages from the beginning of the study period with little transfer observed at older ages (Schnitzer and Krasinski, 1994). A longitudinal study of a Norwegian-English bilingual from the ages of 1;2 to 1;8 revealed a separation of his two languages in the form of differences in the phonetic inventory, differences in accuracy by word position, and a preference for specific word forms in English and others in Norwegian (Johnson and Lancaster, 1998). In a longitudinal study of three German-Spanish children from the ages of 1;0 to 3;0, the bilinguals were found to follow a faster course in vowel acquisition in Spanish, a language with a simpler vowel system, than in German, a language with a larger vowel system (Kehoe, 2002). In a study of voicing contrast acquisition among 4 Spanish-German bilingual children 1;0 to 3;0, the results suggested that the acquisition of this contrast does not occur independently in each language, but rather that the two languages interact resulting in deceleration for some children, and transfer for others (Kehoe, Lleo and Rakow, 2004). In a longitudinal study of a French-English bilingual from 1;8 to 2;6, two language specific processes were observed in his early words: in English, he produced consonant harmony in English, but in French he produced reduplication (Brulard and Carr, 2003). In a fascinating study of two trilingual children between the ages of 1;0 to 1;11,

Faingold (1996) observed different strategies used depending on the language being used: Spanish and Portuguese productions resembled more closely the adult targets, whereas the Hebrew productions were more likely to show syllable reduction.

Studies that focus on 2-year-old children also report on case studies. In a study of a Hungarian-English bilingual 2-year-old child, the researchers focused on phonological mean length of utterance (PMLU) and found that the child consistently matched the complexity of target words in both Hungarian and English, even though Hungarian contains longer words (Bunta, Davidovich and Ingram, 2006). Although evidence was found to support language differentiation at the lexical and segmental level, the child was found to use the same set of phonological features (i.e., marking of voicing, continuant, and sonorant) in both languages (Bunta, Davidovich and Ingram, 2006). The longitudinal study of two Cantonese-English children between the ages of 2;3 and 3;5 years revealed that these children shared a number of features with monolingual children of each language (Holm and Dodd, 1999). These children, however, produced error patterns that were unusual in monolingual development, but were similar to patterns observed among sequential Cantonese-English bilingual children (Holm and Dodd, 1999).

Research that focuses on preschool aged children (i.e., 3- to 5-year-olds) tends to report on groups of children, often measured at a single point in time. The goal of these studies is to identify commonalities across the development of several children rather than identify individual developmental trajectories. A number of these studies focus on Spanish-English bilingual children and will be presented first, followed by the remaining studies across other language pairs. A study of 12 four-year-old Spanish-English bilinguals revealed that the children were quite similar to their monolingual peers with regards to overall consonant accuracy but that they produced phonological patterns that were different from their monolingual English and Spanish peers (Goldstein and Washington, 2001). Gildersleeve-Neuman and her colleagues (2008) studied 33 Spanish-English bilinguals who had either limited or balanced exposure to English by the age of 3 years. These children were found to be similar to their monolingual peers in that they accurately produced most sounds of English and, on average, the children with more exposure to English produced fewer errors. Some cross-linguistic effects were observed for error patterns that reflected less exposure to English for some bilinguals. A series of studies targeting eight Spanish-English bilingual children aged 3 to 4 years revealed patterns of interaction for some abilities but not for others. First, in a study of the acquisition of "early-middle-late" consonants (Shriberg, 1993) by these bilingual Spanish-English speaking children revealed key differences in the order of acquisition between the bilinguals and their monolingual peers in both English and Spanish (Fabiano-Smith and Goldstein, 2010a). They were also found to produce very low incidence of transfer between English and Spanish (Fabiano and Goldstein, 2010b). Although these children showed differences in order of acquisition of consonants, they were found to acquire the phonetic inventories of both languages at the same rate as their monolingual peers and with the same level of complexity (Fabiano-Smith and Barlow, 2010). This trio of studies illustrates that bilingual children may show different types of interactions between their two languages, even within one sphere of their language development. A study of 5 sequential bilinguals learning English in kindergarten revealed that these children acquired the sounds that occurred in their first language and English more quickly than sounds that existed only in English (Anderson, 2004).

Table 13.1. Summary of studies of typical bilingual phonological development including the languages spoken by the children, the number (N) and age of the participants, a summary of the results, and evidence for autonomous and interactions between the language systems

Study	Languages	N	Age	Summary	Evidence for Autonomous Language Systems	Evidence for Interaction between the Language Systems	Type of Interaction Observed
Keshavarz and Ingram (2002)	Farsi-English	1	0;8-1;8	Use of features from one language in the other	Y	Y	
Kehoe (2002)	Spanish-German – 1	3	1;0-3;0	Bilinguals slower to master the more complex vowel contrast		Y	Deceleration in 1 language
Kehoe, Lleo and Rakow (2004)	Spanish-German (2 are the same as Kehoe 2002)	3	1;0-3;0	Dominant language influences VOT		Y	Deceleration and transfer
Schnitzer and Krasinski (1994)	Spanish-English	1	1;1-3;9	No separation of the languages at the earliest ages.	N		
Schnitzer and Krasinski (1996)	Spanish-English	1	1;6-4;6	Consistent separation of languages	Y		
MacLeod, Laukys and Rvachew (2011)	French-English	21	1;6 and 3;0	Bilinguals kept pace with monolingual peers for accuracy and complexity measures.	Y		
Johnson and Lancaster	Norwegian-English	1	1;9	Separation phonetic inventories	Y		
Bunta, Davidovich and Ingram (2006)	Hungarian-English	1	2;0	Match target complexity in each language	Y		
Holm and Dodd (1999)	Cantonese-English	2	2;3-3;5	Error patterns different from monolinguals		Y	
Fabiano-Smith and Goldstein (2010a)	Spanish-English	8	3;0-4;0	Slower rate of acquisition of certain phonemes		Y	Deceleration and Rare transfer

Table 13.1. (Continued).

Study	Languages	N	Age	Summary	Evidence for Autonomous Language Systems	Evidence for Interaction between the Language Systems	Type of Interaction Observed
Fabiano-Smith and Goldstein (2010b)	Spanish-English	8	3;0-4;0	Differences in order of phoneme acquisition from monolinguals		Y	Deceleration?
Fabiano-Smith and Barlow (2010)	Spanish-English	8	3;0-4;0	Similar to monolinguals in phonetic inventory size and complexity	Y		
Gildersleeve-Neumann, Kester, Davis and Peña (2008)	Spanish-English	33	3;1-3;10	Increased exposure to English resulted in fewer errors; phonemes that occur in both languages were acquired quicker		Y	Transfer from L1 to L2
Goldstein and Washington (2001)	Spanish-English	12	4;0	Different types of errors and substitution patterns than monolingual children		Y	
Holm, Dodd, Stow and Pert, (1999)	Mirpuri/Punjabi/Urdu-English	35	4;8-7;5	Patterns in one language not identical across languages: either differences in context or rate		Y	

Studies of other language pairs have revealed a similar pattern. A study of 16 Cantonese-English bilingual children revealed patterns of phonological development that were different from monolinguals (Dodd, Holm and Li, 1996). A study of 21 French-English bilingual children aged 18 and 36 months revealed that the bilinguals kept pace with monolingual children in their dominant language (MacLeod, Laukys, and Rvachew, 2011). Finally, a study of 35 children aged 4 to 7 years who spoke Mirpuri, Punjabi or Urdu prior to starting school and learning English, found that a process present in one language is not always present in the other, and that even when processes occurred in both languages they were not applied in the same way or at the same rate in each language (Holm, Dodd, Stow and Pert, 1999).

Current research supports the Dual System Hypothesis: even at a young age, a bilingual has two language-specific systems. Research, however, is less conclusive regarding the relative autonomy of these two systems: some studies have shown interaction between these systems, while others have found autonomous development (see Table 1 for a summary). Interestingly, it appears that for the same children, one can observe both interactions and autonomy depending on the unit of analysis. During the early word stage, research has focused on longitudinal case studies and covers a broad range of language pairs.

These studies support the hypothesis of separate but interacting linguistic systems: bilingual children produce different sounds and exhibit different levels of mastery across their two languages but also some signs of interaction such as similar voicing patterns. In their second year, bilinguals were found to produce language specific strategies; for example, achieving more accurate word production in each language by increasing the complexity of productions (e.g., number of syllables produced) for one language. The strategies used by bilingual children are not always used by monolingual children of the same language. In children age 3 to 5 years, researchers have observed that bilingual children show three main differences compared to monolingual children. First, some children use strategies to differentiate between their two languages, possibly reducing the chance that the two languages interfere with one another in the phonological planning stages or to facilitate the categorization of the phoneme for listeners. Second, some children produce unexpected phonological patterns when compared to monolingual peers; however, these patterns are similar to other bilingual children acquiring the same languages. Finally, some children produce phonemes or errors that can be explained by the influence of one language on the other. Overall, it appears that a bilingual's two languages interact such that the phonological development of bilingual children parallels the development of monolingual children in some aspects (e.g., consonant accuracy), but error patterns that are unique to bilinguals have also been observed.

Speech Sound Disorders among Bilingual Children

Bilingual children may produce different speech patterns in one or both of their languages when compared to monolingual peers. These differences may be typical of their bilingual speech community, may mark membership with a particular ethno-linguistic or socio-linguistic group, or may indicate a speech sound disorder. Distinguishing a speech difference and a speech disorder can be challenging for a SLP. As with typical bilingual development, research on bilingual children with speech sound disorders supports the hypothesis that they have language-specific phonological systems that interact. Research documenting speech sound disorders among bilingual children is in its infancy: there are few studies and they tend to focus on a small number of children. The following is a review of studies that describe speech sound disorders (SSD) among bilingual children, change following intervention for bilinguals with SSD, and recommendations for evaluation and treatment of bilinguals with SSD.

Burrows and Goldstein (2010) reported on eight Spanish-English bilingual children with speech sound disorders and found that they resembled monolingual children with speech sound disorders. Specifically, the bilingual children were found to have consonant accuracy, measured by Percent Consonants Correct and Phonological Mean Length of Utterance, comparable to English and Spanish monolingual peers. Holm, Dodd, Stow and Pert (1999) highlighted the importance of comparing bilingual children to bilingual norms through a case study of two children who spoke English and Urdu or Mirpuri. The first child produced inconsistencies that were not observed in typical bilingual or monolingual development; the second child produced errors that were atypical of monolingual children but commonly observed in typical bilingual development. Holm and Dodd (1999) reported on two case studies of Italian-English children who presented with speech sound disorders. One child produced variable speech errors in both languages, 6 of 10 phonological patterns were common to both languages, and only 3 phonemes were present in one language but absent in the other. The second child's speech was characterized by delayed development: she produced inventories and phonological processes that were similar to younger monolingual children in both languages. These authors drew three conclusions based on this data: (1) the bilinguals had separate phonological systems for each language, (2) each language needs to be assessed to obtain a clear picture of the phonological system, and (3) the same underlying phonological disorder may present with different errors in each language.

Two bilingual children were studied in a treatment study (Holm and Dodd, 2001): one child spoke English and Cantonese and the other English and Punjabi. The children were evaluated in both of their languages and a series of treatment goals were established. The English-Cantonese speaking child produced an inter-dental lisp and a number of phonological processes in both languages. Although the intervention for the lisp was provided only in English, this boy's productions improved in both languages. The authors hypothesized that this error was tied to the motor level (i.e., articulation) of speech production rather than the linguistic level, and thus cross-language generalization was possible. In contrast, the phonological pattern intervention was not found to generalize from English, the treated language, to Cantonese. This supported the authors' hypothesis that phonological patterns are tied to the linguistic level of speech production and thus should be treated in each language. The second child in this study presented with inconsistent error patterns in both languages. The treatment provided in English (i.e., Core Vocabulary Approach: Dodd, Holm, Crosbie and McIntosh, 2010) resulted in increases in consistency and accuracy that generalized to Punjabi. As with the first child, this finding supports the hypothesis that motor-level difficulties (i.e., motor planning) will generalize across languages. The research on treatment of speech sound disorders among bilingual children sheds light on the dual systems hypothesis. The findings described above suggest that motor-level abilities may be shared across a bilingual's two languages, but that phonological-level abilities are language specific.

Although there are few studies of bilingual children with speech sound disorders, experts have expressed their concern regarding the SLP services available to these children (e.g., Stow and Dodd, 2003). Research suggests that establishing a differential diagnosis is difficult and this difficulty results in having an over-representation of bilingual children on SLP caseloads (Stow and Dodd, 2003), or an under-representation of these children (Yavas and Goldstein, 1998). Yavas and Goldstein (1998) proposed the following key elements to consider in assessment. First, it is important to consider the child's socio-cultural background including his family structure, child socialization and play routines, and length of residency in the country. They note the importance of evaluating both of the child's languages: this may require collaborating with a bilingual SLP colleague or bilingual SLP aid, working with an interpreter, or working with other bilingual professionals or community members. In addition to the typical phonological assessment, it is important to describe the phonological patterns that are expected among monolingual speakers of that language (see Chapters 9 through 12 for a sample of cross-linguistic monolingual data), and those that are not common among monolingual speakers of either language. Finally, they suggest that the SLP identify "bilingual patterns." These patterns may include an error pattern that normally occurs in monolingual development in one of the child's languages but that the child also produces in his other language where the pattern is unusual among monolingual children. These patterns also include differences in the rate of pattern use when compared to monolinguals. The authors propose the following guidelines for choosing treatment targets for phonological intervention: (1) prioritize phonological error patterns that occur in both languages at a similar rate; (2) next, target phonological error patterns that are present in both languages, but at different rates; (3) last, target phonological error patterns only present in one language. When combined with the findings of Dodd and colleagues, it would be reasonable to also prioritize motor-level (i.e., articulation or motor planning) errors since these are more likely to transfer across both languages.

CONNECTIONS

In this chapter, I have provided an overview of the theoretical frameworks used to study bilingual development among children and adults. I have also described phonological development among bilingual children who have learned their languages simultaneously or sequentially. Chapter 8 provided a description of how adults learn to speak a second language. Chapter 9 describes the similarities and differences in monolingual phonological development across various languages. Chapters 10 through 12 provide detailed cross-linguistic descriptions of monolingual phonological development. Chapter 14 provides a fascinating example of phonological development in children who speak Spanish and who have just begun to learn English in kindergarten.

CONCLUDING REMARKS

Understanding phonological acquisition among bilingual children is a crucial component in the advancement of our theoretical frameworks and clinical applications in the field of phonological development. The study of bilingual phonological development has been gaining ground in the past 15 years and a number of important studies have been published. Most studies focus on children learning English and another language, but other language pairings have also been studied. Bilingual children are faced with the complex task of learning two languages at once, yet despite the challenges posed by this task they have been found both to develop separate systems from a young age, and to develop each system at a rate that is within the range of typical monolingual development. Research on phonology supports the hypothesis that bilinguals have separate but interacting linguistic systems – the nature of the interactions is not always easy to qualify, but certain linguistic features may develop in an accelerated or decelerated fashion, and others may be subject to transfer from one language to the other. The course of bilingual phonological development can make it difficult to distinguish between differences and disorder. Two key features have begun to emerge from the available research: (1) the observation of delays and errors in both languages may indicate a disorder; and (2) the observation of patterns that are not common to typical bilingual or monolingual development may indicate a disorder. Finally, it is important to assess a bilingual in both of their languages since bilingual children have separate phonological systems and the underlying phonological disorder may present with different errors in each language.

Sidebar 13.1. Code-Switching

Code-switching is a linguistic act of changing the language spoken within or between utterances and is motivated by contextual factors such as the *interlocutor,* the context, or the topic (Mishina, 1999). Although on the surface code-switching may look like the indiscriminate use of two languages, careful linguistic study has revealed that it is a linguistic ability that is governed by pragmatic and syntactic factors (Köppe and Meisel, 1995; Genesee, 2001). Code-switching depends on a number of factors including the context of the conversation (school, home, community center), the speakers involved in the conversation (monolinguals, bilinguals), and the subject of conversation (math homework, sports team, family event). A bilingual's language choice may reflect ethno-linguistic group membership, allegiance with modernity, or a willingness to respect another's language choice and ability (O'Driscoll, 2001).

Early in bilingual language development, children have been found to code-switch more often when speaking in their non-dominant language and when they don't know the word in the language they are speaking (Genesee, Nicoladis and Paradis, 1995). These types of code-switching (sometimes called "code-mixing" to reflect the lack of systematicity) diminish with age. Children can make the appropriate language choice based on the language context as young as 1;8 (Deuchar and Quay, 1999).

In addition, children as young as 2 years of age have been found to be sensitive not only to the language choice made by others, but to the amount of code-switching the adult produces (Commeau, Genesee and Lapaquette, 2003; Mishina, 1999). In fact, bilingual children have been found to adjust the frequency of code-switching they produce in response to the frequency produced by an adult (Commeau, Genesee and Lapaquette, 2003). This pragmatic function, switching according to the interlocutor, is thought to develop first; followed by the syntactic function around the ages of three or four, since it relies syntactic development (Köppe and Meisel, 1995).

Sidebar 13.2. Why is Understanding Bilingual Speech Development Important to SLPs?

There are two main reasons that an understanding of bilingual speech and language development is essential to SLPs. First, SLPs are experts in the area of speech and language development and disorders. Parents, teachers, and other specialists turn to us for information regarding these issues. It is essential that the advice and information we give be based on the most up-to-date data and approaches. Second, an SLP must be able to establish a differential diagnostic to distinguish between errors due to the process of learning a new language and errors that characterize a delay or disordered speech or language development.

Sidebar 13.3. What are the Advantages of Bilingualism?

Bilingual language learning has a number of advantages for cognitive development in addition to educational, socio-cultural, and economic benefits. At the cognitive level, researchers have demonstrated that bilingual children have an earlier understanding of the arbitrary nature of word-object associations (De Houwer, Bornstein and De Coste, 2006). Bilingual children have also been found to outperform age-matched monolingual peers in executive function tasks (Bialystok, 1999)—an effect observed as early as 2 years of age (Poulin-Dubois, Blaye, Coutya and Bialystok, 2011). In education, researchers have found that a systematic support of a child's first language during preschool years has a positive effect on success at school when learning occurs in the child's second language (Campos, 1995). For many children, bilingualism allows a child to preserve their cultural identity and maintain important ties with their family and community on one hand, and allows the child to integrate into the greater society leading to more professional options on the other (Kohnert, Yim, Nett and Duran, 2005; Moore and Pérez-Méndez 2006).

Chapter Review Questions

1. What is the difference between simultaneous and sequential bilingual development? Why is this distinction important?
2. Describe the Unitary System Hypothesis and identify five studies that do not support the hypothesis.
3. Describe the three main approaches to studying bilingual phonology among children and adults.

Suggestions for Further Reading

Kohnert, K., Yim, D., Nett, K., Kan, P. F., and Duran, L. (2005). Intervention with linguistically diverse preschool children: A focus on developing home language(s). *Language, Speech, and Hearing Services in Schools*, *36*(3), 251-63.

Moore, S. M., and Pérez-Méndez, C. (2006). Working with linguistically diverse families in early intervention: Misconceptions and missed opportunities. *Seminars in Speech and Language*, *27*(3), 187-98.

Kohnert, K., and Medina, A. (2009). Bilingual children and communication disorders: A 30-year research retrospective. *Seminars in Speech and Language*, *30*(4), 219-33.
Pearson, B. Z. (2007). Social factors in childhood bilingualism in the United States. *Applied Psycholinguistics*, *28*(03), 399-410.

SUGGESTIONS FOR STUDENT ACTIVITIES

1. Reflect on your own language learning experiences to describe your bilingual profile by identifying your second (or third, etc) language, the age that you first began learning this language, the context of language learning, the context of ongoing language use, and your proficiency across different tasks (i.e., understanding and producing speech and written language). Compare your profile to a classmate.

ANSWERS TO CHAPTER REVIEW QUESTIONS

1. What is the difference between simultaneous and sequential bilingual development? Why is this distinction important?

These terms refer to differences in the age of exposure to the second language. In simultaneous bilingual development, children are exposed to both languages simultaneously or nearly so; in sequential development, children are exposed to their second language later in childhood. The distinction is important for a number of reasons. For example, when trying to understand the way children learn their languages: in simultaneous acquisition, children acquire both of their languages at once; whereas in sequential acquisition, children can make use of structures and abilities in one language to help the acquisition of their second language. When trying to understand the social context of language learning, the distinction is also important since children who acquire their second language sequentially often do so in school – a context that is quite different from the home or early daycare environments of simultaneous development.

2. Describe the Unitary System Hypothesis and identify five studies that do not support the hypothesis.

The Unitary Hypothesis proposes that bilingual children begin with a shared linguistic system and that this system gradually becomes differentiated resulting in two language-specific systems. Among the seven studies of bilingual children under the age of 2 years, only one study supports this hypothesis: Schnitzer and Krasinski (1994); the remaining 6 studies found differentiation of the two languages.

3. Describe the three main approaches to studying bilingual phonology among children and adults.

The three main approaches for studying bilingual phonology among children and adults are the age-effect approach, the monolingual-approach, the shared-separate approach.

REFERENCES

Anderson, R.T. (2004). Phonological acquisition in preschoolers learning a second language via immersion: a longitudinal study. *Journal of Clinical Linguistics and Phonetics,* 18(3), 183-210.

Bialystok, E. (1999). Cognitive complexity and attentional control in the bilingual mind. *Child Development*, 70(3), 636-644.

Birdsong, D. (2006). Age and second language acquisition and processing: A selective overview. *Language Learning*, 56, 9-49.

Birdsong, D. (2007). Native-like pronunciation among late learners of French. In E-S. Bohn and M.J. Munro (Eds.) Language experience in L2 Speech Learning, pgs 99-116. Philadelphia, PA: John Benjamins.

Birdsong, D., and Molis, M. (2001). On the evidence for maturational constraints in second-language acquisition. *Journal of Memory and Language*, 44(2), 235-249.

Brulard, I. and Carr, P. (2003). French-English bilingual acquisition of phonology: One production system or two? *The International Journal of Bilingualism,* 7(2), 177-202.

Bunta, F., Davidovich, I., and Ingram, D. (2006). The relationship between the phonological complexity of a bilingual child's words and those of the target languages. *International Journal of Bilingualism*, 10(1), 71-88.

Burrows, L., and Goldstein, B. A. (2010). Whole word measures in bilingual children with speech sound disorders. *Clinical Linguistics and Phonetics*, 24(4-5), 357-68.

Campos, S. J. (1995). The Carpentería preschool program: A long-term effects study. In E. E. Garcia and B. McLaughlin (Eds.), Meeting the challenge of linguistic and cultural diversity in early childhood education (pp. 34-48). New York: Teachers College Press.

Comeau, L., Genesee, F. and Lapaquette, L. (2003). The modelling hypothesis and child bilingual codemixing. *International Journal of Bilingualism,* 7(2), 1130-1126.

De Houwer, A., Bornstein, M. H., and De Coster, S. (2006). Early understanding of two words for the same thing: A CDI study of lexical comprehension in infant bilinguals. *International Journal of Bilingualism*, 10(3), 331-347.

Deuchar, M., and Quay, S. (1998). One vs. Two systems in early bilingual syntax: Two versions of the question. *Bilingualism: Language and Cognition*, 1(03), 231-243.

Dodd , B., So, L. and Li, W. (1996). Symptoms of disorder without impairment: The written and spoken errors of bilinguals. In B. Dodd, R. Campbell and L. Worrall (Eds), Evaluating theories of language, pp. 119-139. London: Whurr.

Dodd, B., Holm, A., Crosbie, S., and McIntosh, B. (2010). Core vocabulary intervention for inconsistent speech disorder. In L. Williams, S. McLeod, and R. McCauley (Eds.), *Interventions for speech sound disorders in children.* (pp. 117-136). Baltimore: Brookers.

Fabiano-Smith, L., and Barlow, J. A. (2010). Interaction in bilingual phonological acquisition: Evidence from phonetic inventories. *International Journal of Bilingualism*, *13*(1), 81-97.

Fabiano-Smith, L., and Goldstein, B. A. (2010a). Phonological acquisition in bilingual Spanish-English speaking children. *Journal of Speech, Language, and Hearing Research. JSLHR*, 53(1), 160-178.

Fabiano-Smith, L., and Goldstein, B. A. (2010b). Early-, middle-, and late-developing sounds in monolingual and bilingual children: An exploratory investigation. *American Journal of Speech-Language Pathology*, 19(1), 66-77.

Faingold, E. D. (1996). Variation in the application of natural processes: Language-Dependent constraints in the phonological acquisition of bilingual children. *Journal of Psycholinguistic Research,* 25(5), 515-526.

Fishman, J.A. (1980). Bilingualism and biculturalism as individual and as societal phenomina. *Journal of Multilingual and Multicultural Development,* 1(1), 3-15.

Flege, J. E., and Davidian, R. D. (1984). Transfer and developmental processes in adult foreign language speech production. *Applied Psycholinguistics*, *5*(04), 323-347.

Flege, J.E., (1988). The production and perception of foreign language speech sounds. In H. Winitz (Ed.), Human Communication and It's Disorders-A review, pgs 224-401. Norwood, NJ: Ablex.

Flege, J. E., Yeni-Komshian, G. H., and Liu, S. (1999). Age constraints on second-language acquisition. *Journal of Memory and Language*, 41, 78-104.

Genesee, F. (2001). Bilingual first language acquisition: Exploring the limits. *Annual Review of Applied Linguistics,* 21 153-168.

Genesee, F., Nicoladis, E., and Paradis, J. (1995). Language differentiation in early bilingual development. *Journal of Child Language,* 22(3), 611-631.

Gildersleeve-Neumann, C. E., Kester, E. S., Davis, B. L., and Peña, E. D. (2008). English speech sound development in preschool-aged children from bilingual English-Spanish environments. *Language, Speech, and Hearing Services in Schools*, 39(3), 314-28.

Glennen, G. (2009). Speech and language guidelines for children adopted from abroad at older ages. *Top Lang Disord Topics in Language Disorders*, 29(1), 50-64.

Glennen, S., and Masters, M. G. (2002). Typical and atypical language development in infants and toddlers adopted from eastern europe. *American Journal of Speech-Language Pathology*, 11(4), 417.

Goldstein, B. and Washington, P.S. (2001). An investigation of phonological patterns in typically developing 4-year-old Spanish-English bilingual children. *Language, Speech and Hearing Services in Schools,* 32, 153-164.

Grosjean, F. (1982). *Life With Two Languages: An Introduction to Bilingualism.* Cambridge, MA: Harvard University Press.

Holm, A. and Dodd, B. (2001). Comparison of cross-language generalisation following speech therapy. *Folio Phoniatrica et Logopaedica,* 53(3), 166-172.

Holm, A., and Dodd, B. (1999). A longitudinal study of the phonological development of two Cantonese-English bilingual children. *Applied Psycholinguistics*, 20(03), 349-376.

Holm, A., Dodd, B., Stow, C., and Pert, S. (1999). Identification and differential diagnosis of phonological disorder in bilingual children. *Language Testing*, 16(3), 271-292.

Johnson, C.E. and Lancaster, P. (1998). The development of more than one phonology: A case study of a Norwegian-English bilingual child. *International Journal of Bilingualism* 2, 265-300.

Johnson, J.S., and Newport, E.L. (1989). Critical period effects in second language learning: The influence of maturational state on the acquisition of English as a second language. *Cognitive Psychology*, 21, 60-99.

Kehoe, M. (2002). Developing vowel systems as a window to bilingual phonology. *International Journal of Bilingualism*, 6(3), 315-336.

Kehoe, M. M., Lleó, C., and Rakow, M. (2004). Voice onset time in bilingual German-Spanish children. *Bilingualism: Language and Cognition*, 7(01), 71-88.

Kohnert, K. J., and Bates, E. (2002). Balancing bilinguals II: Lexical comprehension and cognitive processing in children learning Spanish and English. *Journal of Speech, Language, and Hearing Research : JSLHR*, 45(2), 347-359.

Kohnert, K., and Medina, A. (2009). Bilingual children and communication disorders: A 30-year research retrospective. *Seminars in Speech and Language*, 30(4), 219-33.

Kohnert, K., Yim, D., Nett, K., Kan, P.F., and Duran, L. (2005). Intervention with linguistically diverse preschool children: A focus on developing home language(s). *Language, Speech and Hearing Services in Schools,* 36, 251-263.

Köppe, R. and Meisel, J. (1995). Code switching in bilingual first language acquisition. In L. Milroy and P. Muysken (Eds.) *One speaker, two languages: Cross disciplinary perspectives on code-switching.* pp. *276-301.*

Kuhl, P. K. (2000). A new view of language acquisition. Proceedings of the National Academy of Sciences of the United States of America, 97(22), 11850-11857.

Mack, M. (2003). The Phonetic Systems of Bilinguals. In M.T. Banich and M. Mack (Eds), *Mind, Brain, and Language Multidisciplinary Perspectives.* pp. 309-349. Mahwah: Lawrence Erlbaum Associates.

MacLeod, A.A.N., and Stoel-Gammon, C. (2009). Comparing bilingual and monolingual production of Voice Onset Time in Canadian English and Canadian French. *Applied Psycholinguistics,* 30, 53-77.

MacLeod, A.A.N., Laukys, K., Rvachew, S. (accepted). Impact of bilingual language learning on whole-word complexity and segmental accuracy among children aged 18 and 36 months. *International Journal of Speech Language Pathology.*

MacLeod, A.A.N., Stoel-Gammon, C., and Wassink, A.B. (2009). Production of high vowels in Canadian English and Canadian French : A comparison of early bilingual and monolingual speakers. *Journal of Phonetics,* 37, 374-387.

MacWhinney, G. (2005). Extending the competition model. *International Journal of Bilingualism,* 9, *69-84.*

Mishina, S. (1999). The role of parental input and discourse strategies in the early language mixing of a bilingual child. *Multilingual,* 18(4), 317-342.

Moore, S.M. and Pérez-Méndez, C. (2006). Working with linguistically diverse families in early intervention: Misconceptions and missed opportunities. *Seminars in Speech and Language,* 27(3), 187-198.

Moyer, A. (1999). Ultimate Attainment in L2 acquisition: The critical factors of age, motivation and instruction. *Studies in Second Language Acquisition,* 21, 81-108.

Munro, M., Flege, J.E., and MacKay, I.R.A. (1996). The effect of age of second-language learning on the production of English vowels. *Applied Psycholinguistics,* 17, 313-334.

O'Driscoll, J. (2001). A face model of language choice. *Multilingua 20,* 245-268.

Paradis, J., and Genesee, F. (1996). Syntactic acquisition in bilingual children. *Studies in Second Language Acquisition*, 18(01), 1-25.

Pearson, B. Z. (2007). Social factors in childhood bilingualism in the United States. *Applied Psycholinguistics*, 28(3), 399-410.

Pearson, B. Z., Fernandez, S. C., Lewedeg, V., and Oller, D. K. (1997). The relation of input factors to lexical learning by bilingual infants. *Applied Psycholinguistics*, 18(01), 41-58.

Poulin-Dubois, D., Blaye, A., Coutya, J., and Bialystok, E. (2011). The effects of bilingualism on toddlers' executive functioning. *Journal of Experimental Child Psychology*, 108(3), 567-579.

Richard, T. (1999). A global perspective on bilingualism and bilingual education. Washington, DC: ERIC Clearinghouse on Language and Linguistics.

Schnitzer, M. L., and Krasinski, E. (1994). The development of segmental phonological production in a bilingual child. *Journal of Child Language*, 21(03), 585-622.

Shriberg, L. D. (1993). Four new speech and prosody-voice measures for genetics research and other studies in developmental phonological disorders. *Journal of Speech and Hearing Research*, 36(1), 105-40.

Stow, C., and Dodd, B. (2003). Providing an equitable service to bilingual children in the UK: A review. International Journal of Language and Communication Disorders / Royal College of Speech and Language Therapists, 38(4), 351-377.

Volterra, V., and Taeschner, T. (1978). The acquisition and development of language by bilingual children. *Journal of Child Language*, *5*(02), 311-326.

Watson, I. (1991). Phonological processing in two languages. In E. Bialystok (Ed.)., *Language Processing in Bilingual Children* (25-48), Cambridge: Cambridge University Press.

Werker, J., and Lalonde, C. (1988). Cross-language speech perception: Initial capabilities and developmental change. *Developmental Psychology,* 24(5), 672-683.

Yavas, M. and Goldstein, B. (1998). Phonological assessment and treatment of bilingual speakers. *American Journal of Speech-Language Pathology*, 7(2), 49-60.

In: Comprehensive Perspectives …
Editors: Beate Peter and Andrea A. N. MacLeod
ISBN: 978-1-62257-041-6

Chapter 14

Acquisition of the English Voicing Contrast by Native Spanish-Speaking Children: Phonological Development in Voice Onset Times

Eugene H. Buder, Linda Jarmulowicz and D. Kimbrough Oller

Introduction

In Chapter 13, MacLeod introduces a number of definitive concepts regarding bilingual speech acquisition. She distinguishes the term bilingualism as applied to societies and to individuals. She points out that sequential acquisition, in which a child learns one language first and a second one later, is likely to show different phonological development patterns than simultaneous acquisition, in which a child is exposed to two languages from birth and acquires both simultaneously. MacLeod also reviews findings indicating that childhood acquisition of a second language typically leads to higher levels of phonetic accuracy (e.g. lack of accentedness) than adult acquisition—see also Chapter 8 by Franklin.

General theoretical frameworks reviewed by MacLeod, distinguish between "Unitary System" hypotheses in which a single language system develops that is later differentiated by experience with the sounds and rules of the separate languages, and "Dual System" hypotheses in which separate language systems develop concurrently. Dual system development is now generally accepted as a better description of the facts and allows for the possibility of complex interactions between the languages. Such interactions can result in inter-linguistic transfer effects, implying that bilingual children develop along different lines than monolinguals. When there is early exposure to the second language, transfer effects may occur between the first and second language (L1 and L2, respectively) at many levels of speech and language. Such effects are likely to be seen earlier in development in phonological and phonetic skills rather than in morphological and syntactical skills which are generally mastered later. Phonological effects specific to Spanish-English bilingual 4-year-old children have been summarized by Goldstein and Washington (2001), supporting the clinically important observation that bilingual children can exhibit normal patterns of development that are nonetheless distinct from those seen in children learning either language monolingually. At this same early age it is also highly likely that specific phonetic effects will be found, and because these are acoustically measurable it is possible that very subtle phenomena may be uncovered even if sound substitutions are not reliably heard. See Chapter 2 by Hodge and Pollock for further review of ways in which acoustic phonetic analysis are generally used to augment transcriptional and phonological analyses in documenting and understanding developmental patterns.

Here we present a phonetic approach to Spanish-English sequential bilingual acquisition of two different voicing systems for obstruent consonants, presenting some case study examples to illustrate inter-linguistic effects. We examined the early acquisition of English as L2 by a child with Spanish as L1 during the child's initial exposure to English schooling in kindergarten. The evidence we present suggests that patterns of development in this domain may be even more complex and subtle than the distinction between unitary and dual hypothesis implies. First, a review of the importance of Voice Onset Time (**VOT**) as a cue to the phonetic voicing **contrast** is in order.

REVIEW OF VOICE ONSET TIMES IN STOP PRODUCTION

English and Spanish stop consonants such as /d/ and /t/ require a full valving of the expiratory flow of air during speech production so that it "stops" long enough to allow a buildup of pressure that is then released; the audible consequences of this behavior include either a silence or very low amplitude/low frequency **periodic energy** sound during the stop gap, and usually a **burst** of audible turbulence when the pressure is released. In addition to the lingui-alveolar (or sometimes dental) place for this valving in /d/ or /t/, these languages also require stopping at the lips (the bilabial /b/ or /p/) or with the tongue at the velum (for /g/ or /k/, with allophonic variants at the palate). Pairs such as /d/ and /t/, which share the stop manner of production and the alveolar or dental place of production, differ by voicing. A key acoustic feature that distinguishes voiced from voiceless stops is the Voice Onset Time (VOT). VOT is the time from the instant of the burst release to the onset of full voicing. In the figure discussed below, it is relatively long, with a voice onset after the burst release at +94 ms. It is marked with a positive sign here and in the figure to emphasize that voicing could also have begun prior to the burst, in which case the VOT would have been negative.

Figure 14.1 depicts the **waveform** and **spectrogram** for the word "secure" ([sɪk^{h}juɹ], spoken by an adult, female, native speaker of English. The waveform (along the top of the figure) is pressure variation over time, while the spectrogram (along the bottom of the figure) reveals the frequency-specific energies in this sound, with time along the horizontal (aligned with the waveform), frequencies along the vertical (0 to 11 kHz is displayed here), and intensity coded by darkness.

This is actually one of the stimulus words used to elicit pronunciations by the children whose VOT patterns we will review below. In this word, all the phases of voiceless obstruent production can be seen in a word-medial velar stop /k/ preceding a stressed syllable (but the specific case examples to be reviewed below will focus on word-initial coronal stops /d/ and /t/). Four phases in the production of this phoneme are stop gap, burst, **aspiration**, and voicing. These are labeled in Figure 1, and are further explained as follows:

1. First there must be a **stop gap**, during which time pressure is built up behind the place of closure. In this case, for [k^h], closure is achieved by the tongue placed in contact with the soft palate ("velum"), and because it is an unvoiced stop there is no voicing evident during the stop gap. As we will see later, it is possible for there to be voicing during a stop gap for a time, as long as air can flow past the vocal folds and continue to expand the supraglottal cavities to provide the transglottal pressure difference needed to maintain **phonation**. When such stop gap voicing is seen in a word-initial stop (i.e. not as a continuation of the voicing of some preceding phoneme, like a vowel), the duration of that voicing can be measured and referred to as negative voice onset time. In this particular production, it is spectrographically evident that the speaker enhanced the silent interval associated with the stop gap by ceasing phonation much earlier: this is why the bracket marking the stop gap is placed only after the cessation of low frequency energy and some abrupt low-energy marks probably associated with glottal stopping and the accomplishment of the oral cavity closure. Such details can often be seen in spectrograms of a high-quality recording such as this. Strictly speaking, a glottal stop might then also have been transcribed here after the first vowel, but it is not clear that such detail would have been audible to a transcriber.
2. The pressure built up during the stop gap is released, producing a brief burst of energy. This audible and visible burst is formed by the turbulence that arises when air particles are accelerated through a narrow channel, producing vortices (i.e., eddies or swirls) at the anterior exit of this channel. Because this is the same aerodynamic mechanism that produces fricatives, the burst is often dubbed a "frication" interval, but as a **plosive** this production is clearly transient in comparison to the sustained turbulence produced in a fricative ([+continuant]) phoneme. It is important to note that the burst is necessarily brief (just the relatively intense vertical mark appearing between the intervals marked stop gap and aspiration, in this figure, essentially lasting only about 10 ms). The acoustic filtering effect of **resonance**, in the portion of the oral cavity anterior to this sound source location at the velum, shapes the spectrum of the burst. In this token, that resonance is seen as peaking of the energy in the spectrogram in the region between the horizontal 3 and 4 kHz lines.
3. Following the release of the built up pressure for this American English long-lag stop [k^h], the glottis is maintained in a position that is neither fully open nor adducted for phonation (a glottal feature called [+spread]), also creating a narrow channel through which rushing air produces turbulence: this interval is marked aspiration in the figure. Normally, aspiration is produced as soon as air begins flowing again after the stop gap so it arises concurrently with the burst turbulence, but continues much longer (essentially the same as in the glottal fricative /h/, hence the diacritic ^{h}). Due to its location at the glottis, the source energy of aspiration is also more evenly spread across all the frequencies, and may display some of the formant resonances of the vocal tract (though usually not F1, as this low frequency resonance is heavily damped by the relatively open glottis).
4. Finally, the periodic energy of voicing at the glottis (i.e. phonation) becomes evident as the speaker transitions into the vowel segment.

From the definition of VOT and the precision with which it must be measured, it may be understood why differences between voiced and voiceless stop consonants were not very well established prior to the development of tools for spectrographic inspection in the late 1940s/early 1950s (and hence, the advent of modern acoustic phonetics). The primacy of VOT in this **contrast** was established historically by Leigh Lisker and Arthur Abramson (1964), who analyzed the measure from American English word-initial /b d g/ and /p t k/ and their cognates from ten other languages, including Spanish.

Lisker and Abramson's goal was to determine whether this measure adequately distinguished voicing-related contrasts across different languages. While English and Spanish essentially distinguish only two voicing categories amongst such stops (disregarding allophonic variation), other languages, such as Thai and Hindi, distinguish three or even four. They also noted that a variety of more or less ambiguously defined features had been used in association with these distinctions, including aspirated/unaspirated and **fortis/lenis** (also called tense/lax for consonants, a contrast used in Korean and described in Chapter 12, associated articulatorily with the degree of "force" with which the plosive was executed), and they hypothesized that VOT would be an adequate basis by itself for such featural contrasts.This relatively well-defined acoustic measure did indeed clearly contrast voicing for two- and three-category languages, although the results were not so clear cut for the three categories of Korean stops and did not adequately distinguish four category systems (Hindi and Marathi), in which one of the categories was both voiced and aspirated. Their work was the foundation for the modern consensus that VOT makes possible clear distinctions between (1) "lead" or **prevoiced** phones, with negative VOTs, (2) "**short-lag**" phones, with VOTs ranging from 0 up to about 40 ms, typically unaspirated, and (3) "**long-lag**" phones, with VOTs much longer than 40 ms, typically ranging from 60 to 100 ms or longer, usually with aspiration. The clarity provided by this measure has shed much light on cross-linguistic comparisons, allowing other researchers such as Cho and Ladefoged (1999), examining altogether 18 languages, to further discern that systematic variation with place of articulation seems to be the default across many languages of the world. Most relevant to the current chapter, this work established that the two categories used in English (word-initial) were the short-lag unaspirated vs. long-lag aspirated but that the two categories used in Spanish (again, word-initial) were lead, or prevoiced, and short-lag unaspirated. For clarity, we will follow the strict modern IPA system of representing the Spanish prevoiced and short-lag phonemes as [d] and [t], respectively, and will transcribe the English orthographic "d" and "t" as [t] (short-lag) and [t^h] (long-lag aspirated), respectively. Note that in broadly referring to the phonemes that indicate minimal contrasts in a language, linguists always using slashes (virgules) to enclose phonemes, but when referring narrowly to the actual sounds more universally and in full detail, square brackets are used to enclose the phonetic representations. With this in mind, it is even more critical to keep the IPA symbols and what they represent separate from the letters used in traditional orthography, especially when adopting the truly international perspective required for cross-linguistic and bilingual research purposes—the reader may wish to refer to Table 14.1 and note carefully that the voiced sound we usually think of as a "d" is actually a [t]! Finally, note that a lot of variation may occur in actual pronunciations: English "short-lag" word-initial stops may freely be prevoiced.

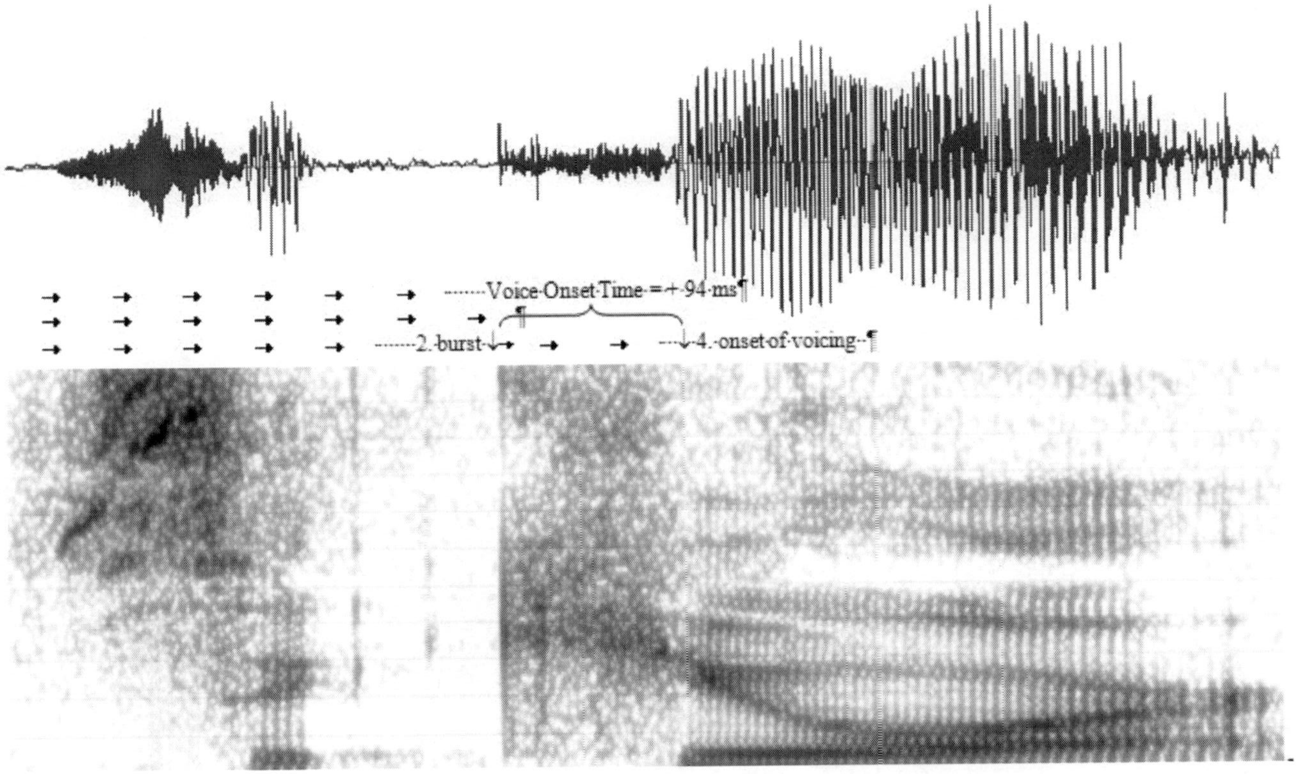

Figure 14.1. The word “secure” spoken by a female adult who is a native speaker of English.

Table 14.1. Understanding the International Phonetic Alphabet system for Universal Transcription of Voicing Contrasts in English and Spanish

	Orthographic	IPA
English	dough	[toʊ]
	toe	[tʰoʊ]
Spanish	di (tr. say)	[di]
	ti (tr. you)	[ti]

This is the essential fact of interest for our consideration of Spanish-English bilingual development: Although these two languages both have two phonemic categories contrasting stop consonants by voicing, they utilize different phonetic categories from the VOT continuum to implement them. The possibilities this has afforded for study of phonological development of these consonantal phones, which are among the earliest acquired, came to the attention of the Stanford Child Phonology Project headed by Charles Ferguson, leading to work conducted by Marcy Macken and David Barton which tracked toddlers and young children's development of the voicing contrast in English (Barton and Macken, 1980; Macken and Barton, 1979) and in Spanish (Macken and Barton, 1980).

The third author of this chapter also co-authored a paper (Eilers, Oller, and Benito Garcia, 1984) detailing the early acquisition of the Spanish voicing system by toddlers. Meanwhile, the extensive interest in Spanish-speaking children learning English as their L2 has included studies of differential acquisition of these voicing systems as reflected in VOT or heard in productions contrasting voiced and voiceless stops (Deuchar and Clark, 1996; Goldstein and Washington, 2001; Konefal and Fokes, 1981). In general, this line of work has supported the fact that bilingual children can acquire and master these two voicing systems concurrently and distinctively. However, when the voicing cue was first explored in English development, it was observed that the short-lag production was the typical default and likely the easiest to produce (Zlatin and Koenigsknecht, 1976). Applied to development in languages which include the prevoicing category, others speculated that later acquisition of that category may be explained by its relative difficulty to produce and perceive (Konefal and Fokes, 1981).

What do young native Spanish-speaking children do when faced with the task of acquiring a second voicing system in which the contrast is accomplished by different phonetic categories than in their L1? Do any transfer effects interfere with this acquisition, or does interference develop with mastery of L2 during the first period of exposure? When they are pre-literate, children will likely not be confused by the orthographic conventions by which "t" in Spanish is supposed to be phonetically the same (or nearly the same) sound as "d" in English, but the fact that the two languages share this category is still a potential source of interference in these bilinguals' phonological development. To demonstrate some of the possibilities, we review a case study in the next section that traces one pathway through this phonological dilemma. The study speaks to some of major themes of bilingualism introduced by MacLeod, and parallels findings reported by others who have investigated this basic scenario in the same and other languages where different VOT-based systems must be acquired.

SPANISH-ENGLISH BILINGUALISM: EARLY ACQUISITION AND L1 EFFECTS

We have conducted a project in Memphis headed by Kimbrough Oller with Linda Jarmulowicz and Eugene Buder as co-investigators, titled "Phonology and Literacy in Early Bilinguals." To assess early phonological skills and the impact of immersion in English schooling, the project has accumulated acoustical and transcriptional data on native Spanish speaking children just entering kindergarten, along with similar data from Spanish and English monolingual children. We also tracked the development of the English Language Learners' word productions in both English and Spanish after approximately six months of English schooling, allowing for the investigation of possible longitudinal exposure effects on both L1 and L2 systems.

Materials. Two word lists were created—one in English, the other in Spanish. The words we chose included coronal phonemes in word initial, medial, and final positions, in both Spanish and English. The words ranged in length from one to three syllables in English, with a mean syllable length of 2.1. In Spanish, the words ranged in length from two to four syllables, with a mean syllable length of 2.4. Spanish has fewer one-syllable words and has a less complex syllable structure than does English.

For each language, the words were recorded in isolation (without a carrier phrase) by native-speaking women. It was important to use recorded stimuli in order to maintain consistency of the stimuli that the children heard. Each word list was randomized in three different orders and the lists were rotated, so that the order of presentation was balanced across participants. The stimulus words were presented to the children over headphones, and the children's repetitions of the words were recorded using high-quality headset microphones to digital compact flash card recorders (these recordings were conducted in whichever reasonably quiet rooms could be found in the school settings). English words selected for further analysis of word-initial coronal stops "d" [t] and "t" [t^h] were "disappear," "divide," "dizzy," "donut," "tardy," "teacher," "ticket," and "toot." Spanish words were "*dedos*" ("fingers"), "*depende*" (he/she/it-"depends"), "*diario*" ("daily"), "*dinero*" ("money"), "*tarde*" ("late"), *tazas* ("cups"), and *torta* ("cake").

Figures 14.2 through 14.5 display waveforms and spectrograms from selected Spanish and English stimulus words ("*depende*," "*tazas*," "dizzy," "tardy"). As labeled in these figures and discussed above, Spanish employs the first and second VOT categories [d] and [t] for the word-initial voicing contrast, while English employs the second and third VOT categories [t] and [t^h]. As can be seen by the resemblance between the VOT segments for Spanish "*tazas*" and English "dizzy," the languages share the middle category with a short-lag VOT, yet this is contrasted against prevoiced VOT in Spanish and against long-lag aspirated VOT in English. Can Spanish-speaking children manage these two systems, shortly after having been immersed in English language schooling? Does anything happen to their L1 and L2 voicing systems after many months of this immersion?

L1 acquisition and L2 development. To present a phonologically informative pattern that we have been observing, we now display spectrograms of words produced by a typically developing Spanish girl ["SF1"] who was learning English. She was five years and four months of age at the time of her first sample early in Kindergarten. Although she had been born in Memphis, her home was a monolingual Spanish-speaking environment, and she had not been pre-schooled in English, so her Kindergarten enrollment was her first English learning experience. Her second sample was recorded 6 months later.

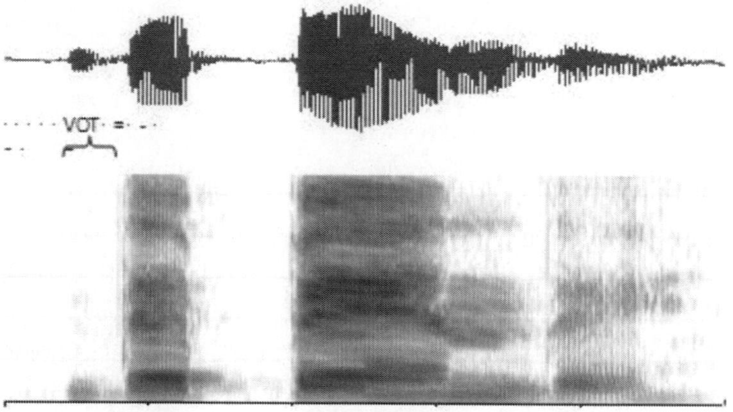

Figure 14.2. Stimulus word "*depende*": Spanish word-initial "d" [d] is prevoiced.

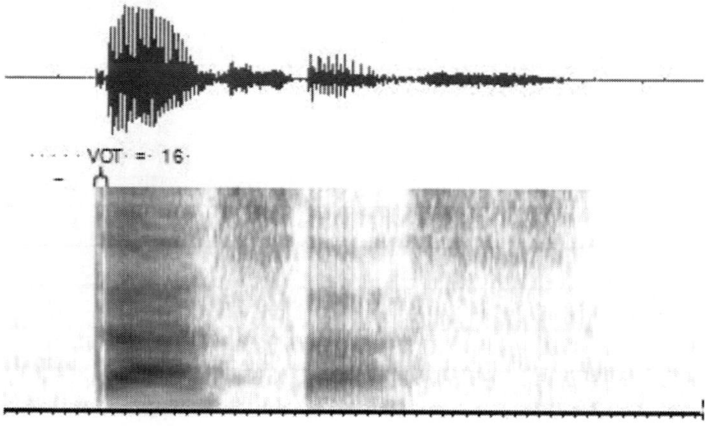

Figure 14.3. Stimulus word "*tazas*": Spanish word-initial "t" [t] is short-lag unaspirated.

Figures 14.6 and 14.7 display two spectrograms of words that SF1 spoke in English at the first stage of our sampling; it should be clear that the word-initial consonants are, in terms of VOT, virtually perfect exemplars of the English-appropriate categories, including short-lag unaspirated for the [t] target ("d") in "donut" and the long-lag aspirated for the [t^h] ("t") target in "toot," even though the latter sound is not found in her native Spanish. She did not, however, demonstrate full mastery of English pronunciation at this time: Among the "d" target sounds, she avoided saying "disappear," pronounced the onset of "divide" with a sound that looked and sounded more like the homorganic nasal /n/, and even the onset of the word "donut" could be heard as the nasal /n/, apparently because the burst itself was quite weak. (Such weakening processes are often called "lenition" in reference to the fortis/lenis feature that was historically associated with the voiceless/voiced contrast). Among the "t" target sounds in English, however, all were heard to be produced with clear long-lag aspirated [t^h], and the average VOT from these words' onsets was 100 ms.

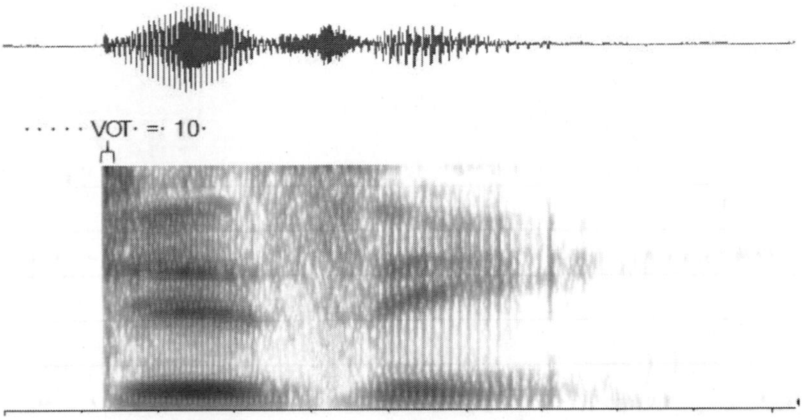

Figure 14.4. Stimulus word "dizzy": English word-initial "d" [t] is short-lag unaspirated.

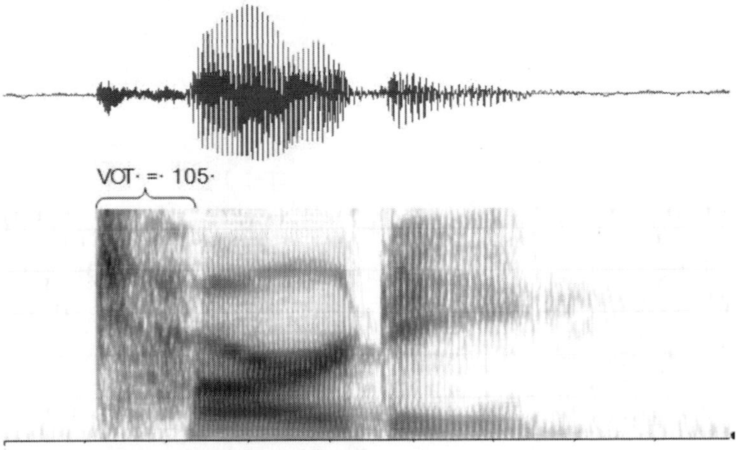

Figure 14.5. Stimulus word "tardy": English word-initial "t" [tʰ] is long-lag aspirated.

At the same time, SF1 also exemplified her Spanish VOT system quite well. Figures 14.8 and 14.9 display the words "*dedos*" and "*tarde*" from the same early Kindergarten session at which the above English words were recorded: the first word with a [d] target shows the prevoicing appropriate for this Spanish phoneme, and the second word with a [t] target shows the correct short-lag unaspirated form.

Here also there is some variation probably attributable to her young age: of the four "d" target words, she pronounced "*dinero* " with an /n/ sound and so its VOT was not measurable (but note that this was also a substitute sound in her English "d" words), and the word "*diario*" was pronounced and measured with a short lag unaspirated [t].

All three "t" target words were heard and measured with the appropriate short-lag unaspirated [t] VOTs.

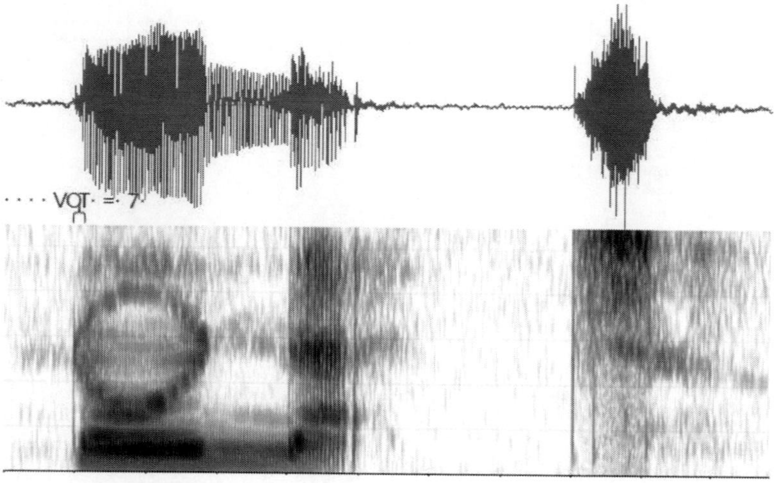

Figure 14.6. "Donut" produced by SF1 at age 5;4: English word-initial "d" [t] is correctly produced with short-lag unaspirated VOT.

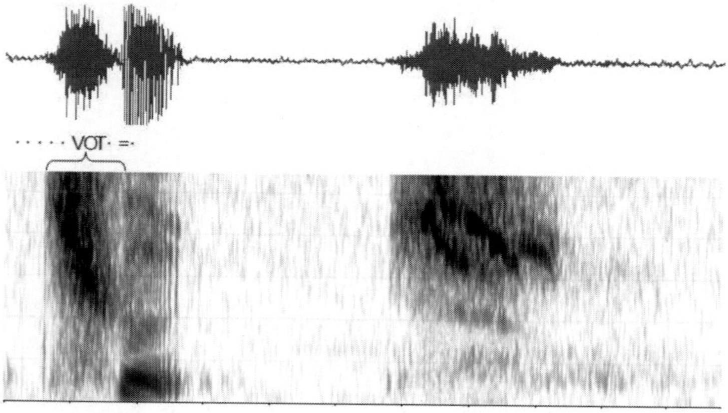

Figure 14.7. "Toot" produced by SF1 at age 5;4: English word-initial "t" [t^h] is correctly produced with long-lag aspirated VOT.

After six months of English schooling, however, there were some changes in SF1's bilingual phonologies. Her English words retained the appropriate voicing categories and some improvement was also evidenced at this later session by the facts that all "t" target words were (again) measured and heard with the appropriate long-lag aspirated VOTs, but more importantly, her "d" target words included "disappear" and "divide" at this session; "dizzy" was pronounced with a [z] onset, but all the other words were heard and measured as the correct short-lag unaspirated [t] sound.

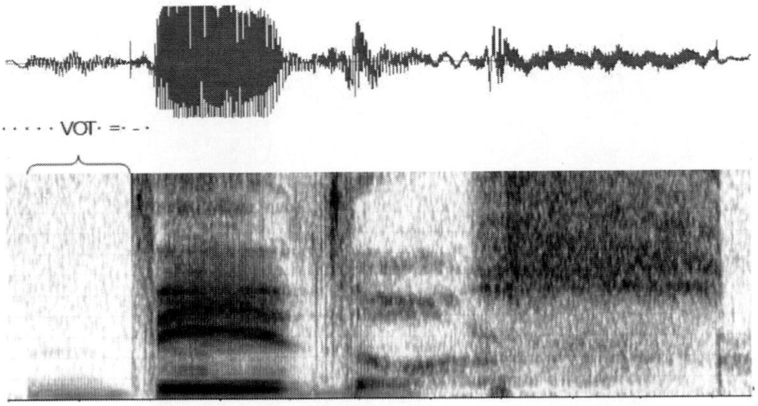

Figure 14.8. "*Dedos*" produced by SF1 at age 5;4: Spanish word-initial "d" [d] is correctly produced with prevoicing.

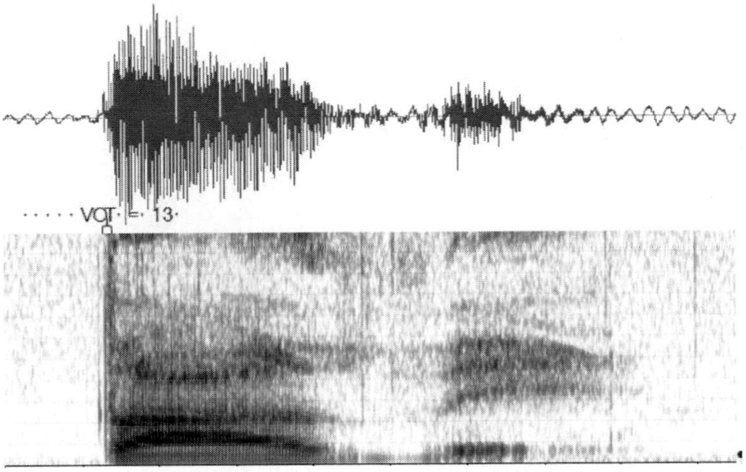

Figure 14.9. "*Tarde"* produced by SF1 at age 5;4: Spanish word-initial "t" [t] is correctly produced with short-lag unaspirated VOT.

The most noticeable change, however, was in SF1's L1 Spanish "d" target words: *All four were pronounced with short lag VOTs and heard as* [t], and none were pronounced with the prevoiced [d] sounds as presented in the native stimuli and which had dominated her productions at the beginning of Kindergarten. Her Spanish "t" target words were all still pronounced quite acceptably with positive VOTs under 30 ms.

Figures 14.10 and 14.11 display the words "*depende*" and "*dedos*" from this session, showing clearly the short-lag form she now apparently preferred over prevoicing. In summary, this is an example of L1 deterioration apparently resulting from L2 interference: she seems to have lost, at least temporarily, her native prevoicing category.

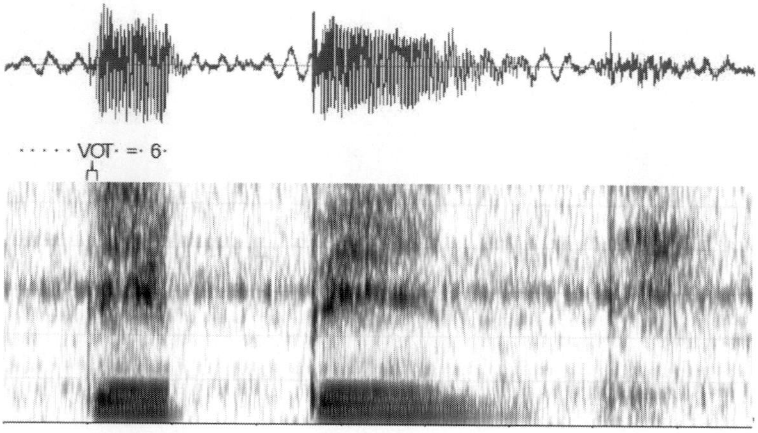

Figure 14.10. "*Depende*" produced by SF1 at age 5;10: Spanish word-initial prevoiced [d] is now produced with short-lag unaspirated VOT.

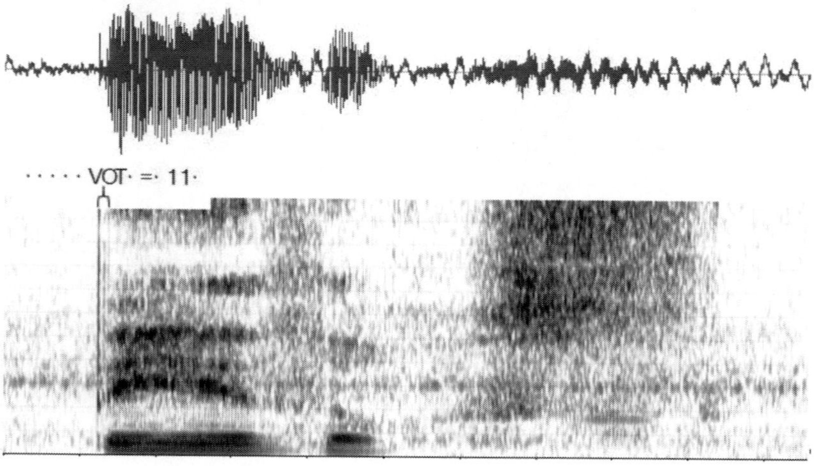

Figure 14.11. "*Dedos*" produced by SF1 at age 5;10: Spanish word-initial prevoiced [d] is now produced with short lag unaspirated VOT.

We recorded at least one other Spanish-speaking child learning English in this project who similarly showed prevoicing of Spanish "d" initial words at the beginning of kindergarten schooling in English, but no prevoicing at all on the same words after 6 months of schooling. However, this child ["SF2"] also exhibited a possibly related development over this time interval in L2. At the beginning of Kindergarten, her English "d" words were all produced with the short-lag [t] sound, essentially with the same VOTs as her appropriately short-lag unaspirated Spanish "t" words. This suggests that the same phonetic category was serving both languages, having been drawn from one end of the voicing contrast for L1 and the other end of the contrast for L2. However, after 6 months of exposure, *about half of SF2's English "d" onset words were now pronounced with prevoicing,* even though at this time there was no longer any prevoicing found in her Spanish "d" onsets!

A possible interpretation is that early in second language acquisition, an existing phonetic category, such as the [t] stop with short-lag VOT found in both Spanish and English, could be adopted to functionally serve both languages as long as it was contrastive from the new L2 category (i.e., long-lag aspirated [t^h]). In both children we saw subsequent deterioration of the L1 category not found in both languages, and some loss of **contrastivity** in this native language, but in this second child we also saw an *enhancement* of the contrast in L2 by the optional pronunciation of English "d" sounds with prevoicing.

In summary, this is consistent with the notion that a unified phonetic system may have been underlying the VOT system in early sequential bilingualism, but with just 6 months of immersion and some of L2 advancement, the phonological contrasts serving the two languages had begun to diverge, as if the prevoiced category was now "released" from service for L1 and hence free to serve contrastivity in the L2 that now dominated the child's schooling environment.

Sidebar 14.1. L1 Language Degradation

Is this L1 interference phenomenon effect limited to VOT of stops? No! Research at the University of Memphis has illustrated that Spanish-speaking children who enter English-only Kindergarten show very low expressive vocabulary in Spanish within three months (Gibson, Oller, Jarmulowicz, and Ethington, 2012; Oller, Jarmulowicz, Pearson, and Cobo-Lewis, 2010). Rapid shift from L1 to L2 has been described as language loss or language attrition (Oller and Jarmulowicz, 2007), and Anderson (Anderson, 2004) notes that children are particularly affected by language loss. A primary characteristic of language loss is a reduction, regression, or stagnation of L1 skills, particularly expressive language skills (Anderson, 1999). This pattern suggests a general loss of access to the native language although receptive skills appear to be maintained to a much greater extent.

INTERPRETING THE CROSSLINGUISTIC EFFECTS

The main findings from the two children reviewed above are (1) the English short-lag/long-lag voicing system can be acquired early as a second language, as a different system from the first language Spanish pre-voiced/short-lag voicing system, and (2) with increased exposure and practice with English, prevoicing in native Spanish may deteriorate, trending towards short-lag productions. Do these findings make sense given what has been reported in other literature on acquisition of voicing?

One affirmation comes from a recent report investigating acquisition of the English voicing system by a 3-year-old child whose native Dutch voicing system, like Spanish, also employs prevoicing for voiced stops and short-lag voice onsets for unvoiced stops (Simon, 2010). Although Simon investigated a younger child, her findings are essentially like ours. With initial exposure to English, her subject quickly acquired short-lag and long-lag voice onsets for English word-initial stops while concurrently retaining prevoiced and short-lag stops in Dutch. Additionally parallel to our results, Simon's subject also shifted his Dutch prevoiced stops in the direction of short-lag productions over the seven-month period following initial English L2 acquisition. In Simon's work, this longitudinal trend can be seen to occur gradually over 11 sessions recorded during this period.

Note also that in our work, the children's Spanish productions were elicited as imitations of the same recorded adult stimuli for both sessions. Even while hearing and repeating

Spanish words spoken with pre-voicing on the initial voiced stops, the children in our study produced these words mostly with short-lag productions in the later session. Thus, it appears that the children's phonological systems were shifting and that the L2, English, was influencing the L1, Spanish. Indeed, it appears that kindergarten children are beginning to lose some of their L1 categories with only a short period of L2 immersion.

Figures 14.10 and 14.11 display the words "*depende*" and "*dedos*" from this session, showing clearly the short-lag form she now apparently preferred over prevoicing. In summary, this is an example of L1 deterioration apparently resulting from L2 interference: she seems to have lost, at least temporarily, her native prevoicing category.

Connections

This chapter illustrates and extends themes reviewed by MacLeod in Chapter 13 on "Bilingual Speech Acquisition," and it also exemplifies techniques introduced in detail by Hodge and Pollock in Chapter 2, "Describing and Measuring Children's Speech Sound Abilities in Clinical and Research Settings: From Articulation Tests to Acoustic Analysis." Chapter 8 by Franklin, "Acquisition of a Phonological System in Adulthood" also covers related themes.

Concluding Remarks

In conclusion, we have illustrated how the initial discovery of VOT as an acoustic-phonetic cue to phoneme categories has evolved into a method by which questions about the nature and course of bilingualism and the emergence of language-specific categories can be examined.

Recall that early work in VOT acquisition speculated that short-lag productions were easier to produce than prevoiced (Konefal and Fokes, 1981; Zlatin and Koenigsknecht, 1976). While that may explain the deterioration of this category we observed in both these children's L1 productions, it does not explain why more prevoicing was observed with time in at least one child's *English* voiced stops. It therefore seems, as others have argued for phonological contrasts of this nature (Davis, 1995), that acoustic contrastiveness itself, and not necessarily the direct targeting of specific sounds, drives acquisition.

As a summary point regarding VOT in particular, we would like to emphasize that fine-grained details of L2 acquisition and L1 interference effects were most clearly documented by close inspection of the acoustic phonetic detail represented by this simple number, fairly easy to see and measure on spectrograms and waveforms. Furthermore, the quantitative nature of this measure can be summarized over large numbers of tokens and/or children, affording large-scale statistical analyses, and work is underway in our labs in Memphis to verify the findings of this chapter at that level of analysis.

CHAPTER REVIEW QUESTIONS

1. What are the four main phases in American English word-initial, or stressed syllable-initial, unvoiced stop production?
2. How do Spanish and English divide the VOT continuum into distinct phonetic categories? How do these phonetic categories correspond to the voiced/voiceless contrast in each language?
3. In our case studies, what was the key difference observed in the Spanish VOTs between early and late kindergarten?

SUGGESTIONS FOR FURTHER READING

One of the most prolific and authoritative figures in phonetic aspects of second-language acquisition has been Dr. James L. Flege. His work on a large variety of speech and language effects has spanned several decades, giving special attention to factors related to age and duration of L2 exposure and accentedness. An example of such work with special relevance to this chapter was titled "Age of learning affects the authenticity of voice onset time (VOT) in stop consonants produced in a second language" (Flege, 1991). All his work is collected with personal commentaries at his website jimflege.com, and a festschrift of articles by important researchers influenced by his seminal contributions was recently published (Bohn and Munro, 2007).

SUGGESTIONS FOR STUDENT ACTIVITIES

Obtain a program that lets you record your own voice and display spectrograms. PRAAT is a free but extremely capable program used by a lot of phoneticians, found at http://www.fon.hum.uva.nl/praat/, but it requires a bit of study and orientation to begin using. TF32 "Demo version" is another free program that is very intuitive to use, but you will need to use a separate recording utility (such as Windows Sound Recorder) to acquire your speech samples. The commercial version of TF32 was used to make the spectrograms in this chapter, and the free version can be found at http://userpages.chorus.net/cspeech/. Then you can study your own voice onset times, trying the following activities (which do not assume that you know Spanish):

1. Record some productions of words that differ only in the voicing of the initial stop consonant, like "pat" and "bat", "tip" and "dip", "got" and "cot." You should observe short-lag and long-lag aspirated productions, but you might also find yourself producing some of the voiced stops with prevoicing.
2. Try and produce voiced stops with prevoicing; this can happen especially if you try to say the word extra clearly, as if teaching a child. Confirm that you are producing these Spanish phonemes by inspection of the waveform and spectrogram.
3. Although English makes use of the short-lag versus long-lag aspirated contrast as the voiced and voiceless phonemes in word initial positions (e.g., the phonemes /b/ and

/p/ are realized as [p] in big and [p^h] in pig), what we hear as a voiceless stop in a word initial blend (e.g., the ‘p’ in spin) is actually similar to the short-lag voicing onset that we hear in “bin”. In fact, if you were to splice the /s/ off of the word “spin” you would perceive “bin” not “pin”. You can use the programs to try this on your own recordings by listening to portions of s-cluster words using segment-specific playback (e.g. cursor selections in TF32) to exclude the /s/ sound.

ANSWERS TO CHAPTER REVIEW QUESTIONS

1. What are the four main phases in American English word-initial, or stressed syllable-initial, unvoiced stop production?

First, there must be a stop gap, during which pressure is contained and built up behind a closure at the place of articulation. Second, the pressure is released suddenly by the opening of the closure at this place, releasing a brief burst of turbulence noise. Third, American English unvoiced stops in these positions will be aspirated, so there will also be an episode of sustained turbulence at the glottis, lasting typically nearly as long as the VOT itself (i.e. starting shortly after the burst and lasting to the onset of voicing). Fourth, voicing then begins at the glottis as the speaker begins to articulate a following vowel.

2. How do Spanish and English divide the VOT continuum into distinct phonetic categories? How do these phonetic categories correspond to the voiced/voiceless contrast in each language?

Between Spanish and English, all three major VOT categories can be observed. The target for Spanish voiced stops is a negative VOT, meaning that voicing begins during the stop gap and before the release. The target for Spanish unvoiced stops is a zero or slightly positive (<25-40 ms) VOT: voicing begins with or shortly after the release and there is no aspiration. This short-lag VOT is actually the target for English voiced stops, however. For English stops to be perceived as unvoiced in most positions they must be produced with a VOT longer than 40 ms, and in word- or stressed syllable-initial positions there will also be aspiration in the interval between the burst and onset of voicing. Note in summary that the English "voiced" stop is phonetically comparable to the Spanish "voiceless" stop!

3. In our case studies, what was the key difference observed in the Spanish VOTs between early and late kindergarten?

The key difference that our study observed in young Spanish speakers, between the onset of English immersion school at the beginning of Kindergarten and approximately 6 months later, was some loss of the pre-voicing in their Spanish voiced stops: acquisition of L2 English apparently began to interfere with this aspect of L1 pronunciation.

References

Anderson, R. T. (1999). Impact of first language loss on grammar in a bilingual child. *Communication Disorders Quarterly, 21*, 4-16.

Anderson, R. T. (2004). First language loss in Spanish-speaking children: Patterns of loss and implications for clinical practice. In B. A. Goldstein (Ed.), *Bilingual language development and disorders in Spanish-English speakers* (pp. 187-212). Baltimore: Brookes.

Barton, D., and Macken, M. A. (1980). An instrumental analysis of the voicing contrast in word-initial stops in the speech of four-year-old English-speaking children. *Language and Speech, 23*, 159-169.

Bohn, O.-S., and Munro, M. J. (Eds.). (2007). *Language experience in second language speech learning: In honor of James Emil Flege*. Philadelphia, PA: John Benjamins Publishing.

Cho, T., and Ladefoged, P. (1999). Variation and universals in VOT: Evidence from 18 languages. *Journal of Phonetics, 27*, 207-229.

Davis, K. (1995). Phonetic and phonological constrasts in the acquisition of voicing: voice onset time production in Hindi and English. *Journal of Child Language, 22*, 275-305.

Deuchar, M., and Clark, A. (1996). Early bilingual acquisition of the voicing contrast in English and Spanish. *Journal of Phonetics, 24*, 351-365.

Eilers, R. E., Oller, D. K., and Benito Garcia, C. R. (1984). The acquisition of voicing contrasts in Spanish and English learning infants and children: A longitudinal study. *Journal of Child Language, 11*, 313-336.

Flege, J. E. (1991). Age of learning affects the authenticity of voice onset time (VOT) in stop consonants produced in a second language. *Journal of the Acoustical Society of America, 89*, 395-411.

Gibson, T.A., Oller, D. K., Jarmulowicz, L., and Ethington, C. (2012). The receptive-expressive gap in the vocabulary of young second-language learners: Robustness and possible mechanisms. *Bilingualism: Language and Cognition. 15(1)*, 102-116.

Goldstein, B. A., and Washington, P. S. (2001). An initial investigation of phonological patterns in typically developing 4-year-old Spanish-English bilingual children. *Language, Speech, and Hearing Services in Shools, 32*, 153-164.

Konefal, J. A., and Fokes, J. (1981). Voice onset time: The development of Spanish/English distinction in normal and language disordered children. *Journal of Phonetics, 9*, 437-444.

Lisker, L., and Abramson, A. S. (1964). A cross-language study of voicing in initial stops: Acoustical measurements. *Word, 20*, 384-422.

Macken, M. A., and Barton, D. (1979). The acquisition of the voicing contrast in English: A study of voice onset time in word-initial stop consonants. *Journal of Child Language, 7*, 41-74.

Macken, M. A., and Barton, D. (1980). The acquisition of the voicing contrast in Spanish: A phonetic and phonological study of word-initial stop consonants. *Journal of Child Language,* 7, 433-458.

Oller, D. K., and Jarmulowicz, L. (2007). Language and literacy in bilinguals. In E. Hoff and M. Shatz (Eds.), *Handbook of language development* (pp. 368-386). Oxford, UK: Blackwell.

Oller, D. K., Jarmulowicz, L., Pearson, B. Z., and Cobo-Lewis, A. B. (2010). Rapid spoken language shifts in early second language learning. In A. Durgunouglu and C. Goldenberg (Eds.), *Dual langauge learners: Their development and assessment in oral and written language* (pp. 94-120). New York: Guilford.

Simon, E. (2010). Child L2 development: A longitudinal case study on voice onset times in word-initial stops. *Journal of Child Language, 37*, 159-173.

Zlatin, M., and Koenigsknecht, R. (1976). Development of voicing contrast: A comparison of voice onset time in perception and production. *Journal of Speech and Hearing Research, 19*, 93-111.

IV. Disordered Speech Development

In: Comprehensive Perspectives …
Editors: Beate Peter and Andrea A. N. MacLeod
ISBN: 978-1-62257-041-6

Chapter 15

SUBTYPES OF PRIMARY SPEECH SOUND DISORDERS: THEORIES AND CASE STUDIES

Beate Peter

INTRODUCTION

Suppose you acquire a large number of miscellaneous books and wish to organize them into a library. What should your principle of organization be? There are several options. For instance, you could simply sort the books by size and designate a category for the large, coffee-table books, another category for small paperbacks, and a third for the remainder. Another organizing principle could be the age of the targeted readership, with divisions for various children's groupings and one division for adults. Subject area, language, literary genre, publication date, and alphabetical order of the author's last name are other ways to organize the books. Perhaps you would combine several classification schemes and have five sections of children's books by age and within each section, you organize by subject area and then by the author's last name, whereas in the books for adults, you organize by subject matter first, genre second, and alphabet last. Which is the best way to organize miscellaneous books? Different libraries use different systems, for instance the Dewey system with its ten broad subject categories or the Library of Congress system with its 21 subject categories. Some libraries use one system for part of their collection and another for the remainder. The fact that different organizational principles for library books coexist is a hint that sorting miscellaneous items into some logical arrangement is a complex process for which several different solutions can emerge. The problem is really one of classification, and the question is which classification scheme is best suited to provide easy access (practical relevance) and to capture the essence of each category (theoretical relevance).

The problem of classification applies to many areas including animals, plants, words in a language, and, of course, human diseases, also frequently called disorders. For plants and animals, the term **taxonomy** refers to a hierarchically categorized set of entities, whereas for diseases, the analogous term is **nosology.** The goal is to "carve nature at its joints," to borrow from Plato the metaphor of expertly butchering an animal. The best classification system for human diseases, consequently, would be one that mirrors some natural divisions inherent in the disorders. It would group cases into subtypes that share an **etiology**, observable characteristics, and/or recommended interventions (clinical relevance) while also maximally capturing the differences between subtypes and the similarities within subtypes (statistical relevance). Why does it matter how disorders are classified? When a clinical diagnosis is made, a label is applied and that label is taken from an available disorder classification. Across all clinical fields, accurate diagnosis is a highly valued goal and the quest for it is driven by a number of different forces. A diagnostic label has far-reaching implications, including an individual's prognosis and therapy plan, both of which are crucial for the successful management of the disorder in question. Because health care is extremely costly, diagnostic accuracy has gained importance from a public health perspective as well (Katz, 2001). With the paradigm shift from opinion-based to evidence-based practice (Guyatt, Sackett, and Cook, 1994; Oxman and Guyatt, 1993; Oxman, Sackett, and Guyatt, 1993), it has become imperative that both diagnosis and treatment be based on systematically researched data, peer-reviewed results, and meta-analyses. A diagnostic label, however, can only be as authentic and meaningful as the classification scheme that created the label. An example of the clinical relevance of an accurate subtype diagnosis is dystonia, a neurological disease affecting body posture and movement. Primary dystonia can have a genetic etiology, and in very rare cases of **familial** dystonia caused by genetic mutations, patients respond to levadopa, a drug commonly used to treat Parkinson's disease (Ling et al., 2011; Segawa, 2011). A correct diagnosis of this dopa-responsive subtype is crucial for selecting the appropriate therapy. This chapter provides an overview of various ways of subtyping speech sound disorder (SSD) that have been proposed on theoretical grounds. It proceeds to suggest some additional ways of deriving SSD nosologies using empirical and biological approaches. Several case examples throughout the chapter highlight the fact that disordered speech can look and sound very different across affected children.

Proposed Nosologies of Speech Sound Disorders

Speech sound disorder (SSD) is a widely used term generally defined as difficulty developing speech that can be readily understood, due to speech sound omissions, distortions, or substitutions (Pennington and Bishop, 2009). The SSD definition excludes any speech difficulties that result from known causes. Examples of known causes include structural anomalies such as cleft lip and/or palate, chromosomal developmental disabilities such as trisomy 21, and hearing impairment. No universally accepted SSD nosology is currently in use. Over the past few decades, various ways of defining SSD and its subtypes have been proposed. The following text retraces some of these nosologies.

For many years, children who had difficulty learning to talk were simply thought to have a functional **articulation** disorder, a general term without reference to subtypes or causes. As advances were made in understanding the systematic nature of the speech sounds of a language, i.e., its **phonology**, these insights were translated into descriptions of typical and disordered speech development (Ingram, 1976). Consequently, the term phonological disorder was adopted to describe children who struggled with acquiring speech (Shriberg and Kwiatkowski, 1982a, 1982b, 1982c). In the following years, a subdivision into two different levels of representation was proposed, phonological knowledge on one level and motoric or phonetic aspects of speech production on another. An example of an impairment at the phonological level would be typical production of /s/ in "sick" but realization of "stick" as [tɪk] because consonant clusters were reduced to single consonants. A frontal lisp during /s/ or /z/ is frequently cited as an example for a more motor-based or articulatory error. Because children with speech deficits could not always be assigned unambiguously to one of the two proposed levels of impairment (and perhaps also because the two levels themselves cannot always be unambiguously distinguished), some researchers and clinicians proposed integrating the two frameworks into a spectrum (Bauman-Wängler, 2004). Under this approach, a speech error profile would lead to a diagnosis as a primarily phonological disorder, a primarily articulatory disorder, or as a mixed case with elements from both. Dodd's general classification system of child speech disorders is based on a psycholinguistic model that incorporates a dichotomy of articulation and phonology (Dodd, 2005). The subtype characteristics derived from this model are described as follows (Fox, Dodd, and Howard, 2002):

1. Articulation disorder, i.e., the inability to produce a perceptually acceptable instantiation of a particular speech sound. The proposed level of impairment is the phonetic assembly module, where, in the case of a disorder, a faulty articulatory motor sequence has been acquired.
2. Delayed phonological development, i.e., error patterns that typically occur in younger children but are inappropriate for a given child at the time of assessment. No level of impairment is proposed. The errors may resolve spontaneously.
3. Deviant-consistent phonological disorder; i.e., errors that are not typically seen at any age and that are produced consistently. The proposed level of impairment is in the cognitive-linguistic domain and involves faulty acquisition of the phonological contrasts and constraints in the ambient language.
4. Deviant-inconsistent phonological disorder; i.e., atypical errors with inconsistent production. The proposed impairment level is the phonologic assembly module, specifically the processes of selection and sequencing of speech sounds.

Sound file 15S1 is a recording of a boy, age 5;0, with a lateral lisp. This type of speech error would fit under Dodd's subtype of articulation disorder resulting from a faulty articulatory motor program. Sound file 15S2 is a recording of a girl, age 4;11, with multiple phonological processes including occasional affrication whose gliding and fronting processes would fit under Dodd's category of delayed phonological development and whose occasional affrication errors would fit under Dodd's category of deviant-inconsistent phonological disorder.

Access Sound File 1 (Chapter 15)

15S1 Story retell provided by a boy, age 5;0, with a lateral lisp.

Access Sound File 2 (Chapter 15)

15S2 Picture naming provided by a girl, age 4;11, with multiple phonological processes.

In the most recent version of their Speech Disorders Classification System (Shriberg, Fourakis, et al., 2010), first introduced in 1982 (Shriberg and Kwiatkowski, 1982a), Shriberg and colleagues classify speech disorders in two ways. The first, a typology, is based on the type of current and/or previous speech errors. For children age 3 to 9 years, four subtypes are listed. *Normal Speech Acquisition* describes children whose development is within normal limits. *Speech Delay* describes children with substantial speech sound deletions, substitutions, and distortions that usually respond to treatment. *Motor Speech Disorder* describes children whose substantial speech sound deletions, substitutions, and distortions may not completely normalize with treatment. *Speech Errors* includes children with speech sound distortions such as sibilants and/or liquids. The typology has a second tier for children 9 years and older, where the cover term *Persistent Speech Disorder* is concatenated with the history of each of the three types of speech disorder in the younger age bracket.

The second classification in the Speech Disorders Classification System is based on suspected **etiology,** with the most distal category, genetic and environmental influences, acting on the next tier, neurodevelopmental substrates. From this tier on down, differentiation is described in terms of five etiological classes, each of which is associated with one or more SSD subtype labels. The cognitive-linguistic etiology produces *Speech Delay - Generic*, the auditory-perceptual etiology produces *Speech Delay – Otitis Media with Effusion*, the psychosocial etiology produces *Speech Delay – Developmental Psychosocial Involvement*, speech motor control produces *Motor Speech Disorder* which is subdivided into **apraxia** of speech, *dysarthria*, and *not otherwise specified*, and the speech attunement etiology produces *Speech Errors* related to distortions of two classes of sounds, **sibilants** and **rhotics**.

The term **childhood apraxia of speech (CAS)** is a proposed subtype of SSD that is not specific to any given nosology, although it is mentioned in some of them including Shriberg, Fourakis, et al. (2010). CAS is thought to interfere with motor planning and/or motor programming processes. In its position statement on CAS, the American Speech-Language-Hearing Association (http://www.asha.org/docs/html/PS2007-00277.html) describes CAS as a "distinct diagnostic subtype of childhood (pediatric) speech sound disorder" and defines it as follows:

> [CAS] is a neurological childhood (pediatric) speech sound disorder in which the precision and consistency of movements underlying speech are impaired in the absence of neuromuscular deficits (e.g., abnormal reflexes, abnormal tone). CAS may occur as a result of known neurological impairment, in association with complex neurobehavioral disorders of known or unknown origin, or as an idiopathic neurogenic speech sound disorder. The core impairment in planning and/or programming spatiotemporal parameters of movement sequences results in errors in speech sound production and prosody.

This definition implies that CAS is a subtype of SSD even if it was acquired through some disease or injury. Some researchers, however (Potter, Lazarus, Johnson, Steiner, and Shriberg, 2008; Shriberg, Potter, and Strand, 2010; Terband, Maassen, van Lieshout, and Nijland, 2011), hold a more narrow view in which only primary, non-acquired forms of CAS form one SSD subtype. A universally accepted catalogue of diagnostic criteria is not available, although many sources including the American Speech-Language-Hearing Association website cited above mention more difficulty with longer words than with shorter ones, choppy and monotonous prosody, and highly unintelligible speech. The label CAS remains controversial. Sound file 15S3 is an example of conversational speech of a preschooler age 3;2 who was diagnosed with CAS, and sound file 15S4 is an excerpt from articulation testing of a 5-year-old girl with a CAS diagnosis. Chapter 18 in this volume discusses motor-based speech disorders in greater detail.

Access Sound File 3 (Chapter 15)

15S3 Conversational speech of a girl with a CAS diagnosis, age 3;2.

Access Sound File 4 (Chapter 15)

15S4 Articulation test of a girl with a CAS diagnosis, age 5;11.

Strictly speaking, the word "dysarthria" means unable to utter distinctly. In the field of speech-language pathology, the term **dysarthria** refers to impaired production of speech due to disturbances in the muscular control of the speech mechanism. Unlike SSD and CAS, dysarthria is caused by one of several known impairments in the **central nervous system** or **peripheral nervous system**. As described in Chapter 3, the central nervous system includes the the brain and the spinal cord, whereas the peripheral nervous system includes the cranial and spinal nerves once they exit the brain step or spinal cord. Dysarthria in children may be due to injury to the central or peripheral nervous system that occurred during pregnancy or childbirth, or to injury following the normal onset of speech development (i.e., acquired childhood dysarthria). This injury may be related to a genetic syndrome, tumors, or accidental injury. Many children with dysarthria have other developmental delays or disorders as well, including delays in gross and fine motor development, difficulty feeding and dysphagia, cognitive delays, hearing impairment, and visual impairment. These children may also experience important health problems that result in frequent or lengthy stays in hospitals. As a result, speech-language pathologists (SLP) will often find themselves working within an interdisciplinary team in assessment and treatment. In this setting, SLPs need to communicate with the team and parents to understand how to prioritize treatment goals given the general health and development of the child.

Sound file 15S5 was recorded from a 10-year-old boy with severely disordered speech and left hemiparesis, both of which are thought to be related to a stroke he suffered at birth. His speech is characterized by weak pressure consonants, imprecise articulation, and low intelligibility.

Access Sound File 5 (Chapter 15)

15S5 Single words ("spoon," "girl," "ball," "wagon," "shovel") produced by a 10-year-old boy with dysarthria.

Another way of thinking about differences among children with SSD is the idea that underlying deficits may capture clinical differences more meaningfully than observable speech characteristics. Pyscholinguistic models such as that proposed by Stackhouse and Wells (Stackhouse & Pascoe, 2010; Stackhouse & Wells, 1997, 2001) were developed because it was suspected that more traditional diagnostic categories may group individual cases based on superficial similarities even though these cases may not share underlying deficits and may not respond well to the same type of treatment. Psycholinguistic models of speech deficits, by contrast, are built on the processes and elements underlying speech production.

The psycholinguistic model proposed by Stackhouse and colleagues takes its name from the interactions of underlying processes ("psycho-") and the observable speech traits ("-linguistic"). Its components include input-related processes such as peripheral auditory perception, speech/nonspeech discrimination, and phonological recognition; elements of stored knowledge such as phonological and semantic representation, and output-related processes such as motor planning and motor execution. Breakdowns can occur in any of these components and cause speech problems. Careful observation of a child's strengths and weaknesses during a variety of tasks can help pinpoint where in the system a breakdown occurred. For instance, if a child is asked to name some pictures and also to repeat some real words, both tasks may be performed as expected. If performance during naming is poorer than during repetition, this may indicate difficulties with the stored lexicon or with accessing it. If the reverse is the case and performance during repetition is poorer than during naming, this may indicate a breakdown in the input mechanism. A child who has more difficulty repeating nonwords than real words may have a breakdown in the assembly of novel motor programs (Stackhouse and Pascoe, 2010). Once a locus of impairment has been identified, treatment can be tailored to address the underlying deficit rather than treat the speech error observed on the surface.

Although psycholinguistic models have found clinical use in the assessment and treatment planning for individual children, they are useful for thinking about SSD subtypes as well. Children may have difficulty with their speech output for a variety of reasons, and grouping them according to the suspected locus of impairment may have more clinical validity than grouping them according to characteristics of their speech output.

Some inherent technical challenges regarding the classification of speech difficulties into subgroups should be mentioned. A child's speech error profile may change fairly rapidly as a function of treatment and maturation. An 8-year-old child with only /ɹ/ missing from the phonemic inventory may be referred for an assessment for the first time. Another 8-year-old child also currently struggling with /ɹ/ may have had extremely unintelligible speech at age 4 years, received a diagnosis of CAS, and undergone years of intense treatment until only /ɹ/ needed to be addressed further in treatment. In some cases, children have multiple sounds or sound patterns in error, and what initially appeared to be mainly a subtype characterized by phonological processes may resemble an SSD subtype characterized by distortions later on. Many factors can introduce variability, including the age at which a child is first referred for assessment, the speech sound accuracy across structural levels such as single words and conversational speech, and even the approach selected for clinical management of the disorder. The dynamic nature of children's speech abilities over time should be taken into consideration when classification into SSD subtypes is attempted.

The coexistence of several nosologies and the controversy surrounding the validity and specific characteristics of some diagnostic categories, for example those of CAS, explain the fact that children with speech problems do not fit into neatly arranged categories. The nosologies reviewed here were defined largely on theoretical grounds. This leaves two additional options for creating a nosology: (1) empirical classification where cases are clustered based on multivariate data profiles, and (2) classification based on genetic causes. The following sections review recent advances regarding these two approaches.

New Frontiers in Identifying Speech Sound Disorder Subtypes

Empirical Classification

One alternate approach to defining SSD subtypes on theoretical grounds is data-based classification. Toward this goal, one would ascertain a large sample of participants with broadly defined SSD and collect a wide variety of data, then use a multivariate classification **algorithm** that joins cases with similar profiles into subtypes. In the area of language impairment, such an empirical approach to classification has been presented by a team of researchers in the United Kingdom (Conti-Ramsden, Crutchley, and Botting, 1997). The participants were 242 children, age six to eight years, who attended special language units. The input variables for the classification procedure were derived from a receptive grammar test, a number skill test, expressive vocabulary, word reading, an articulation test, a story-telling task, and a measure of nonverbal abilities. The statistical procedure, ***k*-means** clustering, grouped the children into six clusters that were maximally different from each other while the individuals within each cluster were maximally similar. The clusters consisted of (1) participants with low scores on all variables except the articulation test and the naming vocabulary; (2) participants with low scores on the word reading task but average scores on all other tests; (3) participants with low scores on all tests except naming vocabulary; (4) participants with average scores on receptive and expressive language tasks, low average scores on naming vocabulary, number skills, and articulation testing, and low scores on the word reading task; (5) participants with low scores on all tests except the articulation task; and (6) participants with above-average scores on the articulation test, the word reading task, and the naming vocabulary task but poor scores in the story telling information content and in the number skills task.

In the area of SSD, Lewis and colleagues (Lewis et al., 2006) applied **factor analysis**, a statistical tool used to classify variables, not individuals, to a multivariate dataset collected from 185 children with disordered speech. They found two main factors, the first related to articulation and phonology and the second related to semantics and syntax. This indicates that measures of articulation and phonology were strongly cross-correlated and together explained most of the variability in the data, followed by the measures of semantics and syntax. In a study of motor programming in a sample of 100 children between the ages of 3;0 and 5;6 (Ozanne, 1995), six relevant concepts were selected, namely difference in performance on voluntary versus involuntary speech and oromotor tasks, inability to maintain word or syllable phonological structure, non-fluent speech production, increased errors with increased performance load, phonetic adjustments in speech, and slow **diadochokinetic rate**. 18 specific behaviors representing these six concepts were rated as present or absent. This dataset was entered into a clustering procedure resulting in four clusters.

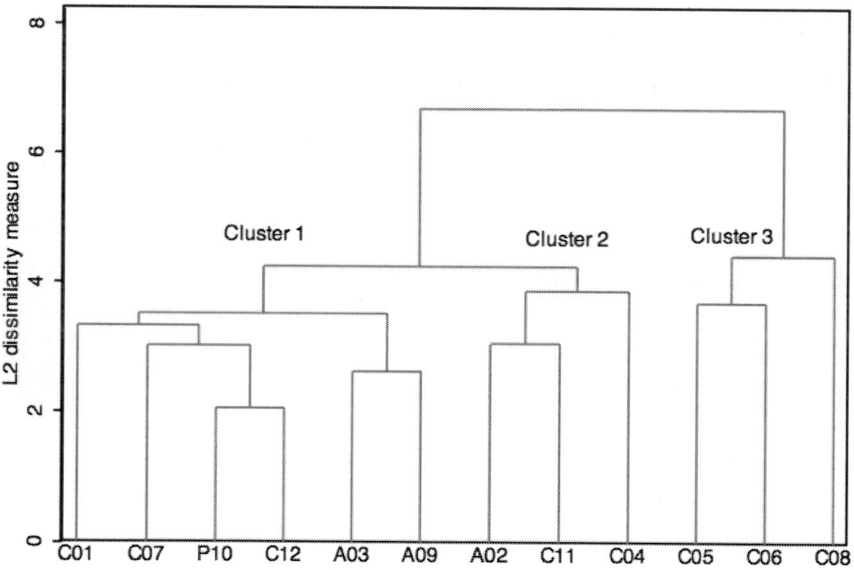

Figure 15. 1 Cluster dendrogram. Endpoints are labeled with participant codes. Letter codes reflect the proposed SSD subtype that best fit the observed speech characteristics. A = articulation disorder, P = phonological disorder, C = childhood apraxia of speech.

One cluster showed primarily deviant inconsistent errors, a second cluster showed deficits in oromotor and motor speech components, a third cluster showed evidence of groping, consonant deletion, and a difference between voluntary and involuntary performance, and a fourth cluster was characterized by prosodic disturbances and a history of no babbling.

In a pilot study of 12 children with SSD (Peter, 2006), variables derived from speech and language testing and variables measuring timing accuracy in oral and hand motor tasks were used to create clusters of children with similar profiles. In two different clustering procedures (**hierarchical agglomerative clustering** and *k*-means clustering), three clusters emerged.

Cluster 1 contained six children who showed overall high scores in all areas except in articulation and phonology testing. These children resembled the cohort of age- and gender-matched controls with typical development except for their low speech and/or phonology scores. Cluster 2 contained three children with intermediate scores in all tested areas except in articulation and phonology testing. Cluster 3 contained three children with overall low scores and clinical deficits in language tests. Figure 15.1 shows a **dendrogram** created with hierarchical agglomerative clustering. The endpoints are labeled with the children's participant codes, which were created prior to clustering based on speech diagnostics. The label "articulation disorder" was selected when a child's standard score from an articulation test was lower than that from a test of phonological processes, and the label "phonological disorder" was selected in the reverse case. The label "childhood apraxia of speech" was selected when at least 8 of 11 proposed characteristics of CAS (Davis, Jakielski, and Marquardt, 1998) were observed, regardless of the results from speech and phonology testing.

To date, a large-scale classification based on a broad spectrum of input variables has not been developed to derive data-based subtypes of SSD. As Ozanne's (1995) clustering study shows, the variables selected as inputs into a clustering procedure determine the dimensions along which the cases are being grouped. To arrive at an empirical SSD nosology with minimal bias, care should be taken to select a balanced and wide variety of variables of clinical relevance. To capture underlying processes and elements, measures such as those developed in psycholinguistic models can be selected as well. Once established, a valid empirical SSD nosology can provide new diagnostic labels and motivate new clinical questions regarding therapy approaches. Such a nosology could potentially describe deficits that are associated with a subtype, for instance in phonology, expressive language, or motor processing, that could become additional targets of therapy.

Genetic Causes

A second alternative to theory-based definitions of SSD subtypes is to group cases based on biological substrates. If certain SSD cases share a genetic mechanism, this mechanism could define an etiological SSD subtype on biological grounds. It is acknowledged here, of course, that disease genes rarely act in a deterministic fashion. Depending on the gene and the disease, the proportion of carriers of a risk gene who also show evidence of the disease can vary greatly, i.e., gene mutations can have various degrees of **penetrance**. Furthermore, environmental factors can substantially influence a disease in terms of presence and severity.

It is well accepted that SSD has a genetic component. Evidence for a genetic etiology is found in higher SSD concordance rates in identical versus fraternal twins (Lewis, 1992), high SSD heritability estimates (Bishop, 2002), and higher susceptibility in biological versus adopted children with affected parents (Felsenfeld and Plomin, 1997). More recently, several studies have addressed the molecular genetics of speech problems. In some cases, speech production difficulties of genetic origin are part of a **syndrome**. Rare mutations in the *FOXP2* gene on chromosome 7 cause severe difficulties with speech, receptive and expressive language, reading, writing, cognition, and oral praxis (Fisher, Vargha-Khadem, Watkins, Monaco, and Pembrey, 1998; MacDermot et al., 2005; Vargha-Khadem, Watkins, Alcock, Fletcher, and Passingham, 1995; Watkins, Dronkers, and Vargha-Khadem, 2002), but changes in this gene do not explain common non-syndromic SSD (MacDermot et al., 2005).

Efforts to identify causal genes for SSD are currently ongoing. Several studies were conducted to evaluate gene regions implicated in other disorders where speech deficits are frequently seen in addition to the core characteristics. In one such study of sibling pairs from 77 families (Stein et al., 2004), measures of phonological memory, phonological representation, articulation, receptive and expressive vocabulary, reading decoding, and reading comprehension were evaluated for **genetic linkage** in a region of interest, 3p12-q13, previously shown to be linked to **dyslexia** (Nopola-Hemmi et al., 2001). Note that these region codes indicate the chromosome number (in this case, 3), the chromosome arm p or q (straddling both in this case), and the chromosomal band. If known variants in certain regions on a chromosome are inherited along with the disorder, they are thought to be genetically linked to each other, presumably because they are located in close vicinity on the same chromosome. Significant evidence for linkage was found for phonological short-term memory and reading decoding. Evidence for a composite factor of articulation skill was suggestive but not statistically significant. Similarly, 15q14-q2 is implicated in dyslexia and autism and harbors genes causing Prader-Willi and Angelman syndromes, all of which are associated with speech deficits. This region was evaluated for linkage in children from 151 families (Stein et al., 2006). In one type of **linkage analysis,** the speed of single syllable repetitions was tentatively linked while other measures of articulation and reading did not show evidence of linkage. A second type of linkage analysis confirmed that the region of interest contains a putative locus influencing articulation, phonological memory, and oral motor functioning. Three dyslexia candidate regions, 1p36, 6p22, and 15q21, were evaluated for linkage in 111 kindergarten children with SSD and 76 siblings (Smith, Pennington, Boada, and Shriberg, 2005) with linkage analyses. The 1p36 region provided only suggestive evidence for linkage to standardized speech scores whereas evidence for linkage to speech scores was seen in 6p22 and 15q21. The candidate locus on chromosome 1, with expanded boundaries to include 1p34-p36, was also evaluated for linkage to SSD in 151 families, each ascertained through a child with SSD (Miscimarra et al., 2007). Measures included standardized articulation testing, nonword repetition, multisyllabic word repetition, difficult-to-articulate phrases, visual perception, and receptive and expressive language. Two types of linkage analysis revealed two narrow genomic regions with high levels of the test statistic in the candidate region, one with suggestive linkage to verbal short-term memory and articulation and the other, with suggestive linkage to language processing skills.

More recently, candidate genes that had been implicated in reading and language disorders were tested for **genetic association** in 52 families with children who had been diagnosed with SSD (Lewis et al., 2011). Markers within three of the six tested candidate genes (*ROBO2* on chromosome 3, *BDNF* on chromosome 11, and *DYX1C1* on chromosome 15, showed evidence of association with SSD with nominal statistical significance. All three of these genes influence brain development.

The molecular genetic studies reviewed here were based on the common disease/common variant (CDCV) model that posits that many genes act together to confer SSD susceptibility on an individual. To test for candidate regions or genes under this model, a large sample of children from different families can be analyzed. This approach is not particularly sensitive to SSD subtypes because a mix of causal gene variants could be contained in the sample. An alternate view, the common disease/rare variant (CDRV) model, posits that in each family with familial SSD, only very few genes are at work. To test for candidate genes or regions under this **heterogeneous** model, multigenerational families with evidence of a familial SSD form can be analyzed. One challenge of applying the CDRV model to SSD is the fact that most adults with a childhood history of SSD have compensated for their disorder and the **expression** of SSD is difficult to observe, so that other residual traits must be identified. The CDRV model was the basis of a recent study of SSD genetics in five multigenerational families (Peter and Raskind, 2011). Participants produced rapid sequences of monosyllables and disyllables and tapped computer keys with repetitive and alternating movements. The hand task was included in this study because in previous studies, timing accuracy and speed were found to be closely associated in oral and hand tasks in families with dyslexia (Peter, Matsushita, and Raskind, 2011) and children with SSD (Peter and Stoel-Gammon, 2008). In two families with children who had previously been diagnosed with CAS, most of the affected children and adults with a history of SSD produced slowed alternating but not repetitive oral movements. Slowed alternating hand movements were also seen in some of the biologically related participants. These results were consistent with a familial SSD subtype that disrupts motor praxis not only in the oral system but also in the hand system, and they provided support for the validity of CAS as a motor-based SSD subtype. In a follow-up study of these motor measures in one family (Peter, Matsushita, and Raskind, 2012), suggestive evidence was found for linkage to four regions including one on chromosome 6 that is also a candidate region for dyslexia (Konig et al., 2011).

Suppose causal genes for SSD subtypes are identified in the near future. What clinical implications would this have for children with SSD? First, as mentioned, genetic mechanisms could define SSD subtypes based on etiology. Second, knowing which gene variant caused SSD in a given child would allow the clinician to make a more precise diagnosis than previously possible. Third, it is possible that children who share the same genetic SSD subtype also share underlying disorder characteristics such as deficits in motor sequencing that could be addressed in therapy in more sophisticated ways. Fourth, infants with risk genotypes can be identified early and become candidates for early preventative intervention, once such early intervention approaches are validated in careful research studies. Lastly, knowing the genetic causes of SSD can motivate biochemical studies leading to pharmaceutical interventions in the future.

No consideration of a genetic etiology would be complete without mentioning the public health perspective. One concern with respect to genetically transmitted disorders is insurability. If a person's genetic profile can be considered a pre-existing condition, then insurances may attempt to deny coverage of therapy services. In the United States, new legislation addressing this concern became effective in 2008. The Genetic Information Nondiscrimination Act (GINA) protects patients from loss of insurance coverage and increased premiums based on their genetic profiles. Another concern regarding genetic research is privacy. An individual's genetic information could potentially be used to identify that person uniquely. Institutional review boards at research institutions place a heavy burden on researchers to protect an individual's privacy in genetics research studies. Ultimately, in cases when there is a family history of SSD, knowing a young child's genetic risk status can help conserve resources because early intervention can be preferentially considered if the child is at risk.

Sidebar 15.1. "Lissa"

Lissa (the names of all children in this chapter were changed to protect their privacy) was a bright sixth-grader whose speech was characterized by vowelization and [w] substitutions of /ɹ/. No other speech sounds were in error. Several of her classroom teachers had referred Lissa for speech evaluations in the past starting in third grade, but her parents had resisted the idea of their gifted daughter receiving speech therapy. Lissa was keenly aware of her inability to produce /ɹ/ and the difference between her speech production and that of her peers. At the beginning of sixth grade, she told her parents that she felt self-conscious and really wanted help for her speech. The parents finally agreed to the evaluation and also to the recommended course of treatment, and Lissa began to see the speech-language pathologist at her school for twice-weekly individual sessions. It took several sessions before Lissa was able to produce her first [ɹ] in isolation. Despite Lissa's good cooperation, her progress was slow and her productions of [ɹ] were variable.

Sidebar 15.2. "Kyle"

Kyle was a first-grader whose parents sought professional help from a private speech-language pathologist service because of concerns regarding his speech. Kyle's speech was characterized by a frontal lisp ([ð] for /z/ and [θ] for /s/). He also substituted [f] for /θ/. In a way, the phonemes in his relational inventory were playing musical chairs: /s, z/ were missing from his sound inventory altogether. Where an /s/ was the target, he produced [θ], and where /θ/ was the target, he produced [f] instead. Kyle's parents were not only aware of his speech production errors but also began to notice that he spelled the way he talked ("teef" for teeth and "thun" for sun). Using a mouth model and a mirror, the clinician showed Kyle the articulatory positions for alveolar, interdental, and labiodental sounds. Kyle learned to sort word cards into bins representing each of these places of articulation. The word cards were created using minimal pairs such as "free" and "three," "sink" and "think," and "sound" and "found." Next, Kyle worked on producing /s, z/, the sounds missing from his inventory, in isolation, syllables, words, and sentences. Using minimal pairs as stimuli, Kyle worked toward eliminating the [f] for /θ/ substitution. In the process of reorganizing his sound inventory, he went through a brief phase of overgeneralization, where he substituted [s] for /θ/. His diligence and his parents' support paid off and he was dismissed from treatment after only four months when all of his target sounds were produced correctly in conversation.

Sidebar 15.3. "Mia"

Mia was a lively Kindergartener who watched the news along with her parents at night and could cogently converse about current political events. While her teacher was very impressed with her precocious intellect, she had concerns about Mia's speech as she consistently substituted [t] for /k/, [d] for /g/, and [n] for /ŋ/. Mia was referred for an evaluation and began twice-weekly sessions with the school's speech-language pathologist. Following perceptual accuracy checks and an introduction to places of articulation using a mouth model as a visual aid, Mia attempted production of /k/ in isolation. She was exuberant when she heard and felt herself produce the sound for the first time. Within two months of treatment, all velars had generalized into conversational speech and Mia was dismissed from treatment.

Sidebar 15.4. "Tom"

As soon as Tom reached his third birthday, his parents referred him for a speech evaluation in the public school district where they lived. They had been concerned about his speech since he was a toddler and they had already obtained a hearing test to rule out hearing loss as a cause. At the time of the evaluation, Tom's parents said that they had difficulty understanding him and frequently asked Tom to confirm whether their guess was correct. Over time, Tom had developed signs of extreme frustration and sometimes acted out or, worse, sometimes gave up trying to talk when he was not understood. Articulation testing and conversational samples showed that Tom's speech was characterized by a frontal lisp, various sound substitutions ([ð] for /j/, [w] for /j/, [w] for /ɹ/, [f] for /θ/), sound omissions ([nopaʊ] for "snowplough"), syllable omissions ([bun] for "balloon"), vowel errors ([to] for "toy"), sequencing errors ([ʃawaf] for "shovel"), and inconsistent productions of the same word ([pɛðɛn, pɛnɛ] for "present").

Tom began to meet with the speech-language pathologist twice per week. His course of treatment was custom-made for him and consisted of elements of various approaches. Tom made rapid progress. By the time he started kindergarten, the only residual speech errors were the frontal lisp and the substitution of [f] for /θ/, and he now eagerly communicated his ideas without any signs of frustration or resignation. His case is discussed in more detail in a book chapter (Peter, 2010).

Sidebar 15.5. "Jenna"

> Jenna was 5;1 when her teacher referred her for a speech assessment. During standardized articulation testing, which involved single-word productions in response to a picture stimulus, the following sound distortions, substitutions, and omissions were noted, among others:
>
> - [θ] for /s/ and [ð] for /z/ (frontal lisp)
> - ʃˡ, ʧˡ, ʤˡ (lateralized airflow on palatal fricatives and affricates)
> - t/k, d/ɡ, n/ŋ (velar fronting)
> - d/ɡɹ, t/kl, θ/sp (cluster reduction)
> - bənunθ/bəlunz (assimilation and final devoicing)
> - wɪn/ɹɪŋ, faʊɜθ/flaʊɚz (gliding and derhotacization)
> - a:f/naɪf (initial consonant deletion and vowel error)
> - bæt/bæθ (stopping)
> - j/ð, v/b, nəʤˡæmən/pəʤæməz (unusual and idiosyncratic errors)
>
> The fact that Jenna had so many errorred speech sounds and patterns, together with concerns about her ability to make herself understood in school and at home, were taken into consideration when the decision was made to qualify her for treatment.

Sidebar 15.6. The "Collins" Family

> Trevor was a second grader who saw the school's speech-language pathologist for twice weekly sessions to address multiple speech errors including a frontal lisp and liquid substitutions. His older sister, a fourth grader, had received speech therapy for similar sound errors and was close to being dismissed from treatment. Two younger children in the family, ages 5 and 3 years, had been assessed and qualified for speech services because of multiple speech sounds in error. The children's mother spoke with a frontal lisp and reported that both she and her brother had had a childhood history of disordered speech; only her brother, however, had received speech services. The speech-language pathologist wrote a family treatment plan in which she outlined some general concepts regarding speech sound production as well as principles of treatment and some suggested activities and materials. This document was helpful in supporting home practice for the children, and the children's mother reported that she herself took a more active role in her children's home speech assignments, which helped her to become more aware of her own distorted speech sounds and to increase correct productions in her own speech.

CONNECTIONS

The SSD nosologies proposed on theoretical grounds mirror the linguistic theories of their time, as recounted in Chapter 1. Just as there are many proposed SSD classification schemes and resulting SSD subtypes, there are many proposed types of, and approaches to,

SSD interventions. Tools for discovering a child's profile of strengths and weaknesses across a variety of tasks are described in Chapter 2 from a general perspective and in Chapter 20 in the context of assessment and diagnosis. Chapter 21 describes many of these intervention types and approaches in detail. One way to classify intervention approaches is to divide them into direct speech production methods, interventions within a broader communicative context, and interventions designed to improve motor functioning (Williams, McLeod, and McCauley, 2010). Multiple approaches are grouped within each category. Some approaches are designed for all SSD subtypes in general whereas others were designed to be used with certain types of children, for instance those with CAS, phonological difficulties, or inconsistent speech errors.

Concluding Remarks

Our field has made great strides in gaining a deeper understanding of SSD and its subtypes. A universally accepted SSD nosology remains elusive at this time, however. Much work lies ahead to determine how observable characteristics and biological markers can be used to define SSD subtypes with clinical and statistical relevance. Progress toward this goal will inform us as we strive to empower individuals with SSD to overcome their communication barriers.

Chapter Review Questions

1. Why is it important to have a valid SSD nosology in general?
2. In the future, how can a better understanding of empirically derived SSD subtypes benefit a child with SSD?
3. What are some fundamental differences between the CDCV model and the CDRV model?
4. How can knowledge of genetic etiologies inform the field of speech-language pathology?
5. In the future, how can a better understanding of genetic causes benefit a child with SSD?

Suggestions for Further Reading

Peter, B., and Stoel-Gammon, C. (2008). Central timing deficits in subtypes of primary speech disorders. *Clinical Linguistics and Phonetics, 22*(3), 171-198.

Thoonen, G., Maassen, B., Gabreels, F., and Schreuder, R. (1999). Validity of maximum performance tasks to diagnose motor speech disorders in children. *Clinical Linguistics and Phonetics, 13*(1), 1 - 23.

Thoonen, G., Maassen, B., Wit, J., Gabreels, F., and Schreuder, R. (1996). The integrated use of maximum performance tasks in differential diagnostic evaluations among children with motor speech disorders. *Clinical Linguistics and Phonetics, 10*(4), 311 - 336.

Volkmar, F. R., State, M., and Klin, A. (2009). Autism and autism spectrum disorders: diagnostic issues for the coming decade. *Journal of Child Psychology and Psychiatry, 50*(1-2), 108-115.

SUGGESTIONS FOR STUDENT ACTIVITIES

1. On the basis of what you know about proposed SSD subtypes, observe several different children or use the case descriptions in the sidebars and attempt to explain all of them with a single taxonomy. Ask yourself: Can I justify fitting all of these cases on Bauman-Waengler's (2004) phonetic/phonemic continuum? Can I fit the observed speech errors into Dodd's taxonomy based on error types? Can I fit all of these cases into Shriberg et al.'s (2010) taxonomy by error types? Can I hypothesize convincing etiologies for all of these cases, following Shriberg et al.'s (2010) taxonomy by etiology?
2. Many children with SSD have siblings or other child relatives who also have SSD and receive therapy from the same service provider. For two or more affected related children, obtain information on current levels of speech competence as well as information from the children's history and evaluate the evidence for a familial form of SSD with similar expression.
3. Obtain current copies of the *Diagnostic Statistical Manual* and the *International Classification of Diseases* and read the disorder definition and criteria for what this book terms speech sound disorder (SSD). Compare and contrast the two views. Now state your own view of how SSD fits into superordinate categories and how SSD should be further subtyped. Draw a tree diagram of your own classification.
4. Compare the study of SSD subtypes to that of autism spectrum disorder (ASD) subtypes. What are the similarities and differences? Consider explaining SSD as a spectrum disorder instead of consisting of distinct subtypes. The following reference discusses the nosology of ASD:

ANSWERS TO CHAPTER REVIEW QUESTIONS

1. Why is it important to have a valid SSD nosology in general?

Accurate diagnosis depends on a valid system of disorder labels that capture the clinical nature of the disorder. A valid nosology also leads to interventions that can address the disorder characteristics more effectively.

2. In the future, how can a better understanding of empirically derived SSD subtypes benefit a child with SSD?

Empirically derived subgroups of children with SSD would capture children with similar profiles of observable traits. Hypothetically speaking, it is possible that one subgroup is distinct from the others because the children in this subgroup were extremely difficult to understand. In another subgroup, the children might struggle with morphology or syntax more than the children in other subgroups. These subtype-specific characteristics may provide clues of associated impairments and suggest therapy targets in addition to speech-related targets.

3. What are some fundamental differences between the CDCV model and the CDRV model?

The CDCV model posits that risk variants of many genes, each of a potentially small effect, must converge on a single individual to confer disease susceptibility. To find the causal genes, one would study many affected individuals from different families. Disease subtypes would be difficult to define, because an affected person would have a mix of causal gene variants. Therapy would address the observed deficits in each affected person but not necessarily any associated or underlying processes. The CDRV posits that in a given family, only one or very few gene variants cause the disease and that different variants can run in different families, causing traits of distinct subtypes. To find the causal genes, one would study entire families. If distinct subtypes emerge from observing the speech characteristics in these families, then these can become biologically defined diagnostic labels and therapy can address underlying processes.

4. How can knowledge of genetic etiologies inform the field of speech-language pathology?

First, as mentioned, genetic mechanisms could define SSD subtypes based on etiology. Second, knowing which gene variant caused SSD in a given child would allow the clinician to make a more precise diagnosis than previously possible. Third, it is possible that children who share the same genetic SSD subtype also share underlying disorder characteristics such as deficits in motor sequencing that could be addressed in therapy in more sophisticated ways. Fourth, children with risk genotypes can be identified early and become candidates for early preventative intervention. Lastly, knowing the genetic causes of SSD can motivate biochemical studies leading to pharmaceutical interventions in the future.

5. In the future, how can a better understanding of genetic causes benefit a child with SSD?

Suppose that one day in the future, a gene is identified that, when disrupted, causes one of the SSD subtypes. Suppose also that in a given family, a child has been diagnosed with this subtype based on his speech profile and also his genotype. This child can now benefit from specially designed therapy targeting the characteristic and associated deficits of this SSD subtype. The parents are concerned about a younger sibling, still an infant. If the infant carries the risk variant, early intervention may be considered. If the infant does not carry the risk variant, it may be reasonable to suspect that early intervention will not be necessary and to adopt a wait-and-see strategy.

References

Bauman-Wängler, J. A. (2004). *Articulatory and phonological impairments: a clinical focus* (2nd ed.). Boston, MA: Pearson/Allyn and Bacon.

Bishop, D. V. (2002). Motor immaturity and specific speech and language impairment: evidence for a common genetic basis. *Am. J. Med. Genet., 114*(1), 56-63. doi: 10.1002/ajmg.1630 [pii].

Conti-Ramsden, G., Crutchley, A., and Botting, N. (1997). The extent to which psychometric tests differentiate subgroups of children with SLI. *J. Speech Lang Hear Res., 40*(4), 765-777.

Davis, B. L., Jakielski, K. J., and Marquardt, T. P. (1998). Developmental apraxia of speech: Determiners of differential diagnosis. *Clin. Ling. Phon, 12*(1), 25-45.

Dodd, B. (2005). Differential diagnosis and treatment of children with speech disorder (2nd ed.). London; Philadelphia: Whurr.

Felsenfeld, S., and Plomin, R. (1997). Epidemiological and offspring analyses of developmental speech disorders using data from the Colorado Adoption Project. *J. Speech Lang Hear Res., 40*(4), 778-791.

Fisher, S. E., Vargha-Khadem, F., Watkins, K. E., Monaco, A. P., and Pembrey, M. E. (1998). Localisation of a gene implicated in a severe speech and language disorder. *Nat. Genet., 18*(2), 168-170. doi: 10.1038/ng0298-168.

Fox, A. V., Dodd, B., and Howard, D. (2002). Risk factors for speech disorders in children. *Int. J. Lang Commun. Disord., 37*(2), 117-131. doi: 10.1080/13682820110116776.

Guyatt, G. H., Sackett, D. L., and Cook, D. J. (1994). Users' guides to the medical literature. II. How to use an article about therapy or prevention. B. What were the results and will they help me in caring for my patients? Evidence-Based Medicine Working Group. *JAMA, 271*(1), 59-63.

Ingram, D. (1976). *P*honological disability in children: Studies in language disability and remediation, 2nd Ed. New York: Elsevier.

Katz, D. L. (2001). Clinical epidemiology and evidence-based medicine: fundamental principles of clinical reasoning and research. Thousand Oaks, Calif.: Sage Publications.

Konig, I. R., Schumacher, J., Hoffmann, P., Kleensang, A., Ludwig, K. U., Grimm, T., . . . Schulte-Korne, G. (2011). Mapping for dyslexia and related cognitive trait loci provides strong evidence for further risk genes on chromosome 6p21. *Am. J. Med. Genet. B Neuropsychiatr. Genet., 156B*(1), 36-43. doi: 10.1002/ajmg.b.31135.

Lewis, B., Qui, F., Freebairn, L., Truitt, B., Joseph, P., Raghavendra, R., . . . Stein, C. (2011). *Candidate genes for speech sound disorders*. Paper presented at the American Speech-Language-Hearing Association Convention, San Diego.

Lewis, B. A. (1992). Pedigree analysis of children with phonology disorders. *J. Learn Disabil, 25*(9), 586-597.

Lewis, B. A., Freebairn, L. A., Hansen, A. J., Stein, C. M., Shriberg, L. D., Iyengar, S. K., and Gerry Taylor, H. (2006). Dimensions of early speech sound disorders: A factor analytic study. *J. Commun. Disord., 39*(2), 139-157. doi: S0021-9924(05)00063-8 [pii] 10.1016/j.jcomdis.2005.11.003.

Ling, H., Polke, J. M., Sweeney, M. G., Haworth, A., Sandford, C. A., Heales, S. J., . . . Lees, A. J. (2011). An intragenic duplication in guanosine triphosphate cyclohydrolase-1 gene in a dopa-responsive dystonia family. *Mov. Disord.*, Epub ahead of print. doi: 10.1002/mds.23593.

MacDermot, K. D., Bonora, E., Sykes, N., Coupe, A. M., Lai, C. S., Vernes, S. C., . . . Fisher, S. E. (2005). Identification of FOXP2 truncation as a novel cause of developmental speech and language deficits. *Am. J. Hum. Genet., 76*(6), 1074-1080. doi: S0002-9297(07)62902-4 [pii] 10.1086/430841.

Miscimarra, L., Stein, C., Millard, C., Kluge, A., Cartier, K., Freebairn, L., . . . Iyengar, S. K. (2007). Further evidence of pleiotropy influencing speech and language: analysis of the DYX8 region. *Hum. Hered., 63*(1), 47-58. doi: 000098727 [pii] 10.1159/000098727.

Nopola-Hemmi, J., Myllyluoma, B., Haltia, T., Taipale, M., Ollikainen, V., Ahonen, T., . . . Widen, E. (2001). A dominant gene for developmental dyslexia on chromosome 3. *J. Med. Genet., 38*(10), 658-664.

Oxman, A. D., and Guyatt, G. H. (1993). The science of reviewing research. *Ann. NY Acad. Sci., 703*, 125-133; discussion 133-124.

Oxman, A. D., Sackett, D. L., and Guyatt, G. H. (1993). Users' guides to the medical literature. I. How to get started. The Evidence-Based Medicine Working Group. *JAMA, 270*(17), 2093-2095.

Ozanne, A. (1995). The search for developmental verbal dyspraxia. In B. Dodd (Ed.), *Differential diagnosis of children with speech disorders* (pp. 91-109). London: Whurr.

Pennington, B. F., and Bishop, D. V. (2009). Relations among speech, language, and reading disorders. *Annu. Rev. Psychol., 60*, 283-306. doi: 10.1146/annurev.psych.60.110707.163548.

Peter, B. (2006). Multivariate characteristics and data-based disorder classification in children with speech disorders of unknown origin: WorldCat Dissertations and Theses.

Peter, B. (2010). Complex disorder traits in a three-year-old boy with a severe speech-sound disorder. In S. Chabon and E. Cohn (Eds.), *Communication disorders: A case-based approach*. Delaware: Pearson.

Peter, B., Matsushita, M., and Raskind, W. H. (2011). Global processing speed in children with low reading ability and in children and adults with typical reading ability: exploratory factor analytic models. *J. Speech Lang Hear Res., 54*(3), 885-899. doi: 1092-4388_2010_10-0135 [pii] 10.1044/1092-4388(2010/10-0135).

Peter, B., Matsushita, M., and Raskind, W. H. (2012). Motor sequencing deficit as an endophenotype of speech sound disorder: A genome-wide linkage analysis in a multigenerational family. *Psychiatric Genetics*. Epub ahead of print. PMID: 22517379.

Peter, B., and Raskind, W. H. (2011). Evidence for a familial speech sound disorder subtype in a multigenerational study of oral and hand motor sequencing ability. *Topics in Language Disorders, 31*(2), 145-167. doi: 10.1097/TLD.0b013e318217b855.

Peter, B., and Stoel-Gammon, C. (2008). Central timing deficits in subtypes of primary speech disorders. *Clin. Linguist. Phon., 22*(3), 171-198. doi: 791036551 [pii] 10.1080/02699200701799825.

Potter, N. L., Lazarus, J. A., Johnson, J. M., Steiner, R. D., and Shriberg, L. D. (2008). Correlates of language impairment in children with galactosaemia. *J. Inherit. Metab. Dis., 31*(4), 524-532. doi: 10.1007/s10545-008-0877-y.

Segawa, M. (2011). Hereditary progressive dystonia with marked diurnal fluctuation. *Brain Dev, 33*(3), 195-201. doi: S0387-7604(10)00278-0 [pii] 10.1016/j.braindev.2010.10.015.

Shriberg, L. D., Fourakis, M., Hall, S. D., Karlsson, H. B., Lohmeier, H. L., McSweeny, J. L., . . . Wilson, D. L. (2010). Extensions to the Speech Disorders Classification System (SDCS). *Clin. Linguist. Phon., 24*(10), 795-824. doi: 10.3109/02699206.2010.503006/

Shriberg, L. D., and Kwiatkowski, J. (1982a). Phonological disorders I: a diagnostic classification system. *J. Speech Hear Disord., 47*(3), 226-241.

Shriberg, L. D., and Kwiatkowski, J. (1982b). Phonological disorders II: a conceptual framework for management. *J. Speech Hear Disord., 47*(3), 242-256.

Shriberg, L. D., and Kwiatkowski, J. (1982c). Phonological disorders III: a procedure for assessing severity of involvement. *J. Speech Hear Disord., 47*(3), 256-270.

Shriberg, L. D., Potter, N. L., and Strand, E. A. (2010). Prevalence and Phenotype of Childhood Apraxia of Speech In Youth with Galactosemia. *J. Speech Lang Hear Res.*. doi: 1092-4388_2010_10-0068 [pii]. 10.1044/1092-4388(2010/10-0068).

Smith, S. D., Pennington, B. F., Boada, R., and Shriberg, L. D. (2005). Linkage of speech sound disorder to reading disability loci. *J. Child Psychol. Psychiatry, 46*(10), 1057-1066. doi: JCPP1534 [pii] 10.1111/j.1469-7610.2005.01534.x.

Stackhouse, J., and Pascoe, M. (2010). Psycholinguistic intervention. In A. L. Williams, S. McLeod and R. J. McCauley (Eds.), *Interventions for Speech Sound Disorders in Children* (pp. 219 - 245). Baltimore: Brookes.

Stackhouse, J., and Wells, B. (1997). Children's speech and literacy difficulties: a psycholinguistic framework. San Diego, Calif. London, England: Singular Pub. Group; Whurr Publishers.

Stackhouse, J., and Wells, B. (2001). Identification and intervention. London Philadelphia;: Whurr Publishers.

Stein, C. M., Millard, C., Kluge, A., Miscimarra, L. E., Cartier, K. C., Freebairn, L. A., . . . Iyengar, S. K. (2006). Speech sound disorder influenced by a locus in 15q14 region. *Behav. Genet., 36*(6), 858-868. doi: 10.1007/s10519-006-9090-7.

Stein, C. M., Schick, J. H., Gerry Taylor, H., Shriberg, L. D., Millard, C., Kundtz-Kluge, A., . . . Iyengar, S. K. (2004). Pleiotropic effects of a chromosome 3 locus on speech-sound disorder and reading. *Am. J. Hum. Genet., 74*(2), 283-297. doi: S0002-9297(07)61839-4 [pii] 10.1086/381562.

Terband, H., Maassen, B., van Lieshout, P., and Nijland, L. (2011). Stability and composition of functional synergies for speech movements in children with developmental speech disorders. *J. Commun. Disord., 44*(1), 59-74. doi: S0021-9924(10)00062-6 [pii] 10.1016/j.jcomdis.2010.07.003.

Vargha-Khadem, F., Watkins, K., Alcock, K., Fletcher, P., and Passingham, R. (1995). Praxic and nonverbal cognitive deficits in a large family with a genetically transmitted speech and language disorder. *Proc. Natl. Acad. Sci. USA, 92*(3), 930-933.

Watkins, K. E., Dronkers, N. F., and Vargha-Khadem, F. (2002). Behavioural analysis of an inherited speech and language disorder: comparison with acquired aphasia. *Brain, 125*(Pt 3), 452-464.

Williams, A. L., McLeod, S., and McCauley, R. J. (2010). *Interventions for speech sound disorders in children*. Baltimore: Brookes.

In: Comprehensive Perspectives …
Editors: Beate Peter and Andrea A. N. MacLeod
ISBN: 978-1-62257-041-6

Chapter 16

INTERACTIONS BETWEEN SPEECH SOUND DISORDER AND DYSLEXIA

Beate Peter

INTRODUCTION

Most children acquire the ability to comprehend and produce spoken language naturally within the first few years of life, but learning to read and write usually requires formal instruction that starts around 5 years of age and can continue into adulthood.

This is true for all types of writing systems, including logographic systems such as that used in China, where a written character represents a unit of meaning; syllabic systems like the Japanese *hiragana* or *katagana* scripts where a written symbol represents a syllable; and alphabetic systems like the Cyrillic script used in Russian or the Latin-based script used in most Western European languages including English, where a written symbol generally represents a speech sound.

In English, speech sounds and their alphabetic representations are related to each other via extraordinarily complex relationships. To become a successful reader and speller, a child needs to not only have a functional mental representation of speech sounds as phonemic units and as sequential strings but also master the complex association patterns between letters and sounds and memorize written word forms that do not follow standard spelling rules. Many children with speech sound disorders (SSDs) struggle with at least one of these basic prerequisites in that their mental representation of speech sounds is deficient.

The goal of this chapter is to explore the interactions between speech sound development and literacy skills. Following a description of English orthography, I outline some of the core and associated traits of dyslexia, cite demographic data on the co-occurrence of SSD and dyslexia, and end with some thoughts about shared substrates and disorder subtypes in both of these disorders. A discussion of speech and literacy development in languages other than English is beyond the scope of this chapter.

The Written Code of English

"Pleaf," "meng," and "shextine" are not real words in English. They convey no meaning, but you can sound them out by applying what you know about rule-based English orthography: As you probably learned when you first were introduced to spelling, many letters have a fixed assigned sound value. For instance, "f" is always pronounced as the voiceless labiodental fricative /f/ and "m" is always pronounced as the bilabial nasal /m/. A little later, you probably also learned that the letter sequence "ng," when seen in word-final position, represents a single sound, the velar nasal /ŋ/, and that the letter sequence "sh" represents a single sound, the voiceless palatal fricative /ʃ/. A sequence of two letters representing one sound is referred to as a *digraph*, and English has several additional ones, e.g., "ee," "ou," "ch", "ck", and "ph." Conversely, the single letter "x" represents a sequence of two sounds, /ks/. Finally, you may have learned rules such as these: The "magic e" makes the vowel before the intervening consonant say its name, and: "When two vowels go walking, the first one does the talking." This is essentially all you need to know to *decode* the nonwords at the beginning of this paragraph.

Orthographic rules predict how strings of letters should be pronounced and, hence, describe the inherent associations between the written symbol (the *grapheme*) and the sound it represents. In that sense, alphabetic languages encode their speech sounds with letters. In English, however, even rule-based spelling is not unambiguous. To cite just a few examples of the variability in the number of graphemes that can represent a single sound, /i/ can be represented with "ea" ("sea"), "ee" ("see"), "ie" ("believe"), "ei" ("receive"), or "e" + consonant (C) + "e" ("cede"). The sound /o/ can be represented with "ow" ("row"), "oe" ("roe"), "oa" ("road"), "o" + C + "e" ("rode"), "oh" ("oh!"), or simply "o" ("so"). There is a bit less variability in how many different sounds can be represented by the same grapheme. For instance, the digraph "th" before a vowel is used to represent both /θ/ ("thistle") and /ð/ ("this"); the digraph "oo" can represent both /ʊ/ ("book") and /u/ ("boot"), and the letter "u" in initial position can represent both /ʌ/ ("uncle") and /ju/ ("unanimous"). Orthographies where individual sounds can be represented by more than one grapheme and, conversely, individual graphemes stand for more than one sound, are referred to as *deep orthographies*, sometimes also referred to as *opaque orthographies*. This is in contrast to *shallow orthographies* or transparent orthographies such as that of Spanish, where letters and their sound values are aligned much less ambiguously.

Not only is the orthography of English deep, it also includes many words that do not follow its standard spelling rules. The word "bread" defies the rule about the two vowels going walking, the word "you" is not pronounced with the diphthong in the word "out," the words "have," "done," and "come" defy the "magic e" rule, and the words "caught," "sought," "draught," "laugh," and "should" are full of silent letters and other irregularities. The "-ue" ending is silent in "tongue" and "vague" but not in "argue." School children must memorize the spelling of these exception words as "*sight words*," a skill that benefits from repeated exposure in terms of automatic recognition. To make spelling these kinds of words a little easier, some teachers provide mnemonics such as "oh you little doggie" to memorize the letter sequence in "should" and "could."

One reason for the complexities in the orthography of English is the fact that English evolved from many diverse linguistic sources – in other words, the English we speak today has many ancestors. From its Anglo-Saxon origins dating back to the 5th century, it inherited words like "answer" (composed of the predecessor words for "against" and "swear") and "strong." Between AD 750 and 1050, invading Vikings imported words like "horse," "wagon," and "sell" to the British Isles. In the 11th century, the Anglo-Normans brought French influences to the Isles and, along with these, words like "indict," "jury," and "sovereign." During the Renaissance, Latin and Greek terms became popular and were incorporated into the language, including, for instance, the class of words ending in "-tion" from Latin and composite words containing the Greek word for life, "*bios*" and animal, "*zoon*." All these diverse influences resulted not only in multiple terms for the same *denotational* content (e.g., "answer," "reply," "respond," "retort," "rejoin") but also in an eclectic amalgam of spelling conventions that coexist as linguistic fossils of their various ancestries. Not only does the English we speak and write today reflect its diverse linguistic ancestry, its orthography has also remained relatively stagnant across time in that it has undergone few attempts to unify and systematize. This results in different spelling conventions in different English-speaking countries and a mismatch between obsolete spelling conventions in the presence of changing pronunciation conventions. For instance, the "k" in "knife," "know," and "knee" was actually pronounced up until the 17th century. Languages such as French or German have overseeing organizations that propose orthographic reforms among other functions at regular intervals, although their implementations have been controversial.The mixed linguistic ancestry of English, together with its stagnant orthography over time, resulted in an alphabetic script that requires considerable effort to master. In his preface to a book on the history of language (Wilson and Shaw, 1942), George Bernard Shaw remarked,

> Thus an intelligent child who is bidden to spell debt, and very properly spells it d-e-t, is caned for not spelling it with a b because Julius Caesar spelt the Latin word for it with a b.

Learning to read and spell any alphabetical language requires *phonemic awareness,* also referred to as *phonological awareness,* defined as a well-specified mental representation of speech sounds. Phonological awareness applies not only to features of isolated units of sounds (/ʃ/ is different from /s/) but also to sequential strings of sounds (the order of the sounds in /lɛft/ and /fɛlt/ distinguishes between two different words; the words "mouse" and "house" rhyme because they share their middle and end sounds; removing the /b/ sound from the word "broom" results in a different word). Other pre-reading skills include understanding that letters represent words and sentences, knowing how to hold a book and which direction the text flows, knowing the meanings of words, and being able to follow a story. To master the orthography of English in particular, children are not only asked to learn the sound value of each letter, where some of the letter names bear little resemblance to the actual sound ("h," "y"), but also to acquire the complex associations among speech sounds and letters used to represent them. In addition, they need to understand some fundamental features of word shapes, for instance the basic facts that a word consists of at least one syllable and that each syllable must contain one vowel sound represented by at least one vowel letter. Furthermore, they must memorize the spelling of word shape classes such as words ending in "-le," "-ce," or "-tion." Lastly, they must memorize the spelling of sight words that do not easily fit into any spelling convention, such as "have," "you," "know," "psyche," and "four"/"fourteen"/"forty." Learning to read and spell English, hence, is a tall order for any child, and it comes as no surprise that spelling bees were invented in the United States.

Dyslexia: Definition, Associated Traits, and Causes

Definition

The International Dyslexia Association (Lyon, Shaywitz, and Shaywitz, 2003) narrowly defines dyslexia as a specific disability that interferes with the acquisition of written language at the word level, characterized by deficits in accurate and/or fluent word recognition, decoding, and spelling. These difficulties are not associated with variations in cognitive ability or quality of reading instruction, and they are thought to have a neurobiological origin. Here are some actual examples of children whose difficulty with reading and/or spelling do *not* meet the dyslexia criteria: A 10-year-old boy whose mother had never sent him to school was finally placed in foster care and began attending a fourth-grade class without any prior reading skills at all. His initial struggles with reading and spelling resulted from lack of access to instruction, not dyslexia. A girl in fifth grade was able to read individual words correctly but had difficulty answering questions about the content in paragraph-level text. Her difficulties were in the area of reading comprehension and could have been caused by a number of underlying problems, for instance short-term memory deficits or difficulty with drawing inferences. A sixth grader with substantial delays in reading grade-level texts also had difficulty comprehending orally presented information. She had a general deficit in comprehension that was not specific to written language. A 16-year-old high school student had recently arrived in the United States from an African country and was still in the process of acquiring spoken and written English. His reading and spelling errors were caused by lack of exposure to English, not dyslexia. In the past, a diagnosis of dyslexia was restricted to cases where reading ability was substantially lower than measures of verbal and/or nonverbal IQ. This so-called IQ discrepancy criterion, however, has been called into question (Fletcher, Francis, Rourke, Shaywitz, and Shaywitz, 1992; Stanovich, 1991). Critics have pointed out, among other things, that poor readers with low IQ and poor readers with average or high IQ have similar difficulties with sounding out unfamiliar words and with phonological processing. An alternate approach to determine the presence and severity of dyslexia is Response to Intervention (RTI), introduced in the 2004 Reauthorization of the Individuals with Disabilities Education Act (IDEA), where a child with difficulties in reading and writing, given adequate classroom instruction, receives additional and/or more individual interventions, and if the difficulties persist, the next level of interventions (usually delivered as special education) is provided.

Associated Behaviorally Observed Deficits

In addition to the core deficits in sounding out orthographically spelled words and recognizing sight words, associated deficits have been observed when groups of individuals with dyslexia were compared with typical controls. An early finding was that children with low reading ability had difficulty with auditory perception of nonspeech sounds when the stimuli were presented rapidly, and that the children's performance on this task was associated with their phonologic decoding skills (Tallal, 1980). Whether or not this temporal auditory deficit is causal to aspects of reading impairment is the subject of debate. As recently reviewed in detail (Catts, Kamhi, and Adlof, 2012), some subsequent studies have replicated the findings in Tallal (1980) whereas others have not, or have reported deficits in the auditory perception of speech but not nonspeech stimuli. One possible explanation for these discrepancies is that only a subset of individuals with dyslexia shows evidence of rapid auditory processing deficits (Boets, Wouters, van Wieringen, and Ghesquiere, 2007; Ramus, 2003).

An extensive body of research shows that individuals with dyslexia have deficits in phonological processing skills. For instance, individuals with dyslexia tend to have difficulty with dissecting words into individual sounds and making changes to their sequence, compared to individuals without dyslexia (Bradley and Bryant, 1983; Fletcher et al., 1994). They also have difficulty with phonological memory, i.e., uploading and storing speech sounds in memory. A task like nonword imitation is frequently used to assess phonological short-term memory. Difficulty with phonological retrieval from long-term memory is also frequently observed in individuals with dyslexia. For instance, during naming tasks where a word was produced in response to a picture, children with dyslexia were slower and less accurate than children without dyslexia (Catts, 1986; Denckla and Rudel, 1976). Producing complex strings of speech sound is also more difficult for individuals with dyslexia compared to controls without dyslexia. For instance, in a naming task where the pictured objects had complicated names and in a word imitation task where the stimuli contained complex speech sound sequences, adolescents with dyslexia made more errors than their controls without dyslexia (Catts, 1986). College students with a history of dyslexia imitated complex words and phrases at a slower rate and with more errors than peers without a history of dyslexia (Catts, 1989). Slower rate has been observed not only in the phonological productions of individuals with dyslexia but also in a wide variety of other tasks. In a cohort of third graders, slower response times were seen during motor, visual, lexical, grammatical, and phonological measures as well as in rapid naming (Catts, Gillispie, Leonard, Kail, and Miller, 2002). A longitudinal study of 27 children, most of whom were at high familial risk for dyslexia, showed that those who received a diagnosis of dyslexia in grade school had substantially slower speaking rates at ages 2 and 3 years, compared to those who did not develop dyslexia (Smith, Smith, Locke, and Bennett, 2008). In a large sample of families with evidence of *familial* dyslexia, we found that scores from a wide variety of timed tasks including motor, rapid naming, executive functioning, and alphabet writing tasks were heavily cross-correlated and children with poor reading scores showed evidence of globally slower processing speeds, compared to children with average or high reading scores (Peter, Matsushita, and Raskind, 2011).

Associated Anatomical and Physiological Deficits

In addition to the behavioral traits often seen in individuals with dyslexia, some physical traits have been observed, in particular with respect to brain anatomy and physiology. One of the earliest anatomical findings was that the brains of individuals with dyslexia contained neuron bodies that were of abnormal size and neurons that had not migrated to their target locations correctly.

As mentioned in Chapter 3, neurons follow a systematic migration pattern during fetal development as the cell layers of the cortex are formed. Subtle deficits in cortical migration patterns were observed in some postmortem studies of adults with a history of dyslexia (Galaburda, Sherman, Rosen, Aboitiz, and Geschwind, 1985). Another discovery that came from these postmortem studies was that the planum temporale, a cortical region located on the superior temporal gyrus that has functional importance for auditory and linguistic processing, was equally large in the left and right hemispheres in the brains of individuals with dyslexia, whereas in typical individuals, the planum temporale in the right hemisphere is smaller than that in the left (Galaburda, Menard, and Rosen, 1994; Livingstone, Rosen, Drislane, and Galaburda, 1991).

This lack of asymmetry in the brains of individuals with dyslexia, however, has not been replicated in some studies (Eckert et al., 2003). More recently, research results suggested that this lack of asymmetry is seen more frequently in individuals with poor reading ability who also have impaired language ability, compared to individuals who fit the narrow definition of dyslexia (Leonard and Eckert, 2008). As reviewed in more detail elsewhere (Catts et al., 2012; M. Eckert, 2004; Peterson, McGrath, Smith, and Pennington, 2007), other structural differences have been described in various other regions including the cerebellum.

A newer body of literature describes structural abnormalities in the brains of individuals with dyslexia with respect to white matter, which is made up of glial cells surrounding and insulating the axons of neurons. White matter deficiencies have been observed in temporoparietal fiber tracts in the left hemisphere (Deutsch et al., 2005; Klingberg et al., 2000; Niogi and McCandliss, 2006) and the corpus callosum (Frye et al., 2008).

Functional brain imaging studies, as extensively reviewed (Peterson et al., 2007; Sandak, Mencl, Frost, and Pugh, 2004), have shown that certain brain regions are actively involved in reading tasks in typical individuals.

These regions include two posterior left-hemisphere regions, 1) the superior temporal gyrus that is thought to process phonological information and associations between letters and sounds (this region is sometimes referred to as the temporoparietal system, which includes the planum temporale and the angular gyrus) and 2) the fusiform gyrus that is thought to process visual word forms (this region is also sometimes referred to as the occipitotemporal system and encompasses areas in the left inferior boundary region of the occipital and temporal lobes).

A third region is located in the inferior frontal gyrus in the frontal lobe (an area encompassing Broca's area) and it is thought to support effortful phonological decoding or articulatory recoding, tapping into the articulatory system. Figure 16.1 shows these areas. Many studies of individuals with dyslexia report underactivation of the left fusiform gyrus, interpreted as being related to impaired word recognition, and underactivation in the superior temporal gyrus, interpreted as related to difficulties with phonologic processing, whereas studies of the inferior frontal gyrus have reported either underactivation or overactivation, where overactivation has been interpreted as compensational activity. To add a caveat, whether or not differences in brain structure and function are the cause or the result of reading difficulties cannot be determined with certainty.

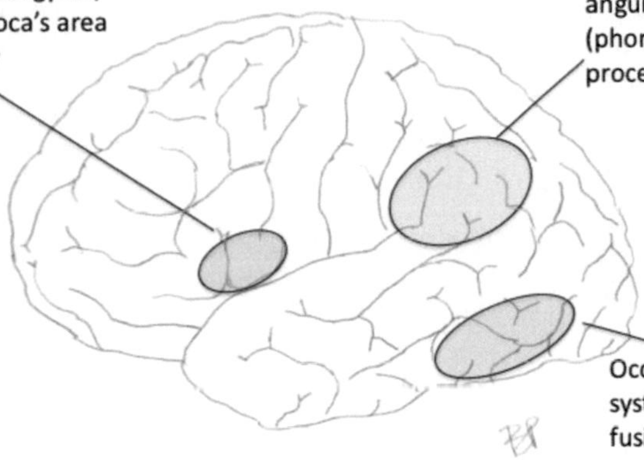

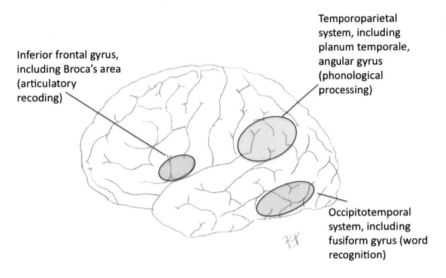

Figure 16.1. Areas of brain activation during reading in typical readers.

Genetic Findings

Dyslexia frequently runs in families and evidence for a genetic etiology is strong. The current assumption is that dyslexia results when many genes are disrupted in the same individual. In this theoretical framework, dyslexia is viewed as a *quantitative trait* where the *expression* and severity of the disorder depend on the number and type of disrupted genes. To date, no causal gene has been identified and validated, but several candidate regions and genes have been found using a variety of molecular and statistical methods. As extensively reviewed elsewhere (Catts et al., 2012; Lewis et al., 2006; Pennington, 1990; Pennington and Bishop, 2009; Peterson et al., 2007), candidate regions include loci on chromosomes 1, 2, 3, 6, 15, 18, and X. New candidate regions continue to emerge. For instance, a locus on chromosome 6p21 was identified in a genome-wide study in a sample of children with dyslexia and their siblings, using a rapid naming task of objects and colors (Konig et al., 2011). The list of candidate genes that are located within the candidate regions includes one called *ROBO1*, located on chromosome 3, that functions as an axon guidance receptor gene, and another one called *DCDC2*, located on chromosome 6, that is involved in the migration of cortical cells during prenatal development. New candidate genes continue to be proposed. For instance, in a large German sample of children with dyslexia (Roeske et al., 2009), a measure of brain response to speech sounds called mismatch negativity was found to be associated with a marker on chromosome 4q32.1. This region does not code for proteins but was found to be functionally associated with a gene on chromosome 12, *SLC2A3*, that facilitates glucose transport in neurons.

Demographics of Speech Sound Disorder and Dyslexia

Miles (all real names in this chapter have been changed) was a first grader who had been referred to the speech-language pathologist (SLP) at his public school for an evaluation of his speech. His teacher was concerned that his speech was very difficult to understand. The SLP conducted an assessment and concluded that Miles had a severe speech sound disorder (SSD) with evidence of many phonological processes, especially involving consonant clusters. Some of his speech sound errors were quite unusual. For instance, both /s, t/ were in his phoneme inventory, but he reduced /st/ clusters to the component singleton [s] instead of [t], which is more commonly found in children who reduce clusters, and he reduced /pl/ and /fl/ clusters to the singleton [ʃ], a sound not even part of the target cluster and resembling the cluster only in that it is voiceless like the stop consonant in the target clusters and continuant like the liquid consonant in the target cluster. Language testing did not reveal clinical deficits in the areas of vocabulary, comprehension, or expression. Miles began twice weekly speech sessions, where he made steady but slow progress.

In addition to qualifying for speech services at his school, Miles also received special support in the area of reading. He had extreme difficulty with learning to read and his progress, even with a lot of extra help, was slow. Clearly, Miles struggled in the two areas of speech and literacy. Was this just a coincidence, or were the two deficits somehow causally related?

Before we venture a guess, let's explore the associations between speech production and literacy skills from a demographic perspective. Prevalence estimates of SSD range from approximately 1% to 15.6% and are not only influenced by age and gender but also by the quantitative criteria selected to identify children with SSD. For example, using a criterion of 75% intelligible productions in spontaneous speech, Campbell and colleagues (Campbell et al., 2003) estimated that 15.6% of three-year-old children have SSD. Using a standard score of -1.14 in a 20-item articulation test, Shriberg and colleagues (Shriberg, Tomblin, and McSweeny, 1999) reported a prevalence rate of 3.8% in six-year-old children. Using a four-stage process of identification, including teacher report and a speech-language pathologist report, McKinnon and colleagues (McKinnon, McLeod, and Reilly, 2007) identified approximately 1.1% of children in an Australian school-age sample in Kindergarten through 6th grade as having SSD.

SSD prevalence rates differ for males and females. The general consensus is that more boys than girls have this type of disorder, but estimates of the male:female ratio vary. Shriberg et al. (1999), whose population-based study of 1,328 six-year-old children was stratified by gender, racial categories, and socioeconomic factors, reported male:female ratios as low as 1.2:1 (1.2 boys for every girl) and as high as 2.4:1. Campbell et al. (2003) reported that 70 out of 100 study participants with SSD were boys, a male:female ratio of 2.3:1.

Similar to prevalence estimates of SSD, prevalence estimates of reading disability as defined by difficulties learning to read accurately and fluently vary by the criteria used to and the statistical cutoff. Commonly cited prevalence estimates range from 5% (Francks, MacPhie, and Monaco, 2002) to 9% (Pennington and Bishop, 2009; Peterson et al., 2007) of school-age children.

Also similar to the demographics of SSD, poor reading ability in general is seen more frequently in males than in females, with male:female ratios ranging from 1.3:1 to 3.3:1

(Rutter et al., 2004; Shaywitz, Shaywitz, Fletcher, and Escobar, 1990). Recent research suggests that high male:female ratios may be an artifact of over-referrals from school and clinical settings. In a comparison between a researcher-identified sample of poor readers whose reading scores were at least 1.5 standard deviations (SDs) below their IQ and a school-identified sample of poor readers who qualified for special services, the researcher-identified sample had a male:female ratio of 1.3:1 whereas the school-identified sample had a male:female ratio of 4:1 (Shaywitz et al., 1990). The authors suspect that school-referred samples are influenced by behavioral factors that affect boys and girls differently, for instance attention, level of activity, and classroom behaviors.

As with the classification frameworks for SSD described in the chapter on SSD subtypes in this volume, poor reading ability in children has been variously classified.

The Simple View of Reading (Aaron, Joshi, and Williams, 1999; Carver, 1993; Catts, Hogan, and Fey, 2003; Gough and Tunmer, 1986), which is based on a broad definition of reading disability regardless of associated language deficits, sorts poor readers into two binary variables, good vs. poor written word recognition and good vs. poor listening comprehension. Children with good listening comprehension but poor written word recognition fit the narrow dyslexia definition proposed by the International Dyslexia Association (Lyon et al., 2003). Children with poor performance in both listening comprehension and written word recognition fall into the category of mixed comprehension deficit, and children with poor listening comprehension but good word recognition fall into the category of specific comprehension deficit, sometimes also referred to as hyperlexia. The Simple View of Reading includes a fourth category of children who have good word recognition skills and good listening skills and who fail to comprehend when reading but comprehend well when the text is read to them.

In addition to the Simple View of Reading, other frameworks of reading disability have been proposed. Examples include the visual attention span deficit hypothesis (Bosse, Tainturier, and Valdois, 2007) that posits that a limit in the amount of visual information that can be processed in parallel contributes to difficulties with reading, and the auditory hypothesis (Tallal, 1980) that posits a general deficit in processing auditory stimuli including nonlinguistic ones.

Within the narrow definition of dyslexia, the fact that reading involves two different processes, decoding words by applying orthographic rules and recognizing irregularly spelled sight words, has given rise to the question whether specific impairment in either of these two processes presents a clinical dyslexia subtype. Impairment with decoding but not sight word recognition has been termed, among other labels, "phonological dyslexia" whereas the reverse case has been termed "surface dyslexia." Deficits in both areas have been labeled "alexia," "mixed dyslexia," or "deep dyslexia" (Marshall and Newcombe, 1973). It turns out, however, that children do not seem to fall neatly into distinct deficit categories of decoding vs. sight word recognition; instead, most have some difficulty with both of these processes, and impairment in only one of these areas is seen less frequently (Castles and Coltheart, 1993; Stanovich, Siegel, and Gottardo, 1997). It is thought that children who struggle relatively more with sight words than with decoding regularly spelled words originally had difficulties with both types of reading processes but had received interventions that targeted decoding skills more than sight word recognition (Murphy and Pollatsek, 1994; Stanovich et al., 1997). Children who struggle more with decoding regularly spelled words than with recognizing sight words, on the other hand, appear to have a distinct dyslexia disorder subtype characterized by phonological processing deficits (Stanovich et al., 1997) that is likely to have a genetic etiology (Castles, Datta, Gayan, and Olson, 1999).

What follows next is a discussion of *comorbidity*. In general, the proportion of individuals who have two different disorders simultaneously by chance will the product of the two disorder prevalence rates. For instance, in Shriberg et al.'s (1999) demographic study of SSD and *language impairment* in 1,328 six-year-old children in the United States, 3.8% had SSD and 8.1% had language impairment. Under random conditions, one would expect 0.3% of all children in the sample to have both SSD and language impairment, based on the joint probability of both prevalence rates (0.38 X 0.81 = 0.003). It was found, however, that 0.5% of the children had both SSD and language impairment, a proportion rate that is slightly higher than expected under random conditions and is consistent with an association between the two disorder types. Incidentally, studies in younger children have reported higher comorbidity rates (Beitchman et al., 1986; Shriberg and Austin, 1998), perhaps because SSD is substantially more prevalent in younger children, compared to school-age children.

The discrepancy between SSD/language impairment comorbidity among preschoolers and school-age children points to one of the difficulties of estimating disorder comorbidities. When prevalence rates of one or both disorders vary as a function of factors such as age or intervention effects, estimates of comorbidity are automatically affected. This is especially relevant for estimating SSD/dyslexia comorbidity rates, as SSD is frequently diagnosed and treated in preschoolers whereas dyslexia cannot be diagnosed and treated until well after the onset of literacy instruction, typically in the early school years. Therefore, it is possible that a child with SSD during the preschool years shows little evidence of SSD when reading instruction begins. To estimate comorbidity, studies have either used a retrospective design where children with poor reading ability were evaluated for a history of SSD (this type of study is rare), or a prospective design where children with current evidence of SSD were followed to determine whether or not they developed reading problems (a more common type of study). As a caveat, in children with SSD who are being evaluated for dyslexia, it is important to differentiate between true reading errors and reading errors caused by the SSD. An example would be a child who does not have /ɹ/ and who reads [wɪŋ]/ for "ring."

Some of the earliest studies reported that children with speech disorders had an increased risk for developing deficits in written language later on, but the current consensus is that children with SSD are not at risk unless there is also evidence of language impairment and/or deficits in phonological processing. In an early study reporting reading deficits in children with SSD, a mixed sample of 15 children with SSD, 41 children with language impairment, 56 children with both SSD and language impairment, and 30 typically developing children was ascertained (Catts, 1993). The children with SSD obtained slightly lower word reading scores, compared to the typically developing controls, whereas those with language impairment obtained by far the lowest scores and the children with both SSD and language impairment obtained intermediate scores. Similarly, in a study of 5-year-old children with speech difficulties (Bird, Bishop, and Freeman, 1995), phonological awareness problems were observed at age 6 and 7 years and most of these children showed literacy deficits regardless of whether they also had language impairments. In a longitudinal study of preschoolers with moderate to severe SSD, those with evidence of concomitant language impairment went on to have more difficulty with learning to read and spell than those with only SSD; the children with SSD had reading scores that were within normal limits but spelling scores that were below expectation (Lewis, Freebairn, and Taylor, 2000).

More recently, evidence suggests that the risk for developing reading problems in the presence of SSD alone may be negligible. In a study comparing ten children with childhood apraxia of speech (CAS) to 15 children with non-CAS SSD and 14 children with non-CAS SSD and language impairment, the children with CAS showed substantial difficulties with decoding, word recognition, reading comprehension, and spelling, whereas the children with non-CAS SSD had average scores in these tasks and the children with non-CAS SSD and language impairment obtained scores in the low average range (Lewis, Freebairn, Hansen, Iyengar, and Taylor, 2004). As detailed in Chapter 15 about disorder SSD subtypes in this volume, CAS is defined as a motor-based speech disorder with deficits in motor planning and/or motor programming, resulting in difficulties with the sequential movements of speech. In a study of 125 children with SSD, age 3 to 6 years, reading readiness scores and early writing skills were substantially below expectation in those children who also showed evidence of language impairment, whereas reading and writing scores appeared to be unaffected by the presence of SSD alone (Sices, Taylor, Freebairn, Hansen, and Lewis, 2007). Several other studies also reported no elevated risks of reading difficulties in children with SSD only (Bishop and Edmundson, 1987; Snowling, Stothard, Bishop, Chipchase, and Kaplan, 1998).

One proposed explanation why concomitant language impairment increases the dyslexia risk in children with SSD is the "semantic bootstrapping" hypothesis (Snowling, 2005). According to this hypothesis, poor readers rely on semantic cues to compensate for their deficits in word recognition or decoding. Children with language impairment are less able to use these semantic cues, resulting in lower reading performance.

Severity and persistence of SSD involvement may be related to comorbid difficulties with reading, and this may, in part, explain the discrepancies in the reported reading risks for children with SSD. The "critical age hypothesis" (Bishop and Adams, 1990) posits that children whose speech difficulties persist are at a higher risk for reading disabilities compared to those whose speech deficits resolve. Empirical evidence for this hypothesis exists. In a study of 39 7-year-old children with SSD and 35 controls with typical development, those children whose SSD had resolved by the time of the data collection performed as well as the control children in reading, reading comprehension, spelling, and mathematics, whereas those children with persisting SSD obtained lower scores in all areas and especially in spelling, compared to the controls (Nathan, Stackhouse, Goulandris, and Snowling, 2004).

Substrates Common to Speech Production and Literacy Skills

Back to Miles, the first grader with needs in the areas of speech production and literacy. His classroom teacher, SLP, and reading teacher consulted with each other and, following some testing in the area of phonemic awareness, agreed that the underlying difficulty was one of deficient mental representation of phonemes.

Together, they decided to adopt components of a program designed to build phonemic awareness using colored symbols to represent individual sounds, both in isolation and in sequences, the Lindamood Phoneme Sequencing Program for Reading, Spelling, and Speech (Lindamood and Lindamood, 1998), shown to be effective in children with reading disabilities (J. K. Torgesen et al., 2001). The team effort paid off and Miles began to make substantial progress, both in his speech sessions and in his reading program.

Miles is an example of a child who fits the dyslexia subtype characterized by poor decoding skills and, at the same time, a subtype of SSD characterized by multiple and unusual phonologic processes. It is possible that both disorders were caused by his deficits in phonemic awareness. In addition, the fact that his speech difficulties persisted into his early school years is consistent with the "critical age hypothesis." As described in Chapter 15, studies investigating the molecular genetics of SSD (Miscimarra et al., 2007; Smith, Pennington, Boada, and Shriberg, 2005; Stein et al., 2006; Stein et al., 2004) have focused on regions in the genome that had already been identified in dyslexia studies. The fact that these SSD studies found evidence of linkage in the dyslexia candidate regions may imply that SSD and dyslexia are influenced by the same genes in some cases.To illuminate the interactions between speech sound development and literacy development further, studies should investigate the nature and possible subtypes of SSD and dyslexia in more detail. Many questions remain yet to be answered: How are the reading and spelling errors in children with dyslexia and SSD different from those in children with dyslexia only? Similarly, how are the speech errors in children with SSD and dyslexia different from those in SSD only? What is the role of cognitive processes such as sequential processing, speed of processing in general, and visual orientation in space in SSD and dyslexia? Finding shared and unshared cognitive substrates would contribute to our understanding of SSD and dyslexia subtypes.

Sidebar 16.1. How is Learning to Talk Different from Learning to Read and Spell?

Most children learn to talk at a very young age and without explicit instruction, mostly by being around proficient speakers of the language. They listen, watch, talk, receive feedback (including from their own sensory systems), and build their mental and motoric speech abilities based on these natural interactions. Learning to read and spell is different: Written language is acquired much later than spoken language, and most children require explicit instruction to become proficient. Regarding English, a special challenge is that the pronunciation conventions evolved over the centuries but its orthography has remained more stagnant, leading to spelling anomalies such as the "h" in "honor," the "k" in "knee" and "knife," and the "gh" in "although," all silent letters now that, centuries ago, were actually pronounced.

Granted, infants do receive some extra assistance with spoken language. The speech they hear is frequently different from that most older children and adults hear in that infant-directed speech, sometimes referred to as "motherese," exaggerates some of the acoustic properties of speech, for instance speed, intonational range, and vowel space. Written language, on the other hand, offers the advantage that its representation is stable across time, allowing the reader to go back and re-process, whereas a speech event is transient and must be stored in auditory short-term memory for further processing.

Sidebar 16.2. "Jessi"

Jessi was a third grader with severe difficulties in the areas of reading and spelling, but her oral language abilities and her nonverbal processing skills were far above average, and she was also very artistic and creative. The struggle with written language caused her no end of frustration. For instance, she eagerly wished to keep a diary but gave up on the idea because she could not read her own writing. Jessi also struggled with sequential and directional processing. Her 3-ring notebook had two beginnings, front to back and back to front, and she sometimes drew cartoons with speech bubbles in mirror-image writing without noticing the reversal in direction. Mirror image reversals were also seen in her many "b"/"d" and "d"/"b" substitutions. Many of her reading errors showed that she was not processing the graphemes sequentially from left to right. For instance, she read "no"/"on," "claps"/"is glad," "filled"/"lifted," and "left"/"felt." Other errors showed that she payed attention to the beginnings and ends of words but did not process the middles sequentially: "smells"/"smiles," "tested"/"teased," "rafted"/"raved," and "rug"/"rag."

When sounding out words, Jessi found it helpful to use a guide card that she slid across written words so that she could see the letters sequentially from left to right. To help her put her thoughts into writing, she began using a speech-to-text computer program.

Sidebar 16.3. "Insa"

Insa is a 51-year-old woman who had struggled tremendously with learning to speak as a child. She remembers feeling frustrated when others could not understand what she was attempting to say, even at 10 or 11 years of age. Because treatment was not available to her, she tried improving her speech on her own by closely watching others saying certain words, then practicing the words by herself, over and over. In school, she had substantial difficulty learning to read and spell. As an adult, Insa continues to struggle with her speech. Although she can easily produce all speech sounds of English without errors, pronouncing multisyllabic words is difficult for her. Similarly, reading and spelling continues to be challenging for Insa.

Connections

Interactions between speech sound development and literacy development were the focus of this chapter. It is possible that certain SSD subtypes are more susceptible to reading difficulties than others; Chapter 15 provides an overview of current hypotheses regarding SSD subtypes. Chapter 22 considers professional settings where SLPs and other service providers participate in teams that can support children from a multidisciplinary perspective.

CONCLUDING REMARKS

A thorough understanding of the interactions between speech and literacy development has clinical implications. For instance, an SLP who is treating a child for SSD will find it helpful to know whether the child also struggles with reading and/or spelling. If so, the SLP can consult with the child's reading specialist and gain insights into the nature of the deficits in written language. Frequently, a deficit in phonological processing underlies both areas of struggle, and if the members of the professional team co-ordinate their efforts and target the underlying deficit together, they may see faster progress in both areas. It is not known whether or not deficits in sequential processing can underlie comorbid cases of SSD and dyslexia. If this were the case, then new research questions would arise regarding the possibility of treating the sequential processing deficits at a basic level to achieve improvements in speech and reading.

There is strong evidence for a genetic etiology in both SSD and dyslexia, but causal genes have not yet been identified. Once knowledge of risk genotypes for these two disorders in isolation and in comorbidity becomes available, it will be possible to build a more biologically based subtype system and embark on a new journey of discovering the biochemical mechanisms involved in these disorders. Translating this new knowledge back into the clinical world will involve identifying at-risk infants and investigating new approaches to early intervention.

CHAPTER REVIEW QUESTIONS

1. List some of the special challenges in learning to read and spell English words, compared to other alphabetic languages like Spanish.
2. What are the core elements of the dyslexia definition issued by the International Dyslexia Association?
3. What are some of the associated deficits in dyslexia?
4. Why are so many more boys than girls thought to have dyslexia?
5. What type of preschool child with SSD is most likely to also develop dyslexia?

SUGGESTIONS FOR FURTHER READING

Catts, H. W., and Kamhi, A. G. (2005). *The connection between language and reading disabilities.* Mahwah: Laurence Erlbaum.

Kamhi, A. G., and Catts, H. W. (2012). Language and reading disabilities, 3rd Edition. Boston: Pearson.

McGill-Franzen, A. and Allington, R. L. (2011). *Handbook of reading disability research.* New York: Routledge.

Seki. A,, Kassai , K., Uchiyama, H., and Koeda, T. (2008). Reading ability and phonological awareness in Japanese children with dyslexia". *Brain Dev.* 30 (3): 179–88.

Siok, W.T., Niu, Z., Jin, Z., Perfetti, C.A., and Tan, L.H. (2008). "A structural-functional basis for dyslexia in the cortex of Chinese readers" (Free full text). *Proc. Natl. Acad. Sci. U.S.A.* 105 (14): 5561–6.

Access Sound File 1 (Chapter 16)

16S1 Nonword reading test, 8-year-old boy with SSD.

Access Sound File 2 (Chapter 16)

16S2 Story retell, 8-year-old boy with SSD.

SUGGESTIONS FOR STUDENT ACTIVITIES

1. Sound file 16S1 captures a child with SSD reading a list of pseudowords from the Phonemic Decoding Efficiency subtest from the Test of Word Reading Efficiency (TOWRE) (Joseph K. Torgesen, Wagner, and Rashotte, 1999). Sound file 16S2 captures the same child in a story retell task from the Goldman-Fristoe Test of Articulation (Goldman, 2000). Obtain a test protocol for the TOWRE and score the pseudowords for accuracy (one point for each accurate psuedoword). Based on the speech sound errors you notice in the story retell, determine which of the reading errors are true reading errors and which are most likely related to the presence of SSD.
2. Using resources listed under SUGGESTIONS FOR FURTHER READING and other resources of your choice, determine the differences in brain involvement for readers of alphabetic, logographic, and syllabic writing systems.
3. Using online resources, evaluate the hypothesis that the complexities of English orthography lead to higher dyslexia rates in English-speaking countries, compared to countries where languages with shallow orthographies are spoken.

ANSWERS TO CHAPTER REVIEW QUESTIONS

1. List some of the special challenges in learning to read and spell English words, compared to other alphabetic languages like Spanish.

A deep orthography and many irregularly spelled words, some of which include silent letters.

2. What are the core elements of the dyslexia definition issued by the International Dyslexia Association?

Difficulties with written language restricted to the word level; involving the processes of decoding, sight word recognition, and spelling; affects accuracy and/or fluency; not predicted by cognitive impairments or lack of instruction.

3. What are some of the associated deficits in dyslexia?

Deficits in auditory processing, phonemic awareness, structural and functional brain differences, evidence of genetic etiology.

4. Why are so many more boys than girls thought to have dyslexia?

A high male:female ratio may be an artifact of other behavioral differences between boys and girls, such as attention and activity levels.

5. What type of preschool child with SSD is most likely to also develop dyslexia?

A child with SSD (a) whose speech difficulties persist into the school years, (b) who has impaired phonological processing skills, and/or (c) who also shows evidence of language impairment is most likely to also struggle with learning to read and spell when she or he enters school.

References

Aaron, P. G., Joshi, M., and Williams, K. A. (1999). Not all reading disabilities are alike. *J. Learn Disabil, 32*(2), 120-137.

Beitchman, J. H., Nair, R., Clegg, M., Patel, P. G., Ferguson, B., Pressman, E., and Smith, A. (1986). Prevalence of speech and language disorders in 5-year-old kindergarten children in the Ottawa-Carleton region. *J. Speech Hear Disord, 51*(2), 98-110.

Bird, J., Bishop, D. V., and Freeman, N. H. (1995). Phonological awareness and literacy development in children with expressive phonological impairments. *J Speech Hear Res., 38*(2), 446-462.

Bishop, D. V. M., and Adams, C. (1990). A Prospective-Study of the Relationship between Specific Language Impairment, Phonological Disorders and Reading Retardation. *Journal of Child Psychology and Psychiatry and Allied Disciplines, 31*(7), 1027-1050.

Bishop, D. V. M., and Edmundson, A. (1987). Language-Impaired 4-Year-Olds - Distinguishing Transient from Persistent Impairment. *Journal of Speech and Hearing Disorders, 52*(2), 156-173.

Boets, B., Wouters, J., van Wieringen, A., and Ghesquiere, P. (2007). Auditory processing, speech perception and phonological ability in pre-school children at high-risk for dyslexia: a longitudinal study of the auditory temporal processing theory.

Neuropsychologia, 45(8), 1608-1620. doi: S0028-3932(07)00045-0 [pii] 10.1016/j.neuropsychologia.2007.01.009.

Bosse, M. L., Tainturier, M. J., and Valdois, S. (2007). Developmental dyslexia: the visual attention span deficit hypothesis. *Cognition, 104*(2), 198-230. doi: S0010-0277(06)00127-2 [pii] 10.1016/j.cognition.2006.05.009.

Bradley, L., and Bryant, P. E. (1983). Categorizing Sounds and Learning to Read - a Causal Connection. *Nature, 301*(5899), 419-421.

Campbell, T. F., Dollaghan, C. A., Rockette, H. E., Paradise, J. L., Feldman, H. M., Shriberg, L. D., . . . Kurs-Lasky, M. (2003). Risk factors for speech delay of unknown origin in 3-year-old children. *Child Dev., 74*(2), 346-357.

Carver, R. P. (1993). Merging the Simple View of Reading with Rauding Theory. *Journal of Reading Behavior, 25*(4), 439-455.

Castles, A., and Coltheart, M. (1993). Varieties of Developmental Dyslexia. *Cognition, 47*(2), 149-180.

Castles, A., Datta, H., Gayan, J., and Olson, R. K. (1999). Varieties of developmental reading disorder: genetic and environmental influences. *J. Exp. Child Psychol., 72*(2), 73-94. doi: S0022-0965(98)92482-1 [pii] 10.1006/jecp.1998.2482.

Catts, H. W. (1986). Speech Production Phonological Deficits in Reading Disordered Children. *Journal of Learning Disabilities, 19*(8), 504-508.

Catts, H. W. (1989). Speech Production Deficits in Developmental Dyslexia. *Journal of Speech and Hearing Disorders, 54*(3), 422-428.

Catts, H. W. (1993). The relationship between speech-language impairments and reading disabilities. *J. Speech Hear Res., 36*(5), 948-958.

Catts, H. W., Gillispie, M., Leonard, L. B., Kail, R. V., and Miller, C. A. (2002). The role of speed of processing, rapid naming, and phonological awareness in reading achievement. *Journal of Learning Disabilities, 35*(6), 509-524.

Catts, H. W., Hogan, T. P., and Fey, M. E. (2003). Subgrouping poor readers on the basis of individual differences in reading-related abilities. *Journal of Learning Disabilities, 36*(2), 151-164.

Catts, H. W., Kamhi, A. G., and Adlof, S. M. (2012). Causes of reading disabilites. In A. G. Kamhi and H. W. Catts (Eds.), Language and reading disabilities. 3rd edition. Boston: Pearson.

Denckla, M. B., and Rudel, R. G. (1976). Rapid Automatized Naming (Ran) - Dyslexia Differentiated from Other Learning-Disabilities. *Neuropsychologia, 14*(4), 471-479.

Deutsch, G. K., Dougherty, R. F., Bammer, R., Siok, W. T., Gabrieli, J. D., and Wandell, B. (2005). Children's reading performance is correlated with white matter structure measured by diffusion tensor imaging. *Cortex, 41*(3), 354-363.

Eckert, M. (2004). Neuroanatomical markers for dyslexia: a review of dyslexia structural imaging studies. *Neuroscientist, 10*(4), 362-371. doi: 10.1177/1073858404263596.

Eckert, M. A., Leonard, C. M., Richards, T. L., Aylward, E. H., Thomson, J., and Berninger, V. W. (2003). Anatomical correlates of dyslexia: frontal and cerebellar findings. *Brain, 126*(Pt 2), 482-494.

Fletcher, J. M., Francis, D. J., Rourke, B. P., Shaywitz, S. E., and Shaywitz, B. A. (1992). The validity of discrepancy-based definitions of reading disabilities. *J. Learn Disabil., 25*(9), 555-561, 573.

Fletcher, J. M., Shaywitz, S. E., Shankweiler, D. P., Katz, L., Liberman, I. Y., Stuebing, K. K., . . . Shaywitz, B. A. (1994). Cognitive Profiles of Reading-Disability - Comparisons of Discrepancy and Low Achievement Definitions. *Journal of Educational Psychology, 86*(1), 6-23.

Francks, C., MacPhie, I. L., and Monaco, A. P. (2002). The genetic basis of dyslexia. *Lancet Neurol., 1*(8), 483-490. doi: S1474442202002211 [pii].

Frye, R. E., Hasan, K., Xue, L., Strickland, D., Malmberg, B., Liederman, J., and Papanicolaou, A. (2008). Splenium microstructure is related to two dimensions of reading skill. *Neuroreport, 19*(16), 1627-1631. doi: 10.1097/WNR.0b013e328314b8ee.

Galaburda, A. M., Menard, M. T., and Rosen, G. D. (1994). Evidence for aberrant auditory anatomy in developmental dyslexia. *Proc. Natl. Acad. Sci. USA, 91*(17), 8010-8013.

Galaburda, A. M., Sherman, G. F., Rosen, G. D., Aboitiz, F., and Geschwind, N. (1985). Developmental dyslexia: four consecutive patients with cortical anomalies. *Ann. Neurol., 18*(2), 222-233. doi: 10.1002/ana.410180210.

Goldman, R. F., M. (2000). *Goldman-Fristoe Test of Articulation 2*. Circle Pines: American Guidance Service.

Gough, P. B., and Tunmer, W. E. (1986). Decoding, reading, and reading disability. *Remedial and Special Education, 7*, 6 - 10.

Klingberg, T., Hedehus, M., Temple, E., Salz, T., Gabrieli, J. D., Moseley, M. E., and Poldrack, R. A. (2000). Microstructure of temporo-parietal white matter as a basis for reading ability: evidence from diffusion tensor magnetic resonance imaging. *Neuron, 25*(2), 493-500. doi: S0896-6273(00)80911-3 [pii].

Konig, I. R., Schumacher, J., Hoffmann, P., Kleensang, A., Ludwig, K. U., Grimm, T., . . . Schulte-Korne, G. (2011). Mapping for dyslexia and related cognitive trait loci provides strong evidence for further risk genes on chromosome 6p21. *Am. J. Med. Genet. B Neuropsychiatr. Genet., 156B*(1), 36-43. doi: 10.1002/ajmg.b.31135.

Leonard, C. M., and Eckert, M. A. (2008). Asymmetry and dyslexia. *Dev Neuropsychol, 33*(6), 663-681. doi: 905451873 [pii] 10.1080/87565640802418597.

Lewis, B. A., Freebairn, L. A., Hansen, A. J., Iyengar, S. K., and Taylor, H. G. (2004). School-age follow-up of children with childhood apraxia of speech. *Lang Speech Hear Serv. Sch., 35*(2), 122-140.

Lewis, B. A., Freebairn, L. A., and Taylor, H. G. (2000). Follow-up of children with early expressive phonology disorders. *J. Learn Disabil., 33*(5), 433-444.

Lewis, B. A., Shriberg, L. D., Freebairn, L. A., Hansen, A. J., Stein, C. M., Taylor, H. G., and Iyengar, S. K. (2006). The genetic bases of speech sound disorders: evidence from spoken and written language. *J. Speech Lang Hear Res., 49*(6), 1294-1312. doi: 49/6/1294 [pii] 10.1044/1092-4388(2006/093).

Lindamood, P., and Lindamood, P. (1998). The LIndamood phoneme sequencing sequencing program for reading, spelling, and speech. Austin: PRO-ED.

Livingstone, M. S., Rosen, G. D., Drislane, F. W., and Galaburda, A. M. (1991). Physiological and anatomical evidence for a magnocellular defect in developmental dyslexia. *Proc. Natl. Acad. Sci. USA, 88*(18), 7943-7947.

Lyon, G. R., Shaywitz, S. E., and Shaywitz, B. A. (2003). A definition of dyslexia. *Annals of Dyslexia,* (53), 1-14.

Marshall, J. C., and Newcombe, F. (1973). Patterns of paralexia: a psycholinguistic approach. *J. Psycholinguist Res., 2*(3), 175-199.

McKinnon, D. H., McLeod, S., and Reilly, S. (2007). The prevalence of stuttering, voice, and speech-sound disorders in primary school students in Australia. *Lang Speech Hear Serv. Sch., 38*(1), 5-15. doi: 38/1/5 [pii] 10.1044/0161-1461(2007/002).

Miscimarra, L., Stein, C., Millard, C., Kluge, A., Cartier, K., Freebairn, L., . . . Iyengar, S. K. (2007). Further evidence of pleiotropy influencing speech and language: analysis of the DYX8 region. *Hum. Hered., 63*(1), 47-58. doi: 000098727 [pii] 10.1159/000098727.

Murphy, L., and Pollatsek, A. (1994). Developmental dyslexia: Heterogeneity without discrete subgroups. *Annals of Dyslexia, 44*, 120-146.

Nathan, L., Stackhouse, J., Goulandris, N., and Snowling, M. J. (2004). Educational consequences of developmental speech disorder: Key Stage 1 National Curriculum assessment results in English and mathematics. *Br. J. Educ. Psychol., 74*(Pt 2), 173-186. doi: 10.1348/000709904773839824.

Niogi, S. N., and McCandliss, B. D. (2006). Left lateralized white matter microstructure accounts for individual differences in reading ability and disability. *Neuropsychologia, 44*(11), 2178-2188. doi: S0028-3932(06)00023-6 [pii] 10.1016/j.neuropsychologia. 2006.01.011.

Pennington, B. F. (1990). The genetics of dyslexia. *J. Child. Psychol. Psychiatry, 31*(2), 193-201.

Pennington, B. F., and Bishop, D. V. (2009). Relations among speech, language, and reading disorders. *Annu. Rev. Psychol., 60*, 283-306. doi: 10.1146/annurev.psych. 60.110707.163548.

Peter, B., Matsushita, M., and Raskind, W. H. (2011). Global processing speed in children with low reading ability and in children and adults with typical reading ability: exploratory factor analytic models. *J. Speech Lang Hear Res., 54*(3), 885-899. doi: 1092-4388_2010_10-0135 [pii] 10.1044/1092-4388(2010/10-0135).

Peterson, R. L., McGrath, L. M., Smith, S. D., and Pennington, B. F. (2007). Neuropsychology and genetics of speech, language, and literacy disorders. *Pediatr. Clin. North Am., 54*(3), 543-561, vii. doi: S0031-3955(07)00038-7 [pii]10.1016/ j.pcl.2007.02.009.

Ramus, F. (2003). Developmental dyslexia: specific phonological deficit or general sensorimotor dysfunction? *Curr. Opin. Neurobiol., 13*(2), 212-218. doi: S0959438803000357 [pii].

Roeske, D., Ludwig, K. U., Neuhoff, N., Becker, J., Bartling, J., Bruder, J., . . . Schulte-Korne, G. (2009). First genome-wide association scan on neurophysiological endophenotypes points to trans-regulation effects on SLC2A3 in dyslexic children. *Mol. Psychiatry*. doi: mp2009102 [pii] 10.1038/mp.2009.102.

Rutter, M., Caspi, A., Fergusson, D., Horwood, L. J., Goodman, R., Maughan, B., . . . Carroll, J. (2004). Sex differences in developmental reading disability: new findings from 4 epidemiological studies. *JAMA, 291*(16), 2007-2012. doi: 10.1001/jama.291.16.2007 291/16/2007 [pii].

Sandak, R., Mencl, W. E., Frost, S. J., and Pugh, K. R. (2004). The neurobiological basis of skilled and impaired reading: Recent findings and new directions. *Scientific Studies of Reading, 8*(3), 273-292.

Shaywitz, S. E., Shaywitz, B. A., Fletcher, J. M., and Escobar, M. D. (1990). Prevalence of reading disability in boys and girls. Results of the Connecticut Longitudinal Study. *JAMA, 264*(8), 998-1002.

Shriberg, L. D., and Austin, D. (1998). Comorbidity of speech-language disorder: Implications for a phenotype marker for speech delay. In R. Paul (Ed.), *The speech-language connection* (pp. 73-117). Baltimore: Brookes.

Shriberg, L. D., Tomblin, J. B., and McSweeny, J. L. (1999). Prevalence of speech delay in 6-year-old children and comorbidity with language impairment. *J. Speech Lang Hear Res., 42*(6), 1461-1481.

Sices, L., Taylor, H. G., Freebairn, L., Hansen, A., and Lewis, B. (2007). Relationship between speech-sound disorders and early literacy skills in preschool-age children: impact of comorbid language impairment. *J. Dev. Behav. Pediatr., 28*(6), 438-447. doi: 10.1097/DBP.0b013e31811ff8ca 00004703-200712000-00003 [pii].

Smith, A. B., Smith, S. L., Locke, J. L., and Bennett, J. (2008). A Longitudinal Study of Speech Timing in Young Children Later Found to Have Reading Disability. *Journal of Speech Language and Hearing Research, 51*(5), 1300-1314.

Smith, S. D., Pennington, B. F., Boada, R., and Shriberg, L. D. (2005). Linkage of speech sound disorder to reading disability loci. *J. Child Psychol. Psychiatry, 46*(10), 1057-1066. doi: JCPP1534 [pii] 10.1111/j.1469-7610.2005.01534.x.

Snowling, M. J. (2005). Literacy outcomes for children with oral language impairments: Developmental interactions between language skills and learning to read. In H. W. Catts and A. G. Kamhi (Eds.), *The connections between language and reading disabilities*. Mahwah: Laurence Erlbaum.

Snowling, M. J., Stothard, S. E., Bishop, D. V. M., Chipchase, B. B., and Kaplan, C. A. (1998). Language-impaired preschoolers: A follow-up into adolescence. *Journal of Speech Language and Hearing Research, 41*(2), 407-418.

Stanovich, K. E. (1991). Discrepancy Definitions of Reading-Disability - Has Intelligence Led Us Astray. *Reading Research Quarterly, 26*(1), 7-29.

Stanovich, K. E., Siegel, L. S., and Gottardo, A. (1997). Converging evidence for phonological and surface subtypes of reading disability. *Journal of Educational Psychology, 89*(1), 114-127.

Stein, C. M., Millard, C., Kluge, A., Miscimarra, L. E., Cartier, K. C., Freebairn, L. A., . . . Iyengar, S. K. (2006). Speech sound disorder influenced by a locus in 15q14 region. *Behav. Genet., 36*(6), 858-868. doi: 10.1007/s10519-006-9090-7.

Stein, C. M., Schick, J. H., Gerry Taylor, H., Shriberg, L. D., Millard, C., Kundtz-Kluge, A., . . . Iyengar, S. K. (2004). Pleiotropic effects of a chromosome 3 locus on speech-sound disorder and reading. *Am. J. Hum. Genet., 74*(2), 283-297. doi: S0002-9297(07)61839-4 [pii] 10.1086/381562.

Tallal, P. (1980). Auditory temporal perception, phonics, and reading disabilities in children. *Brain Lang, 9*(2), 182-198.

Torgesen, J. K., Alexander, A. W., Wagner, R. K., Rashotte, C. A., Voeller, K. K., and Conway, T. (2001). Intensive remedial instruction for children with severe reading disabilities: immediate and long-term outcomes from two instructional approaches. [Clinical Trial. Comparative Study. Randomized Controlled Trial. Research Support, Non-U.S. Gov't. Research Support, U.S. Gov't, P.H.S.]. *J. Learn Disabil., 34*(1), 33-58, 78.

Torgesen, J. K., Wagner, R. K., and Rashotte, C. A. (1999). *TOWRE, Test of Word Reading Efficiency : examiner's manual*. Austin, Tex.: PRO-ED.

Wilson, R. A., and Shaw, B. (1942). *The miraculous birth of language*. London,: J. M. Dent and sons ltd.

In: Comprehensive Perspectives …
Editors: Beate Peter and Andrea A. N. MacLeod
ISBN: 978-1-62257-041-6

Chapter 17

CLEFT LIP AND PALATE

Amy Skinder-Meredith and Alice Smith

INTRODUCTION

This chapter provides a brief, but comprehensive review of cleft lip and palate. In addition to explaining the nature, consequences and management of cleft, it also addresses the considerations that need to be taken into account when working with internationally adopted children with cleft. This is a growing population that literature has yet to address.

Cleft refers to a split, fissure, or separation. Thus, cleft lip refers to a split of the upper lip, which may go through just part of the lip or up through the nostril; cleft palate refers to a separation of tissues of the soft and/or hard palate.

A cleft lip occurs when there is a disruption in the fusion of the upper lip during the development of the face, which occurs between the 5th and 8th weeks of gestation. Cleft palate occurs when there is disruption during weeks 8 through 12, when the embryonic processes that give rise to the hard and soft palate fuse to separate the oral and nasal cavities. These causes may be genetic or environmental. A child can have a cleft lip, or a cleft palate, or both.

Sidebar 17.1. Harelip

An outdated term for cleft lip is "harelip" because of the resemblance to the lip of a hare. This term was used in American medical journals throughout the 1960s and is still used today in international journals (e.g., Peng and ***Hong-yan***, 2011). When one is aware of the history of this term, it is less likely to be used. While some believed that the cause of cleft was the mother seeing or being frightened by a hare when she was pregnant (Noll, 1983), others believed that witchcraft and/or Satan was involved with the mother, resulting in the baby being born with this animal like characteristic. This belief did not bode well for the mother or child, as mothers could be put to death and children left to die (WideSmiles.org, 1996). Hence, if you hear someone use the term harelip, politely explain that "cleft lip" and "cleft palate" are the terms we use today. Needless to say, no witchcraft or animals are to be blamed for cleft.

The Centers for Disease Control and Prevention (CDC) recently estimated that 2,651 babies in the United States are born with a cleft palate and 4,437 babies are born with a cleft lip with or without a cleft palate each year (Parker et al., 2010). **Incidence** rates vary for different ethnicities. For example, Asian and American Indian populations have the highest reported birth rates (1/500), European-derived populations have intermediate rates (1/1000), and African-derived populations have the lowest rates (1/2500) (Dixon, Marazita, Beaty, and Murray, 2011). The incidence of clefts in general has been quoted to be between one in 600 to one in 750 live births (Cleft Palate Foundation, 1999).

Children who are internationally adopted into the United States are most likely not included in these figures. It is difficult to obtain an exact number, but trends in the number of internationally adopted children with a cleft appear to be on the rise, especially from China. As the number of healthy children available for adoption in China decreases, the number of children adopted with special needs, such as cleft, increases (Dan, 2011). Because these statistics are not readily available in the literature, two large international adoption agencies and craniofacial teams were contacted to obtain estimates of internationally adopted children with cleft. Chinese Children Adoption International (CCAI) reported that of the 580 children, who were adopted in 2010, 358 had special needs and one third of these children had cleft lip and or palate. The Holt International Adoption Agency reportedly placed a total of 550 children with cleft lip and palate, with the majority of the adoptees being from China and South Korea. In 2010 alone, 749 children were placed through Holt, 93 (12%) had cleft lip and/or palate. The Spokane craniofacial team reported that 11% of the children who are seen by the craniofacial team have been internationally adopted while the Cincinnati Medical Center reported an estimate of 20%. Due to the growing number of internationally adopted cleft-affected children, this chapter will later address some of the inherent issues to be aware of when working with internationally adopted children with cleft.

Although relatively rare in the population, cleft palate is the most common birth defect an SLP will come across, as it directly relates to speech, language, feeding, and hearing. One may assume that children born with cleft lip and palate would be very straightforward to treat. However, the saying, "if you've seen one, you've seen them all" does not apply to this population. Given the heterogeneity of children born with cleft, if you've seen one, you've seen one. As noted by Shprintzen, "clefting is not a specific disease, but rather a symptom of many possible disease processes" (Shprintzen, 1995, p. 5). The speech and language performance of children with a cleft can vary greatly due to the severity of the cleft, access to a qualified cleft management team, the success of surgical repairs, and whether the cleft is associated with a **syndrome** or occurred in isolation. A syndrome is a pattern of multiple genetic differences or anomalies thought to have a common cause, such as a gene or chromosomal abnormality.

TYPES OF CLEFT

There are many different types of cleft, as seen in Figure 17.1, and most clefts are clearly observable. There are three primary types of visible clefts: cleft of the lip, cleft of the palate, and cleft of both the lip and palate. Clefts that involve the palate may include the hard palate, soft palate, or both. When the cleft is only of the soft palate, it can easily be overlooked at the time of birth. It may not be noticed until weeks or months later, when the mother is having difficulty feeding her baby. A cleft may involve just one side (unilateral) or both sides (bilateral). A cleft may be incomplete (affect only a portion of the structures involved) or complete (affect all of the structures involved).

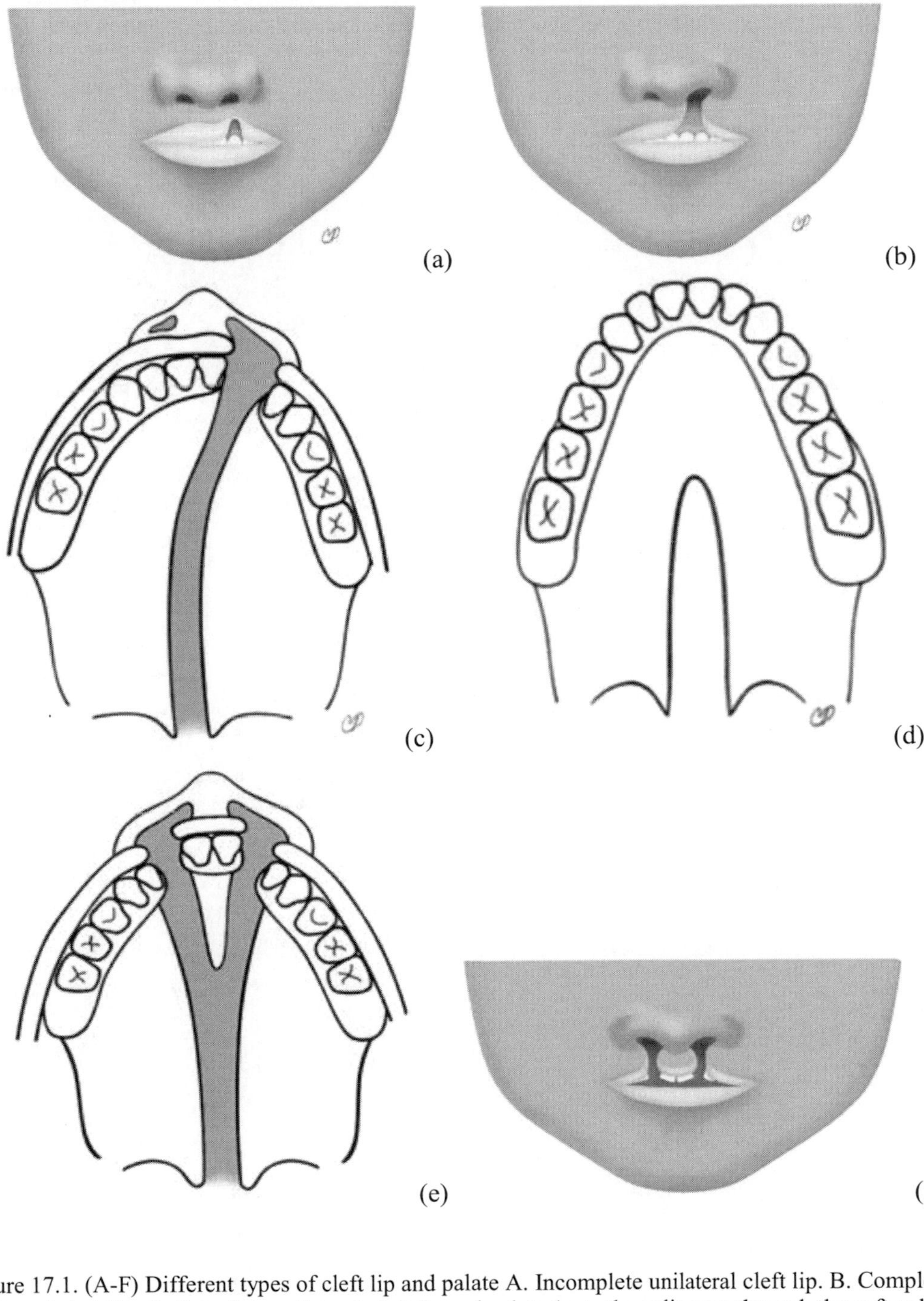

Figure 17.1. (A-F) Different types of cleft lip and palate A. Incomplete unilateral cleft lip. B. Complete unilateral cleft lip. C. Complete unilateral cleft lip and palate (note the split goes through the soft palate, hard palate, alveolus, and lip). D. Cleft of the soft palate only. E. Inferior view of a complete bilateral cleft lip and palate. E. Anterior view of a bilateral cleft lip and palate.

For example, a complete cleft of the lip would include the floor of the nose and, possibly, the dental alveolus (the system of sockets that hold the teeth). The width and length of tissue involved determine the severity of the cleft. For example, a bilateral cleft lip and palate would be considered more severe than a unilateral incomplete cleft lip.

A type of cleft that can be more difficult to see is called a submucous cleft. Submucous cleft refers to when the oral mucosal lining is intact, but the muscles deep to the mucosal lining are not oriented correctly.

Rather than meeting midline as in Figure 17.2A, they may be oriented more vertically as in 17.2B. Children with submucous clefts may experience some of the same difficulties with speech and feeding as children with visible clefts.

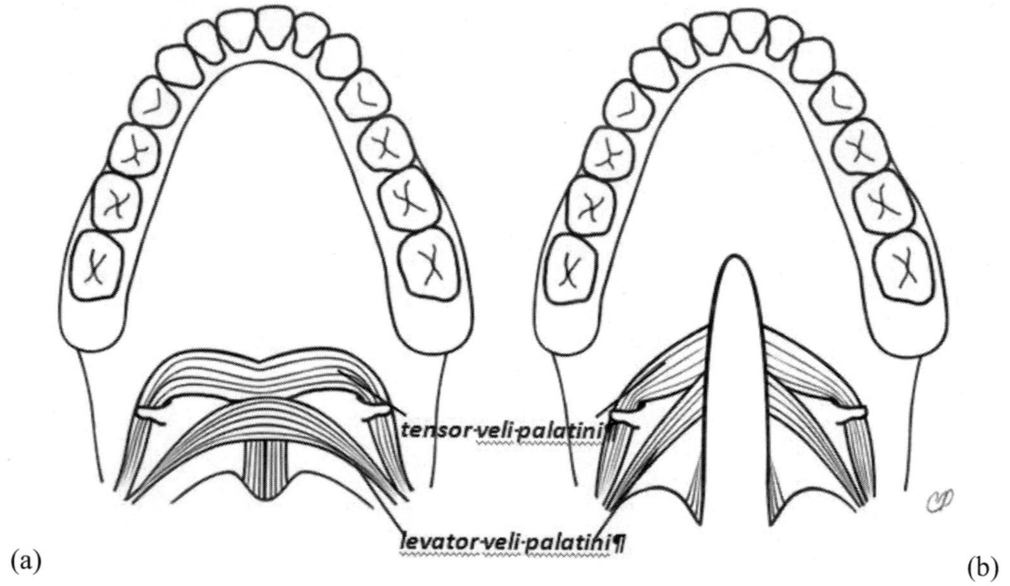

Figure 17.2. (A). Muscle orientation of the *levator veli palatini* (elevates the velum) and *tensor veli palatini* (tenses the velum and dilates the eustachian tubes) in a normal palate. (B). Muscle orientation of the *levator veli palatini* and *tensor veli palatini* in a cleft palate.

The presence of a submucous cleft may not be identified until the child begins to talk with **hypernasal** speech. This type of cleft involves the underlying muscular tissue and is, therefore, not visible to the untrained eye, but may be discovered during a careful intra-oral examination. If a submucous cleft is suspected, it is best to view the nasal side of the velum with **nasendoscopy** for a direct look at the muscles of the soft palate. The following is a list of characteristics one may see with this anomaly. However, any one or all of these characteristics may or may not be present.

- ***Bifid*** uvula with two separate tags (fairly common and not always indicative of a submucous cleft palate)
- Hypoplastic (short and stubby) uvula
- Zona pellucida (a bluish area in the middle of the velum) due to a thin and transparent velum

- Inverted V-shape of velum during phonation due to muscles inserting vertically into the hard palate versus horizontally into each other (see Figure 17.2)

ETIOLOGIES OF CLEFT

"Approximately 70% of cases of cleft lip and palate and 50% of cases of cleft palate only occur as isolated entities with no other apparent cognitive or structural abnormalities; commonly termed 'isolated, non-syndromic CLP' [cleft lip and/or palate]" (Dixon, Marazita, Beaty, and Murray, 2011, p. 2-3). Researchers have been trying to find genetic mutations that may be responsible for non-syndromic clefting. Although progress has been made, the heterogeneity of the disorder makes this difficult. Non-syndromic cleft lip and palate are known to be influenced by exposure to environmental **teratogens** such as smoking, alcohol, environmental toxins, poor nutrition, and anti-seizure medication during embryonic development (Dixon et al., 2011; Kummer, 2008). Other causes may be mechanical, such as inter-uterine crowding or the fetus swallowing an amniotic band. One of the leading explanations for non-syndromic cleft lip and palate is a **multifactorial model of inheritance** where genetic risk factors and environmental factors interact (Dixon et al., 2011).

"Multifactorial disorders can be divided into two categories: traits that demonstrate continuous variation and threshold disorders" (Kummer, 2008, p. 80). Cleft lip and palate fall into the threshold disorder category, where the combination of specific gene variations and environmental factors will make the expression of cleft more likely.

In her 2008 text, Kummer stated that there were 300 recognized syndromes associated with cleft conditions and in 2011; this number was increased to 500, as reported by Dixon and colleagues. This number continually increases as more syndromes are discovered (Cohen, 1978). Some craniofacial syndromes have obvious characteristics, such as malformed ears or eye abnormalities, while others have less visible characteristics, such as heart defects (Kummer, 2008). Craniofacial syndromes may be associated with cleft lip only, cleft palate only, or cleft lip and palate. When parents of a biological child notice more than one anomaly, genetic testing of the family may help the geneticist determine if a syndrome is involved and where the chromosomal or genetic anomaly lies. Adoptive parents are at a slight disadvantage, as they do not have access to genetic information about the birth parents in most cases. Thus, adoptive parents should review the medical history of their child carefully to see if there may be multiple anomalies in addition to a cleft that may signal the presence of a syndrome that will require special care.

One example of a syndrome frequently associated with cleft lip and palate is 22q11.2 deletion syndrome, also referred to as velo-cardio-facial syndrome (VCFS) or diGeorge Syndrome. There are more than 160 identified characteristics of VCFS ranging from mild to severe, primarily including palate, heart, and facial feature anomalies. Language delays, learning and reading disabilities, behavioral concerns, and intellectual disability are also associated with 22q11.2 deletion syndrome (Robin and Shprintzen, 2005; Shprintzen, 2000). Other syndromes that are often associated with cleft lip and palate include Opitz Syndrome, Trisomy 13, Van der Woude syndrome, Stickler syndrome, Treacher Collins syndrome, and fetal alcohol syndrome (Kummer, 2008; Shprintzen, 2000).

Pierre Robin **Sequence** is also a common cause of cleft palate. This condition is associated with micrognathia (small jaw), which does not allow the tongue to descend into the oral cavity during fetal development. The tongue thus stays elevated and interrupts the fusion of the palatal shelves (Cohen, 1999).

How Cleft Palate Affects Speech

Studies of cleft affected speech development and production have provided a variety of results. Earlier studies showed greater differences between speech development between cleft affected and non-cleft affected peers than recent studies (Hardin-Jones, Chapman, and Schulte, 2003; Hattee, Farrow, Harland, Sommerlad, and Walsh, 2001; Trost-Cardomone, 1986). Fortunately, speech outcomes for individuals with cleft palate have improved greatly over the past 50 years due to progress in treatment methods and the timing of palate repair (Howard, 2004).

Especially relevant to a successful speech outcome is early closure of the palate (Lehman, 2008). Prior to palate repair, the child will not be able to close off the nasal cavity from the oral cavity.

See Figure 17.3 for an example of the velopharyngeal port being open versus closed. Inability to seal off the oral cavity causes hypernasal resonance. Hypernasality affects vowels and most consonants and nasal air emission affects the production of high-pressure consonants, such as /p, b, t, d, g, k, s, z, ʃ/. The nasal sounds /m, n, ŋ/ should sound normal.

The child may also sound normal with low-pressure sounds like /h, r, l, w, j/. Even after the palate is repaired, the function of the soft palate may not be adequate to fully close off the nasal cavity in about 20% to 25% of children because of either decreased length of the soft palate or poor mobility.

This is referred to as velopharyngeal insufficiency. Unrepaired cleft of the lip only will solely have an impact on sounds made by bringing the lips together, like /b, p, m/, prior to surgery. These sounds should be readily produced once the lip is repaired and the child has been taught how to make the sounds with the lips.

The following is a list of terms commonly used to refer to aspects of velopharyngeal deficiency (Trost-Cardamone, 1986):

- *Velopharyngeal Inadequacy*: generic term for any abnormal velopharyngeal function.
- *Velopharyngeal Insufficiency*: any structural deficit, such as there not being enough tissue to accomplish closure.
- *Velopharyngeal Incompetence*: movement patterns are inadequate due to neurogenic impairments that result in partial or total paresis of muscles of the velum and pharynx.

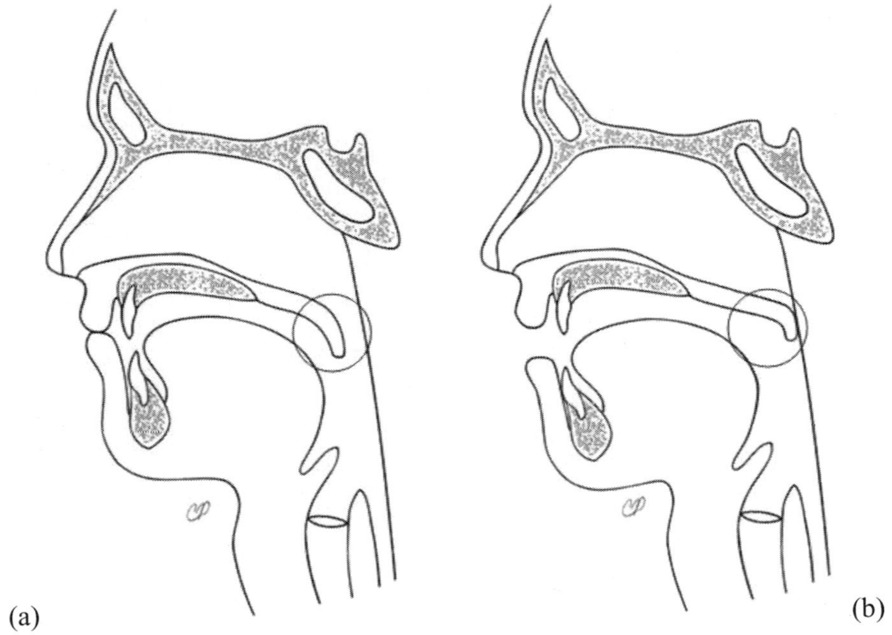

Figure 17.3. (A). Vocal tract with the velopharyngeal (V-P) port open (circled) for nasal consonants. (B). Vocal tract with the V-P port closed (circled) for the production of oral consonants.

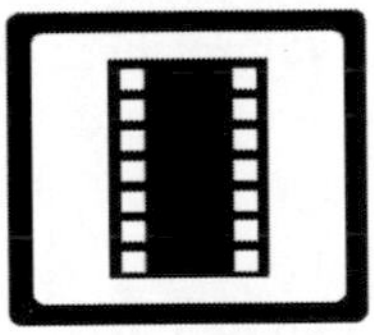

Access Video File 1 (Chapter 17)

17V1 Case Example 1.

Lilly (all names have been changed to protect the individuals' privacy) is a 2 ½ year old girl adopted from China. She was adopted at one year of age and had her lip and palate repaired by two years of age. The surgeon recommended the parents wait for 6 months post palate repair to begin speech therapy. This is a common misconception among surgeons. Therapy can begin even prior to repair to work on correct articulatory placement. In this video, Lilly is interacting with her mother, labeling toys and commenting on pictures in a book. Note Lilly's phonetic repertoire is limited to mainly nasals, vowels, and glottal stops. Her voice quality is also of concern. Therapy is focusing on correct place of articulation, elimination of glottal stops and easy onset.

Speech development of infants with cleft palate has been of particular interest for researchers (Chapman, Hardin-Jones, and Halter, 2003; Chapman, Hardin-Jones, Schulte, and Halter, 2001) as the amount of babbling and different sounds produced can impact the phonological and lexical development of the child. Babies with cleft palate often babble less frequently early in life, have a smaller phonemic repertoire, and produce less complex consonant-vowel sequences as they get older (Chapman et al., 2001; 2003). More specifically, children with cleft produce fewer stops, glides, and velars and more glottals than children without cleft.

In addition, the child is apt to receive less communicative feedback and correct modeling of speech sounds from parents since they may not be initiating as much interaction (Chapman et al., 2003). Stoel-Gammon's (1998a, b) seminal work has shown that during early stages of language development, the phonological system drives lexical acquisition. Similarly, there is a strong relationship between the size of the children's lexicons and the size of their consonant inventories. Thus, babies with cleft palate are at a higher risk for delayed language skills, especially when you add their risk for hearing impairment as explained in the next section.

How Cleft Palate Affects Hearing

Issues related to hearing are a significant threat for children with cleft palate. Prior to palate repair, many children with cleft palate have poor Eustachian tube function. The Eustachian tube connects the middle ear with the nasopharynx and is responsible for middle ear drainage and equalizing pressure in the middle ears (such as when you change altitude in an airplane). The muscle that assists in opening the nasal end of the Eustachian tube, the *tensor veli palatini*, as seen in Figure 17.2, is also attached to the soft palate. This muscle is generally disrupted and non-functional on at least one side in a child with a cleft palate. Thus, the child's ability to drain the middle ear is diminished, placing the child at risk for middle ear infections, also referred to as otitis media, and middle ear effusion (MEE), also referred to as otitis media with effusion (OME), which can lead to a mild to moderate hearing loss (Broen, Devers, Doyle, McCauley, Prouty, and Moller, 1998). For normal hearing to be restored, this fluid must drain adequately. For children without cleft, it is common practice to put the child on antibiotics or antihistamines or wait for the fluid to drain on its own. When a child has a cleft, these are not helpful solutions and the intervention needs to be more direct. Thus, one practice is to make an incision (myringotomy) in the eardrum and place a pressure-equalizing (P-E) tube in each affected ear. It is extremely important that these children are monitored for hearing loss, middle ear infections, and proper functioning of P-E tubes (Broen et al, 1998).

How Cleft Palate Affects Language and Cognition

Children born with cleft are at an increased risk for language delays due to delayed speech development, chronic otitis media, and reduced environmental stimulation due to multiple surgeries (Broen et al., 1998; Fredrickson, Chapman, and Hardin-Jones, 2006; Hardin-Jones et al., 2003; Jocelyn, Penko, and Rode, 1996; Scherer, 1999). When a child's cleft is part of a syndrome, the risk of language delay increases greatly, as in the case of Deletion 22q11.2 Syndrome, which has a well-documented impact on language and cognitive development (Robin and Sphrintzen, 2005). Earlier studies often combined the results of children with syndromic cleft and non-syndromic cleft. Hence, the findings of children with cleft having language delays was carefully questioned and controlled in more recent studies

(Broen et al., 1998; Fredrickson, Chapman, and Hardin-Jones, 2006; Hardin-Jones et al., 2003; Jocelyn, Penko, and Rode, 1996; Scherer, 1999). However, children with non-syndromic clefts have also been found to have expressive language delays. This may be due to the fact that children with cleft lip and palate have a reduced phonetic repertoire as explained earlier. This speech delay does not allow them to practice stringing sounds together to make a variety of words and phrases. In addition, children with cleft have been found to use shorter utterances, have slower vocabulary acquisition, and less verbal output (Broen et al., 1998; Fredrickson, Chapman, and Hardin-Jones, 2006; Hardin-Jones et al., 2003; Jocelyn, Penko, and Rode, 1996; Scherer, 1999). The high incidence of ear infections also puts children with cleft palate at risk for language delays. Early parent interactions in the home may also have an effect. Some parents may not interact with their baby with cleft as easily as a child born without cleft. A study done on parent involvement in therapy for their children with cleft palate and a concomitant language delay found that parent involvement does have a significant positive impact on language development (Scherer and Antonio, 1997).

Cleft may also impact the child's pragmatic skills. Fredrickson and colleagues (2006) studied the conversational patterns of children with cleft lip and palate and found that the group of children with cleft had fewer assertive acts than those without cleft. However, there was no significant difference between the two groups regarding responsive acts. The children with cleft offered fewer topic extensions and more comments focused on topic maintenance than those without cleft, but there was no difference between the two groups regarding initiating remarks. They also found that the children with cleft gave fewer adequate responses to their adult partners, and produced fewer assertive utterances proportionate to the total number of utterances. Lastly, it is important to note that speech intelligibility did affect the speaker's assertiveness, as the children with less articulate speech produced fewer assertive utterances.

Management of Cleft

Team Care Management

Successful management of children with cleft palate requires a team approach. Team members may include any of the following: a plastic surgeon, oral maxillofacial surgeon, dentist, prosthodontist, endodontist, orthodontist, SLP, otolaryngologist, audiologist, geneticist, psychologist or social worker, pediatrician, and nurse. Every team will have a coordinator who may be one of those professionals or someone else on the team.

The frequency with which the child will be seen by the cleft team will depend on the child's medical/surgical needs. Some teams see infants, toddlers, and preschoolers twice a year and older children once a year or less. The decision regarding the frequency of appointments will be made by the family and the team. Similarly, team visits will vary with respect to the number of disciplines seen by the child and the length of time spent with each discipline. Again, this will depend on the child's needs. Generally, the child will always see the otolaryngologist, plastic surgeon or oral maxillofacial surgeon, audiologist, and SLP at each visit until the child reaches school age. At these visits, the child's progress in palate function, hearing, speech, and language will be evaluated. Recommendations for further surgery, speech and language therapy, and hearing health will be made. Further information regarding issues related to surgery, dentistry, and speech and hearing issues is discussed below.

Speech Therapy

When repairs are done in a timely manner (e.g., the palate is repaired by 12 to 18 months of age) there is an 80% chance that the child will use correct speech patterns and will not need the services of a speech therapist. However, the later a child receives their palate repair, the more likely she or he is to develop compensatory strategies and will need speech therapy (Chapman et al., 2001; Trost-Cardomone, 1986). These compensatory strategies are used as substitutions for sounds produced in the front of the mouth to compensate for loss of air through the nose. These strategies are considered learned and maladaptive, meaning they will interfere with good articulation skills and the child will need to be trained not to use them. Generally, the child may try to make the sound in the back of their throat or at the level of the vocal folds (Kuehn and Henne, 2003). This posterior placement for articulation, such as in /h/ or a glottal stop (i.e., the stoppage of air during normal production of "uh oh" is a glottal stop), is exactly the opposite of what is needed to make a good anterior sound, like /t, d, p, b/. Another example of a learned maladaptive strategy is directing the air out of the nose on only one or two sounds, such as /s, z/. This is often called sound specific nasal emission (Kummer, 2008).

Sidebar 17.2. A Note about Potential Misdiagnosis

Because some children born with cleft palate produce speech with a lot of glottal stops and vowels, their parents or speech therapist may think there is something wrong with how their tongue moves and will misdiagnose the child as having childhood apraxia of speech (CAS). CAS is a motor speech disorder due to a problem in the brain (neurogenic).

The part of the brain that helps plan and sequence movement for speech is affected. Thus, these children often get frustrated when they try to speak as they struggle to achieve the correct place to put their tongue, jaw, and lips. Due to these difficulties, children with CAS initially tend to speak with simplified word shapes and sentences (e.g., /ʔæʔ/ for /kæt/). They may sound similar to a child born with cleft who has learned to communicate with glottal stops and vowels.

However, the reason for the speech disorder is neurogenic and due to poor planning for the child with apraxia, versus a learned behavior to compensate for structural differences in the child born with cleft. It is possible for a child to have both a structural cause and a neurogenic cause, especially in some syndromes, where there are both neurological and structural deficits.

The cleft team SLP will identify the use of compensatory and other articulation behaviors and make recommendations for therapy designed to address them. These types of errors cannot be fixed with surgical repair, but will need speech therapy. For example, if the child is saying /ʔap/ for "pop," you could add a breathy "h" to the sound they should be producing, such as modeling "p^{hhhhhhhhhh}op" for "pop" The breathy "h" will keep the child from making a glottal stop. Eventually, the breathy "h" can be faded out (Kuehn and Henne, 2003).

The timing of speech therapy should begin prior to surgery, if possible. Before children turn two years of age, SLPs can be very helpful in teaching parents how to work on sound imitation through vocal play and to recognize maladaptive compensatory strategies. In addition, vocal play can be helpful in introducing the internationally adopted child to the speech sounds of his/her new language. Before the palate is repaired, the child should be able to say all nasal sounds.

The child may even be able to produce /h, j, w, r, l/. Thus, encouraging vocal play with these sounds can be a lot of fun for the child (e.g., mamama, wawa, lala). Prior to palate repair, some early words and phrases to work on include:

Mama	home
my/mine	hey
no	no more
more	wow
now	nana (for "banana" or "grandmother")
hi/hello	

Choosing real words instead of just non-sense words will be more motivating for the child and will help build her or his lexicon. After the palate is repaired, the child can be encouraged to produce words with the high-pressure consonants mentioned earlier. Some of these early developing words include:

Baby	toy
bye-bye	top
boy	duck
Pooh	daddy
Pop	go
put-put-put (while pushing a car along)	girl
cookie	cow

In addition to focusing on simple words with specific phonetic targets for speech, it is also important to work on language. Scherer (1999) examined the effects of working on vocabulary with children with cleft who had a limited consonant inventory as well as delayed expressive language. She used a naturalistic intervention, called milieu intervention. "Milieu intervention combines six components, including environmental arrangement, responsive interaction, modeling, **mand-model**, incidental teaching, and time delay procedures" (Scherer, 1999, p. 83). Results indicated that phonological performance improved as well as expressive language skills. Blowing for the purpose of learning to produce a continuous air stream from the mouth can also be encouraged in a toddler or an older child who has not yet had surgery. Once the palate has been repaired, directing air out the mouth is a new skill the child needs to learn. As soon as the child can achieve this using games such as blowing bubbles, the parent and the speech therapist can work on sounds like /ʃ, s, z/. The child may need some help getting the air to go in the right direction at first. By carefully occluding the nares (blocking the nostrils with the fingers) the child will have the opportunity to see what it feels like to build up intra-oral pressure and will have more success with these sounds. Soon, she or he should be able to produce the sounds without blocking the nose, unless there is need for further surgery, discussed below. In the preschooler or older child who has not yet had a palate repair, many people assume that speech therapy would not begin until after surgical repairs of the palate have been done. However, correct placement of the tongue, jaw, and lips can be worked on even before the palate is repaired. For example, the child could be instructed to put the tongue tip behind the teeth for /t, d/, put the lips together for /p, b/, etc. As noted above, once surgery has taken place, the child will need additional therapy to continue to address the production of any compensatory maladaptive patterns that are still present. After approximately six months of speech therapy focusing on oral placement of sounds, the SLP and the cleft palate team will discuss whether the child needs a secondary palate surgery. It is important to note that there are two main factors that can reduce the effectiveness of speech therapy, thus requiring an adjustment to the six months guideline. The first factor is the child's ability to focus and follow directions in speech therapy. Not every child is willing or able to focus on the task at hand. The other factor is the SLP's knowledge of how to work with children born with cleft palate. Since this is a fairly low-incidence population, many SLPs have little experience treating children born with a cleft condition. Thus, the cleft team has an important role in ensuring that the therapy being provided is appropriate to the child. Some SLPs may have been trained in the past to do exercises that we now know are ineffective for improving the oral pressure for speech, such as blowing and sucking exercises. Although these actions require raising the soft palate as in speech, it is for a different function and does not generalize to speech. However, using blowing as a way to demonstrate that air needs to come out of the mouth versus the nose is appropriate in the early stages of therapy as noted above. In addition to these two factors influencing the effectiveness of treatment, the SLP will investigate whether the child needs additional surgery. This decision should be based on careful evaluation of the child's progress in therapy and function of the soft palate. Persistent air escape through the nose may be due to poor elevation of the soft palate or the soft palate being too short to make contact with the back of the throat. It is helpful to have two important pieces of information when making this decision. The first piece of information comes from the SLP. Speech therapy may be able to remediate inconsistent hypernasality and phoneme specific nasal emission, but it cannot fix speech problems due to velopharyngeal incompetence. After obtaining good articulatory placement, the SLP must then determine if the child continues to sound hypernasal and/or presents with nasal emission of air. Consistent hypernasality, nasal emission, and poor ability to obtain adequate intra-oral air pressure for speech would all suggest that the child would need secondary surgery (Kummer, 2008).

The second piece of information comes from viewing the soft palate and pharyngeal walls (velopharyngeal mechanism). A videonasoendoscopy conducted by an ENT or SLP is a common imaging procedure for this purpose.

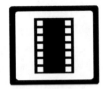

Access Video File 2 (Chapter 17)

17V2 Case Example 2 Pre-Surgery.

Access Video File 3 (Chapter 17)

17V3 Case Example 2 Post-Surgery.

> Jonah is a four-year-old boy who received a secondary palate repair to treat his VPI/C. Prior to the surgery, Jonah was consistently hypernasal with nasal air emissions, nasal grimaces, but good articulatory placement. Three weeks following the pharyngeal flap surgery, Jonah continues to be hypernasal, but with less severity. One may question did the surgery work? We will not know until Jonah is taught how to direct airflow orally. Thus, Jonah will go back to speech therapy to focus on his resonance. If his speech does not change, he may need another surgery to modify the width of the pharyngeal flap. Note the differences prior to and after surgery.

It involves putting a thin tube–like scope through the nose in order to see functioning of the velopharyngeal mechanism (Kuehn and Henne, 2003). Although this procedure does not hurt, it can be awkward and not all children tolerate it on the first attempt. Another imaging method sometimes used is **videofluoroscopy** conducted by a radiologist (Kuehn and Henne, 2003). This method provides a motion X-ray of the structures of the soft palate and pharyngeal walls after a radio-contrastive powder or liquid is placed inside the child's nose to coat the structures of interest. Videofluoroscopy is considered less invasive than **videonasoendoscopy**, but can be challenging because the child's head needs to remain still while talking. During both procedures the child is asked to repeat some sounds and words that require raising the soft palate and constriction of the pharyngeal (throat) walls. For example, the child may be asked to repeat a phrase like, "Buy Bobby a puppy." The chosen phrases have many sounds that need build up of air in the oral cavity and thus closing off of the nasal cavity by closing the velopharyngeal port (the space between the walls of the throat and the soft palate that close the oral cavity from the nasal cavity). The normally talkative daughter of the first author of this chapter refused to speak during her first scoping procedure and hence it needed to be repeated at a later time. Videotaping during either of these procedures allows the cleft palate team to replay and analyze the ability for the soft palate and pharyngeal wall to close off the velopharyngeal port. If the child is using good articulatory placement, but has poor closure, he or she may be a candidate for further surgery. The exact type of surgery recommended will depend on the surgeon and the amount of space remaining in the velopharyngeal port during maximal closure during speech. The surgeon and/or the cleft palate team will discuss the options with the family.

Orthodontia

Although all children require routine dental care, a child with a cleft involving the upper dental arch requires more than normal dental care both to repair the cleft through the gum line and to manage tooth eruption and positioning. The cleft of the dental arch is typically located between the central incisor and the canine, with a missing or malpositioned lateral incisor on the cleft side. In addition, children with clefts of the dental arch may experience one or more of the following difficulties: missing teeth, malformed teeth, malpositioned teeth (ectopic), and extra teeth (supernumerary). Closure of the upper and lower teeth on both sides of the mouth may be affected by the presence of the cleft as well as growth of the upper jaw, both requiring dental or surgical care. (Kummer, 2008). The cleft team that includes a number of dental professionals including: a pediatric dentist to look after tooth health, an orthodontist to look after tooth positioning, an oral surgeon to repair the dental arch cleft (or the plastic surgeon may perform this task), and a prosthodontist to create artificial teeth or dental prostheses. Timelines for treatment will vary from team to team but a typical timeline follows:

- 2-10 weeks of age possible presurgical orthopedic appliance to narrow palatal cleft
- 2-6 years pediatric dental care
- 7-9 years orthodontic care begins
- 9-11 years alveolar cleft repair via bone grafting or distraction
- 11-18 years orthodontia, surgery (orthognathic) to align the upper and lower jaws, and dental restoration via prosthodontics

Surgery

The goals and timeline of surgery to repair the cleft will depend on the severity of the cleft. Generally, "primary surgery" refers to each surgery that is needed to repair the initial cleft condition. Primary surgeries may include repair of the lip (cheiloplasty), the nose (rhinoplasty), and the palate (palatoplasty). "Secondary surgeries" refer to the surgeries needed to repair residual deficits in the lip or palate or surgeries to improve speech production (**pharyngoplasty** or **pharyngeal flap**) due to poor soft palate function. The timeline for surgeries needed by the child will vary among teams. For a good overview of the procedures, see *Cleft Palate Repair and Variations* by Agrawal, 2009.

Many children require multiple primary and secondary surgeries, due in part to the growth of the oral cavity. The following timeline is typical of most teams in North America:

- 3 months of age lip repair
- 6-18 months of age palate repair
- 4-6 years of age secondary surgery for speech (only needed for children with VPI/S post palate repair)
- 4-6 years of age primary nose/lip revision
- 11-18 years of age secondary nose/lip revision
- 13-18 years of age orthognathic surgery-maxillary advancement

The goals of primary lip repair include normal lip and nose appearance and function with minimal scarring.

The goals of primary palate repair include optimal speech development and normal facial growth. The goals of secondary surgery for speech are to improve soft palate function in order to facilitate normal speech resonance (nasality in speech). Secondary surgery speech is only needed by approximately 20% to 25% of the children with cleft palate.

Access Video File 4 (Chapter 17)

17V4 Case example 3.

> Alexander is a nine-year old boy with bilateral cleft lip and palate. He was adopted at 17 months of age and had his lip and palate repaired at 2 years of age. He had a pharyngeal flap at 3 years of age. Prior to the pharyngeal flap, he was producing speech with primarily nasals, glottal stops, and vowels. After receiving speech therapy and the pharyngeal flap, Alexander achieved correct place of articulation, but then became **hyponasal**. This can happen when the flap is made too wide. Over time, his vocal tract will grow, adenoid tissue will atrophy, and he will need advancement of the maxilla, which may increase space in the velopharyngeal port. In addition, he makes obligatory errors (errors made due to structural differences) due to the misalignment of his teeth and the orthodontia in his mouth. Although his speech is not ideal, speech therapy is not advised at this time because his speech errors are obligatory.

This type of surgery is commonly referred to as a pharyngoplasty. Depending on the closure pattern of the V-P mechanism, the surgeon may choose to do a pharyngeal flap or a pharyngeal wall augmentation.

In the first procedure, a flap of tissue is raised from the posterior pharyngeal wall and then sutured into the velum, leaving ports on both sides for nasal breathing (Kummer, 2008). For pharyngeal wall augmentation, the posterior pharyngeal wall is bulked up with tissue to lessen the space needed for V-P closure.

Complications following surgery include the occurrence of a small hole (fistula) somewhere in the hard or soft palate. This fistula may or may not have an impact on speech and will be assessed by the team SLP. Dehiscence, which refers to the breakdown of a surgical repair, is another possibility. When there is dehiscence the tissue may come apart where the sutures were placed, such as where the mucosa was sewn together midline to close the palate. If dehiscence occurs, it is more likely to happen within two to six weeks of the repair.

Special Considerations

Adopted Children with Cleft

Unless the child's cleft was repaired early on in their birth country, the child will most likely have the repairs done once the adoptive family can schedule their surgery when they get her or him home. The adoptive process can be time consuming and thus children who do not receive repairs until they arrive in their adoptive country often receive them much later than children born in the adoptive country.

Thus, the ideal surgery timelines discussed earlier will occur at older ages. As mentioned earlier, roughly one in four to five children who receive surgeries in the United States need speech therapy and/or secondary surgery to produce good speech. The data are not clear about children adopted internationally. However, based on US data it is likely that children who have their cleft repairs after 2 years of age are more likely to need speech therapy and/or secondary surgeries. The authors of this chapter each have two internationally adopted children and all four children needed secondary palate repair surgeries and speech therapy. Further research on average age of cleft repair and its impact on speech development of internationally adopted children are warranted.

Language Implications of Internationally Adopted Children with Cleft Lip and Palate

This last section addresses the risk factors concerning language development for internationally adopted children with cleft lip and palate. Although there is no research on this specifically, this chapter has already discussed language development for children with cleft and there is also a body of literature on language development of internationally adopted children without cleft.

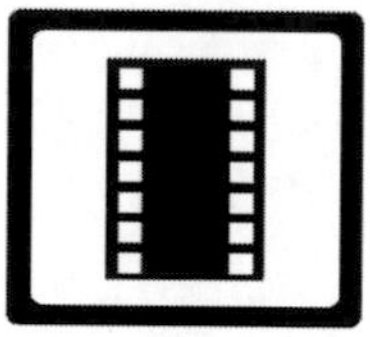

Access Video File 5 (Chapter 17)

17V5: Case Example 4.

> Edward is a six-year-old boy who was adopted from China when he was 25 months old. His lip and palate were repaired in China and he received a pharyngeal flap at four years of age. He has been in speech therapy for four years. Edward continues to work on correct placement of articulation and oral airflow. Compare his performance on fricatives to stops. Also note how his class III malocclusion (retracted maxilla as compared to the mandible) impacts his articulation. This is a common condition for children with bilateral cleft lip and palate.

When one begins to read about the health and development concerns of internationally adopted children it can be quite overwhelming. For example, internationally adopted children often present with stunted growth, abnormal behaviors, and significant motor, speech and language delays. However, the majority of internationally adopted children do catch up within a year of being with their adoptive family (Glennen, 2002; 2008). Nonetheless, parents should be made aware of some of the risk factors associated with children being raised in institutional settings.

Pediatricians who specialized in assessing internationally adopted children estimated that children average one month of developmental delay for ever four to five months spent in an orphanage (Jenista, 1997). This can be due to a myriad of reasons such as low birth weight, poor nutrition, growth failure, lack of consistent human contact, and little language exposure and interaction with caregivers (i.e., lack of adequate stimulation). In addition, internationally adopted children have an increase in hearing loss most likely due to chronic otitis media.

For reasons already mentioned, children with cleft palate are almost guaranteed to have chronic ear infections. This risk factor for children with cleft often seems to get overlooked in institutional settings, and thus the child is further at risk for language delay. Thus, as noted earlier, hearing should be assessed and P-E tubes should be placed if found necessary, as soon as possible.

It is important to be aware of the expected rate of acquiring English language after the internationally adopted child has been brought home. The majority of children adopted into a supportive environment should be acquiring the second language at a rapid rate. Children adopted prior to age two fare better than children adopted after age two (Glennen, 2008). However, the research done on this topic up to date has not addressed internationally adopted children with cleft palate, specifically.

In general, when children are adopted, they transition from their birth language to their adopted language. As this happens, development of their birth language is arrested and ceases to develop, and then attrition of the birth language follows as they begin to learn their new adoptive language (Glennen, 2002).

Interestingly, internationally adopted children follow the same English language development as children raised exclusively in English speaking cultures. English language learning begins soon after the child is brought into their English speaking homes and progresses rapidly. If the child is not making rapid gains in vocabulary within the first few months, the child is likely to be language delayed and will need services. Children adopted at older ages tend to acquire English words more rapidly than children adopted at younger ages (Glennen, 2007).

It could be that an older child is developmentally more ready to acquire new words. However, the older a child is at the time of adoption, the longer it takes him or her to "catch up" with his or her peers. It is important to note that the majority of internationally adopted children who received orphanage care prior to adoption make rapid gains in English and do well by preschool age (Glennen, 2007, 2008).

In general, studies have found that the majority of internationally adopted children perform well within or above the average range of performance after being in the country for two years (Glennen, 2002; 2007; 2008; Scott, Roberts, and Glennen, 2011). Children who are still delayed after two years will need speech therapy services to address language concerns (McConnell, Sylvestre and MacLeod, 2010).

For the child born with cleft, however, it is not recommended to wait two years to see if the child needs intervention. Given that children with cleft palate are already at risk for speech and language delays and hearing loss, it is important that the child begins receiving speech therapy and audiological services as soon as he or she enters the country. If the child is under the age of three when brought him home, parents can contact their local education office about their Birth to Three program and they will come to the home to assess the child's abilities in multiple areas (speech, language, gross motor, fine motor, and cognition). Even though a cleft palate team will see the child, the local school district will also play an important role in providing on-going services for the child.

Sidebar 17.3. Parent Involvement

As noted earlier, parent involvement in therapy is very important. In addition, there are many things that can be done in everyday events to facilitate language development. The following is a list of tips for parents:

- Talk as you bathe and dress your child. Label the different body parts, clothing items, and anything else that is relevant.
- Take your child grocery shopping with you. Label and describe all of the food and drinks you're getting. Allow the child to touch and smell the items that are appropriate.
- Talk about what you are doing, where you are going, what you will do when you arrive, and who and what you will see.
- Look through picture books together. Label the objects and describe what the people are doing. Ask the child to point to the objects you describe.
- Use gestures such as waving goodbye to help convey meaning.
- Identify colors.
- Count everything. "Let's count the steps, 1, 2, 3, 4, …" "How many goldfish do you want?" "Let's count them."
- Introduce environmental sounds to associate a sound with a specific meaning: "The doggie says woof-woof." "The car goes vroom-vroom."
- Acknowledge any attempts to communicate.
- Expand on single words the child uses: "Here is Mama. Mama loves you. Where is baby?"

Children with Multiple Disabilities

As stated earlier, cleft lip and/or palate can occur in over 500 known syndromes. Some of these syndromes also have multiple life-endangering birth defects. For example, Trisomy 13 is a chromosomal disorder associated with severe brain anomalies and congenital heart defects in addition to cleft lip and palate (Kummer, 2008). Wolf-Hirschhorn Syndrome is another chromosomal disorder with severe consequences. It causes **microcephaly**, heart defects, seizures, and severe to profound mental retardation and communication impairments.

The first author of this chapter recently evaluated a child with Wolf-Hirshhorn Syndrome. The client was a delightful 11-year-old boy with an unrepaired cleft of the soft palate. Due to the child's small airway and limited verbal skills, the team suggested to the family when he was younger to wait until the child was speaking in sentences prior to risking palate repair surgery. When the child was 11 years old, the parents believed he was attempting to speak in sentences and wanted to know if he should have his palate repaired so he could be better understood.

The client was given a receptive language evaluation, a motor speech evaluation, and a structural functional exam. He was very animated and successfully got his message across through gestures and word approximations. Word approximations consisted of a few vowels and /m/. He was unable to move his tongue on command and no attempts were made at alveolar sounds, even with maximal prompting.

The client had difficulty sustaining attention, which would have been required for motor learning to occur for correct articulatory placement. After explaining to the parents how speech was produced with the aid of an anatomical model of the vocal tract and all of the structures that would have to work together to make speech intelligible, and the amount of sustained attention it would require for their son to progress in speech, they realized that the benefits to surgery would be limited and that the surgery would most likely not fix their son's speech.

In addition, it was explained that an augmentative communication device (AAC) was recommended for their son to be a more successful communicator. Like many parents who wish for their children to be verbal, these parents were initially hesitant to use an AAC device because they feared that they would be giving up on their child becoming verbal. It is important to educate families on all of the components of communication and that becoming verbal is not the only way. In addition, sometimes AAC devices are used to show the child the power of communication and the use of the AAC device turns into a stepping-stone to more verbal communication. Similar conversations to the one above were had several times on a recent cleft palate mission trip in Guatemala. There were several children with syndromic cleft palate who also had a motor speech disorder and/or intellectual disability. Some of these families traveled a great distance in hopes that surgery would fix their child's communication impairment. It can be heartbreaking, but it is crucial that the SLP educate the family on all of the factors that make communication happen, so that a successful plan can be put in place.

CONNECTIONS

In this book, you have learned about sound productions from birth to babble, transition to first words, and the interactions between speech sound development and other areas of development such as prosody. Now that you have read about the speech development of children with cleft palate, you can see how our understanding of normal speech and language development allows us to better understand the threats to speech and language development when structural anomalies interfere with normal speech production.

The critical ages of speech development make it evident that early intervention and appropriate surgical repairs can have long lasting positive implications. In the next two chapters, you will see how motor speech disorders, hearing impairment, and developmental disabilities can also have an impact on speech development.

CONCLUDING REMARKS

Some instructors in communication disorders and science programs believe that students do not need a class in cleft lip and palate because the information can be covered in anatomy, speech and hearing sciences, and articulation disorders. After reading this chapter, which has only had the chance to touch on a few of the many nuances that come with this population, we hope you see that there is much more to consider. For example, there is interdependence between the cleft palate team members. The surgeon cannot surgically correct a behavioral speech sound disorder just as the SLP cannot correct a speech disorder caused by structural deficits. The client will often have to go between the two to work on both issues. Hearing status needs to be monitored and oral structures and teeth need to be in alignment. The contributions of every team member are crucial for the child affected by cleft to succeed as a verbal communicator.

CHAPTER REVIEW QUESTIONS

1. Why is the use of the term "harelip" incorrect?
2. What are some of the causes of cleft lip and palate?
3. What differences might exist between children born in this country with cleft versus internationally adopted children with cleft?
4. How does cleft palate impact speech and hearing?
5. Why might surgery **not** be recommended for a child with cleft palate?

SUGGESTIONS FOR FURTHER READING

The Center for Children with Special Needs Seattle Children's Hospital, Seattle, WA (2010). Cleft Lip and Palate Critical Elements of Care Fifth Edition.

http://cshcn.org/sites/default/files/webfm/file/CriticalElementsofCare-CleftLipandPalate.pdf retrieved on 9/20/11.

Golding-Kushner, K. (2001). *Therapy Techniques for Cleft Palate-Speech and Related Disorders,* Singular Thompson Learning, San Diego, CA.

Kuehn, D. P. and Moller, K. T. (2000). Speech and language issues in the cleft palate population: The state of the art. *Cleft Palate-Craniofacial Journal*, 37-4, p. 1-35.

Kummer, A.W. (2008). *Cleft Palate and Craniofacial Anomalies: Effects on Speech and Resonance* (2nd Ed.). Clifton Park, NY: Thomson Delmar.

Peterson-Falzone, S., Hardin-Jones, M. and Karnell, M. (2001). *Cleft Palate Speech, 3rd Ed.* Mosby-Elsevier, St. Louis, MO.

Peterson-Falzone, S., Trost-Cardomone, Karnell, M. and Hardin-Jones, M. (2006). *The Clinician's Guide to Treating Cleft palate Speech*, Mosby-Elsevier, St. Louis, MO.

Shprintzen, R.J. (2000). Syndrome Identification for Speech-Language Pathology: An Illustrated Pocket Guide, Singular Publishing.

Websites with General Information about Cleft Lip and Palate

American Cleft Palate-Craniofacial Association
http://www.acpa-cpf.org
American Cleft Palate-Craniofacial Association For Evaluation and Treatment of Patients with Cleft Lip/Palate or Other Craniofacial Anomalies, Revised 2009
http://www.acpa-cpf.org/teamcare/Parameters%20Rev.2009.pdf.
Cleft Palate Foundation Cleftline 1-800-24-CLEFT or
http://www.cleftline.org
Cleft Advocate
www.cleftadvocate.org
Craniofacial Services at Children's Healthcare of Atlanta
http://www.choa.org/Childrens-Hospital-Services/Pediatric-Craniofacial-Center/Programs-and-Services/Cleft-Lip-and-Palate
University of Iowa Cleft Palate and Craniofacial Clinic
http://www.uihealthcare.com/depts/med/otolaryngology/clinics/cleftlippalate/index.html
Wide Smiles
http://www.widesmiles.org
For Evaluation and Treatment of Patients with Cleft Lip/Palate or Other Craniofacial Anomalies, 3rd edition
http://www.acpa-cpf.org/teamcare/Parameters%20Rev.2009.pdf

Suggestions for Student Activities

1. Perform an oral peripheral exam on as many people as possible to view the variability of the oral structures.
2. Look up stories on the Cleft Palate website to learn about the lives of families with children with cleft lip and palate. http://www.cleftline.org/features/story_of_the_month.
3. Find the closest cleft palate/craniofacial team in your area and ask if you can observe for a day.

Answers to Chapter Review Questions

1. Why is the use of the term "harelip" incorrect?

It is an outdated term that has negative connotations. It describes the child as having an animal like characteristic, which was once thought to be associated with witchcraft or relations with Satan.

The term cleft is an objective term that better describes the separation of the lip and/or palate.

2. What are some of the causes of cleft lip and palate?

Causes of cleft lip and palate can include teratogens, such as medications, alcohol, or nicotine the mother takes while pregnant; mechanically induced anomalies, such as intrauterine crowding; and genetic causes, such as Pierre Robin Sequence. Often the cause is unknown.

3. What differences might exist between children born in this country with cleft versus internationally adopted children with cleft?

Children born with cleft in this country typically receive their repairs in a timely manner and are learning to speak the language they were born to.

Internationally adopted children may have a different surgical timeline, depending on the age they were adopted and what surgical management happened in the country they were born in. In addition, depending on the amount of stimulation they were given during development, they could be at higher risk for developmental delays in general.

4. How does cleft palate impact speech and hearing?

Cleft palate impacts speech by causing difficulties with building inter-oral air pressure for high-pressure consonants such as stops, fricatives and affricates.

Cleft impacts hearing because the tensor veli palatine muscles are not in the correct position to dilate the eustachian tubes, which makes the child more susceptible to middle ear infections and conductive hearing loss.

5. Why might surgery not be recommended for a child with cleft palate?

Surgery might not be recommended for a child who has other medical complications. For example, if the airway is compromised, a surgical procedure may be too risky. This can be the case with more severe craniofacial anomalies due to syndromes.

REFERENCES

Agrawal, K. (2009). Cleft palate repair and variations. *Indian Journal of Plastic Surgery, 42* (suppl): S102-S109. http://www.ncbi.nlm.nih.gov/pmc/articles/PMC2825076/ (retrieved 11/11/11).

Broen, P., Devers, M. C., Doyle, S. S., McCauley Prouty, J., and Moller, K. T. (1998). Acquisition of linguistic and cognitive skills by children with cleft palate. *American Speech-Language and Hearing Research*, *41,* 676-687.

Cohen, M. M. (1978). Syndromes with cleft lip and cleft palate. *Cleft Palate Journal*, 15, 4, 306-328.

Cohen, M. M. (1999). Editorial comment: Robin Sequences and complexes: causal heterogeneity and pathogenetic/phenotypic variability. *American Journal of Medical Genetics*, 84, 311-315.

Dixon, M.J., Marazita, M. L., Beaty, T. H., and Murray, J. C. (2011). Cleft lip and palate: synthesizing genetic and environmental Influences. *Nature Reviews Genetics, 12* (3), 167–178.

Frederickson, M. S., Chapman, K. L., and Hardin-Jones M. (2006). Conversational skills of children with cleft lip and palate: A replication and extension. *Cleft Palate-Craniofacial Journal, 43* (2), 179-188.

Glennen, S. (2002). Language development and delay in internationally adopted infants and toddlers: A review. *American Journal of Speech Language Pathology*, 11: 333-339.

Glennen, S. L. (2007). Predicting language outcomes for internationally adopted children. *Journal of Speech, Language, and Hearing Research, 50*, 529-548.

Glennen, S. (2008). Speech and Language "Mythbusters" for Internationally Adopted Children *ASHA Leader,* December 16,2008.

Jenista, J. (1997). Russian children and medical records. *Adoption Medical News*, *3*(7), 1–8.

Jocelyn, L. J., Penko, M. A., Rode, H. L. (1996). Cognition, communication, and hearing in young children with cleft lip and palate and in control children: a longitudinal study. *Pediatrics, 97, 4*, 529-534.

Kuehn, D. P. and Henne, L. J. (2003). Speech evaluation and treatment for patients with cleft palate. *American Journal of Speech-Language Pathology, 12*, 103-109.

Kummer, A.W. (2008). Cleft Palate and Craniofacial Anomalies: Effects on Speech and Resonance (2nd Ed.). Clifton Park, NY: Thomson Delmar.

Lehman, J. (2008). Cleft lip and palate management in the developing world: Primary and secondary surgery and its delivery. In M. Mars, D. Sell, and A. Habel (Eds.) Management of Cleft Lip and Palate in the Developing World, West Sussex, England, John Wiley and Sons Ltd. pp 37-48.

McConnell, Sylvestre and MacLeod (2010). Atypical language development in a child adopted from China: Clinical reasoning and evolution of language abilities. *Canadian Journal of Speech-Language Pathology and Audiology, 34*/1(33-42).

Noll, JD (1983). The origin of the term "harelip". *The Cleft Palate Journal*, vol. 21, 169-171.

Parker SE, Mai CT, Canfield MA, Rickard R, Wang Y, Meyer RE, et al; for the National Birth Defects Prevention Network. Updated national birth prevalence estimates for selected birth defects in the United States, 2004-2006. Birth Defects Research. Part A Clinical and Molecular Teratoly. 2010 Sept 28. [Epub ahead of print]

Peng, J. and Hong-yan, L. (2011). Cleft palate surgery orbicularis oris secondarily provide off type of intraoperative 400 cases clinical application separation summary. Jilin Medical Journal, abstract http://en.cnki.com.cn/Article_en/CJFDTOTAL-JLYX201105012.htm.

Robin, N. H. and Shprintzen, R. J. (2005). Defining the clinical spectrum of deletion 22q11.2. *The Journal of Pediatrics,* 1(47), 90-96.

Scherer, N. J. (1999). The speech and language status of toddlers with cleft lip and/or palate following early vocabulary intervention. *American Journal of Speech-Language Pathology,* 8, 81-93.

Scott, K. A., Roberts, J. A., and Glennen, S. (2011). How Well Do Children Who Are Internationally Adopted Acquire Language? A Meta-Analysis. *Journal of Speech, Language and Hearing Research, 54*, 1153-1169.

Scherer, N. J. (1999). The speech and language status of toddlers with cleft lip/and/or palate following early vocabulary intervention. *American Journal of Speech-Language Pathology, 8*, 81-93.

Scherer, N. J. and Antonio, L. D. (1997). Language and play development in toddlers with cleft lip and/or palate. *American Journal of Speech-Language Pathology: A Journal of Clinical Practice*, *6*, 48-54.

Shprintzen, R. J. (1995). A new perspective on clefting. In R. J. Shprintzen and J. bardach (Eds), Cleft Palate Speech Management: A Multidisciplinary Approach, St. Louis, IL: Mosby.

Shprintzen, R. J. (2000). Syndrome Identification for Speech-Language Pathology: An Illustrated Pocketguide, San Diego: Singular Publishing.

Stoel-Gammon, C. (1998a). Sounds and words in early language acquisition: The relationship between lexical and phonological development. In R. Paul (Ed.), *Exploring the Speech-Language Connection* (pp 22-52). Baltimore: Paul H. Brookes.

Stoel-Gammon, C. (1998b). Role of babbling and phonology in early linguistic development. In A. M. Wetherby, S. F. Warren and J. Reichle (Eds.) Transitions in Prelinguistic Communication (pp. 87-110). Baltimore; Paul H Brookes.

Trost-Cardamone, J. E. (1986). Effects of velopharyngeal incompetence on speech *Communication Disorders Quarterly, 10*: 31-49.

Zucchero, T.M., et al. (2004). Interferon Regulatory Factor 6 (IRF6) gene variants and the risk of isolated cleft lip or palate. *New England Journal of Medicine,* 351 (8), 769-780.

WideSmiles.org (1996) "Harelip" - The Dark History of an Unfortunate Word http://www.widesmiles2.org/cleftlinks/WS-159.html (retrieved 7/25/11).

In: Comprehensive Perspectives …
Editors: Beate Peter and Andrea A. N. MacLeod
ISBN: 978-1-62257-041-6

Chapter 18

MOTOR SPEECH DISORDERS IN CHILDREN

Amy Skinder-Meredith and Andrea A. N. MacLeod

INTRODUCTION

Whereas Chapter 17 discussed speech sound disorders due to structural deficits and Chapter 15 speech sound disorders in otherwise typically developing children, this chapter focuses on speech disorders that specifically affect motor planning, programming, and execution. We refer to these as **motor speech disorders**. This term covers a collection of communication disorders involving the retrieval and activation of motor plans for speech, or the execution of movements for speech production. The two major subcategories of motor speech disorders across all ages are **apraxia** and **dysarthria**. Motor speech disorders may be acquired, as in the case of a stroke, degenerative disease, or brain injury, after speech has already developed, or they may be developmental, where the onset was prior to or during speech development. Developmental motor speech disorders may be caused by inter-uterine stroke, anoxia, seizures, complications before, during, or soon after birth, degenerative diseases, and other known reasons; in addition, for some children the cause of their motor speech disorders remains unknown. The presence of a motor speech disorder in children can influence the development of phonology and other language processes. Thus, children with motor planning, programming, and execution deficits may also exhibit phonologic and perhaps other linguistic deficits (Caruso & Strand, 1999). The goal of this chapter is to outline the key features of developmental dysarthria and childhood apraxia of speech (CAS); we will then outline the key issues to consider in evaluating these children; and finally we will summarize treatment considerations for these children.

Dysarthria

Strictly speaking, the word "dysarthria" means unable to utter distinctly. In the field of speech-language pathology, the term *dysarthria* refers to impaired production of speech due to disturbances in the muscular control of the speech mechanism. Dysarthria is caused by impairment in the **central nervous system** or **peripheral nervous system**. As described in Chapter 3, the central nervous system consists mainly of the brain and the spinal cord, whereas the peripheral nervous system is made up of the cranial and spinal nerves. Dysarthria in children may be due to injury to the central or peripheral nervous system that occurred during pregnancy or childbirth, or to injury following the normal onset of speech development (i.e., acquired childhood dysarthria). This injury may be related to a genetic syndrome, tumors, or accidental injury. Many children with dysarthria have other developmental delays or disorders as well, including delays in gross and fine motor development, difficulty chewing and swallowing food, cognitive delays, hearing impairment, and visual impairment. These children may also experience important health problems that result in frequent or lengthy stays in hospitals. As a result, speech-language pathologists (SLPs) often find themselves working within an interdisciplinary team in assessment and treatment. In this setting, SLPs need to communicate with the team and parents to understand how to prioritize treatment goals given the general health and developmental of the child.

Researchers have found different patterns of dysarthria in children than in adults (van Mourik et al., 1997). Early work describing speech impairment among children has focused on describing speech abilities of children as related to their gross-motor impairment (e.g., Byrne, 1959). This approach, however, has been criticized since considerable overlap has since been observed among children with different gross motor impairments (Ansel & Kent, 1992; Hustad, Gordon & Lee, 2010).

Causes of Dysarthria in Children. In a simplified view, speech production requires a complex coordination between our central and peripheral nervous systems to activate our muscles to produce speech. For children with dysarthria, damage has occurred in the central and/or peripheral nervous system, which does not allow muscles to be activated in a "normal" manner. The abnormal activation affects all the muscles controlled by the damaged part of the nervous system and results in abnormal movement that often goes well beyond the muscles needed to produce speech. Intelligible speech requires a complex coordination between the respiratory, phonatory, resonance, and articulatory systems. In contrast to speech sound disorders described in Chapter 15, children with dysarthria often show difficulty not only with the articulatory system, but also with coordinating their respiratory, phonatory and resonance systems to support speech production. The following paragraphs will summarize the characteristics of dysarthria among children with acquired childhood dysarthria and children with cerebral palsy.

Acquired Childhood Dysarthria. Children with acquired childhood dysarthria have experienced a period of typical development followed by an injury to their central or peripheral nervous system that has resulted in dysarthric speech. Research in this area has focused on case studies and comparisons with dysarthria acquired in adulthood (van Mourik et al., 1997; Morgan & Liégeois, 2010). Research on adults who have suffered injury to their brain or peripheral nervous system has helped to identify subtypes of dysarthria (Darley et al., 1969). These subtypes can be distinguished based on the site of the lesion, and also based on the auditory and visual characteristics of the individuals' speech. Depending on the location of the lesion, the muscles may show weakness, a decreased range of motion, decreased speed, or impaired coordination of the muscles that comprise the respiratory, phonatory, articulatory, and resonance systems (Darley et al., 1969; Duffy & Kent, 2001). Recently, researchers have questioned the applicability of these subtypes based on adults to describe developmental dysarthria (Kent, 2000; van Mourik et al., 2007; Morgan & Liégeois, 2010). The main argument against using adult subtypes is that children have a developing neuromotor system and thus the system may evolve differently from the injury compared to adults (Morgan & Liégeois, 2010; Wit, Maassen, Gabreëls, Thoonen & deSwart, 1994). For children who are born with an injury to the nervous system, it is not simply the execution of speech sounds that is affected but also the ability to acquire these speech sounds (Wit et al., 1994). However, since the adult subtypes are often used clinically to describe dysarthria observed during childhood and a system has yet to be proposed for these children, we will outline the six main subtypes below (see also Table 18.1).

Table 18.1 Summary table of different types of dysarthria (adapted from Duffy, 2005, p. 13)

Type of Dysarthria & Neuromotor Basis	Localization	Speech Characteristics
Flaccid: Flaccidity	Lower motor neuron (LMN)	Slow-labored articulation Hypernasal resonance with nasal emission Hoarse-breathy phonation
Spastic: Spasticity	Bilateral Upper motor neuron (UMN)	Imprecise consonants Monotonous pitch and loudness Harsh or strained/strangled voice quality Poor prosody Hypernasality Decreased rate of speech
Unilateral Upper Motor Neuron Dysarthria (UUMN): Weakness, incoordination, or spasticity	Unilateral UMN	Mild hypernasality Harsh voice quality
Ataxic: Incoordination	Cerebellum (control circuit)	Excess and equal stress Irregular articulatory breakdown Distorted vowels Harsh voice quality Scanning speech
Hyperkinetic or dyskinetic: Abnormal movements	Basal ganglia control circuit	Variable articulatory imprecision Vocal harshness Prosodic abnormalities
Mixed: Any combination of two or more of the above (e.g., spastic-ataxic dysarthria.)	Multiple lesion sites	Variable and depends on the lesion site

*Hypokinetic dysarthria is also due to an imbalance in the basal ganglia control circuit, but is primarily only seen in adults with Parkinsonism, and is thus not listed in this table.

As noted above, children with dysarthria often show difficulty not only with the articulatory system, but also with coordinating between various systems to support speech production. Although all dysarthrias are characterized by imprecise articulation, the specific features for different subtypes depend on which nerves were affected and the resulting degree of weakness. For example, if there was a bilateral lesion of the **vagus nerve**, impaired innervation of the muscles of the **laryngeal** and **velopharyngeal** muscles could result in a breathy voice quality and hypernasal resonance. Likewise, if there was a lesion to the **hypoglossal nerve**, poor tongue movement would result in imprecise articulation. Ataxic dysarthria impacts coordination and synergy of movement of all the subsystems for speech, but tends to have the greatest influence on articulation, phonation, respiration, and prosody. Lastly, hyperkinetic dysarthria (also called dyskinetic dysarthria) includes any motor speech disorder where there is involuntary purposeless movement that interferes with speech production.

Dysarthria in Children with Cerebral Palsy. In contrast to children with childhood acquired dysarthria, children with cerebral palsy sustain damage to their central or peripheral nervous system prior to birth, during birth, or in infancy. Cerebral palsy refers to a group of disorders that is characterized by movement and posture disturbances; is non-progressive; begins within the pre- or neonatal period or in infancy; is caused by damage to the central nervous system; and is accompanied by co-occurring problems with sensation, perception, cognition, communication, and/or behavior (Rosenbaum et al., 2007). Cerebral palsy is the most common cause of severe motor disability in children (Lepage, Noreau, Bernard & Fougeyrollas, 1998) affecting as many as 3.6 per 1000 children (Yeargin-Allsopp et al., 2008), and between 40% and 80% of these children have some level of speech impairment (Odding, Roebroeck & Stam, 2006). In Worster-Drought Syndrome, a subtype of cerebral palsy, speech disorders are consistently present; however, this syndrome is infrequently diagnosed due to the milder gross-motor symptoms (Clark et al., 2010).

In Chapter 2, Hodges and Pollock introduced how we create the sound source for speech by producing voice and noise. Voice requires sustained pressure generated by our respiratory system, which is modulated by our vocal folds and can result in the production of phonation. Noise is created by the articulators, comprised of the muscle groups (vocal folds, soft palate, pharynx, tongue root, tongue body, tongue tip, jaws lips) and the passive structures (hard palate, alveolar ridge, teeth) that stop or constrict the air stream. In the case of a child with dysarthria, the respiratory support for speech may be compromised, as evidenced by inability to produce adequate subglottal pressure (also referred to as tracheal pressure) or by decreased maximum phonation time. Motor disturbances for the phonatory system may be characterized by a breathy, tense, or harsh voice quality, as well as difficulty changing pitch and loudness. If the resonance system is impacted, the child may sound hypernasal and have difficulty building inter-oral air pressure due to impaired movement of the velum and pharyngeal walls. Lastly, weakness, incoordination, and decreased rate and range of motion may impact any or all of the articulators. Thus, the lips may be difficult to close for bilabials and the tongue may not move with adequate speed and force for clear speech.

Many individuals with cerebral palsy who have functional communication abilities are able to accurately produce manner contrasts for stops and nasals but are less accurate in producing fricatives and affricates (Byrne, 1959; Ansel & Kent, 1992). These individuals may also produce less contrastive vowels (Ansel & Kent, 1992; Hustad et al., 2010), as characterized by a weaker vowel height contrast, for example (Ansel & Kent, 1992). Abnormalities in speech breathing, which include irregular breathing, shallow breaths, and difficulty controlling expiration, have been found to negatively impact the speech of those with cerebral palsy (Solomon & Charron, 1998).

Sound file 18S1 is an excerpt from an articulation test administered to a 10-year-old boy with dysarthria. It is suspected that he suffered a stroke at birth. In addition to dysarthria, he has left hemiparesis. Listen for the following target words: "monkey," "banana," "zipper," "scissors," "duck," "yellow," "quack," "vacuum," "watch," "airplane," "swimming," and "watches." In what ways is speech production affected? Also observe the differences between the first and second productions of two of these words when he was asked for a repetition. Chapter 15 contains a different excerpt from this testing session.

Access Sound File 1 (Chapter 18)

18S1 Word productions of a boy, age 10, with dysarthria

Language Considerations for Children with Dysarthria. As noted by Pennington (2008), some children with developmental motor disorders, such as cerebral palsy, have language development that may be delayed due to the severity of their speech disorder. These children may only produce single words, rather than sentences, and may omit grammatical morphemes. These children may have language delays linked to more general cognitive delays or due to reduced interaction with others and their environment. In addition to these expressive language delays, some children may also have impaired language comprehension (Hustad et al., 2010). These findings highlight the importance of considering the child's speech sound abilities *and* her or his language abilities when planning assessments and identifying intervention goals.

Recently, Hustad et al. (2010) proposed four communication profiles to describe the speech and language abilities of children with cerebral palsy: (1) children with no speech-motor involvement with typical or delayed receptive language abilities; (2) children with speech-motor involvement and typically developing receptive language abilities; (3) children with speech-motor involvement and impaired receptive language abilities; and (4) children with no functional speech and with typical, impaired, or unknown receptive language abilities. These four categories were explored through a group study of 34 children with cerebral palsy who were 54 months old. The results supported the presence of the four groups and that speech variables (e.g., the size of the vowel space and speech rate) distinguished the four groups. Children with speech-motor involvement had smaller vowel spaces and slower speech rate than children without speech-motor involvement. Other research has found that children with cerebral palsy and cognitive impairment are more likely to also have impaired speech and language than their peers without cognitive impairment (Pirila et al., 2007).

Childhood Apraxia of Speech

As discussed in Chapter 15, apraxia refers to a problem with the ability to plan movement (praxis). This is usually caused by some determined (acquired) or undetermined (developmental) problem in the central nervous system. The American Speech-Language-

Hearing Association (ASHA) (2007) Position Statement defines it as follows: "*Childhood apraxia of speech (CAS)* is a neurological childhood (pediatric) speech sound disorder in which the precision and consistency of movements underlying speech are impaired in the absence of neuromuscular deficits (e.g., abnormal reflexes, abnormal tone). CAS may occur as a result of known neurological impairment, in association with complex neurobehavioral disorders of known or unknown origin, or as an idiopathic neurogenic speech sound disorder. The core impairment in planning and/or programming spatiotemporal parameters of movement sequences results in errors in speech sound production and prosody" (p. 1). Note that the terms "motor planning" and "motor programming" are used inconsistently in the literature. Generally, there is consensus that speech production requires a stored lexical representation of an intended word or phrase, a stored set of simultaneous and sequential movements necessary to produce the intended utterance, and the finely tuned control of the individual muscles, supported by sensory feedback, that need to contract to achieve the required movements. The two terms have been used variously to refer to these components.

CAS may occur as a result of known neurological impairment, in association with complex neurobehavioral disorders of known or unknown origin, or as an **idiopathic** neurogenic speech sound disorder. In the majority of the cases, CAS is idiopathic, meaning we do not know the cause of the disorder. Evidence of familial deficits in motor sequencing was recently described in multigenerational families where children had a CAS diagnosis. In the first studies investigating the phenotypic expression and molecular genetics in multigenerational families where children had received a CAS diagnosis, the affected children and adults with a history of speech difficulties showed evidence of a motor sequencing deficit, measured as a large discrepancy between monosyllabic and multisyllabic DDK scores (Peter, Matsushita, & Raskind, in press; Peter & Raskind, 2011). The same family members with this DDK discrepancy also showed difficulty with an alternating key tapping task, compared to a repetitive key tapping task. This is consistent with a motor planning deficit that goes beyond the speech production system.

The existence of CAS as a separate speech sound disorder, different from a severe phonological disorder for example, has been questioned for years. In 2007, ASHA published a detailed report that reviewed the research and expert evidence on both sides of this question. The authors of the report concluded that there was sufficient evidence to support the diagnostic category of CAS – however, more research is needed to identify the core characteristics of the disorder and to study treatment approaches. Our goal as clinicians is to be as informed as possible regarding the nature of the motor planning deficit (in relation to any other deficits, such as cognitive, linguistic, and motor execution) so that we may make reasonable clinical decisions as to the relative contribution of the disorder to the child's overall communicative performance (Caruso & Strand, 1999).

In contrast to children with dysarthria, children with CAS do not necessarily show neurological differences. Some subtle signs include fine and gross motor incoordination, difficulties with gait, and difficulties with alternating repetitive movements (Hall, Jordan & Robin, 1993). Studies, however, have not identified a consistent pattern of neurological differences among children with CAS (Crary, 1993; Hall et al., 1993; Yoss & Darley, 1974). However, studies of the KE family (a family where half of the offspring from each generation present with CAS) have shown some morphological differences in brain imaging studies. For example, in a recent study by Liégeois, Morgan, Connelly, and Vargha-Khadem (2011) researchers had four affected members of the KE family and four unrelated age-matched healthy participants repeat nonsense words aloud during functional MRI scanning. Results indicated that "repetition in the affected members was severely impaired, and brain activation was significantly reduced in the premotor, supplementary and primary motor cortices, as well as in the cerebellum and basal ganglia" (p. 283).

Underlying Deficits in CAS. In moving towards a better understanding of CAS, a number of potential underlying deficits have been proposed. It is helpful to keep in mind that as we ponder these different perspectives, we think about what it is that could account for the children's difficulties with both the motor sequencing of articulatory movement, as well as the often concomitant difficulties with phonological awareness and literacy skills. The deficits can be grouped into 3 main categories: (1) a motor planning-programming deficit; (2) a sensorimotor integration deficit, and (3) a linguistic processing deficit. The motor planning-programming deficit suggests that children have difficulty building motor representations for speech sounds (ASHA Technical Report, 2007; Hall, Jordan & Robin, 2007). The underlying source of the symptoms is difficulty with "on-line" planning or programming of elements of the speech and language system into larger organized patterns (Velleman & Strand, 1994). The sensorimotor integration deficit proposes that speech errors are due to impaired sensorimotor integration. Since many children with CAS are reported by their parents to have been "quiet babies," children may be missing the rich sensory feedback and rhythmic coordination provided during the babbling period. The impairment of sensory processing and in particular proprioceptive input leads to a failure to program, organize, and carry out movements necessary for expressive speech (Nelson, 1995). Lastly, the linguistic processing deficit proposes that children with CAS have problems building linguistic representations of their segmental aspects (Marion, Sussman, & Marquardt, 1993; Marquardt, Sussman & Snow, 1998) or **suprasegmental** aspects (Shriberg, Aram, & Kwiatkowski, 1997a, b, c) of their phonological system. They further explain that there may be a subtype of CAS where prosodic errors are a diagnostic marker. In this case, it was posited that the prosodic framework was in error, thus making it difficult for the segments (speech sounds) to be put in place (Shriberg et al., 1997a, b, c). Marquardt and colleagues (1998) proposed that the linguistic integrity of underlying phonological structures may be compromised. There may be dissolution of the neural substrates representing the phonologic framework of the child's speech motor programming performance (Marquardt et al., 1998). In that case, "speech motor output would be severely handicapped as the phonological targets driving articulation may be totally missing or in various states of marginal operational integrity" (Marion et al., 1993, p. 132). This theory is supported by their findings that children with CAS tend to have more difficulty with **categorical perception** of sounds, meaning they do not hear the contrast between sounds as well as typically speaking children do. Groenen, Maassen, Crul, and Thoonen (1996) and Maassen, Groenen & Crul (2003) have also looked at the role of perception. They posit that there is an interdependence of perception and production and thus, if the child doesn't hear the word correctly, he/she won't produce it correctly. They found that although children with CAS did not have difficulty identifying the place of articulation of a consonant, they did have difficulty discriminating consonants with subtle acoustic differences associated with place of articulation. They also had difficulty with identifying and discriminating vowels (Groenen et al., 2003).

Given the controversy and lack of agreement regarding the underlying deficit and the core features of CAS, some may wonder why this term is even used. Despite these issues, the term is useful to delineate a subgroup of children who present with severe articulatory performance deficits and who seem to have a variety of associated characteristics in common. Furthermore, it will significantly impact on how we design our treatment. For example, traditional articulation and phonological approaches will not be adequate.

Observable Characteristics of CAS. In a survey of SLPs, Forrest (2003) identified 50 characteristics that were used by SLPs to identify children with CAS. In contrast to this long list, three core characteristics have been identified in the ASHA report: (1) inconsistent errors on consonants and vowels in repeated productions of syllables or words; (2) lengthened and disrupted coarticulatory transitions between sounds and syllables; and (3) inappropriate prosody, especially in the realization of lexical or phrasal stress. Children with CAS are likely to present with at least one of these core characteristics in addition to secondary characteristics described below. When working clinically, a major challenge is how to evaluate these characteristics in children of different ages and who may have received treatment. For instance, a 3-year-old may produce inconsistent errors, but produce mainly monosyllabic words in isolation. Thus it may be difficult to observe long or disrupted coarticulation, or inappropriate prosody. A description of the secondary segmental, suprasegmental and other characteristis of CAS is essential when evaluating children.

Secondary segmental characteristics have been reported across studies. In contrast to many children with phonological disorders, children with CAS often show a relatively larger independent phonetic inventory compared to their relational inventory. In other words, they can produce many sounds but have difficulty producing the correct sound in the correct place. They show multiple speech sound errors with high frequency of omissions, but also substitutions and distortions. Some children may also add segments to (1) simplify the syllable structure (e.g., "blue" (CCV) (C = consonant, V = vowel) becomes "balue" (CVCV)), or (2) achieve a specific articulatory configuration (e.g., "soap" becomes "tsoap"). In addition to consonant errors, children with CAS often produce vowel errors. Lastly, these children may produce errors that are due to difficulty in coordinating between their phonatory and articulatory system (e.g., voicing errors) or between their resonance and articulatory systems (e.g., hypernasal resonance). Palatometry data and observations suggest that children with apraxia do not develop the more finely tuned speech movements with any specificity or precision, which differentiates them from typically developing children or possibly those with other speech sound disorders (Gibbon, 2002).

Additional prosodic characteristics have also been reported in the literature. Children with CAS often have difficulties in sequencing sounds in both words and non-speech tasks such as **diadochokinetic** (DDK) tasks. They often produce longer word and sentence durations, and produce more errors as words and sentences length increase. Overall, children with CAS show more accurate production of targets at the single word level than when produced in conversational speech.

Lastly, some other characteristics have often been noted in various studies. Children with CAS may have difficulty imitating speech sounds although they have normal anatomy and function of the tongue, lips, jaw and velum. For some children, they may be able to repeat a target more accurately than when that target is produced spontaneously. They may show decreased proprioception of articulator positions causing groping, trial and error behavior, or difficulty achieving certain articulatory configurations. These children, however, often show improved articulatory accuracy when given a simultaneous visual and auditory model. In the video 18V1, we see Jackie (not her real name), an 18-year-old woman with a history of intellectual impairment, phonologic awareness delays, and CAS producing words of increasing length (e.g., "base," "baseball," "baseball player"). Note the increased accuracy with a simultaneous visual and auditory model. Sound file 18S2 was recorded during an articulation test. The child is a 5-year-old girl with severe CAS but no other clinical deficits. Sound file 18S3 was recorded during a conversation and a multisyllabic word imitation task. The child is a 10-year-old girl with a history of severe CAS. Her conversational speech had normalized but she struggled with sequencing the phonemes in the multisyllabic words.

Access Video File 1 (Chapter 18)

18V1: 18-year-old woman with intellectual impairment, phonologic awareness delays, and CAS saying words of increasing length

Access Sound File 2 (Chapter 18)

18S2 Conversational sample and single-word productions of a girl, age 5, with a diagnosis of severe idiopathic CAS

Access Sound File 3 (Chapter 18)

18S3 Conversational sample and multisyllabic word imitations of a girl, age 10, with a history of severe idiopathic CAS

Language Considerations for Children with CAS. For most children with CAS, their receptive language is a relative strength when compared to their expressive language. Their performance may vary according to the task; for example, receptive one-word vocabulary may be age appropriate while comprehension of complex sentences is impaired. As a result, at least three areas of language comprehension should be assessed: semantic comprehension, syntactic comprehension, and the influence of increased length of input (Crary, 1993). Children should also be re-assessed as they age since some children who appeared to have normal language skills early on may demonstrate difficulty with more complex language processes such as categorizing, organizing, and abstracting when they reach the 3rd or 4th grades (Air, Wood, and Neils, 1989). Children with CAS are often reported to have impaired or delayed expressive language abilities. Some observed errors may be related to their limited speech abilities, for instance morpho-syntactic errors such as omission of past-tense "-ed" and omission of plural and possessive "'s". Some children may also omit words to simplify their utterance (Ekelman & Aram, 1983).

With regards to metalinguistic and literacy abilities, children with CAS are at risk for phonological awareness deficits (ASHA Technical Report, 2007; Caspari, 2007). Phonological awareness refers to the ability to reflect on and manipulate the sound structure of a language as distinct from its meaning (Stackhouse, 1997). Specifically, children with CAS may show weaknesses in rhyming, word attack, word identification, spelling, and phonological perception and discrimination (Marquardt, Sussman, Snow & Jacks, 2002).

Although during preschool years, our main concern when treating children with CAS is improving their segmental and suprasegmental production abilities, recent research has shown that our focus may need to shift somewhat when children enter school. In a follow-up of children with CAS who were school-aged, Lewis et al. (2004) noted that their articulation improved, but they had difficulties in syllable sequencing, nonsense word repetition, language abilities, and reading and writing.

ASSESSMENT AND DIAGNOSIS

Differentiating CAS and Dysarthria from Other Speech Disorders

It has been the experience of the first author that CAS is often over-diagnosed while dysarthria is under-diagnosed. For example, when Skinder, Strand & Mignerey (1999) were recruiting participants for a study, they found that only six out of the 24 children referred to the study by practicing speech language pathologists met both the inclusionary and exclusionary criteria for CAS. Four of the children had a history consistent with CAS, yet it seemed to have resolved into a phonologic delay by time of study, six of the children presented with a phonologic delay only, and eight of the children were excluded due to the presence of dysarthria, autism, hearing loss, and/or intellectual impairment. This is not to say that these disorders cannot co-occur with CAS, but when doing research, we need to control for these variables to better identify the core features of CAS and response to treatment among children with CAS. Similar results occurred in a study by Davis, Jakielski & Marquardt, (1997), where only 25% of subjects referred to the researchers fit the CAS criterion. The understanding of dysarthria is typically discussed in much greater detail in both the literature and in the classroom than developmental dysarthria, hence it seems to be overlooked in the pediatric population, particularly for milder forms of dysarthria. Meanwhile, CAS has received much greater recognition in the past ten years (cite ASHA reference used in other manuscript for example).

In Table 18.2., we present key components that differentiate CAS and dysarthria from other speech sound disorders. Children with CAS, dysarthria, and other speech sound disorders show similarities and differences with regards to the consistency of error production, syllable shape, vowel errors, prosody, and muscle status. In addition, these children differ with regards to what helps improve their speech. For clinicians and researchers, part of the challenge of differential diagnosis is that some characteristics often listed for CAS overlap with other speech sound disorders.

Table 18.2. Characteristics Differentiating CAS and Dysarthria from Other Speech Disorders

	Consistency of Errors	Syllable shapes	Vowel Errors	Prosody	Muscle Status	Speech Improves When:
CAS- Difficulty planning the sequence of articulatory movement required for speech	Inconsistent	Reduced	Present	Equal and excessive stress pattern	Normal	Rate is decreased and simultaneous auditory and visual cueing is provided
Dysarthria- Difficulty executing the movement for speech	Generally consistent	Potentially reduced due to decreased physiological support	Present	Decreased rate and difficulty regulating pitch and loudness	Reduced strength, range of motion, and/or coordination	Physiological effort is increased
Phonologic Disorder- Multiple speech errors that fit a pattern	Consistent	Reduced if CR, ICD, or FCD occurs	Not present	Normal	Normal	Phonologic contrasts are used
Articulation delay/disorder- Difficulty in coordinating the articulators in production of a limited set of sounds (e.g., /l, r, s/)	Consistent	Maintained	Only rhotic vowels	Normal	Normal	Traditional articulation therapy is used

(CR= Cluster Reduction, ICD=Initial Consonant Deletion, FCD=Final Consonant Deletion)

When determining the cause for a child's speech impairment, it is important to make sure the child demonstrates **communicative intent**. If a child is selectively mute, has a severe receptive language delay, is deaf, or has autism, these issues will need to be worked on prior to determining the type of speech disorder. Without the child at least attempting to verbalize, we do not have enough evidence to support a speech sound disorder diagnosis.

Case Example 1

> A five-year-old boy was brought in for an assessment to participate in a study on CAS. However, when the examiner tried to test him, he showed no interest in the people in the room. He walked in on his toes, waved his hands, and darted from object to object in the room. When the mother was asked if she had any concerns other than CAS, she reported that this was the only diagnosis that the doctor had mentioned to her.

Framework for Discerning CAS from Dysarthria

When working to discern CAS and dysarthria from other speech sound disorders, it is helpful to include the following components in your assessment:

- Overview of the neuromuscular condition
- Structural-functional examination
- Examination of physiological parameters
- Motor speech examination
- Articulation testing and phonologic analysis of speech errors
- Consistency analysis of errors
- Prosody

These procedures are essential for assessing motor speech disorders. Many children with motor speech disorders have language, phonologic awareness, and literacy deficits as well. Naturally, language and hearing should be assessed as well and a developmental history should be taken.

Overview of the Neuromuscular Condition As we observe the child come into the session, we can make basic observations that will lead us to a hypothesis or prediction regarding the status of the child's speech motor control system. After we have observed the child's gait, examined her/his muscle strength, tone, coordination, and reflexes, and looked for the presence of involuntary movement, we can get a sense of the neurological characteristics that are more consistent with dysarthria versus apraxia. If there were abnormalities noted in any of these areas, it would be indicative of damage to the cerebellum, upper motor neurons, lower motor neurons, or basal ganglia control circuit. If we observe any abnormalities, the child should be referred to the appropriate specialists to conduct a thorough evaluation of the neuromuscular system. Damage to these areas are more typically associated with dysarthria, not CAS.

Structural-Functional Examination. Where the overview of the neuromuscular condition looks at the whole body, the structural-functional exam, otherwise known as the oral peripheral exam, allows the clinician to evaluate the structures of the speech mechanism more specifically. Examination of the mouth, tongue, lips, jaw, teeth, and hard and soft palate will show if the structures are adequate for speech. Structural differences, such as cleft palate, should be obvious. Observations of asymmetry, atrophy, or involuntary movement of any of the structures at rest are consistent with dysarthria. Difficulty with strength, coordination, speed, range of motion, and ability to vary tension of the tongue, lips, jaw, and/or soft palate are also indicative of dysarthria.

DDK tasks are also important when assessing motor speech impairments, especially when comparing the performance of single syllable repetition, as in “pa-pa-pa” or “ta-ta-ta” to variegated syllable repetition, as in “pa-ta-ka” or “patticake.” Children with dysarthria may present with weak articulatory contacts, decreased rate, breathy or strangled voice quality, and voicing errors that are consistent across all syllable repetition tasks. They may also be dysrhythmic, especially in the case of ataxic dysarthria. Children with CAS may perform slowly, but correctly produce the sounds in a single syllable repetition task, but will noticeably struggle when they try to sequence different syllables. For example “pa-ta-ka, pata-ka, pa-ta-ka" turns into "pa-pa--ta, ta ---ta-pa, pa-ka-kuk." See Robbins, J. and Klee, T. (1987) for further guidelines. The sound file 18S4 illustrates an 8-year-old boy with galactosemia and apraxia producing mono- and multisyllables in rapid succession during DDK testing.

Access Sound File 4 (Chapter 18)

18S4 Eight-year-old boy with CAS and galactosemia attempting the DDK task

Examination of Physiological Parameters. The clinician will also need to assess a few basic physiological parameters needed for speech. This relates back to the source-filter function discussed in Chapter 2. In order for speech to occur, adequate pressures and flows need to be generated and regulated appropriately. For example, the client will need to be able to produce 5 cmH2O pressure (i.e., 5 centimeters of water pressure) below the level of the vocal folds for phonation to begin (Hixon, Hawley, & Wilson, K. J., 1982). There is a task called the five for five rule. This task involves having the child blow into a straw with the bottom of the straw 5 centimeters below the surface of the water for five seconds (Hixon et al., 1982). If the child can do this, she or he has enough respiratory power for speech production. If the soft palate is not able to close the airflow from going out the nose, the nares will need to be occluded so that the clinician can differentiate between a velopharyngeal valving issue versus a "power supply" problem (i.e., inadequate respiratory support).

The clinician also needs to see that the vocal folds can be adducted, hence we ask the child to sustain phonation as we listen to the voice quality and measure how long phonation can be sustained. (For norms on maximum phonation duration for children, go to Kent, Kent & Rosenbek, 1982.) If the child has reduced duration, but adequate respiratory support, she or he may be having difficulty coordinating respiration with phonation. This is more common in dysarthria than apraxia. In addition, if the voice quality sounds breathy or strangled, this would also be an indication of dysarthria.

Assessing the functioning of the soft palate is also important. If cleft palate has been ruled out and the child is consistently hypernasal and has nasal emissions, the clinician should examine the soft palate during a sustained "ah" and a quick staccato "ah-ah-ah." If the velum does not rise, is asymmetrical as it rises, or is slow to rise, there is most likely impairment in the innervation of the muscles that close the velopharyngeal port, which is indicative of dysarthria. Sometimes children with CAS may also sound as if they have disordered resonance. However, when motor planning impacts nasal resonance, it tends to be mild, inconsistent, and without nasal emissions (Skinder-Meredith, Graff, & Carkowski, (2004).

Motor Speech Evaluation. As discussed in Chapter 2, a motor speech evaluation examines the ability to sequence phonetic segments in various contexts. The stimuli are systematically made longer. For example, elicited syllable shapes go from V to CV to VC, then to CVC and beyond. It is important to sample all vowels in these syllable shapes, especially diphthongs, as children with motor speech impairments may produce vowel errors. Children with severe dysarthria may only be able to produce a centralized schwa or a limited set of vowels, but they are fairly consistent. Children with CAS tend to also produce vowel errors but are less consistent. However, they do show a pattern early in their speech production of reducing diphthongs to monophthongs (e.g., /a/ for /aɪ/). Observations of the effect of increasing syllable and phrase length is also helpful. As noted in the summary chart, children with dysarthria are fairly consistent in their general imprecise articulation of all speech sounds, while children with CAS make markedly more errors as the length increases. The exact level where the break down occurs depends on the age of the child and the severity of their apraxia. For example, where a three-year old may break down at the CVC level, a ten-year-old may break down at the multisyllabic word level. It is also important to compare automatic speech, such as counting or the alphabet, to novel utterances, such as a picture description. Children with CAS perform better on automatic speech tasks than novel tasks, whereas children with dysarthria do not show a notable difference.

Lastly, it is important to examine the child's ability to produce particular phonetic sequences while varying the temporal relationship between stimulus and response (Strand, 1995). First have the child repeat the stimulus after you. If the child is unable to produce it, have her or him say it with you (simultaneously) with a decreased rate as they watch your articulators go from one configuration to the next. If it is still difficult for the child, add tactile cues. Children with CAS benefit from watching the sequence of the movement needed for speech and hence improve when given these cues. Children with dysarthria may benefit from the decreased rate, but their articulatory contacts may still be weak.

Articulation/Phonologic Analysis

Children with CAS can be difficult to distinguish from children with a severe phonologic delay. They also may have a phonologic delay in addition to their motor planning deficit. For this reason it is very help administer a standardized articulation test that allows for careful analysis of the speech sound error patterns. The clinician should also get a speech sample that yields a relational and independent phonetic inventory, as discussed in Chapter 2. Children with CAS typically have a higher independent phonetic inventory, compared to the relational phonetic inventory.

A syllable shape inventory at various word lengths can also be helpful. Children with CAS may be able to produce a CVC in a single syllable word, but may not be able to produce it in bisyllabic or multisyllabic words. For example, they can say “cat” but when asked to say “caterpillar” it turns into “ca-a-pa.” Comparing percent of consonants correct (PCC) and percent of vowels correct (PVC) in a single word task versus a sentence task also provides important information. Children with CAS typically have lower PCC and PVC scores in sentences than they do in single words.

Consistency of Errors. As previously stated, inconsistency of errors is one of the core features that allows us to differentiate between CAS and other speech sound disorders. Dodd (1995) explains that inconsistent error patterns indicate a deficit in phonological planning, which results in the articulatory parameters being too broad. Furthermore, the inconsistent speech output may be due to the child needing to make a new plan for each word they produce (Bradford & Dodd, 1996). This may also relate to why the children often sound like they are speaking syllable-by syllable (**Skinder-Meredith, Stoel-Gammon, Wright, & Betz, 2000**). There are several ways one can examine consistency. For a full review see Betz &

Stoel-Gammon, 2005. One method described by Betz and Stoel-Gammon was to elicit five words six times each and then calculate consistency of the most frequently used error type. They propose the following calculation: number of productions of the most frequently used error type minus 1, divided by the number of erred productions minus 1, multiplied by 100 to obtain the percentage score.

Dodd (1995) has proposed a more detailed method for measuring consistency of errors. Children are asked to name 25 pictures in three separate trials and an activity is inserted between trials. The clinician should avoid using imitation, but can use semantic cues or teach the name of the item and then ask what it is called later. If a child cannot produce all of the words spontaneously, a percentage score can be derived. Dodd notes that variable production of ten or more words on two of the three trials (or a score of more than 40% variability) suggests an "inconsistent disorder". When calculating errors, both consonants and vowels are included. It is important to note that Dodd does not equate inconsistent disorder with CAS, but her measure is helpful in determining if inconsistent error production is one characteristic of the child's speech sound disorder. Children with dysarthria, phonologic delay and articulation disorders are unlikely to produce high amounts of variability in their speech sound errors.

Prosody. Lastly, observations of prosody are also important for differential diagnosis. One can observe prosody in conversational speech, as well as the ability to imitate prosodic contours of phrases. When listening to speech, SLPs are more apt to hear the segmental errors than the suprasegmental errors. For this reason, it can be helpful to listen through sentence imitation tasks to see if the child stresses the appropriate words and syllables. As children get older, one can see whether they are able to use contrastive stress (e.g., **I** want to go home vs. I want to go **home**.) It can also be helpful to have the child repeat words that have a trochaic stress pattern (strong-weak as in BA-by) and iambic stress patterns (weak-strong as in gui-TAR). Children with CAS tend to have more difficulty with iambic stress patterns (Skinder-Meredith, Stoel-Gammon, Wright, & Strand, 2001) The prosodic pattern of children with CAS when they are trying to use the correct articulatory sequences is often observed to be robotic (Shriberg, Aram & Kwiatkowski, 1997 a,b,c). The disordered prosody of children with dysarthria is related to impaired physiology. For example, if respiratory support is reduced, children have difficulty modifying levels of loudness and if the phonatory system is impaired, they have difficulty varying pitch. Chapter 7 discusses typical and disordered development of prosody in more detail.

This section on assessment has provided you with ways to differentiate CAS from dysarthria and other speech sound errors. There are also several tests that can help SLPs with the task of differential diagnosis, such as the *Verbal Motor Production Assessment for Children (VMPAC)* (Hayden & Square, 1999), the *Screening Test for Developmental Apraxia of Speech-2* (Blakely, 2000), the *The Apraxia Profile/Checklist* (Hickman, 1997) and *The Kaufman Speech Praxis Test for Children* (1995). With the exception of the *VMPAC*, these tests target only CAS. McCauley & Strand (2008) have provided a thorough review of motor speech tests that can be a great resource for clinicians.

Principles of Motor Learning and Their Application to Treatment

When treating children with motor speech disorders, it is important to be aware of the principles of motor learning. Principles of motor learning were initially applied to limb motor learning activities, such as sports (Schmidt & Lee, 2005). Although we have been applying principles of motor learning to treatment of motor speech disorders for over a decade (Strand & Skinder, 1999), it has only been recently that studies have investigated these principles to motor speech skills specifically (e.g., Edeal & Gildersleeve-Neumann, 2011; Mass & Farinella, 2009; Maas, Robin, Austemann-Hula, Freedman, Wulf, Ballard, Schmidt, 2008). In order for motor learning to occur for speech, the child needs to be motivated to communicate verbally, have focused attention, and know what the movement goal will be (pre-practice) (Schmidt & Lee, 2005; Strand & Skinder, 1999; Strand, Stoeckel, & Baas, 2006).

Other pertinent issues include *goal setting* and *instructions*. Goal setting may take the form of getting the child's input on what words and phrases she or he wants to be able to say intelligibly. Having the child be part of the goal setting should also help increase motivation. In regards to instructions, the clinician needs to be mindful of being specific about how to accomplish the articulatory movement needed, but use words the child will understand. Often direct modeling can be more effective than verbal instructions, especially for the child with CAS, where the more volitional the movement is, the harder it becomes.

Three issues especially relevant to treatment of motor speech disorders are the use of *repetitive practice* and the concepts of *mass versus distributed practice* and *random versus blocked practice*. Repetition is one of the most important principles for motor learning. There need to be enough trials per session in order to allow motor learning to occur and become habituated toward more automatic processing (Velleman, 2005). A recent study done by **Edeal & Gildersleeve-Neumann** (2011) examined the difference between providing higher production frequency treatment (e.g., over 100 productions in 15 minutes) to moderate-frequency treatment (30-40 productions in 15 minutes). Although all of the participants improved, children who received the higher production frequency treatment were able to acquire the skills (e.g., speech targets) more quickly and had better generalization to **untrained probes**.

The concept of mass versus distributed practice has been interpreted in different ways. Schmidt & Lee (2005) describe mass practice as working on the same skill continuously without taking breaks versus practicing the skill in shorter periods of time with breaks in between. Some may equate this with providing speech therapy to a child in one long session per week instead of in several shorter sessions per week (e.g., one 60 minute session versus three 20 minute sessions per week). Maas and colleagues (2008) describe mass practice as giving a number of trials in a small period of time and distributed as giving a number of trials over a longer period of time. Kinesiology research on limb motor skills has shown that mass practice yields quick development of the skill but poor generalization; in contrast, distributed practice requires more time to develop the skill, but achieves better motor learning. This practice distribution, however, has not been studied well in acquisition of speech skills (Maas et al., 2008). The conditions of blocked versus random practice works in a similar way: In blocked practice, all practice trials of a given stimulus are practiced together before moving on to the next; in random practice the order of presentation of the stimuli are randomly mixed throughout the session. Blocked practice leads to better performance but random practice seems to result in better retention, or motor learning, which has been observed in both nonspeech and speech skills (Maas et al., 2008).

Given that it can be difficult to obtain multiple repetitions and get the focused attention one needs in therapy, a behavior plan may be warranted. The behavior plan should ensure that the child looks at the model for articulatory placement cues, listens to the model, and verbally attempts to repeat the target the model (SLP) has provided. An extrinsic reward, such as a sticker, may be necessary initially, but as the child learns that repetitive practice of the target phrase brings about the desired response (e.g., "Can I have a turn?" said intelligibly actually gives them a turn with their peers), extrinsic rewards can be faded.

Case Example 2

The role of motivation is extremely important. If a child has met a lifetime of verbal communicative attempts with little success, he or she may understandably want to give up. Annabel was a bright 6-year-old girl with dysarthria and apraxia. She wanted to be a verbal communicator, but this was very difficult for her motorically. It was made clear to Annabel from the onset that she had three jobs in speech therapy; to watch the therapist's mouth, listen to the therapist, and try to say what the therapist asked her to say. If she did these three things enough times in a session, she would earn a prize. During one therapy session she was asked to work on her speech and she turned her back to the therapist and signed, "no." She did not earn her prize on this particular day, which made her very upset. However, she came back to the next therapy session willing to work hard on her speech again. Extrinsic reinforcement may be necessary initially. However, the intrinsic reinforcement of successful verbal communication should soon take over once the child has put the work in to see the gains that can be made in speech therapy.

How a client is given feedback has also been examined. The terms used for this are **knowledge of results (KR)** and **knowledge of performance (KP)**. KR refers to general feedback (e.g., correct versus incorrect production) and KP refers to specific feedback (e.g., "put your lips together"). Morehouse and Cornish (2004) found KP to be more effective than KR, but others (Maas et al., 2008) feel that this is more often the case when a child is just beginning to learn the skill. Once the child has more ability, KR is considered more time efficient. In addition, the feedback needs to be faded, so that the child is not dependent on the clinician, thus fading the specificity of feedback to KR (Maas et al., 2008), as well as the frequency of the feedback changes over time. We may begin with 1:1 feedback ratio, then when appropriate decrease to 1:5 (Golding-Kushner, 2001; Schmidt & Lee, 2005). Specific and intensive feedback may assist the child in acquiring a new skill, but general feedback given less frequently allows for more motor learning and retention to occur. The responsibility is essentially shifting from the clinician to the client and as soon as it is appropriate to achieve the goal that the child begins to monitor her or his own performance. Increased pause time after the client's response has also been found to be more effective in studies of acquired apraxia of speech (Austermann Hula, Robin, Maas, Ballard, & Schmidt, 2008)

Decreasing rate is another tool the therapist can use to assist in increasing accuracy (Rosenthal, 1994). If the child has dysarthria, it may take more time to achieve articulatory contact and if she or he has CAS, it may take more time to map the spatiotemporal parameters for sequencing the movements for speech. Varying rate can be an effective tool to vary during repetitive practice of targeted utterances, in order to allow habituation of articulatory movement accuracy while working toward natural rate and prosody. For a more comprehensive tutorial on principles of motor learning in the treatment of motor speech disorders, see Maas et al., 2008).

TREATMENT OF DYSARTHRIA IN CHILDREN

Treatment of developmental dysarthria is variable and depends on the type of dysarthria the child has (e.g., ataxic, spastic, flaccid, hyperkinetic, mixed), the subsystems involved (e.g., articulatory, phonatory, respiratory, and resonance), and if the condition is static (e.g., cerebral palsy) or progressive (e.g., Friedreich's ataxia). Children with dysarthria may or may not also have intellectual impairment, which will further influence treatment approaches. Therefore, the reader is encouraged to research the most effective treatment for individual clients and to work with a team of therapists as the motor difficulties most likely also impact fine and gross motor skills. Treatment for dysarthria often consists of increasing physiological drive and effort, increasing articulatory precision, managing velopharyngeal dysfunction, and developing compensatory strategies, such as using an augmentative communications system when necessary. Results from the assessment should guide the therapist in their treatment goals, as it will alert them as to which subsystems are most compromised for speech. See Table 18.3 for treatment examples. In addition, it is extremely important to make sure the child is seated in an appropriate position. Optimal positioning allows the child trunk stability and the best possible respiratory kinematics. For a tutorial on functional seating, see Costigan & Light (2011). In addition, non-speech oral motor exercises (NSOMEs) for strengthening the physiology needed for speech needs to be carefully examined. A review of Clark (2003) will assist the clinician in examining the efficacy for NSOMEs.

If the strategies in Table 18.3 are not allowing the child to have intelligible speech, use of compensatory strategies is also recommended. For example, an alphabet-topic board can be used for the speaker to point to the topic being discussed and then the first letter of each intended. Improving listener's knowledge of the context in this way can greatly increase understanding. If motor skills and intelligibility are severely impaired, a comprehensive assessment for an augmentative system that can grow with the child's linguistic needs is recommended.

Table 18.3. Examples of Treatment from a Systems Approach

System	Examples of Treatment
Articulatory	• Decrease rate to allow the articulators to reach the correct articulatory configuration • Increase articulatory precision through drill and phonetic contrasts in terms of place, voice, and manner (e.g., /d/ vs. /g/, /p/ vs. /b/, and /s/ vs. /t/) • Use a bite block to stabilize the jaw if the child is having difficulty coordinating lip, jaw, and tongue movements
Phonatory	• Increase phonatory effort to increase overall loudness (Fox & Boliek, 2012) • Use relaxation techniques for clients with over adduction (i.e., tense voice quality) • Use lifting and pushing during phonation for clients who need increased adduction of the vocal folds (i.e., breathy voice quality)
Respiratory	• Encourage taking in a larger breath before speaking • Use impedance of airflow exercises such as holding out an /s/ as long as possible • Work with a respiratory therapist to strengthen respiratory muscles and increase vital capacity • Work on efficient coordination of breath and phonation • Work on linguistically appropriate breath groups • (See Hixon & Hoit (2004) for the most thorough information on management of the respiratory system for speech)
Resonance	• Increase jaw opening for increased oral resonance • Consider prosthetic management such as palatal lift or speech bulb for improved velopharyngeal closure • Consult with an otololaryngologist (ENT) to see if surgical intervention, such as a pharyngeal flap, would assist in adequate velopharyngeal closure
Prosody	• Work on varying pitch with sustained vowels • Work on varying loudness with sustained vowels • Work on contrastive stress exercises in words (e.g.,ADDress-addRESS) and phrases (I want to go HOME vs. I WANT to go home.)

TREATMENT OF CHILDHOOD APRAXIA OF SPEECH

Just as results from the structural functional exam assists the clinician in determining goals for the child with dysarthria, the motor speech exam will help determine the goals for the child with CAS. The therapist should target words and phrases that are motivating to the client and within the client's ability given the appropriate support (e.g., simultaneous and tactile cuing). The targets should also contain sounds that are already in the child's repertoire or are easily stimulable. Lastly, the syllable shape, syllable length and phrase length also need to be considered.

Let's look at the motor speech and articulation exam results for a hypothetical client, Josiah, and then determine appropriate target phrases. Josiah is a 3 year-old-boy. He is able to correctly produce CVs, VCs, and CVCs with the /b, p, k, m, n, t, d, s, l/ sounds and all vowels with simultaneous and/or tactile cuing. In spontaneous speech, he can produce these sounds, but not always where they belong. For example, he says /pʌ/ for "cup." He also tends to speak in one- to two-word phrases, but is intelligible only 25% of the time if the context is known with a familiar listener. He also uses predominantly V and CV syllable shapes. Josiah would like to exert his will and his mother is tired of his emotional outbursts. We have chosen the following phrases for him to begin with:

1. Oh no
2. Hi Mom
3. I do
4. *My turn
5. Open ____
6. *More ____
7. All done

***We don't necessarily expect a perfect rhotic vowel, but we will accept approximations**

As we use these principles of motor learning and a hierarchical systematic approach to Josiah's motor speech skills, he improves and thus we make the phrases a little harder by increasing phonetic complexity, word length, and syllable length.

1. No more _____
2. I want _____
3. I do it
4. May I have ____?
5. My turn please
6. I'm all done
7. I love Mommy.

Let's take a step back and determine how to make this kind of progress occur. There are many treatment techniques that are used to improve the speech of children with developmental motor planning deficits, such as *PROMPTs for Restructuring Oral Muscular Phonetic Targets (PROMPT)* (Grigos, Hayden & Eigen, 2010), the *Nuffield Dyspraxia Programme* (Bowen, 2009), and the Kaufman approach (see the link to the Kaufman website under "Helpful Websites" at the end of this chapter). Although there is no one perfect program for all children, there are some basic principles that should be integrated in our treatment approach.

- Use of a bottom up approach with careful construction of hierarchies of stimuli: Start simple and build on success.
- Use of intensive paired auditory and visual stimuli: The child should watch and listen to the clinician prior to having attempting the target utterance on his or her own.

- Prioritize the production of sound combinations rather than isolated phoneme training: Producing diphthongs in isolation, like /aɪ/ is acceptable, as it carries meaning, but move to sound combinations as soon as possible.
- Focus on movement performance drill: Elicit the meaningful words with the correct articulatory movement sequence. If the correct movement is not achieved, provide more cues for better accuracy to occur or simplify the target stimulus to something the child is capable of with cuing.
- Use of repetitive production and intensive systematic drill: The child will need to repeat the target utterances enough times for motor learning to occur. As the child's productions improve, cues can be faded.
- Use of decreased rate, with proprioceptive monitoring.
- Use of carrier phrases to gradually expend the child's communicative effectiveness.
- Pair movement sequences with suprasegmental facilitators such as stress, intonation and rhythm, especially with young children.
- Focus on a core and functional vocabulary, especially for the nonverbal child.

It is also important that the treatment technique incorporates the principles of motor learning that were discussed earlier. *Dynamic Temporal and Tactile Cueing (DTTC)* (Strand et al., 2006) is a motor-based hierarchical speech treatment adapted from Rosenbek, Lemme, Ahern, Harris & Wertz (1973) that incorporates these principles and has been supported by evidence-based practice research (Edeal & Gildersleeve-Neumann, 2011; Strand & Debertine, 2000; Strand et al., 2006). The *DTTC* method has been designed to build on successful utterances, emphasize extensive practice, use meaningful and useful utterances for motivation and functional communication, and maximize proprioceptive input. The therapist adds and fades cues as necessary for correct speech production. The first step is for the therapist to say the utterance while the child watches the clinician's face and then the child repeats. If the child is unsuccessful, the clinician moves to simultaneous production and adds tactile or gestural cues as necessary while maintaining auditory and visual stimuli for several repetitions. This step is typically done with a decreased rate of speech so that the child is able to obtain the correct order and precision of the articulatory targets. The clinician continues until the child can easily produce the utterance with the therapist at a more normal rate. As the child becomes more successful, the clinician fades the cues by reducing the loudness of her or his voice and removes tactile cues. Once the child is successful at this level, the clinician will go back to eliciting the target word or phrase in immediate repetition, where the therapist says the target utterance and the child repeats. The therapist can mouth the utterance if additional support is needed, and then fades this cue as well. The next step in this cuing hierarchy is the addition of a short delay, where the clinician says the utterance and then after about a three second delay, the child says the utterance. After the child is successful at this level, the target will be repeated by the child several times without intervening stimuli from the clinician. Lastly, the utterance is elicited spontaneously. Throughout all stages of the hierarchy, the clinician also needs to be mindful of prosody. It is easy to slip into a robotic prosody when saying phrases simultaneously and using a decreased rate. Hence, it is helpful to practice the target phrases with natural and varying intonation patterns. When the child is able to say the phrase without support but is still struggling with prosody, it can be helpful to work on prosody by asking questions that prompt different lexical stress patterns.

For example:

- Target phrase: "I have football on Fridays."
- Clinician: Do you have **ballet** on Fridays?
- Client: No, I have **football** on Fridays.
- Clinician: Do you have football on **Mondays**?
- Client: No, I have football on **Fridays**.
- Clinician: Does your sister have football on Fridays?
- Client: No, **I** have football on Fridays.

Adding Motor Speech to Phonological Awareness. It has been well documented that children with persistent speech sound disorders are at high risk for delays in phonologic awareness and literacy skills (Anthony, Greenglatt Aghara, Dunkelberger, Anthony, Williams, & Zhang, 2011; Bird, Bishop, & Freeman, 1995; Gillon & Moriarty, 2007; Lewis, Freebairn, Hansen, Iyengar, & Taylor, 2004; Snowling, Goulandris, & Stackhouse, 1994; Stackhouse & Snowling, 1992). Hence, recent studies have looked at using a phonological awareness approach for children with CAS and argued that "written language development of children with CAS must also be fostered in intervention" (McNeill, Gillon, & Dodd, 2009, p. 342). The benefits of addressing these skills are twofold. If the neurological substrates of phonemes are in varying levels of operational integrity, as Marion and colleagues (1993) suggest, supplementing motor speech therapy with phonologic awareness activities could strengthen the neural substrates of phonemes and thus improve the clarity of the phonetic targets that drive articulation. Furthermore, by teaching the motor conceptualization of phonemes as represented by graphemes, we will be able to use the printed word to assist the child in sequencing the movements for speech. McNeill and colleagues (2009) incorporated phonological awareness tasks such as letter-sound knowledge, phoneme identity, segmentation, blending, and manipulation into their therapy sessions. Results indicated that the children not only made gains in their literacy skills, but also had improved speech.

There are many methods and programs available for working on these types of skills. Children who struggle with reading can benefit from a multisensory, systematic, and explicit instruction approach (Berninger & Fayol, 2008; Lindamood & Lindamood, 2011). One such program is the *Lindamood Phoneme Sequencing® for Phonemic Awareness, Reading and Spelling (LiPS®)* (Lindamood & Lindamood, 2011*)*. In this program, phoneme and grapheme labels are used to describe the dynamic aspects of the sound. For example, the bilabial sounds, /p, b/ are called "lip poppers" and /t, d/ are called "tip tappers." There are mouth pictures and letter tiles to go with each label and sound. The clinician can overlay the mouth pictures with the letter tiles, hence cuing the child with the articulatory position needed to make the sound with the grapheme. By using both the mouth shapes and the letter tiles, the clinician can show the child that when the sounds change, the word will change as well. 18V2 shows the18-year-old women you met in 18V1 using the *LiPS* program.

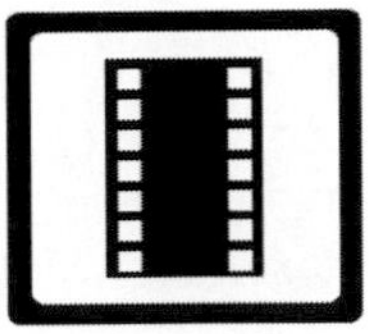

Access Video File 2 (Chapter 18)

18V2 Jackie learning the kinesthetic, auditory, visual, and graphemic cue for /k/ and /g/ with *LiPS®*. Note how the client is paying attention to all elements of this sound. This is the first time she has been able to establish a grapheme phoneme relationship.

This program, like other programs (e.g., Orton-Gillingham) also uses manipulatives (colored blocks) for the child to work on other concepts important to developing phonologic awareness. The colored blocks are used to track syllable changes that include *omission* (taking away a block when the sound went away, e.g., changing "vop" to "op"); *substituting* (switching sounds, e.g., changing "vop" to "vip"); *addition* (adding a sound, e.g., changing "vip" to "vips"); *shifting sounds* (e.g., changing "ip" to "pi") and *repeating* sounds (e.g., change "sop" to "sops"). This program can be very effective for children once they understand the concepts of same and different, can track from left to right, and recognize patterns (Lindamood & Lindamood, 2011). It is primarily designed for school-aged children and adults.

Another multimodal program designed to help children learn the phoneme to grapheme relationship is called *Phonic Faces* (Norris, 2003). This program is appropriate for pre-school and kindergarten age children. In *Phonic Faces* the letters are illustrated in a characters mouth to look like the lips or tongue making the sound. For example, Peter Pops is a character with "P" coming off the lips to help teach the phoneme-grapheme relationship for /p/. With this program each sound is introduced one at a time and each sound has a picture card, a story, and activities. After a group of sounds has been introduced, the sounds can be blended. For example, the clinician introduces the first group of sounds: /p, b, k, g, a, e, ɪ / (vowels are taught with both lax and tense counterparts). Once this set of sounds is learned, the child can then begin blending sounds into /CVC/ words, such as "big," "pig," and "dig." This can lead to other important phonological awareness skills, like rhyming. After *Phonic Faces* has been used to teach the grapheme-phoneme relationships, the phonic face can be faded out and just traditional letters can be used, and then print can be used to facilitate speech in addition to the tactile, visual, and auditory cues. One of the positive aspects of *Phonic Faces* is that each sound comes with a story and the stories provide multiple repetitions for each sound. The pictures and stories can be engaging for the child and are especially helpful for children with attention issues who learn best visually. Phonic Faces is also available in Spanish.

One does not necessarily need to use either of these programs, but just be aware that there are many ways to incorporate phonological awareness skills with a variety of methods. When working with children with persistent speech sound disorders, we know they are at risk for reading and writing deficits (Lewis et al., 2004) and hence it is crucial to incorporate phonological awareness activities into speech therapy (McNeill et al., 2009).

CONNECTIONS

Motor speech disorders, as described in this chapter, are often considered separately from idiopathic articulation and phonological disorders. Motor speech disorders are mentioned briefly in Chapter 15 in the context of various ways to classify childhood speech disorders. Chapter 20 discusses general principles of assessment and diagnosis in these speech sound disorders and Chapter 22 addresses treatment design and implementation, whereas we provide information on assessment, diagnosis, and treatment that is more specifically geared to motor speech disorders.

CONCLUDING REMARKS

To summarize, children with motor speech disorders are a very heterogeneous group. The fact that their motor speech skills are impaired early in development implies that there will most likely be an impact on other skills as well, such as language and literacy. The goal of assessment is to carefully discern between dysarthria, apraxia, phonologic delay, language delays, and intellectual impairment. Any one or a combination of the above issues could be impacting the child. It is the SLP's job to determine the relative contribution of each factor to the child's communication impairment. When motor execution (dysarthria) and/or motor planning (apraxia) is the major contributor to the speech disorder, the child will generally benefit the most from one-on-one therapy to address the motor speech skills. Multiple productions of the target phrases are crucial for motor learning to occur. Mass blocked practice with frequent feedback may help initially, but distributed random practice with lower frequency of feedback will give better retention. It is also important to be mindful of working on appropriate prosody as well as correct articulation. When targeting utterances, build stimuli carefully (e.g., increasing phonetic complexity, syllable shape, number of syllables, and length of utterance) as the child progresses. When organizing your therapy session, carefully plan therapy time to address all of the child's communication needs.

This chapter focused on motor speech and literacy skills. However, expressive language, receptive language, and pragmatic skills may also need to be addressed.

CHAPTER REVIEW QUESTIONS

1. What is the difference between developmental dysarthria and childhood apraxia of speech (CAS)?
2. How do children with phonologic delay differ from children with childhood apraxia of speech (CAS)?
3. Why is it important to incorporate phonologic awareness skills into your speech therapy with children with CAS?

SUGGESTIONS FOR FURTHER READING

Armbruster, B., Lehr, F., & Osborn, J. (2001). *Put reading first: The research building blocks for teaching children to read.* Washington, DC U.S. Department of Education: National Institute for Literacy and National Institute of Child Health and Human Development. Retrieved on July 2, 2006 *http://www.nifl.gov/partnershipforreading/publications/reading_first1.html*

Bowen, C. (2009). *Children's Speech Sound Disorders*. New Dehli, India; Wiley-Blackwell Publishing Co.

Caruso, A. J., & Strand, E. (1999). *Clinical Management of Motor Speech Disorders in Children*. New York: Thieme Publishing Co.

Crary, M. A. (1993). *Developmental Motor Speech Disorders*. San Diego, Singular Publishing Group.

Duffy, J. (2005). *Motor Speech Disorders: Substrates, Differential Diagnosis, and Management 2nd edition*. St. Louis, Mosby.

Gillon, G. (2004). *Phonological Awareness from Research to Practice*. New York, NY, Guilford Publications

Hixon, T., & Hoit, J. (2004). *Evaluation and Management of Speech Breathing Disorders: Principles and Methods,* Plural Publishing

Williams, L., McLeod, S. & McCauley, R. (2010). *Interventions for Speech Sound Disorders in Children*, Brooks Publishing

Workinger, S. M. (2005). *Cerebral Palsy Resource Guide for Speech-Language Pathologists*, Thompson Delmar Learning

Helpful Websites

Apraxia-Kids Web site by the Childhood Apraxia Association of North America (CASANA): *http://www.apraxia-kids.org/index.html*

Gail Gillon's Phonological awareness and other resources: *http://www.education.canterbury.ac.nz/people/gillon/resources.shtml*

Kaufman Children's Center for speech, language, sensory-motor, & social connections inc. *http://www.kidspeech.com/*

Nuffield Centre Dyspraxia Programme 3rd edition: *http://www.ndp3.org/*

The PROMPT Institute: *http://promptinstitute.com/index.php?page=history*

SUGGESTIONS FOR STUDENT ACTIVITIES

1. Based on the tasks typically used for the assessment of a child whose speech is difficult to understand described in this chapter, Chapter 2, and Chapter 20, select two tasks that would help you conduct a differential diagnosis of phonological disorder, CAS, and dysarthria. What adjustments should you make to the tasks? What results would help you distinguish between these disorders?

2. You are working with a 4-year-old girl with CAS whose consonant production is limited to stops. She can produce labio-dental fricatives in simple syllables, with lots of cues. Your goal is to expand this stop-fricative contrast. What principles of motor learning should you incorporate into your treatment to achieve this goal? Provide specific examples – and remember to keep if fun!
3. Go to each of the websites listed above and compare and contrast the treatment methods described by the following programs: The Kaufman approach, PROMPT, and the Nuffield dyspraxia program.

Asnwers to Chapter Review Questions

1. What is the difference between developmental dysarthria and childhood apraxia of speech (CAS)?

Although both are motor speech disorders, children with dysarthria have an injury to their central or peripheral nervous system that results in impairments in respiration, phonation, resonance or articulation. The impairments to their speech is relatively constant despite changes to utterance length or complexity. In contrast, children with CAS do not necessarily have a neurological injury, but have important deficits in motor planning for speech production. This difficulty in motor planning is more marked when utterance length or complexity increases.

2. How do children with phonologic delay differ from children with childhood apraxia of speech (CAS)?

Based on Table 17.2, we can compare children with phonological delay (PD) to those with CAS across the following areas: consistency of errors (CAS – inconsistent, PD-consistent; vowel errors (CAS-present, PD-not present); prosody (CAS-equal and excessive stress, PD-normal); speech improves under the following conditions, CAS-decreased rate and simultaneous audio and visual cuing, PD-using phonological contrasts.

3. Why is it important to incorporate phonologic awareness skills into your speech therapy with children with CAS?

Phonological awareness can help strengthen the neural substrates of phonemes resulting in improved clarity of phonetic targets that drive articulation. These skills can also be used to serve as a visual cue in helping the child to sequence movements for speech.

References

American Speech-Language-Hearing Association (2007a). *Childhood Apraxia of Speech* [Position Statement]. Available from *www.asha.org/policy* Retrieved January 21, 2009.

American Speech-Language-Hearing Association. (2007b). *Childhood Apraxia of Speech* [Technical Report]. Available from *www.asha.org/policy*. Retrieved January 21, 2009.

Ansel, B. M., & Kent, R. D. (1992). Acoustic-Phonetic contrasts and intelligibility in the dysarthria associated with mixed cerebral palsy. *J Speech Hear Res*, 35(2), 296-308.

Anthony, J., Greenblatt Aghara, R., Dunkelberger, M., Anthony, T., Williams, J., & Zhang, Z. (2011). What factors place children with speech sound disorders at risk for reading problems? *American Journal of Speech-Language Pathology,* 20, 146-160.

Austernmann-Hula, S. N., Robin, D., Mass, E., Ballard, K., & Schmidt, R. (2008). Effects of feedback frequency and timing on acquisition, retention, and transfer of speech skills in acquired apraxia of speech, *Journal of Speech, Language, and Hearing Research,* 51, *1088-1113.*

Ballard, K. J., Robin, D. A., McCabe, P., & McDonald, J. (2010). A treatment for dysprosody in childhood apraxia of speech. *Journal of Speech and Hearing Disorders,* 53, 1227-1245.

Berninger, V. & Fayol, M. (2008). Why spelling is important and how to teach it effectively. Encyclopedia of Language and Literacy Development (pp.1-13). London, ON: Canadian Language and Literacy Research Network. Retrieved (2/13/13) from *http://www.literacyencyclopedia.ca/pdfs/Why_Spelling_Is_Important_and_How_To_Teach_It_Effectively.pdf*

Betz, S. & Stoel-Gammon C.(2005). Measuring articulatory error consistency in children with developmental apraxia of speech. *Clinical Linguistics and Phonetics,* 19(1), 53-66.

Bird, J., Bishop, D. V. M., & Freeman, N. H. (1995). Phonological awareness and literacy development in children with expressive phonological impairments. *Journal of Speech and Hearing Research*, 38, 446-462.

Bowen, C. (2009). *Children's Speech Sound Disorders*. (pp. 269-275). West Sussex, UK, John Wiley & Sons.

Bradford, A. & Dodd, B. (1996). Do all speech-disordered children have motor deficits? *Clinical Linguistics and Phonetics*, 10, 77-101.

Byrne, M. C. (1959). Speech and language development of athetoid and spastic children. *The Journal of Speech and Hearing Disorders*, 24(3), 231-40.

Caruso, A., & Strand, E. (1999). *Clinical Management of Motor Speech Disorders in Children*. New York: Thieme.

Caspari, S. (2007). Working Guidelines for the Assessment and Treatment of Childhood Apraxia of Speech: A Review of ASHA's 2007 Position Statement and Technical Report. Available from *http://www.speechpathology.com/articles/article_detail.asp?article_id=328* Retrieved January 27, 2009.

Clark, H. M. (2003). Neuromuscular Treatments for Speech and Swallowing: A Tutorial. *American Journal of Speech-Language Pathology,* 12, 400-415.

Clark, M., Harris, R., Jolleff, N., Price, K., & Neville, B. G. (2010). Worster-Drought syndrome: Poorly recognized despite severe and persistent difficulties with feeding and speech. *Developmental Medicine and Child Neurology*, 52(1), 27-32.

Costigan, F. A. & Light, J. (2011). Functional seating for school-age children with cerebral palsy: An evidence-based tutorial, *Language, Speech, and Hearing Services in Schools*, 42, 223-236.

Crary, M. A. (1993). *Developmental motor speech disorders*. San Diego, CA: Singular.

Crary, M. A. (1995). Clinical evaluation of developmental motor speech disorders. *Seminars in Speech and Language*, 16(2), 110-125.

Darley, F.L., Aronson , A.E., & Brown, J.R. (1969). Differential diagnostic patterns of dysarthria. *Journal of Speech and Hearing Research,* 12, 246-269.

DeThorne, L., Johnson, C. J., Walder, L., and Jamie Mahurin-Smith, J. (2009). When "Simon Says" doesn't work: Alternatives to imitation for facilitating early speech development, *America Journal of Speech Language Pathology,* 18, 133-145.

Dodd, B. (1995). Procedures for classification of subgroups of speech disorder. In B. Dodd (Ed.), *The Differential Diagnosis and Treatment of Children with Speech Disorder* (pp. 65-80). San Diego, CA: Singular Publishing Group.

Duffy, J. R. (2005). *Motor speech disorders: Substrates, diferential diagnosis, and management* (2nd ed.). St. Louis, MO: Mosby.

Duffy, J. R., & Kent, R. D. (2001). Darley's contributions to the understanding, differential diagnosis, and scientific study of the dysarthrias. *Aphasiology*, 15(3), 275-289.

Edeal, D. M. & Gildersleeve-Neumann, C. (2011).The importance of production frequency in therapy for Childhood Apraxia of Speech *American Journal of Speech-Language Pathology*, 20, 95-110.

Ekelman, B. L., & Aram, D. M. (1983). Syntactic findings in developmental verbal apraxia. *Journal of Communication Disorders,* 16, 237–250.

Forrest, K. (2002). Are oral-motor exercises useful in the treatment phonological/articulatory disorders? *Seminars in Speech and Language*, 23(1), 15-26.

Forrest, K. (2003). Diagnostic criteria of developmental apraxia of speech used by clinical speech-language pathologists. *American Journal of Speech-Language Pathology,* 12, 376-380.

Fox, C. & Boliek, C. (2012) Intensive voice treatment (LSVT LOUD) for children with spastic Cerebral Palsy and dysarthria. *Journal of Speech-Language Hearing Research*, Papers in Press. Published January 9, 2012, as doi: 10.1044/1092-4388(2011/10-0235)

Gibbon, F. (2002) Features of impaired motor control in children with articulation/phonological disorders. In Windsor, F., Kelly, L. and Hewlett, N (Eds.) *Investigations in Clinical Linguistics and Phonetics*. Lawrence Erlbaum: London, 299-309.

Grigos, M, Hayden, D. & Eigen, J. (2010).Perceptual and articulatory changes in speech production following PROMPT treatment. *Journal of Medical Speech Pathology*(18) 4, 46-53.

Groenen, P., Maassen, B., Crul, T. & Thoonen, G. (1996). The specific relation between perception and production errors for place of articulation in developmental apraxia of speech. *Journal of Speech and Hearing Research,* 39, 468-482.

Hall, P. K., Jordan, L. S. & Robin, D. A. (1993). *Developmental Apraxia of Speech.* Austin, TX: Pro-ed.

Hall P. K., Jordan L, & Robin D.A. (2007). *Developmental Apraxia of Speech: From Theory to Clinical Practice (2nd Edition),* Austin, TX: Pro-ed.

Hixon, T.J., Hawley, J.L., & Wilson, K. J. (1982). An around-the-house- device for the clinical determination of respiratory driving pressure: a note on making the simple even simpler. *Journal of Speech and Hearing Disorders*, 47, 413-416.

Hixon, Weismer, & Hoit (2008). Preclinical Speech Science anatomy Physiology Acoustics Perception. Plural Publishing, San Diego, CA.

Hodge, M. (1993). Assessment and treatment of a child with a developmental speech disorder: A biological behavioral perspective. *Seminars in Speech and Language,* 14(2) 128-140.

Hodge, M. & Wellman, L. (1999) Management of children with dysarthria. In A. J. Caruso and E. A. Strand, (Eds.) *Clinical Management of Motor Speech Disorders of Children* (pp., 209-280). New York: Thieme Publishing Co.

Hustad, K. C., Gorton, K., & Lee, J. (2010). Classification of speech and language profiles in 4-year-old children with cerebral palsy: A prospective preliminary study. *Journal of Speech, Language, and Hearing Research,* 53(6), 1496-513.

Kent, R., Kent, J., and Rosenbek, J. (1987) Maximum performance tests of speech production. *Journal of Speech and Hearing Disorders,* 52, 367-387.

Lepage, C., Noreau, L., & Bernard, P. M. (1998). Association between characteristics of locomotion and accomplishment of life habits in children with cerebral palsy. *Physical Therapy*, *78*(5), 458-469.

Lewis B.A., Freebairn L.A., Hansen A.J., Iyengar S.K., Taylor H.G. (2004). School-age follow-up of children with childhood apraxia of speech. *Language Speech and Hearing Services in Schools,* 35(2), 122-140.

Liégeois, F., Morgan, A. T., Connelly, A., & Vargha-Khadem, F. (2011). Endophenotypes of FOXP2: Dysfunction within the human articulatory network. *European Journal of Paediatric Neurology*, 15(4), 283-288.

Lindamood, P. & Lindamood, P. (2011). *Lindamood Phoneme Sequencing® for Phonemic Awareness, Reading and Spelling (LiPS®)*, 4th edition. Gander Publishing Educational Materials
http://www.lindamoodbell.com/programs/lips.html

Maas, E., Robin, D. A., Austermann-Hula, S. N., Freedman, S. E., Wulf, W., Ballard, K. J., & Schmidt, R. A. (2008). Principles of motor learning in treatment of motor speech disorders. *American Journal of Speech-Language Pathology*, 17, 277–298.

Maassen, B. & Terband, H. (2010). Speech motor development in childhood apraxia of speech: generating testable hypotheses by neurocomputational modeling. *Folia Phoniatrica et Logoaedica,* 62, 134-142.

Maassen, B., Groenen, P., & Crul, T. (2003). Auditory and phonetic perception of vowels in children with apraxic speech disorders. *Clinical Linguistics and Phonetics, 17*, 447–467.

Marion M. J., Sussman H. M., Marquardt, T.P. (1993). The perception and production of rhyme in normal and developmentally apraxic children. *Journal of Communication Disorders*, 26(3), 129-60

Marquardt T. P., Sussman, H. M., Snow, T., & Jacks, A. (2002). The integrity of the syllable in developmental apraxia of speech. *Journal of Communication Disorders* 35(1):31-49

Mass, E. & Farinella , K. (November, 2009). Practice Schedule Effects in Treatment for Childhood Apraxia of Speech (CAS), Session presented at the *American Speech Language and Hearing Association Convention,* New Orleans, LA.

McCauley, R. J. & Strand, E. A. (2008). Review of standardized tests of nonverbal oral and speech motor performance in children, *America Journal of Speech Language Pathology* 17: 81 - 91.

McCauley, R. J., Strand, E., Lof, G. L., Schooling, T., & Frymark, T. (2009). Evidence-based systematic review: Effects of nonspeech oral motor exercises on speech. *American Journal of Speech-Language Pathology*, 18, 343–360.

McNeill, B.C., Gillon, G. T., & Dodd, B. Effectiveness of an integrated phonological awareness approach for children with childhood apraxia of speech (CAS) (2009) *Child Language Teaching and Therapy,* 25(3), 341-366.

Morgan, A. T., & Liégeois, F. (2010). Re-thinking diagnostic classification of the dysarthrias: A developmental perspective. *Folia Phoniatrica Et Logopaedica,* 62(3), 120-126.

Moriarty, B. & Gillon, G. (2006). Phonological awareness intervention or children with childhood apraxia of speech. *International Journal of Language & Communication Disorders*, 42 (6), 713-734.

Norris, J. (2003). *Phonic Faces Manual*, 2nd Ed. Baton Rouge, LA: EleMentory. *http://www.elementory.com/index.html*

Odding, E., Roebroeck, M. E., & Stam, H. J. (2006). The epidemiology of cerebral palsy: Incidence, impairments and risk factors. *Disability and Rehabilitation*, 28(4), 183-191.

Orton-Gillingham Institute for Multi-Sensory Education *http://orton-gillingham.com/frmMain.aspx*

Pennington, L. (2008). Cerebral palsy and communication. *Paediatrics and Child Health*, 18(9), 405-409.

Peter, B., Matsushita, M. & Raskind W.H. (in press), Motor sequencing deficit as an endophenotype of speech sound disorder: A genome-wide linkage analysis in a multigenerational family. *Psychiatric Genetics*.

Peter, B., & Raskind, W.H. (2011). Evidence for a familial speech sound disorder subtype in a multigenerational study of oral and hand motor sequencing ability. *Topics in Language Disorders* 31(2), 145-167.

Pirila, S., van der Meere, J., Pentikainen, T., Ruusu-Niemi, P., Korpela, R., Kilpinen, J., & Nieminen, P. (2007). Language and motor speech skills in children with cerebral palsy. *Journal of Communication Disorders*, 40(2), 116-28.

Robbins, J. and Klee, T. (1987). Clinical assessment of oropharyngeal motor development in young children. *Journal of Speech and Hearing Disorders. Vol.52, 271-277.*

Rosenbaum, P., Paneth, N., Leviton, A., Goldstein, M., Bax, M., Dan, B., & Jacobsson, B. (2007). A report: The defini-tion and classification of cerebral palsy. *Developmental Medicine & Child Neurology,* 109 (Suppl.), 8-14.

Rosenbek, J. C. (1985). Treating apraxia of speech. In D. Johns, (Ed.) *Clinical Management of Neurogenic Communicative Disorders* (pp., 267-312). Boston: Little, Brown & Co.

Rosenbek, J. C. Lemme, M., Ahern, M. Harris, E., & Wertz, T. (1973). A treatment for apraxia of speech in adults. *Journal of Speech and Hearing Disorders,* 38, 462-472.

Rosenthal, J. B. (1994). Rate control therapy for developmental apraxia of speech. *Clinical Communication Disorders,* 4(3), 190-200.

Schmidt, R. & Lee, T. (2005). *Motor control and learning: A behavioral emphasis* (4th ed.) Champaign, IL: Human Kinetics.

Shriberg., L., Aram, D., & Kwiatkowski, J. (1997a). Developmental apraxia of speech: I. Descriptive and theoretical perspectives. *Journal of Speech, Language, and Hearing Research*, 40, 273-285.

Shriberg., L., Aram, D., & Kwiatkowski, J. (1997b). Developmental apraxia of speech: II. Toward a diagnostic marker. *Journal of Speech, Language, and Hearing Research,* 40, 286-312.

Shriberg., L., Aram, D., & Kwiatkowski, J. (1997c). Developmental apraxia of speech: III. A subtype marked by inappropriate stress. *Journal of Speech, Language, and Hearing Research,* 40, 313-337.

Skinder-Meredith, A, Graff, N., & Carkowski, S. (2004). Comparison of nasalance measures in children with childhood apraxia of speech and repaired cleft palate, to their typically developing peers. *SpeechPathology.com*

Skinder-Meredith, A, Stoel-Gammon, C, Wright, R, & Betz, S. (2000).Relationship of prosodic and articulatory errors in developmental apraxia of speech. *American Speech Language Hearing Association Convention,* Washington, DC.

Skinder-Meredith, A., Stoel-Gammon, C. Wright, & Strand, (2001). The effect of articulatory accuracy on prosody in children with developmental apraxia of speech. *American Speech-Language and Hearing Association Convention*, New Orleans, Louisiana.

Skinder, A., Strand, E. & Mignerey, M. (1999). Perceptual and acoustic analysis of lexical and sentential stress in children with developmental apraxia of speech, *Journal of Medical Speech-Language Pathology*, 7, 133-144.

Snowling, M. Goulandris, N. & Stackhouse, J. (1994) Phonological constraints on learning to read: evidence from single-case studies of reading difficulty. In *Reading Development and Dyslexia: Selected Papers from the Third International Conference of the British Dyslexia Association Dyslexia: Towards a Wider Understanding* (pp., 86-104), Manchester England.

Solomon, N. P., & Charron, S. (1998). Speech breathing in able-bodied children and children with cerebral palsy: A review of the literature and implications for clinical intervention. *American Journal of Speech-Language Pathology*, 7(2), 61-78.

Stackhouse, J. (1997). Phonological awareness: Connecting speech and literacy problems. In B. Hodson and M.L. Edwards (Eds.), *Perspectives in Applied Phonology* (pp. 157-196). Gaithersburg, MD: Aspen Publication.

Strand E, Stoeckel R, Baas B. (2006). Treatment of severe childhood apraxia of speech: a treatment efficacy study. *Journal of Medical Speech-Language Pathology* 14, 297-307.

Strand, E. & Debertine, P. (2000). The efficacy of integral stimulation intervention with developmental apraxia of speech. *Journal of Medical Speech-Language Pathology,* 8, 295-300.

Strand, E. A., (1995). Treatment of motor speech disorders in children. *Seminars in Speech and Language.* 16(2), 126-139.

Strand, E. A., & Skinder, A. (1999). Treatment of developmental apraxia of speech: Integral stimulation methods. In A. J. Caruso and E. A. Strand, (Eds.) *Clinical Management of Motor Speech Disorders of Children* (pp., 109-148). New York: Thieme Publishing Co.

Van Mourik, M., Catsman-Berrevoets, C. E., Paquier, P. F., Yousef-Bak, E., & van Dongen, H. R. (1997). Acquired childhood dysarthria: Review of its clinical presentation. *Pediatric Neurology*, 17(4), 299-307.

Velleman, S. & Strand, K. (1994). Developmental verbal dyspraxia. In J. Bernthal (Ed.), *Phonological Characteristics of Special Populations* (pp., pp. 110-139) New York: Thieme Medical Publishers.

Velleman, S. (2005). *Childhood Apraxia of Speech Resource Guide.* Clifton Park, NY: Singular Thompson Delmar Learning, United States.

Wit, J., Maassen, B., Gabreëls, F., Thoonen, G., & de Swart, B. (1994). Traumatic versus perinatally acquired dysarthria: Assessment by means of speech-like maximum performance tasks. *Developmental Medicine and Child Neurology*, 36(3), 221-229.

Yeargin-Allsopp, M., Van Naarden Braun, K., Doernberg, N. S., Benedict, R. E., Kirby, R. S., & Durkin, M. S. (2008). Prevalence of cerebral palsy in 8-year-old children in three areas of the United States in 2002: A multisite collaboration. *Pediatrics*, 121(3), 547-554.

Yoss, K. A., & Darley, F. L. (1974). Developmental apraxia of speech in children with defective articulation. *Journal of Speech and Hearing Research,* 17, 399–416.

In: Comprehensive Perspectives …
Editors: Beate Peter and Andrea A. N. MacLeod
ISBN: 978-1-62257-041-6

Chapter 19

Hearing Impairment and Developmental Disabilities

Kiyoshi Otomo

Introduction

Children typically begin to communicate verbally around their first birthday, and they acquire a full repertoire of phonological constituents during their first few years (see Chapters 4 through 6 for a full description). Children with hearing impairments and other developmental disabilities exhibit a delay and/or follow a unique path of phonological development. Their characteristic progress reflects various factors, such as their sensory, motor, and cognitive traits. Examination and understanding of the developmental patterns of these populations provide insight into the contributions of these variables to phonological development and offer information for facilitating the phonological development of these children. In this chapter, we will review recent findings concerning phonological development in children with hearing impairments, Down syndrome, Autism Spectrum Disorders, and Fragile X syndrome, and discuss factors associated with phonological development in these populations.

Hearing Impairment

Hearing children acquire the phonological system of the language that they are learning by relying heavily on auditory input. They also use auditory feedback from their own speech productions to adjust their output to match the target sounds. Hearing impairment, however, breaks the chain connecting environmental speech sounds to the creation of a phonological representation, and then to the reproduction of target sounds. Children with a hearing impairment or deafness must rely on frequency information that is distorted due to the characteristics of **residual hearing** or the output of the devices worn to improve hearing. These children may therefore be more reliant on visual information such as the speaker's lip movements, and tactile and kinesthetic feedback from their own articulatory movements.

Early Speech Development in Infants with Hearing Impairments

We will first examine how loss of hearing affects the preverbal vocalizations of infants. Beginning from cries at birth, infants gradually refine their vocal output to approximate the more patterned speech productions in the linguistic environment. Hearing children typically experience several stages of vocal development that begin with reflexive vocalizations and some vowel-like sounds, then move into a gradual increase in the production of immature syllabic forms, and into the production of well-formed syllables with true consonants, a stage called canonical babbling (see Chapter 4). Infants with and without hearing impairments demonstrate both similarities and differences in these patterns. Both deaf and normally hearing infants produce non-speech-like vocalizations such as raspberries, squeals, and growls (Oller, Eilers, Bull, & Carney, 1985; Stoel-Gammon & Otomo, 1986). However, a longitudinal examination of one deaf infant showed that the speech-like vocalizations of this infant, unlike those of hearing infants, became less frequent during the first 30 weeks of life (Maskarinec, Cairns, Butterfield, & Weamer, 1981). Differences have also been found in the syllable structure of those with and without hearing impairments. A deaf infant observed by Oller and colleagues produced no repetitive canonical babbles from 8 to 13 months, whereas hearing infants produced many consonant-vowel canonical syllables during this period (Oller et al., 1985). In other reports, profound hearing loss did not totally suppress the expression of well-formed canonical syllables, but the onset of the expression of canonical syllables tended to be substantially delayed (Eilers & Oller, 1994; Oller & Eilers, 1988). Thus, audition played a significant role in vocal development, but the authors of these studies also suggested that the perception of speech sounds through vision and residual hearing with amplification promoted canonical babbling in even deaf infants. A significant positive correlation between age at the initiation of auditory amplification and age at onset of canonical babbling (Eilers & Oller, 1994) appeared to support this view. The delay in the onset of canonical productions was also consistent with the finding that 12-month-old children with hearing loss produced fewer multisyllabic utterances including consonants than did children with normal hearing at the same age (McGowan, Nittrouer, & Chenausky, 2008).

In terms of the segmental aspect of production, the size of the consonantal inventory has been reported to be smaller among hearing impaired infants (Stoel-Gammon, 1988; Stoel-Gammon & Otomo, 1986). Furthermore, the number of consonant types appeared to remain constant or decrease over time among hearing-impaired infants aged 4–28 months, which contrasted with the expanding repertoire observed in normally hearing infants aged 4–18 months (Stoel-Gammon & Otomo, 1986).

With respect to the place of consonant articulation, Smith (1982) reported that velar consonants tended to dominate the early productions of hearing impaired infants during the 3–6-month period, but that alveolar/dental consonants became dominant during a few months around the first birthday. This pattern coincided with the results of his earlier study among normally hearing infants (Smith & Oller, 1981). A notable difference, however, was that the proportion of labial consonants sharply increased among hearing impaired infants after 15–18 months of age, and this labial dominance persisted until after their third birthday. This prominence of labial consonants, also reported by Stoel-Gammon (1988), contrasted with the declining proportion of labial consonants observed among normally hearing children after 12 months of age (Smith & Oller, 1981). As Smith (1982) and Stoel-Gammon (1988) suggested, children with profound hearing loss may rely more on visually perceived lip movements to reproduce speech sounds than do their normally hearing peers.

When vowels are the targets of analysis, acoustical analysis can provide additional insight. Formant frequencies during vowel-like productions are indicative of the range of articulatory space. Infants' vowel-like productions are generally characterized by expanding vowel space with increasing age, as revealed by the **F1–F2 range** during approximately the first 2 years. Kent and colleagues (Kent, Osberger, Netsell, & Hustedde, 1987) investigated the formant frequencies of vowels of identical (monozygotic) twin boys, one with normal hearing and the other with a profound bilateral hearing loss. The formant frequency range or the size of the vowel space would be expected to increase with age, but the expansion in F1–F2 space was found only in the twin with normal hearing through 18 months of age. In another study, the range of F2 was also found to be greater in normally hearing children than in children with hearing loss at 12 months of age (McGowan et al., 2008). These findings showed that the reduced auditory experience of vowel variations and auditory feedback likely restricted the range of tongue movements during vowel production, which also likely reduced the intelligibility of speech.

Meaningful Speech of Children with Hearing Impairments

The speech of children with hearing impairments who have acquired language is generally characterized by the low levels of intelligibility (Gold, 1980; Paterson, 1994; Yoshinaga-Itano, 1998). Although some children who are profoundly deaf may develop intelligible speech, the speech of most children with **profound hearing loss** is very difficult to understand (Yoshinaga-Itano, 1998). In addition to problems with prosody, errors in the articulation of both vowels and consonants contribute to difficulties in understanding the speech of those with hearing impairments. Both Gold (1980), in a review of previous studies, and Calvert (1982) noted that voicing errors and the omissions of consonants in the initial or final positions of words were common in the speech of individuals who were deaf. Voicing errors, such as the devoicing of final voiced consonants, were particularly frequent, although no fixed patterns were found with regard to whether voiced consonants were substituted for their voiceless consonants in the same place of articulation or vice versa. When producing consonant clusters, children may insert an additional, brief neutralized vowel between two consonants, or omit one consonant, thereby adding a syllable or reducing the cluster. Children with hearing impairment have been reported to show greater accuracy in their production of bilabial consonants than other consonants (Nober, 1967). This is consistent with the aforementioned finding that labial consonants become prominent in the speech of young children with hearing impairments (Smith, 1982; Stoel-Gammon, 1988).

Another type of error in the speech of children with hearing impairments concerns vowel substitutions (Calvert, 1982; Gold, 1980). Although vowel errors may take various forms, they often occur in the form of substituting either another vowel with a similar articulatory position or a neutral /ə/ or /ʌ/. The neutralization of vowels is also consistent with the aforementioned findings of the reduced formant frequency range of the vowels produced by young infants with hearing loss (Kent et al., 1987; McGowan et al., 2008).

Sound files 19S1, 19S2, and 19S3 were provided by a woman who experienced moderate to severe sensorineural hearing loss as a young child and was fitted with hearing aids. The first two sound files are examples of read speech, and in the third, she tells the story of how she lost her hearing and how she was helped by hearing aids.

Access Sound File 1 (Chapter 19)

19S1 The Rainbow Passage read by a woman who wears hearing aids

Access Sound File 2 (Chapter 19)

19S2 The Stella Passage read by a woman who wears hearing aids

Access Sound File 3 (Chapter 19)

19S3 Personal story told by a woman who wears hearing aids

Speech of Children with Otitis Media with Effusion

The effects of hearing impairment on speech development are more pronounced when hearing loss is severe or profound, but many children experience mild to moderate hearing loss due to otits media with effusion (OME), or middle ear infections in which liquid accumulates in the middle ear space. Although this condition is usually temporary, a fluctuating hearing loss may persist for some time in cases of OME. Shriberg, Friel-Patti, Flipsen, & Brown (2000) showed that elevated **hearing thresholds** associated with OME can be a prognostic factor for speech delay. More specifically, 33% of children who had experienced an average hearing loss greater than 20 dB at 12–18 months of age exhibited some kind of speech disorder, whether clinical or subclinical, at 3 years of age. This contrasted with the 2% risk for children with an average hearing loss of less than 20 dB during 12–18 months of age (Shriberg et al., 2000). However, no strong consensus concerning whether a history of OME in early childhood causes later speech problems has been reached. Roberts and colleagues (Roberts, Rosenfeld, & Zeisel, 2004) conducted a systematic review and reanalysis of data from 14 published studies and found no convincing association between OME and speech development. This finding reminds us that hearing status, but not necessarily history of OME, constitutes the primary predictor of speech development.

Speech Perception in Individuals with Hearing Impairments

It has been speculated that the distortion and reduction in speech sound input associated with hearing impairment hinders children from perceiving target sounds and from forming the appropriate phonological representations of words. Consonant recognition studies have shown that adult listeners with sensorineural hearing impairment exhibit significant recognition errors in quiet as well as noisy settings (Bilger & Wang, 1976; Dubno, Dirks, & Langhofer, 1982; Gordon-Salant, 1985). In these studies, patterns of consonant confusion varied in terms of both the degree and the configuration of hearing loss. Place-of-articulation errors were most frequent, irrespective of the listener's audiometric configuration; when an error was made, the listener tended to confuse the stimulus with a syllable that was produced with the same manner of articulation, but with a different place of articulation (Dubno et al., 1982). Such difficulties in consonant recognition should have a significant impact on young children learning the phonological system of the language used in their environments.

To compensate for the loss of hearing sensitivity, a **hearing aid** is usually provided to children with hearing impairment for purposes of amplification. With the aid of amplification, the speech perception of hearing-impaired children can be comparable to that of normally hearing peers in quiet settings (Stelmachowicz, Hoover, Lewis, Kortekaas, & Pittman, 2000). However, the accuracy of word recognition seems to deteriorate for children with hearing loss wearing hearing aids when speech is presented under conditions of competing noise (Hicks & Tharpe, 2002). This difficulty in discriminating speech sounds due to the weakening and distortion of auditory signals may be mitigated by watching how the lips and jaw move and by feeling the vibrations. Nevertheless, it is a challenging task for a child with hearing impairment to become proficient in speech production.

Cochlear Implants

The hypothesis that deprivation of auditory input and auditory feedback hinders children from acquiring adequate phonological skills can be examined by investigating children who, despite profound hearing loss, have had an opportunity for auditory compensation via technological aids. Cochlear implantation is one such technology that is increasingly gaining acceptance. Cochlear implants collect speech and environmental sounds with a microphone and transmit these sounds via a speech processor to tiny wires surgically inserted into the cochlea. Instead of physical vibrations, the electrodes directly stimulate the remaining basal ganglion cells of the auditory nerve fibers with electrical pulses that convey temporal, frequency, and durational information. Figure 19.1 illustrates the components of a cochlear implant. We should note that the auditory sensation gained from such electrical signals is considerably different from the auditory sensation of hearing individuals who receive richer temporal and frequency resolution information from acoustic hearing. Nevertheless, many cochlear implanted children with **congenital** and **prelingual deafness** have experienced significant improvements in speech perception (Calmels et al., 2004; Fryauf-Bertschy, Tyler, Kelsay, Gantz, & Woodworth, 1997).

Numerous studies have reported the positive effects of cochlear implantation on speech production (Allen, Nikopoulos, & O'Donoghue, 1998; Calmels et al., 2004; Flipsen & Colvard, 2006). Examination of changes in intelligibility constitutes one measure for evaluating the effects of implantation. Flipsen and Colvard (2006), for example, reported that intelligible speech emerged rapidly in the conversational speech of six children who received implants before 3 years of age, although their speech was not necessarily as intelligible as the speech of normally hearing children.

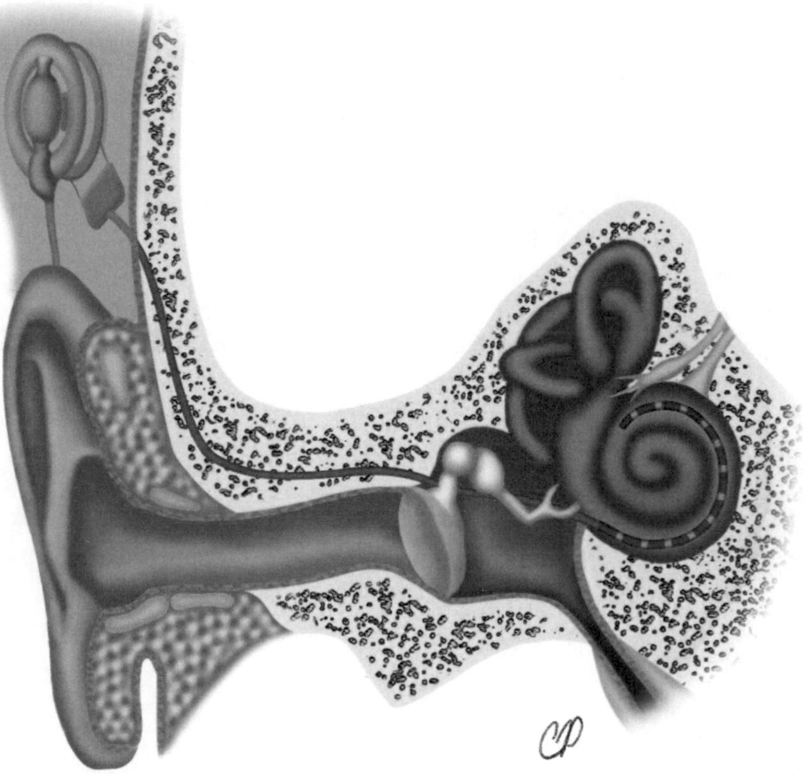

Figure 19.1. The components of a cochlear implant device.

Significant improvements in consonant production have also been demonstrated (Ertmer & Mellon, 2001; Grogan, Barker, Dettman, & Blamey, 1995; McCaffrey, 1999; Warner-Czyz & Davis, 2008). Ertmer and Mellon (2001) discussed a deaf toddler whose multichannel cochlear implant was activated at 20 months. Examination of her speech productions showed that canonical and postcanonical prelinguistic forms increased after 5 months of implant use. The initial dominance of labial consonants was also gradually supplemented by the consonants with other place features, such as alveolar and velar, by 12 months after implantation. A case study conducted by McCaffrey (1999) also demonstrated increased variation following implantation in terms of consonant types, particularly alveolars, after the initial dominance of labial stops and nasals. The accuracy of consonant productions with respect to intended targets also improved over time (Warner-Czyz & Davis, 2008).

Cochlear implantation also promotes the development of a vowel system in congenitally deaf children. Prelingually deaf children who received implants increased their vowel inventories and the production accuracy of their spontaneous speech (Ertmer, 2001; Grogan et al., 1995; McCaffrey, 1999; Tye-Murray & Kirk, 1993; Warner-Czyz & Davis, 2008). This expansion of vowel range was verified with acoustical analyses of formant structures (Ertmer, 2001). In terms of prosody, cochlear implants also offered benefits in some aspects such as phrasing and pitch, although some noticeable deviance in the quality of resonance and the placement of stress tended to persist (Lenden & Flipsen, 2007).

Although children fitted with cochlear implants are able to expand their phonological repertoire and produce highly intelligible conversational speech, these children also produce errors. Some consonants and vowels may be missing, non-English sounds may occur, and several sounds that are unstable with respect to their intended words across productions in their developing phonological system (Chin & Pisoni, 2000). Flipsen and Parker (2008) analyzed the speech of six young implanted children, and found that major error patterns included cluster reduction, stopping, liquid simplification, final consonant deletion, unstressed syllable deletion, and velar fronting. These children also exhibited non-developmental patterns, such as vowel substitution and initial consonant deletion. Longitudinal comparisons of phonetic inventories after cochlear implantation have shown that the rate of improvement decreased as a function of years after implantation, suggesting that a plateau in performance had been reached (Blamey, Barry, & Jacq, 2001).

The age at which a child receives a cochlear implant has been demonstrated to be an important predictor of his or her speech outcomes (Connor, Craig, Raudenbush, Heavner, & Zwolan, 2006; Ertmer, Young, & Nathani, 2007; Fryauf-Bertschy et al., 1997; Tye-Murray, Spencer, & Woodworth, 1995). Ertmer and colleagues (2007) examined speech samples of children who received implants between 10 and 36 months of age. Their results suggested that although children implanted at younger ages may take longer to complete the process of vocal development than children implanted at later ages, the younger group nevertheless tended to reach the highest level of vocalization, which included diphthongs, jargon, and complex syllables, at younger chronological ages. In the study conducted by Tye-Murray, et al. (1995), three groups based on age at implantation (2–5 years, 5–8 years, and 8–15 years) were compared, and children who received cochlear implants before the age of 5 improved the accuracy of their productions more rapidly than did children who received implants at older ages. Thus, the relationship between age at implantation and speech outcome appears to be fairly well established. The benefit of earlier implantation presumably stems from the **neural plasticity** of the brain, which renders it better suited for early language learning (Tomblin, Barker, Spencer, Zhang, & Gantz, 2005). However, a number of additional factors also accounted for variability in children's performance; these included the amount of daily use of the implanted device, the technology of the device, and the degree of educational emphasis on **aural–oral communication** (Fryauf-Bertschy et al., 1997; Geers, 2002).

Sound files 19S4 and 19S5 are examples of read speech provided by a woman who has worn cochlear implants since adolescence. In sound file 19S6, she tells her personal story.

Access Sound File 4 (Chapter 19)

19S4 The Rainbow Passage read by a woman who wears cochlear implants

Access Sound File 5 (Chapter 19)

19S5 The Stella Passage read by a woman who wears cochlear implants

Access Sound File 6 (Chapter 19)

19S6 Personal story told by a woman who wears cochlear implants

Down Syndrome

Down syndrome is probably the most well documented chromosomal syndrome. It occurs 1 in about 800 births in the United States (National Institutes of Child Health and Human Development, 1997), although the incidence rises with increasing maternal age (Carothers, Hecht, & Hook, 1999). Over 90 percent of the cases are Trisomy 21, which is a condition caused by the presence of an extra copy of chromosome 21. Due mostly to the intellectual disabilities associated with Down syndrome, children with this syndrome have slower language development. One of the most prominent features of the speech of persons with Down syndrome is its low intelligibility. Over 95% of the 937 parents of children with Down syndrome who answered a questionnaire indicated that their children, aged 0 to over 40 years, had at least some difficulty in being understood (Kumin, 1994). Since typically developing children also have lower intelligibility during the preschool years (see Chapter 5 for more details), excluding children below the age of 4 years may provide a more typical picture of this syndrome. Even this reanalysis showed that approximately 56% of respondents reported that their children experienced "frequent" difficulties being understood. More objective measurements of intelligibility utilizing the Children's Speech Intelligibility Measure (Wilcox & Morris, 1999) also yielded similar results, suggesting that about half the words produced by children with Down syndrome were unintelligible (Cleland, Wood, Hardcastle, Wishart, & Timmins, 2010).

Prelinguistic Speech Development in Children with Down Syndrome

Before discussing the features affecting intelligibility, we will first address the development of babbling in infants with Down syndrome. Early studies found that the prelinguistic vocalizations of infants with Down syndrome were similar to those of typically developing infants. For example, Dodd (1972) compared the spontaneous babbling patterns of 10 infants with Down syndrome with those of 10 typically developing infants aged 9–13 months and observed no significant differences between the two groups in terms of numbers of vowel utterances, numbers of consonant utterances, and numbers of different vowel and consonant types. In the study conducted by Smith and Oller (1981), the vocal development of infants with Down syndrome and that of normally developing infants were found to be very similar during about the first 15 months. Both groups began to produce reduplicated babbling, which represent sequences of identical or nearly identical syllables such as /dadada…/ at 8–81/2 months of age. The data gathered by Steffens and colleagues also showed both similarities and differences between these groups (Steffens, Oller, Lynch, & Urbano, 1992). Production of canonical babbling increased from 4 to 18 months of age in both groups, but normally developing infants tended to produce a higher ratio of canonical babbling to the total number of syllables than did infants with Down syndrome throughout this period.

Group differences were also reported by Lynch and colleagues (Lynch et al., 1995) in their longitudinal investigation of infants 4 to 18 months of age, 13 of whom were diagnosed with Down syndrome, and 27 of whom were developing typically. First, infants with Down syndrome as a group began canonical babbling about 2 months later than did typically developing infants. Second, canonical babbling appeared less consistently after its onset in infants with Down syndrome. Their finding that infants who began canonical babbling and earlier in life tended to have higher social communication skills at 27 months also suggested a link between vocal development and communicative behaviors and social cognition.

Meaningful Speech of Children with Down Syndrome

Speech production skills can be examined in terms of the consonantal repertoire in speech. Stoel-Gammon (1980) investigated the spontaneous speech of four children with Down syndrome aged 3–6 years and found that they were able to produce most of the phones of English. The consonantal inventory may also be estimated using a set of target words. Consistent with the findings noted above, Van Borsel (1988) reported that nearly all phonemes occurred in the picture-naming speech samples of five Dutch-speaking adolescents with Down syndrome. However, longitudinal records of the speech of 60 children with Down syndrome showed great individual variation in the age at which specific consonants emerged in spontaneous speech (Kumin, Councill, & Goodman, 1994). For example, the age of emergence of /p/ and /s/ ranged from 1 to 8 years.

Another aspect of speech that has been attracted research attention concerns the patterns of errors in the speech of individuals with Down syndrome. Their error patterns have generally appeared to be the same as those observed in typically developing younger children. To summarize the findings of previous studies, children and adolescents with Down syndrome have been shown to frequently exhibit the following phonological processes: final consonant deletion, cluster reduction, devoicing, stopping, gliding, palatal and velar fronting, and syllable deletion (Bleile & Schwarz, 1984; Cleland, Wood, et al., 2010; J. Roberts et al., 2005; Rupela & Manjula, 2007; Smith & Stoel-Gammon, 1983; Stoel-Gammon, 1980; Van Borsel, 1988, 1996). All of these processes are relatively common among typically developing young children who produced phonological errors. Furthermore, both typically developing children and children with Down syndrome were more accurate in producing word-initial than word-final stop consonants (Smith & Stoel-Gammon, 1983). However, the phonological development of individuals with Down syndrome lags behind that of their typically developing peers. When the frequency of occurrence of phonological processes were compared between groups, children with Down syndrome were found to be delayed by 1 to 2 years at age three and by about 4 years at the age of six to seven (Smith & Stoel-Gammon, 1983).

In contrast, more recent reports have stressed that children and adolescents with Down syndrome present with variable and idiosyncratic phonological processes. For example, the data reported by Cleland and colleagues (Cleland, Wood, et al., 2010) indicated that atypical processes such as initial consonant deletions also frequently occurred in the speech of children and adolescents with Down syndrome. When relatively infrequent errors were included, 18 of the 29 processes observed were atypical. The phonotactic structure of the speech productions of those with and without Down syndrome may also differ. An analysis of the imitation of words uttered by children speaking Kannada, a Dravidian language used in part of India, showed that those with Down syndrome produced significantly fewer multisyllabic word shapes consisting of four syllables or more (Rupela & Manjula, 2007). These findings contrasted with those obtained from non-Down syndrome children, who were matched for IQ, and with those obtained from 4–5-year-old normally developing children who produced multisyllabic word shapes within the expected range. Overall, the errors in the speech of individuals with Down syndrome can be characterized primarily in terms of typical phonological processes plus several added irregular error patterns.

Inconsistency of Productions in Children with Down Syndrome

One characteristic often pointed out in the speech of children with Down syndrome is inconsistency of errors in repeated productions of the same words. Dodd and Thompson (2001) showed that children with Down syndrome and those without Down syndrome who exhibited inconsistent phonological errors did so to comparable degrees. In another study, participants were asked to name pictures and imitate the experimenter's productions of the names (Dodd, 1976). Children and adolescents with Down syndrome produced more inconsistent errors than did both typically developing peers matched according to **mental age** and children without Down syndrome with intellectual disabilities. Furthermore, the individuals with Down syndrome were more accurate when imitating than when spontaneously naming. At least two factors may account for the phenomenon of inconsistency. One concerns motor planning and the other relates to incomplete phonological representations of words (Dodd & Thompson, 2001). These factors are discussed later.

Hearing of Children with Down Syndrome

Individuals with Down syndrome often have problems with hearing. Nearly two-thirds of toddlers with this syndrome have either unilateral or bilateral hearing loss, with more children suffering from bilateral hearing loss than from unilateral hearing loss (Roizen, Wolters, Nicol, & Blondis, 1993). Due to physical anomalies and immune system deficiencies, children with Down syndrome are more likely to be affected by recurring otitis media. Thus, a majority of the hearing loss associated with Down syndrome is conductive, but cases of mixed or sensorineural hearing loss also occur. The sensorineural hearing loss of those with Down syndrome may be related to the smaller inner ear structures of these individuals compared with those of normally hearing individuals (Blaser et al., 2006). Based on studies of the phonological development of children with hearing loss, we would expect that many children with Down syndrome would also face some obstacles in acquiring phonological skills.

When hearing impairment is diagnosed in a child with Down syndrome, a hearing aid may be used by when appropriate. Recent advances in cochlear implantation have included children with Down syndrome or other types of intellectual disabilities as candidates for this procedure when they have severe to profound sensorinerural hearing loss (Hans, England, Prowse, Young, & Sheehan, 2010; Lee, Kim, Jeong, Kim, & Chung, 2010). Although the effects of cochlear implants on the speech output of these recipients remains somewhat unclear, the speech intelligibility of children with mild intellectual disabilities may improve (Lee et al., 2010). Application of cochlear implants to individuals with multiple disabilities is expected to expand, and we need to wait for future studies to evaluate how this technology may improve the acquisition of phonology in this population.

Oral Structures of Children with Down Syndrome

Children with Down syndrome may also exhibit a variety of anatomical and physiological differences that can have an impact on their production of speech. These differences include weak facial muscles and general hypotonicity (Bodensteiner, Smith, & Schaefer, 2003). Some children with Down syndrome have an open-mouth stance and their tongues may protrude somewhat. Their tongues are not necessarily enlarged (Ardan, Hardker, & Kemp, 1972), but the smaller palatal dimensions make their oral pathways relatively narrow. More specifically, their palates are "narrower in width, shorter in depth, and lower in height" (Westerman, Johnson, & Cohen, 1975). The height and volume of the oral cavity of those with Down syndrome are significantly smaller than are those of typically developing peers (Bhagyalakshmi, Renukarya, & Rajangam, 2007). These characteristics lower the resonance quality of vowels and may restrict precise palatal contact with the tongue in the articulation of consonants, reducing the overall intelligibility of speech.

Motor Skills of Children with Down Syndrome

Clumsiness in the gross and fine movements constitutes one of the major features of Down syndrome. Children with Down syndrome show a wide range of poor motor skills, such as engaging in steady circular movements and repetitive tapping with a finger (Frith &

Frith, 1974). The oral-motor functions of children with Down syndrome have also been found to be impaired during their first 3 years of life (Spender et al., 1995). They were found to have greater difficulty in the use of the lips, tongue, and jaw for feeding compared with their unaffected twin brothers. Barnes and colleagues (Barnes, Roberts, Mirrett, Sideris, & Misenheimer, 2006) examined oral-motor functions more directly related to speech and found that children with Down syndrome had significantly greater difficulty than typically developing peers with those functions involving the lips, tongue, velopharynx, and larynx.

Some researchers (e.g. Kumin & Adams, 2000) have also maintained that children with Down syndrome demonstrated the characteristics of speech consistent with **Childhood Apraxia of Speech** (CAS) (Kumin & Adams, 2000). CAS is an inability to voluntarily program, combine, organize, and sequence the movements necessary for speech-related tasks. It can be defined as an impairment in planning and/or programming the spatio-temporal parameters of movement sequences that results in errors in speech sound production and prosody (American-Speech-Language-Hearing-Association, 2007). Kumin and Adams (2000) showed that children with Down syndrome displayed characteristics such as decreased intelligibility with increased length of utterances and inconsistency in errors, which were also commonly observed in the speech of children diagnosed with CAS. Thus, inaccurate speech production in children with Down syndrome appears, at least in part, to result not only from oral motor weakness but also from some degree of motor planning and coordination deficits.

Verbal Short-Term Memory and Phonological Awareness in Children with Down Syndrome

Individuals with Down syndrome have demonstrated weakness in verbal short-term memory (Jarrold, Baddeley, & Phillips, 2002; Kay-Raining Bird & Chapman, 1994). For example, when participants were asked to repeat a series of auditorily presented numbers, individuals with Down syndrome were significantly less accurate than controls matched for level of receptive vocabulary (Jarrold et al., 2002). This pattern did not change even when the participants were simply asked to judge whether a list of digits presented immediately after the initial list was the same or different. These results suggested that poor verbal short-term memory performance in those with Down syndrome did not result from the demands of speech production. Although the contribution of verbal short-term memory to phonological development has not been elucidated thus far, phonological representations may be created with greater efficiency and precision when the learner has a stronger verbal short-term memory.

Phonological awareness constitutes another area of verbal information processing often impaired in individuals with Down syndrome. Phonological awareness refers to explicit awareness of the phonological structure of spoken language and can be assessed with tasks such as segmenting a word into syllables and finding words that contain a target syllable or rhyme with a target word. Weakness in phonological awareness has often been linked with phonological disorders in non-Down syndrome children (Carrol & Snowling, 2004; Preston & Edwards, 2010; Rvachew, Ohberg, Grawburg, & Heyding, 2003). For example, Rvachew and colleagues (2003) examined the phonological awareness of 4-year-old children with moderately or severely delayed expressive phonological skills but age-appropriate receptive vocabulary skills. These children demonstrated significantly poorer phonemic perception and phonological awareness skills than did normally developing peers. Weakness in phonological awareness has also been linked with atypical sound changes such as initial consonant deletion, addition of consonants, and labialization of back sounds (Preston & Edwards, 2010).

Children with Down syndrome have been shown to demonstrate reduced phonological awareness. For example, they performed more poorly in syllable segmentation, rhyme detection, and phoneme detection than did younger typically developing children with similar reading levels (Snowling, Hulme, & Mercer, 2002). Thus, phonological awareness is often targeted by intervention programs aimed at improving speech production and literacy skills (Gillon, 2000; Kennedy & Flynn, 2003). Currently, however, there is little evidence that phonological awareness training improves intelligibility of the speech of children with Down syndrome. Three children with Down syndrome who participated in a phonological awareness intervention program showed a discernable improvement in consonant production, but their overall percentage consonant correct (PCC) did not significantly rise from the pre-intervention period (Kennedy & Flynn, 2003).

Phonological Representation

Two characteristics of the speech of persons with Down syndrome, greater accuracy of imitative than spontaneous productions and inconsistent errors in repeated productions of the same words, are of theoretical interest. In terms of the first, imitation may reduce the cognitive load involved in retrieving a phonological form, allowing the speaker to focus more on articulatory accuracy. In terms of the second, dyspraxia may be involved in inconsistent word forms. Alternatively, both characteristics may be ascribed to another factor, namely incompletely specified phonological representations at the level of the mental lexicon. An underspecified blueprint for a word would be expected to yield fluctuating output, and production would be more accurate if auditory input temporarily restored the insufficient specifications. Furthermore, if phonological representations were vague or not specified to the level of a phoneme, the child would be expected to have difficulty in correctly dividing words into syllabic units, finding rhyming words, and identifying words that have a specified phoneme. Therefore, the relatively poor performance of children with Down syndrome in phonological awareness tasks (Snowling et al., 2002) may also be attributable to vague or underspecified phonological representations.

Mild to moderate hearing loss may lead to such incomplete phonological representations. However, questions persist about why typically developing children with similar degrees of hearing loss did not exhibit inconsistent errors and why individuals with Down syndrome did not sustain and generalize correct productions already achieved under imitation to later occasions. We need to assume the influence of cognitive deficits as an additional factor underlying persistent underdeveloped phonological representations.

Sound file 19S7 was recorded from a boy age 3;6 (years;months) with Down syndrome during a treatment session targeting expressive language. During this session, most of the child's utterances consisted of one-word utterances and were elicited with a request for a label ("What's this?") or for an imitation. The few spontaneous utterances he produced consisted of single words as well. The following utterances were isolated: 1. Spontaneous utterance ("Balloon. A ballon."); 2. Elicited utterance ("Baseketball.") 3. Elicited utterance ("A duck."); 4. Imitated utterance ("Skates."); 5. Elicited utterance ("Elephant."); 6. Imitated utterance ("Piggy"). Note the following speech errors: weak syllable deletion, onset deletion, consonant sequence simplification, and imprecise articulation.

Access Sound File 7 (Chapter 19)

19S7 Six utterances produced by a 3-year-old boy with Down syndrome

AUTISM SPECTRUM DISORDERS

Another major type of developmental disability among children is autism, which is described in terms of three characteristics: 1) impaired social interactions, 2) deficits in communication skills, and 3) restricted repetitive and stereotyped patterns of behaviors, interests, and activities. A broader concept encompassing autism is autism spectrum disorders (ASD), which includes high functioning autism and Asperger syndrome. With respect to the second characteristic, impaired communication, children at one end of the autism spectrum may be nonverbal, whereas those at the other end of the continuum may have vocabulary and syntactic skills within the normal range. Even verbal children may exhibit particular deficits in pragmatics, i.e., the use of appropriate language according to the context.

Speech Characteristics of Children with Autism Spectrum Disorders

In the speech domain, inadequacies in suprasegmentals, such as pitch, intonation, and volume, have often been noted, but the phonological domain has been identified as a relative strength in children with ASD (e.g., Kjelgaard & Tager-Flusberg, 2001). It is often the case that autistic children with limited verbal skills engage in echolalia without any articulatory errors. On the other hand, case reports of autistic children with intellectual disabilities exhibiting idiosyncratic error patterns as well as persistent phonological processes that are common in typical development have also been published (Wolk & Edwards, 1993; Wolk & Giesen, 2000). Furthermore, recent studies have shown that a significant percentage of children with ASD, including those with high functioning autism and Asperger syndrome, exhibited speech output errors (Cleland, Gibbon, Peppe, O'Hare, & Rutherford, 2010; Rapin, Dunn, Allen, Stevens, & Fein, 2009). Compared with typically developing speakers, more adolescents and adults with ASD produced residual distortion errors (Shriberg et al., 2001). Such subphonemic changes in articulation included dentalized sibilants and derhotacization. The number of error types a child with ASD demonstrates may be minimal, and in most cases such inaccuracies do not severely affect intelligibility. Particularly noteworthy, however, is the proportion of children with ASD presenting with some kind of error. Cleland et al. (2010), reported that as many as 41% of 69 children with high functioning autism or Asperger syndrome produced at least some speech errors. The errors primarily involved developmental phonological processes such as gliding and cluster reduction, but a few represented individualized patterns. These errors may arise from unique characteristics of individuals with ASD in social cognition. Social referencing, or the use of emotional or behavioral cues provided by others in responding to certain stimuli or situations, is a particular weakness in children with ASD. Children with ASD may not notice differences between phonetic forms used by the others and themselves, or may be less motivated to correct their own misarticulations to match the productions of others due to their limitations in social recognition.

Auditory Processing in Children with Autism Spectrum Disorders

Irregularities in the auditory perceptions of individuals with autism have been reported. Toddlers with ASD showed a reduced preference for child-directed speech, which was found to correlate with their concurrent and later receptive language skills (Paul, Chawarska, Fowler, Cicchetti, & Volkmar, 2007). Individuals with ASD also showed greater difficulty than typically developing controls in tasks requiring the identification of appropriate stress patterns in a given linguistic context (Paul, Augustyn, Klin, & Volkmar, 2005). Another piece of evidence indicating their unique speech-specific perception was provided by a study examining their sensory and early attentional processing of sounds based on event-related brain potentials (ERP) (Čeponiené et al., 2003). When a synthesized vowel was manipulated to have a deviant quality, high functioning children with autism did not detect the change via involuntary orienting. These findings contrasted with these children's normal processing of changes in simple and complex tones. Nieto Del Rincón (2008) concluded that disturbances in various auditory structures, including the brainstem, the cerebellum, and the temporal cortex may alter how individuals with autism attend to auditory information, identify speech sounds, and make decisions about speech signals. Such unique auditory processing associated with autism may impede the mastery of precise articulation and the correction of erroneously learned speech patterns.

Motor Skills of Children with Autism Spectrum Disorders

Some researchers (e.g., Cleland et al., 2010) have noted that errors may arise from underlying neuromotor difficulties. However, data on whether children with autism have neuromotor deficits are inconsistent. Some studies have reported that children with autism were significantly less skillful than typically developing children in tasks involving fine and gross motor functioning of the hands and body, but significant differences in oral-motor functions were not observed between the groups (Noterdaeme, Mildenberger, Minow, & Amorosa, 2002). Other studies have documented motor difficulties in hand and orofacial systems (Amato & Slavin, 1998). It is not known whether oral-motor difficulties are characteristic of ASD or whether cases of children with relatively severe speech difficulties, such as those reported by Koegel and colleagues (Koegel, Camarata, Koegel, Ben-Tall, & Smith, 1998), are simply a combination of ASD and other types of speech disorders such as CAS. Compared with the long history of research on the apparent intelligibility problems associated with hearing impairment and Down syndrome, comprehensive investigations of speech errors in children with ASD have begun relatively recently. More detailed testing may reveal qualitative differences in children with ASD who manifest speech errors.

FRAGILE X SYNDROME

Another condition often associated with speech difficulties is Fragile X syndrome. Fragile X syndrome is second only to Down syndrome as a genetic or chromosomal cause of intellectual disabilities (Reiss & Dant, 2003). Fragile X syndrome is caused by the loss of the fragile X mental retardation 1 protein (FMRP). This genetic disorder is linked to the X chromosome, one of the two sex-determining chromosomes, and males are more affected than are females, with a prevalence 1 in 4,000 for males and 1 in 8,000 for females (Jin & Warren, 2003; Reiss & Dant, 2003). Fully affected males typically have moderate intellectual disability, whereas fully affected females have either a mild intellectual disability or cognitive function at borderline levels. Because the IQ levels of males who are fully affected by Fragile X syndrome are similar to those of individuals with Down syndrome, these two syndromes are often compared with each other. Additionally, males with Fragile X syndrome tend to exhibit autistic features such as reduced eye contact and repetitive behaviors, and to have relatively shy and withdrawn personalities (Kerby & Dawson, 1994; Reiss & Freund, 1992). Several cognitive skills considered important for language learning, such as auditory short-term memory and attention, have also been reported to be impaired in people with this syndrome (Abbeduto, Brady, & Kover, 2007).

Intelligibility and Fluency of the Speech of Children with Fragile X Syndrome

The conversational speech of children with Fragile X syndrome is generally less intelligible than that of their typically developing peers (Barnes et al., 2009; Paul, Cohen, Breg, Watson, & Herman, 1984). In early case reports of three young boys with Fragile X syndrome, Paul and colleagues (1984) noted that 10–14% of their utterances were unintelligible. Their intelligibility scores were significantly lower than those of younger typically developing peers who had similar nonverbal developmental ages (Barnes et al., 2009). One factor affecting intelligibility is speaking rate. The speech of boys with Fragile X syndrome has often been characterized as rapid and impulsive (Borghgraef, Fryns, Dielkens, Pyck, & Van Den Berghe, 1987; Zajac, Harris, Roberts, & Martin, 2009). Hanson and colleagues (Hanson, Jackson, & Hagerman, 1986) also reported that **cluttering** was observed in many boys with this syndrome, noting that these individuals presented with a rapid and fluctuating rate of speech and tended to repeat sounds, words or phrases. This impression of rapid speech, however, may be attributable to other speech characteristics, such as the use of shorter utterances and fewer pauses compared with the speech of typically developing peers (Zajac et al., 2006).

Phonological Inaccuracies in the Speech of Children with Fragile X Syndrome

Phonological errors also reduce speech intelligibility. Three 10–14-year-old boys observed by Paul and colleagues commonly exhibited liquid simplification and one also occasionally deleted final consonants and demonstrated stopping (Paul et al., 1984). More recent studies compared speech characteristics among three groups of boys: those with Fragile X syndrome, with Down syndrome, and typically developing boys matched for **mental age**. Phonological errors were much less common in boys with Fragile X syndrome than in boys with Down syndrome who were matched for nonverbal mental age (Roberts et al., 2005). Roberts and colleagues (2005) reported that cluster reduction occurred in only 8% of the boys with Fragile X syndrome compared with 53% of the boys with Down syndrome, and final consonant deletion occurred in 2% of the boys with Fragile X syndrome compared with 12% of the boys with Down syndrome. Boys with Fragile X syndrome were delayed in their speech development, but their errors were comparable to those exhibited by younger typically developing children, as assessed by a single-word articulation test (Roberts et al., 2005) or by phonological analysis of connected speech samples (Barnes et al., 2009). However, as these authors stressed, we must remember that the production accuracy of children with this syndrome shows considerable individual variation.

Possible Factors Affecting the Speech of Children with Fragile X Syndrome

Hagerman and colleagues (1987) showed that boys with Fragile X syndrome experienced otitis media infections significantly more frequently during their first 5 years than did their unaffected siblings or children with developmental disabilities without Fragile X syndrome (Hagerman, Altshul-Stark, & McBogg, 1987). Also similar to those with Down syndrome, boys with Fragile X syndrome have been reported to display delays and variability in oral motor development compared with typically developing children. They experience difficulty repeating non-reduplicated multisyllabic sequences, such as "pa-ta-ka" (Paul et al., 1984). They also perform less proficiently than typically developing peers in speech function tasks involving the lips, tongue, and velopharynx and in those involving coordinated speech movements (Barnes et al., 2006). The scores for lip structures were also comparatively low in this group. How these factors affect the speech of children with this syndrome remains to be determined.

Sidebar 19.1 Cochlear Implantation and Language Development

The benefits of cochlear implants have been shown to extend beyond speech perception and production. Studies have now shown significant gains among children with cochlear implants in the overall language domain including lexical and grammatical skills, to degrees that equal or exceed the benefits of hearing aids (Geers & Moog, 1990; Miyamoto, Svirsky, & Robbins, 1997; Svirsky, Robbins, Kirk, Pisoni, & Miyamoto, 2000; Tomblin, Spencer, Flock, Tyler, & Gantz, 1999), with earlier implantation yielding greater benefits to expressive language development (Nikopoulos, Dyar, Archbold, & O'Donoghue, 2004; Tomblin et al., 2005). Early use of cochlear implants has also been associated with better reading comprehension skills (Connor & Zwolan, 2004).

Sidebar 19.2 Phonology in Signing

Phonology is not exclusive to spoken languages, but is important in sign languages as well (Morgan, Barrett-Jones, & Stoneham, 2007; Stokoe, 1960). Stokoe (1960) demonstrated that the signs in the lexicon of American Sign Language (ASL) can be divided into a small number of meaningless units, such as handshapes, movements, and locations. These segments are combined to produce a large lexicon. The sign for DRY and SUMMER have the same handshape and outward movement, but are distinguished by location: the finger is placed at the chin for DRY and at the forehead for SUMMER. This is analogous to minimal pairs that differ by a single phoneme in spoken languages.

Connections

This chapter describes the effects of hearing loss and several developmental disabilities on speech development in childhood. The importance of hearing screens in assessments is underscored in Chapter 20 on diagnostic guidelines. You can read more about the speech of children with autism spectrum disorder in Chapter 7 on the development of prosody.

Concluding Remarks

This chapter reviewed the impact of hearing impairment, Down syndrome, Autism Spectrum Disorders, and Fragile X syndrome on speech development. The effect of hearing impairment on phonological development is comparatively straightforward. The other developmental disabilities, however, involve multiple variables, such as sensory, motor, cognitive, and social parameters. The extent to which each variable contributes to the unique patterns of phonological development characteristic of individual disorders remains in question. Besides hearing impairment and the developmental disorders discussed in this chapter, there are other conditions that affect phonological development. For example, children born with a weight of less than 1,500 g and/or a gestational age of less than 32 weeks are known to be at risk for speech and language problems. Children with this condition, known as very low birth weight, tend to have smaller consonant repertoires and lower phonological mean lengths of utterance at the outset of language development (Van Noort-van der Spek, Franken, Wieringa, & Weisglas-Kuperus, 2009). The influence of an environmental factor has also been raised. The English-Spanish environments may increase English speech sound errors, influenced by Spanish phonological properties, in 3- to 4-year-old children with bilingual English-Spanish backgrounds (Gildersleeve-Neumann, Kester, Davis, & Peña, 2008). Each of these conditions illuminates the factors affecting phonological development, and information of this sort contributes to the theoretical understanding of phonological development. Understanding each parameter, in turn, can lead to specific intervention strategies to help children improve their phonological skills and overall communication. Regarding the atypical phonological development due to non-environmental factors, thc goals of such cfforts do not always involve the acquisition of age-appropriate phonological skills. Improvement may be defined in terms of reducing limitations, for instance with the use of hearing aids, cochlear implants, and augmentative and alternative communication (AAC) devices. Important clinical decisions must be made based on appropriate hypotheses about why the child demonstrates the speech characteristics of interest. Thus, studies of the phonological development of children with disabilities offer both theoretical and clinical implications.

Chapter Review Questions

1. For each disorder described in this chapter, identify ways that children's meaningful speech differs from typical development. What factors are thought to explain these differences?
2. What is Otitis Media with Effusion and what impact does it have on speech sound development?
3. What are cochlear implants and how have they been found to help the speech development of children with hearing impairments?
4. What are some key similarities and differences between the speech of children with Down syndrome and those with Fragile X syndrome?

Suggestions for Further Reading

Hearing Impairment

Gold, T. (1980). "Speech production in hearing-impaired children." *Journal of Communication Disorders* 13: 397-418.

Paterson, M. M. (1994). Articulation and phonological disorders in hearing-impaired school-aged children with severe and profound sensorineural losses. *Child Phonology: Characteristics, Assessment, and Intervention with Special Populations*. J. E. Bernthal and N. W. Bankson. New York, Thieme: 199-224.

Stoel-Gammon, C. and M. M. Kehoe (1994). Hearing impairment in infants and toddlers: identification, vocal development, and intervention. Child Phonology: *Characteristics,*

Assessment, and Intervention with Special Populations. J. E. Bernthal and N. W. Bankson. New York, Thieme: 163-181.

Down Syndrome

Cleland, J., S. Wood, et al. (2010). "Relationship between speech, oromotor, language and cognitive abilities in children with Down's syndrome." *International Journal of Language & Communication Disorders* 45(1): 83-95.

Roberts, J.E., J. Price, et al. (2007). "Language and communication development in Down syndrome." *Mental Retardation and Developmental Disabilities* 13: 26-35.

Autism

Shriberg, L. D., R. Paul, et al. (2001). "Speech and prosody characteristics of adolescents and adults with high-functioning autism and Asperger syndrome." *Journal of Speech, Language, and Hearing Research* 44: 1097-1115.

Wolk, L. and J. Giesen (2000). "A phonological investigation of four siblings with childhood autism." *Journal of Communication Disorders* 33: 371-389.

Fragile X Syndrome

Abbeduto, L. and R. J. Hagerman (1997). "Language and communication in fragile X syndrome." *Mental Retardation and Developmental Disabilities* 3: 313-322.

Suggestions for Student Activities

1. Choose one of the disorders described in this chapter and compare the speech sound development to the typical development of babbling (Chapter 4), first words (Chapter 5), or phonology (Chapter 6).
2. The sound files provided with this chapter include standard text (the Rainbow Passage and the Stella Passage), recorded from two adults with hearing impairment. Select a phrase that contains various vowels and high-frequency fricative consonants, e.g., /s, ʃ/ (consider "six spoons of fresh snowpeas" from the Stella Passage) and record someone without hearing impairment producing it. As you listen to all three samples, what are your perceptual impressions of the vowels and fricatives? Now import the sound files into acoustic analysis software and compare the vowels for F1 and F2 frequencies and the consonants for center frequencies. Formulate a hypothesis to explain your findings that includes place of articulation and acoustic changes in the speech sounds.

ANSWERS TO CHAPTER REVIEW QUESTIONS

1. For each disorder described in this chapter, identify ways that children's meaningful speech differs from typical development. What factors are thought to explain these differences?

Hearing Impairment

Reported characteristics
-Fewer multisyllabic utterances including consonants in early speech productions
-Relative dominance of labial consonants in early speech productions
-Restricted range of tongue movements during vowel production
-Low intelligibility
-Phonological errors such as voicing errors, consonant deletions, and vowel additions

Possible factors
-Reduced auditory input
-Auditory input with distorted frequency information
-Difficulty in discriminating speech sounds and reduced accuracy of word recognition
-Reduced auditory feedback from their own speech productions

Down Syndrome

Reported characteristics
-Large individual variation in the emergence of specific consonants
-Slower phonological development
-Low intelligibility
-Mostly typical phonological processes with some idiosyncratic processes
-Infrequent productions of word shapes consisting of several syllables
-Inconsistent errors in repeated productions
-Greater accuracy of imitative than spontaneous productions

Possible factors
-Influence of hearing loss
-Weak muscles and hypotonicity
-Smaller oral cavity relative to the tongue size
-Weak oral motor planning and coordination
-Reduced verbal short-term memory
-Incomplete phonological representations
-Reduced phonological awareness

Autism Spectrum Disorders

Reported characteristics
-Typical as well as some idiosyncratic processes, but reserved intelligibility
-Inadequacies in suprasegmentals

Possible factors
-Lower awareness of own production errors and lower motivation to correct errors
-Irregularities in auditory perception
-Weak oral motor skills

Fragile X Syndrome

Reported characteristics
-Reduced intelligibility with rapid and impulsive speaking rate
-Typical phonological processes

Possible factors
-Higher occurrences of otitis media infections
-Weak oral motor skills
-Reduced auditory short-term memory and attention

2. What is Otitis Media with Effusion and what impact does it have on speech sound development?

In otits media with effusion (OME), liquid accumulates in the middle ear space due to infections. This condition is usually temporary, but a fluctuating hearing loss may persist for some time. There is no strong consensus concerning whether a history of OME in early childhood causes later speech problems. Some recent data suggest, however, that about one-third of the children who experienced a mild hearing loss from OME at about 1 years of age exhibit some kind of speech errors at 3 years of age (Shriberg et al., 2000).

3. What are cochlear implants and how have they been found to help the speech development of children with hearing impairments?

A cochlear implant is an electroacoustic device which consists of a microphone, a speech processor, and electric wires. Speech and environmental sounds collected with a microphone are converted to electrical pulses that convey their temporal, frequency, and durational information. The electric signals directly stimulate the basal ganglion cells of the auditory nerve fibers via tiny wires surgically inserted into the cochlea. Early implantation has been demonstrated to increase the production of canonical babbling for prelinguistic children, and to improve accuracies and increase repertoires of vowel and consonant productions for verbal children. Improvements in suprasegmental aspects have also been demonstrated. Early implantation appears to be essential for the recipient to obtain the maximum benefits.

4. What are some key similarities and differences between the speech of children with Down syndrome and those with Fragile X syndrome?

Both the conversational speech of children with Fragile X syndrome and that of children with Down syndrome are generally less intelligible than the speech of their typically developing peers. However, the reduced intelligibility is often associated with rapid and fluctuating rate of speech in the children with Fragile X syndrome. The children with Down syndrome as a group exhibit more frequent phonological errors than those with Fragile X syndrome, whose errors are comparable to those exhibited by younger typically developing children. While both groups have atypical oral structures and oral-motor functions, the discrepancies in these respects from the typical development are greater for Down syndrome.

REFERENCES

Abbeduto, L., Brady, N., & Kover, S. T. (2007). Language development and fragile X syndrome: Profiles, syndrome-specificity, and within syndrome differences. *Mental Retardation and Developmental Disabilities,* 13, 36-46.

Allen, M. C., Nikopoulos, T. P., & O'Donoghue, G. M. (1998). Speech intelligibility in children after cochlear implantation. *American Journal of Otology,* 19, 742-746.

Amato, J., & Slavin, D. (1998). A preliminary investigation of oromotor function in young verbal and nonverbal children with autism. *Infant-Toddler Intervention,* 8, 175-184.

American-Speech-Language-Hearing-Association. (2007). Childhood Apraxia of Speech [Position Statement].

Ardan, G. M., Hardker, P., & Kemp, F. H. (1972). Tongue size in Down syndrome. *Journal of Mental Deficiency Research,* 16(3), 160-166.

Barnes, E., Roberts, J., Long, S. H., Martin, D., Berni, M. C., Mandulak, K. C., & Sideris, J. (2009). Phonological accuracy and intelligibility in connected speech of boys with fragile X syndrome or Down syndrome. *Journal of Speech, Language, and Hearing Research,* 52, 1048-1061.

Barnes, E. F., Roberts, J., Mirrett, P., Sideris, J., & Misenheimer, J. (2006). A comparison of oral structure and oral-motor function in young males with fragile X syndrome and Down syndrome. *Journal of Speech, Language, and Hearing Research,* 49, 903-917.

Bhagyalakshmi, G., Renukarya, A. J., & Rajangam, S. (2007). Metric analysis of the hard palate in children with Down syndrome - a comparative study. *Down Syndrome Research and Practice,* 12(1), 55-59.

Bilger, R. C., & Wang, M. D. (1976). Consonant confusions in patients with sensorineural hearing loss. *Journal of Speech and Hearing Research,* 19, 718-749.

Blamey, P. J., Barry, J. G., & Jacq, P. (2001). Phonetic inventory development in young cochlear implant uses after 6 years postoperation. *Journal of Speech, Language, and Hearing Research,* 44, 73-79.

Blaser, S., Propst, E. J., Martin, D., Feigenbaum, A., James, A. L., Shannon, P., & Papsin, B. C. (2006). Inner ear dysplasia is common in children with Down syndrome (trisomy 21). *The Laryngoscope,* 116, 2113-2119.

Bleile, K., & Schwarz, I. (1984). Three perspectives on the speech of children with Down's syndrome. *Journal of Communication Disorders,* 17, 87-94.

Bodensteiner, J. B., Smith, S. D., & Schaefer, G. B. (2003). Hopotonia, congenital hearing loss, and hypoactive labyrinths. *Journal of Child Neurology,* 18(3), 171-173.

Borghgraef, M., Fryns, J. P., Dielkens, A., Pyck, K., & Van Den Berghe, H. (1987). Fragile (X) syndrome: a study of the psychological profile in 23 prepubertal patients. *Clinical Genetics,* 32, 179-186.

Calmels, M. N., Saliba, I., Wanna, G., Cochard, N., Fillaux, J., Deguine, O., & Fraysse, B. (2004). Speech perception and speech intelligibility in children after cochlear implantation. *International Journal of Pediatric Otorhinolaryngology,* 68(3), 347-351.

Calvert, D. R. (1982). Articulation and hearing impairment. In N. J. Lass, L. V. McReynolds, J. L. Northern & D. E. Yoder (Eds.), *Speech, Language, and Hearing: Volume II, Pathologies of Speech and Language* (pp. 638-651). Philadelphia: W.B. Saunders.

Carothers, A. D., Hecht, C. A., & Hook, E. B. (1999). International variation in reported livebirth prevalence rates of Down syndrome, adjusted for maternal age. *Journal of Medical Genetics,* 36, 386-393.

Carrol, J., & Snowling, M. (2004). Language and phonological skills in children at high risk of reading difficulties. *Journal of Child Psychology and Psychiatry,* 45, 631-640.

Čeponiené, R., Lepistö, T., Shestakova, A., Vanhala, R., Alku, P., Näätänen, R., & Yaguchi, K. (2003). Speech-sound-selective auditory impairment in children with autism: They can perceive but do not attend. *PNAS,* 100(9), 5567-5572.

Chin, S. B., & Pisoni, D. B. (2000). A phonological system at 2 years after cochlear implantation. *Clinical Linguistics & Phonetics,* 14(1), 53-73.

Clark, J. G. (1981). Uses and abuses of hearing loss classification. *Asha,* 23, 493-500.

Cleland, J., Gibbon, F. E., Peppe, S. J. E., O'Hare, A., & Rutherford, M. (2010). Phonetic and phonological errors in children with high functioning autism and Asperger syndrome. *International Journal of Speech-Language Pathology,* 12(1), 69-76.

Cleland, J., Wood, S., Hardcastle, W., Wishart, J., & Timmins, C. (2010). Relationship between speech, oromotor, language and cognitive abilities in children with Down's syndrome. *International Journal of Language & Communication Disorders,* 45(1), 83-95.

Connor, C. M., Craig, H. K., Raudenbush, S. W., Heavner, K., & Zwolan, T. A. (2006). The age at which young deaf children receive cochlear implants and their vocabulary and speech-production growth: Is there an added value for early implantation? *Ear and Hearing,* 27(6), 628-644.

Connor, C. M., & Zwolan, T. A. (2004). Examining multiple sources of influence on the reading comprehension skills of children who use cochlear implants. *Journal of Speech, Language, and Hearing Research,* 47(3), 509-526.

Dodd, B. (1972). Compariton of babbling patterns in normal and Down-syndrome infants. *Journal of Mental Deficiency Research,* 16, 35-40.

Dodd, B. (1976). A comparison of the phonological system of mental age matched, normal, severely subnormal and Down's syndrome children. *British Journal of Disorders of Communication,* 11, 27-42.

Dodd, B., & Thompson, L. (2001). Speech disorder in children with Down's syndrome. *Journal of Intellectual Disability Research,* 45(4), 308-316.

Dubno, J. R., Dirks, D. D., & Langhofer, L. R. (1982). Evaluation of hearing-impaired listeners using a nonsense-syllable test II. Syllable recognition and consonant confusion patterns. *Journal of Speech and Hearing Research,* 25, 141-148.

Eilers, R. E., & Oller, D. K. (1994). Infant vocalizations and the early diagnosis of severe hearing impairment. *Journal of Pediatrics,* 124(2), 199-203.

Ertmer, D. J. (2001). Emergence of a vowel system in a young coclear implant recipient. *Journal of Speech, Language, and Hearing Research,* 44, 803-813.

Ertmer, D. J., & Mellon, J. A. (2001). Beginning to talk at 20 months: Early vocal development in a young cochlear implant recipient. *Journal of Speech, Language, and Hearing Research,* 44, 192-206.

Ertmer, D. J., Young, N. M., & Nathani, S. (2007). Profiles of vocal development in young cochlear implant recipients. *Journal of Speech, Language, and Hearing Research,* 50, 393-407.

Flipsen, P., Jr., & Colvard, L. G. (2006). Intelligibility of conversational speech produced by children with cochlear implants. *Journal of Communication Disorders,* 39, 93-108.

Flipsen, P., Jr., & Parker, R. G. (2008). Phonological patterns in the conversational speech of children with cochlear implants. *Journal of Communication Disorders,* 41, 337-357.

Frith, U., & Frith, C. D. (1974). Specific motor disabilities in Down's syndrome. *Journal of Child Psychology and Psychiatry,* 15, 293-301.

Fryauf-Bertschy, H., Tyler, R. S., Kelsay, D. M. R., Gantz, B. J., & Woodworth, G. G. (1997). Cochlear implant use by prelingually deafened children: The influence of age at implant and length of device use. *Journal of Speech, Language, and Hearing Research,* 40, 183-199.

Geers, A. E. (2002). Factors affecting the development of speech, language, and literacy in children with early coclear implantation. *Language, Speech, and Hearing Services in Schools,* 33, 172-183.

Geers, A. E., & Moog, J. (1990). Spoken language results: Vocabulary, syntax, and communication. *Volta Review, 96*, 131-148.

Gildersleeve--Neumann, C. E. Kester, E. S., Davis, B. L., & Peña, E. D. (2008). English speech sound development in preschool-aged children from bilingual English-Spanish environments. *Language, Speech, and Hearing Services in Schools*, Vol 39(3), 314-328.

Gillon, G. T. (2000). The efficacy of phonological awareness intervention for children with spoken language impairment. *Language, Speech, and Hearing Services in Schools,* 31, 126-141.

Gold, T. (1980). Speech production in hearing-impaired children. *Journal of Communication Disorders, 13*, 397-418.

Gordon-Salant, S. (1985). Phoneme feature perception in noise by normal-hearing and hearing-impaired subjects. *Journal of Speech and Hearing Research,* 1985, 87-95.

Grogan, M. L., Barker, E. J., Dettman, S. J., & Blamey, P. J. (1995). Phonetic and phonologic changes in the connected speech of children using a cochlear implant. *Annals of Otology, Rhinology, and Laryngology, Supplement,* 166, 390-393.

Hagerman, R. J., Altshul-Stark, D., & McBogg, P. (1987). Recurrent otitis media in the fragile X syndrome. *American Journal of Diseases of Children,* 141(2), 184-187.

Hans, P. S., England, R., Prowse, S., Young, N., & Sheehan, P. Z. (2010). UK and Ireland experience of cochlear implants in children with Down Syndrome. *International Journal of Pediatric Otorhinolaryngology,* 74, 260-264.

Hanson, D. M., Jackson, I., A.W., & Hagerman, R. J. (1986). Speech disturbances (cluttering) in mildly impaired males with the Martin-Bell/fragile X syndrome. *American Journal of Medical Genetics,* 23, 195-206.

Hicks, C. B., & Tharpe, A. M. (2002). Listening effort and fatigue in school-age children with and without hearing loss. *Journal of Speech, Language, and Hearing Research,* 45, 573-584.

Jarrold, C., Baddeley, A. D., & Phillips, C. E. (2002). Verbal short-term memory in Down syndrome: A problem of memory, audition, or speech? *Journal of Speech, Language, and Hearing Research,* 45, 531-544.

Jin, P., & Warren, S. T. (2003). New insights into fragile X syndrome: from molecules to neurobehaviors. *Trends in Biochemical Sciences,* 28(3), 152-158.

Kay-Raining Bird, E., & Chapman, R. S. (1994). Sequential recall in individuals with Down syndrome. *Journal of Speech and Hearing Research,* 37, 1369-1380.

Kennedy, E. J., & Flynn, M. C. (2003). Training phonological awareness skills in children with Down syndrome. *Research in Developmental Disabilities,* 24, 44-57.

Kent, R. D., Osberger, M. J., Netsell, R., & Hustedde, C. G. (1987). Phonetic development of identical twins differing in auditory functioning. *Journal of Speech, Language, and Hearing Research,* 52, 64-75.

Kerby, D. S., & Dawson, B. L. (1994). Autistic features, personality, and adaptive behavior in males with the fragile X syndrome and no autism. *American Journal of Mental Retardation,* 98(4), 455-462.

Kjelgaard, M. M., & Tager-Flusberg, H. (2001). An investigation of language impairment in autism: Implications for genetic subgroups. *Language and Cognitive Processes,* 16(2), 287-308.

Koegel, R. L., Camarata, S., Koegel, L. K., Ben-Tall, A., & Smith, A. E. (1998). Increasing speech intelligibility in children with autism. *Journal of Autism and Developmental Disorders, 28*(3), 241-251.

Kumin, L. (1994). Intelligibility of speech in children with Down syndrome in natural settings: Parents' perspective. *Perceptual and Motor Skills,* 78, 307-313.

Kumin, L., & Adams, J. (2000). Developmental apraxia of speech and intelligibility in children with Down syndrome. *Down Syndrome Quarterly,* 5(3), 1-7.

Kumin, L., Councill, C., & Goodman, M. (1994). A longitudinal study of the emergence of phonemes in children with Down syndrome. *Journal of Communication Disorders,* 27, 293-303.

Lee, Y.-M., Kim, L.-S., Jeong, S.-W., Kim, J.-S., & Chung, S.-H. (2010). Performance of children with mental retardation after cochlear implantation: Speech perception, speech intelligibility, and language development. *Acta Oto-Laryngologica,* 130, 924-934.

Lenden, J. M., & Flipsen, P., Jr. (2007). Prosody and voice characteristics of children with cochlear implants. *Journal of Communication Disorders,* 40, 66-81.

Lynch, M. P., Oller, D. K., Steffens, M. L., Levine, S. L., Basinger, D. L., & Umbel, V. (1995). Onset of speech-like vocalizations in infants with Down syndrome. *American Journal of Mental Retardation,* 100(1), 68-86.

Maskarinec, A. S., Cairns, G. F., Butterfield, E. C., & Weamer, D. K. (1981). Longitudinal observations of individual infant's vocalizations. *Journal of Speech and Hearing Disorders,* 46, 267-273.

McCaffrey, H. A. (1999). Multichannel cochlear implantation and the organization of the early speech. *Volta Review, 101*(1), 5-30.

McGowan, R. S., Nittrouer, S., & Chenausky, K. (2008). Speech production in 12-month-old children with and without hearing loss. *Journal of Speech, Language, and Hearing Research,* 51, 879-888.

Miyamoto, R. T., Svirsky, M. A., & Robbins, A., M. (1997). Enhancement of expressive language in prelingually deaf children with cochlear implants. *Acta Oto-Laryngologica,* 117(2), 154-157.

Morgan, G., Barrett-Jones, S., & Stoneham, H. (2007). The first signs of language: Phonological development in British Sign Language. *Applied Psycholinguistics, 28*, 3-22.

National Institutes of Child Health and Human Development. (1997). *Facts about Down syndrome*. Washington DC: Health Information and Media Publications.

Nieto Del Rincón, P. L. (2008). Autism: Alterations in auditory perception. *Reviews in the Neurosciences,* 19, 61-78.

Nikopoulos, T. P., Dyar, D., Archbold, S., & O'Donoghue, G. M. (2004). Development of spoken language grammar following cochlear implantation in prelingually deaf children. *Archives of Otolaryngology-Head & Neck Surgery,* 130, 629-633.

Nober, E. H. (1967). Articulation of the deaf. *Exceptional Children,* 33, 611-621.

Noterdaeme, M., Mildenberger, K., Minow, F., & Amorosa, H. (2002). Evaluation of neuromotor deficits in children with autism and children with a specific speech and language disorder. *European Child & Adolescent Psychiatry,* 11, 219-225.

Oller, D. K., & Eilers, R. E. (1988). The role of audition in infant babbling. *Child Development,* 59, 441-449.

Oller, D. K., Eilers, R. E., Bull, D. H., & Carney, A. E. (1985). Prespeech vocalizations of a deaf infant: A comparison with normal metaphonological development. *Journal of Speech, Language, and Hearing Research,* 28, 47-63.

Paterson, M. M. (1994). Articulation and phonological disorders in hearing-impaired school-aged children with severe and profound sensorineural losses. In J. E. Bernthal & N. W. Bankson (Eds.), *Child Phonology: Characteristics, Assessment, and Intervention with Special Populations* (pp. 199-224). New York: Thieme.

Paul, R., Augustyn, A., Klin, A., & Volkmar, R. (2005). Perception and production of prosody by speakers with autism spectrum disorders. *Journal of Autism and Developmental Disorders,* 35(2), 205-220.

Paul, R., Chawarska, K., Fowler, C., Cicchetti, D., & Volkmar, F. (2007). "Listen my children and you shall hear": Auditory preferences in toddlers with autism spectrum disorders. *Journal of Speech, Language, and Hearing Research,* 50, 1350-1364.

Paul, R., Cohen, D. L., Breg, W. R., Watson, M., & Herman, S. (1984). Fragile X syndrome: Its relations to speech and language disorders. *Journal of Speech and Hearing Disorders,* 49, 326-336.

Preston, J., & Edwards, M. L. (2010). Phonological awareness and types of sound errors in preschoolers with speech sound disorders. *Journal of Speech, Language, and Hearing Research,* 53, 44-60.

Rapin, I., Dunn, M. A., Allen, D. A., Stevens, M. C., & Fein, D. (2009). Subtypes of language disorders in school-age children with autism. *Developmental Neuropsychology,* 34(1), 66-84.

Reiss, A. L., & Dant, C. C. (2003). The behavioral neurogenetics of fragile X syndrome: Analyzing gene-brain-behavior relationships in child developmental psychopathologies. *Development and Psychopathology, 15*, 927-968.

Reiss, A. L., & Freund, L. (1992). Behavioral phenotype of fragile X syndrome: DSM-III-R autistic behavior in male children. *American Journal of Medical Genetics,* 43, 35-46.

Roberts, J., Long, S. H., Malkin, C., Barnes, E., Skinner, M., Hennon, E. A., & Anderson, K. (2005). A comparison of phonological skills of boys with fragile X syndrome and Down syndrome. *Journal of Speech, Language, and Hearing Research,* 48, 980-995.

Roberts, J. E., Rosenfeld, R. M., & Zeisel, S. A. (2004). Otitis media and speech and language: A meta-analysis of prospective studies. *Pediatrics,* 113(3), e238-e248.

Roizen, N. J., Wolters, C., Nicol, T., & Blondis, T. A. (1993). Hearing loss in children with Down syndrome. *Journal of Pediatrics,* 123(1), S9-12.

Rupela, V., & Manjula, R. (2007). Phonotactic patterns in the speech of children with Down syndrome. *Clinical Linguistics & Phonetics,* 21(8), 605-622.

Rvachew, S., Ohberg, A., Grawburg, M., & Heyding, J. (2003). Phonological awareness and phonemic perception in 4-year-old children with delayed expressive phonology skills. *American Journal of Speech-Language Pathology,* 12, 463-471.

Shriberg, L. D., Friel-Patti, S., Flipsen, P., Jr., & Brown, R. L. (2000). Otitis media, fluctant hearing loss, and speech-language outcomes: A preliminary structural equation model. *Journal of Speech, Language, and Hearing Research,* 43, 100-120.

Shriberg, L. D., Paul, R., McSweeny, J. L., Klin, A., Cohen, D. L., & volkmar, F. R. (2001). Speech and prosody characteristics of adolescents and adults with high-functioning autism and Asperger syndrome. *Journal of Speech, Language, and Hearing Research,* 44, 1097-1115.

Smith, B. L. (1982). Some observations concerning premeaningful vocalizations of hearing-impaired infants. *Journal of Speech and Hearing Disorders,* 47, 439-442.

Smith, B. L., & Oller, D. K. (1981). A comprative study of pre-meaningful vocalizations produced by normally developing and Down' syndrome infants. *Journal of Speech and Hearing Disorders,* 46, 46-51.

Smith, B. L., & Stoel-Gammon, C. (1983). A longitudinal study of the development of stop consonant production in normal and Down's syndrome children. *Journal of Speech and Hearing Disorders,* 48, 114-118.

Snowling, M. J., Hulme, C., & Mercer, R. C. (2002). A deficit in rime awareness in children with Down syndrome. *Reading and Writing,* 15, 471-495.

Spender, Q., Dennis, J., Stein, A., Cave, D., Percy, E., & Reilly, S. (1995). Impaired oral-motor function in children with Down's syndrome: A study of three twin pairs. *European Journal of Disorders of Communication,* 30, 77-87.

Steffens, M. L., Oller, D. K., Lynch, M., & Urbano, R. C. (1992). Vocal development in infancts with Down syndrome and infants who are developing normally. *American Journal of Mental Retardation,* 97(2), 235-246.

Stelmachowicz, P. G., Hoover, B. M., Lewis, D. E., Kortekaas, R. W. L., & Pittman, A. L. (2000). The relation between stimulus context, speech audibility, and perception for normal-hearing and hearing-impaired children. *Journal of Speech, Language, and Hearing Research,* 43, 902-914.

Stoel-Gammon, C. (1980). Phonological analysis of four Down's syndrome children. *Applied Psycholinguistics,* 1, 31-48.

Stoel-Gammon, C. (1988). Prelinguistic vocalizations of hearing-impaired and normally hearing subjects: A comparison of consonantal inventories. *Journal of Speech and Hearing Disorders,* 53, 302-315.

Stoel-Gammon, C., & Otomo, K. (1986). Babbling development of hearing-impaired and normally hearing subjects. *Journal of Speech and Hearing Disorders,* 51, 33-41.

Stokoe, W. (1960). Sign language stucture: An outline of the visual communication systems of the American deaf *Studies in linguistics: Occasional papers* (Vol. No. 8). Buffalo: Dept. of Anthropology and Linguistics, University of Buffalo.

Svirsky, M. A., Robbins, A., M., Kirk, K. I., Pisoni, D. B., & Miyamoto, R. T. (2000). Language development in profoundly deaf children with cochlear implants. *Psychological Science,* 11(2), 153-158.

Tomblin, J. B., Barker, B. A., Spencer, L. J., Zhang, X., & Gantz, B. J. (2005). The effects of age at cochlear implant inital stimulation on expressive language growth in infants and toddlers. *Journal of Speech, Language, and Hearing Research,* 48, 853-867.

Tomblin, J. B., Spencer, L., Flock, S., Tyler, R., & Gantz, B. (1999). A comparison of language achievement in children with cochlear implants and children using hearing aids. *Journal of Speech, Language, and Hearing Research,* 42, 497-511.

Tye-Murray, N., & Kirk, K. I. (1993). Vowel and diphthong production by young users of cochlear implants and the relationship between the Phonetic Level Examination and spontaneous speech. *Journal of Speech, Language, and Hearing Research,* 36, 488-502.

Tye-Murray, N., Spencer, L., & Woodworth, G. (1995). Acquisition of speech by children who have prolonged cochlear implant experience. *Journal of Speech and Hearing Research,* 38, 327-337.

Van Borsel, J. (1988). An analysis of the speech *of* five Down's syndrome adolescents. *Journal of Communication Disorders, 21*, 409-421.

Van Borsel, J. (1996). Articulation in Down's syndrome adolescents and adults. *European Journal of Disorders of Communication,* 31, 415-444.

Van Noort-van der Spek, I. L., Franken, M. C., Wieringa, M. H., & Weisglas-Kuperus, N. (2009). Phonological development in very-low-birthweight children: an exploratory study. *Developmental Medicine & Child Neurology,* 52, 541-546.

Warner-Czyz, A. D., & Davis, B. L. (2008). The emergence of segmental accuracy in young cochlear implant recipients. *Cochlear Implans International,* 9(3), 143-166.

Westerman, G. H., Johnson, R., & Cohen, M. M. (1975). Variations of palatal dimensions in patients with Down's syndrome. *Journal of Dental Research,* 54(767-711).

Wilcox, K., & Morris, S. (1999). *Children's Speech Intelligibility Measure (CSIM)*. London: Psychological Corporation.

Wolk, L., & Edwards, M. L. (1993). The emerging phonological system of an autistic child. *Journal of Communication Disorders,* 26, 161-177.

Wolk, L., & Giesen, J. (2000). A phonological investigation of four siblings with childhood autism. *Journal of Communication Disorders, 33*, 371-389.

Yoshinaga-Itano, C. (1998). Early speech development in children who are deaf or hard of hearing: Interrelationships with language and hearing. *Volta Review,* 100(5), 181-211.

Zajac, D. J., Harris, A. A., Roberts, J. E., & Martin, G. E. (2009). Direct magnitude estimation of articulation rate in boys with fragile X syndrome. *Journal of Speech, Language, and Hearing Research,* 52, 1370-1379.

Zajac, D. J., Roberts, J. E., Hennon, E. A., Harris, A. A., Barnes, E. F., & Misenheimer, J. (2006). Articulation rate and vowel space characteristics of young males with fragile X syndrome: Preliminary acoustic findings. *Journal of Speech, Language, and Hearing Research,* 49, 1147-1155.

V. The Path from Diagnosis to Therapy

In: Comprehensive Perspectives …
Editors: Beate Peter and Andrea A. N. MacLeod
ISBN: 978-1-62257-041-6

Chapter 20

DIAGNOSTIC GUIDELINES

Amy Glaspey

INTRODUCTION

A comprehensive assessment of speech sound disorder involves several tasks that occur prior to treatment and throughout the treatment process. Assessment is a cyclical process that allows the clinician to establish whether a disorder is present, to document changes over time, and to document a child's response to the intervention that is implemented. Assessment includes diagnostics, evaluation of the individual treatment session, evaluation of treatment outcomes over time, and generalization of skills that are acquired in treatment and applied to new contexts. This chapter presents potential components of a preliminary diagnostic assessment and an introduction to assessment as it relates to treatment. A case study is provided to illustrate different aspects of the diagnostic process. The client is a 3-year-old boy with a phonological disorder.

DIAGNOSTIC ASSESSMENT

Prior to initiating a treatment program, a clinician must determine whether a speech sound disorder is present, thus making a diagnosis. Clinicians must carefully choose appropriate terms to describe the characteristics of the disorder. For more information regarding classification systems for speech sound disorder, please see Chapter 15. However, no matter the system that is selected or the nature of the speech sound disorder, several core measures will help the clinician best identify skills that should be targeted in treatment or identify skills in need of further testing. The diagnostic process involves synthesis of information from several tasks: (1) child history, (2) standard assessment, (3) dynamic assessment, (4) connected speech sample with phonetic inventory and intelligibility, (5) structural-functional evaluation (with supplemental motor screening), (6) phonological awareness, (7) hearing screening, and (8) supplemental measures. Each of these tasks will be discussed in detail below.

Child History

Prior to administering any tests or collecting speech samples, clinicians begin by gathering information about the child's developmental, educational, and medical **history**. The child's history may be collected by speaking directly with the caregivers and also by reviewing the child's records. First, clinicians may seek answers to a specific set of questions (see Sidebar 20.1 for partial list). The answers to these questions can be collected with a written questionnaire that lists the questions. Although this process is useful for gathering relevant information, it is additionally beneficial to conduct an oral interview with the caregivers. At times, the written questions may be interpreted differently than intended and the additional interview provides clarification. The questions that are asked may differ based on the age of the child; for example, a two-year old who stays at home with a parent or caregiver may have different language experiences than a six-year-old in first grade who is in a more academic setting.

Cultural differences should be considered in the interview process as not all people respond in the same way to this type of questioning and many families differ in communication styles (Goldstein, 2000; p. 69-73). If a child is from a different cultural background than the clinician, it may be necessary to determine which individual family member should be addressed or possibly a group of family members. Some families may be hesitant to respond, whereas others may be quite directive. Religious beliefs and views on disability may also influence the collection of a case history. Ethnographic strategies may need to be followed using observation as a primary source of information. Furthermore, language proficiency of the parents or caregivers should be taken into account and the clinician may need to determine whether an interpreter should be present. Care should be taken to meets the needs of individuals and their extended relationships.

Sidebar 20.1 Sample Questions that Clinicians May Ask a Parent or Caregiver with a Child with Suspected Speech Delay

What are your concerns regarding your child's speech and language?
Did any complications occur during pregnancy or birth?
Has your child met developmental milestones?
When did your child say his/her first words?
Has the child experienced any health or medical concerns?
Does the child have a history of ear infections?
Has the child had a recent hearing screening?
How is the child performing in school?
How is the child interacting with peers?
How well do others understand the child's speech?
Do you have any concerns about academic achievement?
Is there a family history of speech, language, or reading problems?

With the permission of the caregivers, educational or medical records may also be reviewed to inform the clinician about the child's history. The clinician may look for supplemental information to answer the questions from Sidebar 20.1. Furthermore, the child may exhibit a medically related disorder that affects speech and language development and a better understanding of the disorder and medical history may come from record review.

Once the history is complete, clinicians are more knowledgeable about what types of tests and procedures should be selected to gather the most helpful information about the child's needs and skills. The following section describes the core components of a speech evaluation; however, it is not unusual for a child to exhibit additional needs across developmental domains. Thus, supplemental assessments should be considered for some children.

Standard Assessment

Assessing a child's phonological system often begins with the administration of a **standard assessment** (also referred to as **standardized test**). Insurance companies, billing agencies, or school districts typically require a standard score for the child to qualify for insurance coverage or provision of services. Standard assessments are published tests that generally provide all necessary materials (e.g. manipulatives or pictures books) and an established protocol for elicitation, scoring, and analysis of target speech productions (Velleman, 1998; Williams, 2000). Elicitation may include spontaneous or imitated naming tasks using single words or sentences; the data collected includes a small number of opportunities to produce a wide range of skills. The administration procedures are typically easy to administer and only take a short time to complete. Results provide information that is frequently used to make inferences about severity levels, make a differential diagnosis, or even guide treatment.

Many benefits of standard assessment are also related to measuring *single-word* productions. The clinician points to a picture or object and the child names it. Single-word productions allow the clinician to impose a certain amount of control in the form of size and type of words selected. As a result, the target word is known, and the child's production can easily be compared to it. The same measure may be repeatedly given to the same child or across children for a group comparison. Most published tests come with norms tables that allow for easy comparison, and time is optimized for administration and transcription (Bernhardt & Holdgrafer, 2001). With a standard measure, a child's performance may be compared to other children based on descriptive statistics such as standard scores relative to the population mean or a percentile ranking, and this comparison can be used to determine whether the child's skill levels match the expected progression. Children's productions may fall within, below, or above the expected range. If comparisons reveal skills that are substantially below expectation, then referral for treatment may be made. See Appendix 3 for additional information about the statistical properties of standardized tests.

In contrast, disadvantages of using standard assessments are also apparent. The **ecological validity** (i.e., the ability to reflect real-life activities) may be questioned because productions for many assessments are only at the single word level; some children with speech disorders may easily produce single-words that they are not able to produce in connected speech. Furthermore, Morrison and Shriberg (1992) compared standard assessments and conversational speech samples and found an increased frequency of errors and types of errors on conversational speech samples that were not evident on the assessments evaluating single-word performance. For some standard assessments, the analysis is quite complex and large time commitments are necessary to master the procedures. Perhaps the biggest disadvantage of a standard assessment is the length of time required for scores to change and document significant improvements; standard assessments do not readily allow for measurement of small incremental changes that may occur prior to transfer of skills from treatment to the assessment.

Clinicians need to carefully choose a particular standard assessment based on the needs of the individual child because tests may differ in what they measure. In general, most standard assessments of speech ability administered in current clinical practice either evaluate consonant production or **error patterns** (also referred to as **phonological processes** or **phonological patterns**). See Chapter 2, Chapter 3, and Appendix 2 for more details on error patterns. For clinicians working with English speaking children in North America, several standardized assessments exist. If a clinician is interested in how a child produces consonants in initial, medial, and final position, then a test such as the Goldman-Fristoe Test of Articulation-Second Edition (Goldman & Fristoe, 2000) or the Arizona Articulation Proficiency Scale-Third Edition (Fudala, 2000) should be administered. In contrast, if a clinician is interested in how the child is producing patterns in relation to syllable and word structures, then a phonological assessment such as the Hodson Assessment of Phonological Patterns (HAPP) (Hodson, 2004) should be administered. Some tests include materials to evaluate both articulation and phonology such as the Clinical Assessment of Articulation and Phonology (CAAP) (Secord & Donahue, 2002).

A standard assessment is typically the primary measurement component included in a diagnostic evaluation; sometimes, however, it is not appropriate to administer a standard assessment. Some children may have disabilities or behavioral qualities that do not allow for completion of this type of test. Furthermore, some individuals may come from cultural or linguistic backgrounds that differ from the normative population used to create the test and thus comparative results may not be valid. In these situations, non-standard assessments are beneficial in gathering information about the child's sound system. The assessments described in the following sections can be used to complement a standard assessment or as a primary measure when a standard assessment is not appropriate.

20V1 is the first of several video clips, from a case study that illustrates this chapter. Here, you will see the clinician administer the Hodson Assessment of Phonological Patterns. Scores from the HAPP are summarized in the Sample Diagnostic Report provided at the end of the chapter.

Access Video File 1 (Chapter 20)

20V1 Standard assessment using the Hodson Assessment of Phonological Patterns

Dynamic Assessment

Once the standardized assessment has been completed, the results include documentation of error phonemes or patterns. Typically, the errors that are documented have been elicited using a picture or object identification task where no assistance has been given. The next step in the assessment process is to make some judgments about how the child performs when given assistance from the clinician for these error productions. These judgments can be made by completing a **dynamic assessment**.

Dynamic assessment, as it applies to phonology, is an assessment procedure that measures the support that a child needs to be successful in the production of sounds and patterns. The test administration may be different for each child because the clinician will modify the presentation of test items based on the responses given by the child. Dynamic assessment is complementary to standard assessment. Typically, this type of measure is **criterion based**, which means that the clinician is looking for a specific set of skills that need to be acquired rather than a **normative score** achieved.

Most practitioners begin the dynamic assessment process by giving the child a verbal model of the target within a word. This process is called **stimulability** testing, a very basic form of dynamic assessment used to determine whether the child can be stimulated to produce the target sound (Glaspey & Stoel-Gammon, 2007). In the past, clinicians have evaluated differences in stimulability by comparing single-word productions to an imitated-word production and to an imitated-syllable production (Carter & Buck, 1956). The child was considered "stimulable" for a particular sound if the target was produced either with the verbal model in words, or at the syllable level. For some practitioners, stimulability testing may also include repeating a target multiple times to see if a repeated verbal model facilitates production. These are examples of the most basic forms of stimulability testing; however, some clinicians also add assessment of stimulability with a verbal model in phrases or in sentences. Often, however, stimulability testing is an informal process that is used to make judgments about the child's potential response to intervention.

Building on past work in stimulability, clinicians can expand the approach by using dynamic assessment to measure **speech adaptability** (Glaspey & MacLeod, 2010). Speech adaptability builds from the foundational concept of stimulability by measuring a child's response to verbal models, but also additionally considers how a child may respond when given additional instructions and cues. Furthermore, if a child easily produces a target at the word level, then clinicians should also consider how the targets can be produced in phrases, sentences, and connected speech. This concept is not new, as VanRiper (Secord, 1989) developed a systematic approach and sequence for treatment design that manipulated linguistic environments; yet, when used systematically during assessment the conceptual framework is applied in a different manner.

The clinician provides cues and manipulates the linguistic environment for the child in a systematic hierarchy. This type of support is often referred to as scaffolding. If we think of scaffolding in a literal manner—it is a temporary structure that is used during construction to support workers in completion of a project. As the project is completed, the scaffolding is gradually removed and can be adapted to meet the changing needs of the workers. In the end when the project is finished, the scaffolding is completely removed. When working with children with speech delays we can act in the same manner. We can support a child in the production of speech sounds. We do this by giving cues, which can be instructions, models, or manipulations of the target to make the target more salient. In addition, we can change the linguistic environment for the child by modifying from syllables, to words, to different sentences, and ultimately to connected speech. As clinicians, we layer the cues along with the environmental changes (much like the sway bars that cross on a construction scaffold). Over time, children need less support and can produce sounds and patterns independently.

Using the Glaspey Dynamic Assessment of Phonology (GDAP) (Table 20.2), speech adaptability is first measured by assessing a child's production at the word level without any cues (Score 10). If the child is successful in producing a target at the word level then the linguistic environment is made increasingly more complex (production in a 3-word sentence with the target word at the end of the utterance, Score 6); however, if the child produces the target in error, then the clinician adds cues to support production (Score 11). Cues are systematically added starting with target-specific instructions and a verbal model. Next, the clinician may add prolongation or segmentation (depending on the nature of the target whether it is a stop or continuant sound, Score 12). Finally, if these cues are still not successful, then the clinician adds visual-tactile modeling, which may involve a visual representation of the target or a placement cue to an oral structure (Score 13). If the child is still not successful given all of these types of cues, the linguistic environment is modified to isolation (Score 14); finally, if the child is still not successful, then the child is considered to be not-adaptable for the target (Score 15). A score ranging from 1-15 is documented for each target. The scale can be applied to single phonemes or patterns such as consonant clusters; scores across sound classes can be averaged; or all errors can be added together and averaged for a composite score. The video example 20V2 shows a clinician administering the GDAP to a 3-year-old child.

Table 20.2 Glaspey Dynamic Assessment of Phonology (GDAP)
A 15-point scale of speech adaptability

Environments	**Cue Level 0** No Instruction or verbal model	**Cue Level 1** Instruction & Verbal model	**Cue Level 2** + prolongation, segmentation	**Cue Level 3** + visual-tactile representations
Connected Speech	1			
2-Target Sentence	2	3		
4-word Sentence	4	5		
3-word Sentence	6	7	8	9
Word	10	11	12	13
Isolation				14
Not adaptable				15

Note that a low score is better and shows that the child needs less scaffolding to produce a target

Dynamic assessment presents many advantages and a few disadvantages over other types of assessments. First, it is individualized to each child, it is modifiable as needed and only the test items produced in error need to be evaluated rather than all sounds and patterns. Dynamic assessment helps the clinician gather more information about cueing and linguistic levels to determine which targets should be selected for treatment. Once treatment is implemented, dynamic assessment is typically more sensitive to change over time than traditional tests. It is helpful to the clinician to know how the child is responding to the treatment being administered so that changes can be made if needed. Using a scale such as the GDAP in Table 20.2 allows clinicians to systematically track a child's progress and easily explain this progress to caregivers and other professionals. In contrast, there are also disadvantages to dynamic assessment. Dynamic assessment depends upon the relationship between the clinician and the child. The scores, in part, may rely on the clinician's ability to motivate the child and administer cues. Administration may take a little more time because the clinician is presenting different types of cues and linguistic environments, though the analysis occurs simultaneously, so there is little follow-up analysis involved.

Given the advantages and disadvantages of dynamic assessment, it is complementary to standard assessment. Both are informative assessments that will help guide the clinician in the decision-making process. Advantages and disadvantages have been described for both types of assessment—the best option is to conduct both procedures and compare the results. To further increase knowledge about the child, it is important to conduct additional assessments as well.

The case study continues with video clip 20V2 showing a portion of the dynamic assessment conducted with the 3-year-old child. Scores from the GDAP are summarized in the Sample Diagnostic Report provided at the end of the chapter.

Access Video File 2 (Chapter 20)

20V2 Dynamic assessment using the Glaspey Dynamic Assessment of Phonology (GDAP)

Connected Speech Sample

Another type of assessment is a **connected speech sample**, which involves recording speech as it is produced in a natural speaking environment such as telling a story, holding a conversation, or talking while manipulating toys. The sample may be glossed, transcribed, and analyzed using various measures of interest. The purpose of collecting a connected speech sample is to give a more naturalistic view of the child's speech production by providing a representative picture of the child's functional speech abilities (also called ecological validity). Most standardized tests only evaluate phonemes or patterns within a word or perhaps sentence level production; however, it is important to compare how a child produces targets within words or sentences to a connected speech sample. Thus, to best understand a child's productive abilities, clinicians should collect a connected speech sample for comparison with the standard assessment and dynamic assessment. Overall, samples of connected speech can provide a significant amount of information without requiring a lengthy transcription.

With a connected speech sample, a variety of different measures can be applied, as described in more detail in Chapter 2 on describing and measuring children's speech abilities. Some children may accurately produce targets in single-words; however, when they speak in connected speech without the support of models, many errors and difficulties with production may become evident. Lexical effects such as less frequent use of certain words, coarticulation, and phrase positioning may change the accuracy of phonemes and patterns. Additionally, prosody (rate, rhythm, pitch, and loudness) analysis requires sentence level productions and is better assessed in connected speech. See Chapter 7 for a detailed account of how children acquire prosody and how prosodic aspects of speech can be described and measured. Intelligibility can be more directly assessed with a connected speech sample, unlike the use of indirect correlations obtained using single-word productions. Furthermore, evidence may surface regarding interactions between phonology and semantics (Bernhardt & Holdgrafer, 2001).

With a connected speech sample, the clinician must decide what sort of analysis will be most helpful in determining the child's difficulties and preparing for treatment. When listening to the child, clinicians should try to identify errors in the sample. Is the child having problems with only a few consonant substitutions? Is the child deleting parts of words? Is the child only producing basic syllables shapes? This careful thought process guides decisions in choosing the best analysis of the sample. For a child who is only producing simple syllable shapes, an analysis of all consonants by word position may not be very informative; rather, it may be helpful to know if the child can produce consonant (C) - vowel (V) combinations along with VC or CVC shapes, and how often certain shapes occur. In contrast, for a child with more advanced skills (e.g., syllables structures are intact, deletions are rare, but substitutions are common), an analysis of consonants by position may be the most helpful. Clinicians must use good listening skills to guide decisions in the evaluation process.

Phonetic Inventory

The connected speech sample can be used to document a child's **phonetic inventory**, an independent analysis that relies on the presence or absence of phonemes in a selected sample of speech production (Stoel-Gammon, 1985). The phonemes present in the sample are simply listed. A sound is considered to be part of the child's inventory when it is produced at least twice regardless of whether it is used correctly. For example, if a child says [wid] for /ɹid/, [wek] for /ɹek/, and consistently produces initial /ɹ/ with [w] and deletes all other opportunities for /ɹ/, the child could be said to have /w/ in the inventory, but not /ɹ/. Comparisons can then be made across time as a child acquires more phonemes and/or word positions in the inventory. A phonetic inventory can be formed as soon as a child produces phonemes. Its popularity stemmed from work with infants with emerging sound systems where the variety of a child's productions rather than just accuracy may better document development. This approach is also very useful for children with severe phonological disorders. Although inventories have been used predominantly in relation to phonemes, inventories may also be generated to determine the presence of features, vowels, syllable shapes, and stress patterns.

Accuracy Measures

Many measures may be applied to the connected speech sample to evaluate the **accuracy** of the child's production when compared to the target production. These measures may also be termed relational analysis as discussed in Chapter 2. For the clinician who is most interested in consonant production, a *Percentage of Consonants Correct* (Shriberg and Kwiatkowski, 1982) or its variants (Shriberg, Austin, Lewis, McSweeney, & Wilson, 1997) may be most informative, or if the vowels are in question, then a *Percentage of Vowels Correct* can be calculated. If the errors appear to be more complex beyond omissions and substitutions, then evaluation of the word structures may be a better choice.

Whole Word Measures

Aspects of the word may influence production and multiple errors may occur within one word (Ingram, 2002). It is important to consider production at the word level because some children may seem to be intelligible, when in fact they may be speaking with simple words. When the child is prompted to produce words of greater complexity, intelligibility is significantly compromised. On the other hand, some children may use words that are quite complex for their current level of phonology; in turn, this may make them appear less intelligible. Thus measures at the word level may also be beneficial.

Several measures may be selected. *Syllable Shape Accuracy* measures consonant and vowel sequences and may be most beneficial with younger children (Stoel-Gammon, 1996). The number of CV syllables, consonant clusters, and the overall number of syllables or words produced can also be calculated (Velleman, 1998). *Whole-Word Accuracy* (WWA) may be used to calculate how many words are produced correctly in terms of all phonemes within the word (Ingram & Ingram, 2001). The Bankson-Bernthal Test of Phonology (BBTOP) (Bankson & Bernthal, 1990) incorporates this measure into its assessment. In addition, scores from the WWA correlate with articulation scores from the Arizona Articulation Proficiency Scale-3 (Fudala, 2000). The *Phonological Mean Length of Utterance* (PMLU) (Ingram & Ingram, 2001; Ingram, 2002) metric was developed to factor in complexity within word productions. The PMLU provides a broad and preliminary perspective on a child's phonological skills much like the *Mean Length of Utterance* (MLU) does for language skills. The PMLU compares the complexity of the child's productions with the complexity of the target words produced by tallying the number of segments (consonants and vowels) in the word and the number of correct consonants. The child's score increases when more consonants and longer words are used, even when the consonants are not correct. Ingram & Ingram (2001) further compared the calculation of PMLU to the calculation of Mean Length of Utterance (Brown, 1973) by proposing stages of PMLU. The *Proportion of Whole-Word Proximity* (PWP) divides the child's PMLU score by the PMLU score of the words attempted. This measure attempts to correlate proximity with intelligibility; the authors state that this is intuitive but has yet to be proven. PWP is calculated by dividing the PMLU of the child's production by the PMLU of the adult production being compared. The last metric is the *Proportion of Whole-Word Variability* (PWV)(Ingram, 2002). PWV evaluates the inconsistencies used when a child produces the same word multiple times. For example, given five repetitions of the same word, a child may produce the word in three variable ways (in other words, three forms).

Intelligibility

One last area of analysis that can be documented using the connected speech sample is evaluation of **intelligibility.** Intelligibility is defined as the degree to which a speaker's utterance (or utterances) can be understood by a listener (Niclosi, Harryman, & Kresheck, 1989). As noted in Chapter 6, during typical development, a child's intelligibility increases with age and is expected to reach 75% by age 3 and 100% by age 4. Intelligibility does not imply that consonants are 100% accurate by 4 years of age, because small and systematic developmental errors do not impede the understanding of the child's message.

Levels of intelligibility are influenced by speaker-related variables such as articulation, rate, fluency, vocal quality, and intensity; intelligibility is also influenced by listener-related variables such as the familiarity with the speaker, the ability to decode error productions, and the ability to extract meaning from context (Shriberg & Kwiatkowski, 1982). For children with phonological disorders, the focus of treatment is to increase the child's intelligibility, and thereby improve the relationship between the speaker and listener. The ultimate goal of treatment is to increase the child's intelligibility in any speaking situation, even those situations with the most impoverished communicative context.

Although increased intelligibility is the ultimate goal of treatment, a universally agreed upon measure of intelligibility is absent from the literature (Bauman-Waengler, 2000). Because of the large number of interacting variables, several types of intelligibility measures have been designed. The most common clinical approach to measuring intelligibility includes a subjective score such as a percentage judgment (Morris, Wilcox, & Schooling, 1995; Kent, Miolo, & Bloedel, 1994). For example, after listening to a speech sample the clinician may make a statement such as, "I understand about 50% of the child's connected speech." Judgments are quickly made and frequently used in the qualification process for speech services, however, clinicians may not agree upon the same percentage judgments of the same speech sample (Flipsen, Hammer, & Yost, 2005). The variability may not pose problems for children who are severely unintelligible, clearly disordered, or those highly intelligible and typically developing; however, the children with borderline skills may be inappropriately over- or under-estimated. A second problem with intelligibility ratings has to do with judgments across time (Kent, Miolo, & Bloedel, 1994). Because only gross measures of intelligibility can be made with this method, documentation of progress from an intelligibility judgment is problematic. An improvement from an initial judgment of 30% intelligibility to a subsequent judgment of 60% intelligibility may be considered significant; however, improving from 50% to 60% may just be a factor of judgment error. A clinician who documents small differences in intelligibility ratings must question whether a change has occurred at all. Three alternative intelligibility measures that may provide a more quantitative perspective include: percentage estimates of glossed conversations, scores based on naming tasks, and rating scales.

Somewhat less subjective are percentage estimates based on glossed conversations. Connected speech is recorded and glossed by the clinician with notation of words that could not be identified (Kwiatkowski & Shriberg, 1992). A percentage of intelligibility is calculated by summing intelligible words and dividing by the total words attempted. A percentage from a written form may help with reliability; yet, a great amount of subjectivity remains. Clinicians may think they know what the child is saying, but the phrase may not be the child's actual intent and can lead to a misrepresentation in the calculation. This approach is also influenced by listener familiarity.

A second type of intelligibility measure generates scores from single-word naming tasks. Single-word measures have been used most frequently in the adult disorders population, but are also now being applied with children. Morris, Wilcox, & Schooling (1995) developed one such assessment, the Preschool Speech Intelligibility Measure (later published as the Children's Speech Intelligibility Measure, Wilcox & Morris, 1999) that is based on the Assessment of Intelligibility of Dysarthric Speech (Yorkston & Beaukelman, 1981). The test includes 50 sets of 12 phonetically similar forms allowing the clinician to choose different word sets for each administration. A clinician models single-words for the child and then the child repeats each word, which is audio recorded. From the recording, the child's productions are judged by an unfamiliar listener. The listener may be given a list of possible word productions where the listener circles the word that is heard (i.e. a closed set) or the listener may guess the target words without a list (i.e. an open set) (Gordon-Brannan, 1994). For either type of task, a percentage is generated for total words accurately understood divided by the total of words possible.

A third type of intelligibility assessment includes rating scales. Rating scales allow single-words, individual sentences, or connected speech to be assigned a qualitative rating through listener judgments. Compared to the 100-point percentage judgment described above, rating scales use a slightly more specified descriptive comparison. For example, Strand & Skinder (1999) used a 7-point scale to rate the quality of speech samples; scores spanned from one (no noticeable differences from normal) to 7 (unintelligible). Shriberg & Kwiatkowski (1982) used a four-level ordinal scale for "severity of involvement" in conjunction with the PCC metric. Using scores from the PCC, a child's intelligibility is said to be mild, mild-moderate, moderate-severe, or severe. When a rating scale is used to evaluate connected speech, the functional aspects of speech productions can be measured. Personal judgments such as these are most frequently used by parents and families to determine progress. Rating scales may reflect a correlation to parents' own judgments about whether their child is understood by others. Progress is often indicated when parents report that Grandma, or some other distant relative, can finally understand the child when having a conversation on the telephone.

Increased severity of phonological disorder creates additional problems when using intelligibility measures based on connected speech samples. Kent, Miolo, and Bloedel (1994) suggested that children with severe phonological impairments are not good candidates for conversational speech samples or rating scales because reliability of the intelligibility measure is questionable. First, speech samples may be inaccurately glossed because the clinician makes poor assumptions about what the child has said. Second, a child with a severe impairment maintains a low intelligibility score or rating for a long period of time before changes occur and intelligibility improves, and clinicians may falsely assume that no progress has been made. Third, lack of control of the speech sample produced poses problems for making comparisons of pre/post testing. The child may exhibit higher intelligibility on a sample containing simple word forms and sound combinations (Morris, Wilcox, & Schooling, 1995). As a solution, Kent and colleagues (1994) recommended using closed-set procedures instead of conversational samples or using at least two alternative measures of intelligibility. Careful consideration should guide selection of specific intelligibility measures for children with a severe to profound phonological disorder.

20V3 shows a speech sample that was collected from this three-year-old boy in the case study. In the sample diagnostic report at the end of this chapter, evaluations are provided for phonetic inventory, syllable shape inventory, and intelligibility.

Access Video File 3 (Chapter 20)

20V3 Connected Speech Sample

Phonological Awareness

Assessment of **phonological awareness** is an important component of a diagnostic evaluation for speech disorder. Phonological awareness is a broad term that encompasses listening strategies related to speech sounds. It includes "an awareness of sensitivity to speech sounds and the ability to manipulate the sound structures (i.e., the syllables and phonemes) in words" (Hart Paulson & Moats, 2010 p. 52). Children with phonological disorders are at risk for difficulties with phonological awareness and later literacy development. Thus, clinicians must identify those children who have deficits in phonological awareness and embed development strategies into the treatment sessions. These strategies will support skills necessary for literacy development. For more details about interactions between speech sound disorders and reading impairments, see Chapter 15.

The clinician can assess phonological awareness by screening the following key tasks: rhyming, alliteration, blending, and segmenting (Hart Paulson & Moats, 2010, p. 53). Rhyming involves the child's ability to match the **rime** at the ends of words (e.g. "mat" and "rat"). Alliteration is a skill that requires the child to be able to identify different words that all begin with the same first sound (e.g. My mother makes mittens). Blending involves the ability to combine sounds into words when given separate segments (e.g. What word is m-a-t?) Segmenting is the opposite of blending and requires the child to pull apart words into sounds or syllables (e.g. What are the sounds in "mat"?) The complexity of these tasks can be varied depending on the age of the child.

Structural-Functional Examination

A **structural-functional examination** provides the clinician with the opportunity to observe the oral-structures and the functioning of the articulators. The purpose of the evaluation is to determine whether any structural or functional abnormalities are contributing to a child's speech errors. Many children who are assessed do not show any deficits in structure or function. The examination is conducted by viewing the articulators and requiring the child to complete both non-verbal and verbal motor tasks. The clinician will watch for any differences in symmetry, structural anomalies, and movement abilities, particularly during speech production. This section provides a quick overview of a structural-functional examination; however, if any structural or functional differences are apparent, then a more extensive examination should be completed and a referral to a medical specialist may be considered. Chapter 17 provides details regarding assessing and working with children with structural deficits, such as cleft palate.

The structures of interest include the lips, teeth, the hard palate, the soft palate, the pharynx, and the tongue. When looking at each of the structures, the clinician generally looks for symmetry and any readily apparent anomalies. For the lips, the clinician also looks for lip closure, rounding, protrusion, retraction as an oral function, and then as part of speech sounds, /m, o, u, i/. An evaluation of the teeth includes dentition and mandibular/maxillary positioning. The clinician should look for evidence of misaligned teeth, gaps or missing teeth, decay, and malocclusion. Moving further into the oral cavity, the clinician evaluates the hard palate for height and discoloration that may indicate submucous cleft palate. Moving further back in the oral-cavity, the clinician views the soft palate and checks elevation, the size of the tonsils, and symmetry of the uvula. The tongue is also evaluated and the clinician should look at the size of the tongue, protrusion, elevation to the alveolar ridge, movement from front to back within the oral cavity, and production of sounds that rely on these movements including /θ, t, l, k/.

As part of the structural-functional examination, clinicians will also assess diadochokinesis. This assessment involves the rapid repetition of syllables, first individually, and then in succession. The clinician asks the child to say /pʌ.pʌ.pʌ . . . /, next / tʌ.t.ʌ.tʌ . . /, and / kʌ.kʌ.kʌ . . . /. Then the clinician asks the child to repeat /pʌ.tʌ.kʌ . . ./ (or with young child "peekaboo" or "buttercup"). As children grow older, their speed of repetition increases. Slow rate or uneven repetitions may indicate a more severe motor speech disorder such as childhood apraxia of speech or dysarthria rather than a speech sound disorder. Rates for these repetitions can be found in Robbins & Klcc (1987) for 2:6 to 6:11 ycar olds, and Fletcher (1972) for 6-13 year olds.

Hcaring Scrccning

A **hearing screening** should be conducted as part of a comprehensive evaluation. A basic hearing screening includes a pure-tone screening at 500, 1000, 2000, and 4000 Hz at 20dB. A hearing screening is beneficial because it is important to rule-out hearing loss as a potential cause of the speech sound disorder. It is not unusual for children with speech delays to have a history of otitis media with effusion (OME) (i.e. ear infection), though a direct relationship between the hearing loss and speech delay is controversial. Past studies have suggested that there is not a relationship between OME and phonology, but did not take into account sensorineural hearing loss. Newer studies are beginning to associate hearing loss with language delay and speech delay. For instance, it was shown that days of effusion was not significantly associated with clinical or sub-clinical speech disorders; however, hearing loss at 12-18 months was associated with 10-21 times increased risk for later speech disorder (Shriberg, Friel-Patti, Flipsen, & Brown, 2000). Abraham et al. (1996) documented the effect of OME on phonology and articulation in the presence of expressive language delay. Two groups, one with a history of OME and one without such a history, demonstrated the same receptive language skills. Results of phonological analysis at age 24 months showed similar developmental tendencies in speech sound acquisition between groups; however the OME group had established significantly fewer initial consonant phones and produced them less accurately than the OME free subject group. In addition, fewer back consonants were produced. Similar phonological error patterns of deletion and class deficiency occurred; however, the OME group demonstrated the error patterns more frequently. For a comprehensive review of the literature on hearing impairment and its role in disordered speech, consult Chapter 19.

Supplemental Assessment

Once these core measures have been completed, the clinician should have a good overview of the child's overall speech skills. However, if the child appears to have difficulties in speech sound production that are unusual or show added complexity, the clinician should consider supplemental testing. For example, the core measures may indicate that a motor speech disorder is present and the clinician should further evaluate the motor system in detail (see Chapter 18). As another example, the clinician may observe that the language system is also impaired and further language testing, particularly in expressive language, is warranted. The Sample Diagnostic Assessment Report at the end of this chapter gives an example of supplemental language testing that was conducted.

Completing the Evaluation and Making a Diagnosis

Given all of these choices for assessment, the new clinician may feel overwhelmed or uncertain about which tests and measures to include. A core evaluation should include: at least one standardized assessment, an assessment of speech adaptability of phonemes or patterns in error, a connected speech sample (with phoneme inventory and one measure of intelligibility), a phonological awareness screening, a structural-functional examination, and a hearing screening. If the child's speech is more involved, then adaptations and additional analysis should be applied.

As you have now read about many different measures of articulation and phonology, you may be wondering, "Wow, how long does that take to finish?" The answer depends on the age and behavior of the child and the severity of the disorder. A younger child or a child with a more severe disorder is likely to take longer. Generally, most standardized tests can be administered in 20-30 minutes and a connected speech sample can be collected in 5-10 minutes if the child is cooperative. Speech adaptability testing is variable depending on how many error productions the clinician evaluates. Overall, the time spent with the child can range from 1-2 hours when all of these components are collected. An additional time investment occurs at the stage of analysis when the clinician reviews the samples and completes the procedures for standard assessments. The good news for the new clinician, however, is that with practice and experience in behavior management strategies, the administration and analysis becomes much faster and automated.

The evaluation is complete and comprehensive, but now what does the clinician do with all of this information? The clinician must interpret the measures to determine the next step—diagnosis. To make a **differential diagnosis**, the clinician considers all relevant possibilities and selects the most probable one, given the results of the assessment and any supplemental testing. The following procedures follow Dodd's general classification system (Dodd, 2005). See Chapter 15 for further detail in classification systems and the supplemental testing mentioned in the present chapter. To arrive at a diagnosis using Dodd's system, the clinician asks: Does the child have an articulation or phonological problem? In the case of a phonological problem, is it a delay or disorder? Are the errors consistent or inconsistent? Is the delay or disorder severe enough to warrant intervention? And do the errors qualify for services given the guidelines of the clinician's work setting?

First, the clinician may consider whether the child is exhibiting production errors that reflect an articulation or phonological disorder. Typically, an articulation disorder refers to the articulatory ability of the child (Can the child physically produce the sound?), and a phonological disorder refers to the child's language skills and ability to use the patterns when the motor system is intact. This dichotomy can be documented for some children; however, many young children, particularly those with severe disorders, exhibit difficulties with both articulation and phonology. This categorization can be rather complex and some clinicians and researchers prefer to avoid this step.

Next, does the child have a delay or a disorder? The clinician must look over the results and evaluate whether the child is following the normative sequence of acquisition (see Chapter 6 for more on what to expect at different ages). If a child follows the normative sequence but appears to be functioning at younger age, then we may use the term "delay"; conversely, if the child's development does not seem to be following a typical developmental trajectory and unusual sounds or patterns are produced, then we may use the term "disordered." Further observation may also reveal whether the disordered productions are consistent or inconsistent. Overall, prognosis may be of greater concern for a child who is producing atypical patterns that appear disordered rather than delayed.

Third, the clinician needs to evaluate the severity of involvement. Is the impairment mild, severe, or profound? Administration of a standard assessment with normative data can be helpful in this decision-making process because the scores that are generated can be compared with the scores of other children who are the same age. Developmental continua can also be used for comparison, but there is a range of results when looking across the studies. In some situations, if the delay is mild, it may be appropriate to wait and monitor the child before intervention is implemented.

Another important perspective is the role of the child's speech errors in her or his daily life. For instance, some children with speech deficits do not participate as actively as their peers in classroom discussions and may prefer physical activities, whereas other children may want to participate in the lead role in school plays, yet may not be selected because of speech errors. Some children may develop a deep sense of frustration when their speech is not easily understood by others, whereas other children may show less concern. The complex social and academic impact of a speech disorder or delay should be considered when decisions about treatment are made.

Importantly, the clinician needs to follow the guidelines established by the work setting. For example, some school districts require that the child perform greater than 1.5 standard deviations below the norm on a standardized test in order to receive speech services, or another school district may require a certain number of phonemes to be in error across classes. Even more stringent guidelines have been recommended where some school districts do not provide speech services at all because certain speech errors are viewed as not interfering with academic success. In contrast, some school districts are providing short-term speech services through the response-to-intervention model. In other service environments, insurance coverage may impose certain restrictions such as a limitation of the number of sessions covered. Some insurance companies may also only cover specific diagnosis; for example, a developmental disorder may not be covered, whereas an organic disorder would be covered. The clinician must be cautious that the guidelines reflect new information regarding evidence-based practice and may need to advocate for some children, relying on clinician judgment for determining the need for intervention.

Once the presence of a speech disorder has been confirmed and its nature characterized, the clinician's task is to select an approach to treatment that is appropriate for the child. Dozens of different approaches have been proposed, and it is crucial to select not only one that has shown to be effective but also one that is a good fit, given the disorder characteristics of the child. Chapter 21 describes the pathway from diagnosis to treatment selection.

Connections

This chapter outlines the process of gathering and interpreting information when a child is referred for an initial evaluation because of concerns regarding speech production. Chapter 2 provides a detailed overview of tools for describing and measuring children's speech abilities for clinical as well as research purposes. Chapters 4, 5, and 6 outline various aspects of speech development in typically developing, English-speaking children, providing a reference against which to compare disordered development. Chapter 7 focuses on the acquisition of prosody and ways to assess it. The pathway from diagnosis to treatment selection, design, and implementation is covered in Chapter 22.

Concluding Remarks

While these measures will lead the clinician through a diagnostic process, assessment should also be considered a continuous process throughout treatment. Additional assessment procedures must be completed to test daily and ongoing progress. Treatment data are generated throughout the documentation of practiced skills. Generalization data are collected periodically to assess transfer of skills beyond the treatment room. The assessments will also reflect the clinician's theoretical framework and treatment approach. The above procedures should also be repeated periodically over the course of treatment to support the continuation of intervention.

Chapter Review Questions

1. What are the core components of a diagnostic assessment?
2. How does a Diagnostic Assessment differ from other forms of assessment?
3. What is the difference between a standard assessment and a dynamic assessment?
4. What is the primary benefit of collecting a connected speech sample that may not be assessed on other types of assessments?
5. What are three different types of intelligibility measures?
6. Why is it necessary to conduct a structural-functional examination, hearing screening, and phonological screening when these assessments do not measure speech sound production?

Suggestions for Further Reading

For more information on dynamic assessment:

Glaspey, A. M., & Stoel-Gammon, C. (2007). A Dynamic approach to phonological assessment. *Advances in Speech Language Pathology, 9,* 286-296.

For more information on assessment with cultural and linguistic diversity:

Goldstein, B. (2000). *Cultural and linguistic diversity resource guide for speech-language pathologists.* San Diego: Thomson Delmar Learning.

Lynch, E.W. & Hanson, M. J. (2011). *Developing Cross-Cultural Competence,* 4th Edition. Baltimore: Brookes.

For more information on phonological awareness and literacy:

Gillon, G. T. (2004). *Phonological Awareness from Research to Practice.* New York: The Guilford Press.

Hart Paulson, L. & Moates, L. C. (2010). *LETRS (Language essentials for teachers of reading and spelling) for early childhood educators* (pp. 51-67). Boston, MA: Cambium Learning.

Suggestions for Student Activities

1. Video 20V1 provides an example of a standardized assessment, the Hodson Assessment of Phonological Patterns. Transcribing disordered speech takes practice. Transcribe the words that you hear. If the HAPP is available to you, transcribe and score the test.
2. Video 20V2 provides an example of using the GDAP with child. Using the 15-point scale that is provided in the text, score each phoneme. What scores does the child achieve?
3. Video 20V3 provides an example of a connected speech sample. Document the child's phonetic inventory and complete an intelligibility measure that would be appropriate for the sample.
4. Once you have completed the previous activities, view the Sample Diagnostic Report to see how the results of these measures are combined for a comprehensive Diagnostic Assessment.

The following sample diagnostic report for the case study is provided as a model of the concepts discussed in this chapter. The names, identifying information, and content have been modified.

Sample Diagnostic Assessment Report

Child: Carter Williams
Parents: Bo and Angie Williams
Address: 18 Dogwood Drive,
Missoula, MT 59802
Phone: 000-000-0000

Date of Birth: 1/8/XXXX
Age: 5 years, 3 months
Date(s) of Evaluation: April 15, XXXX
Clinician: Amy M. Glaspey, Ph.D., CCC-SLP

Child History

Carter is a 5 year, 3 month old boy who was evaluated at the Ritecare Speech, Language, and Hearing Clinic on April 15 and 17, XXXX. He was referred for speech and language testing by his preschool teacher, Kathy Jones, because of concerns that he has difficulty making specific speech sounds and being understood by others. Carter's mother, Angie Williams, attended sessions with him and provided the following history.

Developmental history: Carter's birth history was unremarkable. He met all developmental milestones within a typical timeframe. *Medical history:* Carter has no history of major illness, current health concerns, medications, or allergies. He has no history of ear infections. *Social/Educational History:* Carter lives with his parents and two brothers age 7 and 1. He currently attends the Daisy Childcare Center. Mrs. William's also reported a family history of speech and language delays; she participated in speech treatment as a child.

Test Environment and General Behavior

The assessment took place in a quiet room at the University of Montana Ritecare Clinic. Carter was receptive to the novel situation and very cooperative. Test results were judged to be valid.

Hearing Screening

Carter's hearing was screened on 4/15/XXXX at the Ritecare Speech, Language, and Hearing Clinic. Carter passed a pure tone audiometry screening of 500, 1000, 2000, and 4000 Hz at 20 dB and tympanometry revealed acoustic reflex in each ear.

Structural-Functional Evaluation

An oral-motor assessment was administered using techniques from Robbins & Klee (1987) and Strand & McCauley (1999). The assessment was completed with a structural score of 24/24 and a functional score of 100/112. All structures appeared to be within normal limits. Carter could repeat /p/ an average of 3.48 times per second and /t/ 4.4 times per second, indicating average repetition rates for his age. He could not produce the /k/ sound. Carter repeated "patticake" substituting [t] for /k/ at a rate of 1.2 times per second and could sustain a vowel for 3.13 seconds. He could imitate words of increasing length and could maintain the correct number of syllables in multisyllabic words and phrases.

Voice and Fluency

Carter's rate of speaking, fluency, and voice quality were judged to be within normal limits.

Language Assessment

The **Preschool Language Scale IV (PLS-4)** was administered to assess receptive and expressive language skills. This measure uses pictures and objects as prompts to assess the understanding and use of language. A standard score of 85-115 reflects the average range. The following scores were obtained.

PLS-4	Standard Score	Percentile Rank	Age Equivalent
Receptive Language	93	32	4:9
Expressive Language	96	39	5:0
Total Language Score	94	34	5:1

Scores on the PLS-IV place Carter's overall language skills in the average range when compared to other children of the same age. Carter could understand the time concepts of seasons and *first/last*, order pictures from largest to smallest, and identify body parts such as *elbow* and *wrist*. Carter had difficulty understanding quantity concepts *three* and *half*, passive voice sentences, the quantitative concept *each*, and rhyming sounds. Carter could segment words, define words, and name items in categories. Carter had difficulty using past tense forms, formulating grammatical statements and questions, repairing grammatical errors, and rhyming words.

The **Peabody Picture Vocabulary Test-4 (PPVT-4)** was administered to assess vocabulary skills, which are correlated with cognitive skills. Children are asked to choose a picture (one out of four) that best represents the word they hear. A standard score of 85-115 reflects the average range. The following scores were achieved:

PPVT	Standard Score	Percentile Rank	Age Equivalent
Receptive vocabulary	108	70	5;11

Scores on the PPVT place Carter's overall receptive vocabulary skills in the average range when compared to other children of the same age.

Speech Assessment

The **Hodson Assessment of Phonological Patterns-3 (HAPP-3)** was administered using objects as prompts. Scores for each phonological pattern are summarized in the second part of the table. Scores may range between 0 and 100 with low scores being best.

HAPP-3	Score
Total Occurrences of Major Phonological Deviations (TOMPD)	75
Consonant Category Deficiency Sum	52
Percentile Rank	<1
Standard Deviation	≥2
Severity Interval	Moderate
Word Structures	
Syllables	0

HAPP-3	Score
Consonant Sequences/clusters	49
Prevocalic singletons	0
Intervocalic singletons	0
Postvocalic singletons	12.5
Consonant Categories	
Liquids	58
Nasals	0
Glides	20
Stridents	40
Velars	64
Anterior nonstridents (backing)	27

Scores and percentages indicate that Carter demonstrates a moderate phonological disorder. In single word productions he can produce the correct number of syllables, sounds at the beginning and middle of words, and nasals /m, n, ŋ/. Carter had difficulties producing consonant clusters ("sw" in swimming), sequences, anterior/palatal stridents /s, z, ʃ, v/, velars /k, g, ŋ/, and liquid /l/. He sometimes had difficulties producing consonants at the ends of words.

The **Glaspey Dynamic Assessment of Phonology (GDAP)** was administered to obtain a dynamic score of speech adaptability. Scores on the GDAP range from 1 to 15 with a low score being best. A low score indicates that the child needed little assistance to produce a sound. A high score indicates that the child needed many cues and assistance to produce the sound or pattern. See attached scale.

Scores on the GDAP indicate that Carter produced the correct number of syllables and the sounds /j-, w-, m-, -m, n-, -n, p-, -p, b-, -b, t-, -t, d-, -d/. He was highly adaptable for /tʃ-, ð-, r-, -r/, moderately adaptable for /-k, f-, -f, v-, -v, s-, -s, z-, -z, ʃ-, -ʃ, -ʒ, -tʃ, ʤ-, -ʤ, -θ, -ð, l-, sp-, tr-, -ts/, slightly adaptable for /k-, -g, -ŋ, θ-, -l, pl-/, and not adaptable for /g-/.

Sound/pattern	Score	Sound/pattern	Score
Syllables		Stridents	
1. wSw potato	1	23. /f-/ fin	9
2. SwSw macaroni	1	24. /-f/ leaf	8
Glides and /h/		25. /v-/ van	8
3. /j-/ yawn	1	26. /-v/ hive	8
4. /w-/ wood	1	27. /s-/ sing	9
5. /h-/ hug	1	28. /-s/ kiss	7
Nasals (front)		29. /z-/ zip	9
6. /m-/ mop	1	30. /-z/ hose	8
7. /-m/ beam	1	31. /ʃ-/ chute	9
8. /n-/ net	1	32. /-ʃ/ bush	7
9. /-n/ bean	1	33. /-ʒ/ beige	8
Stops		34. /tʃ-/ chop	3
10. /p-/ pin	1	35. /-tʃ/ match	7
11. /-p/ map	1	36. /ʤ-/ jam	9
12. /b-/ boat	1	37. /-ʤ/ badge	8

Sound/pattern	Score	Sound/pattern	Score
13. /-b/ web	1	Interdentals	
14. /t-/ ten	1	38. /θ-/ thumb	12
15. /-t/ bat	1	39. /-θ/ tooth	8
16. /d-/ dad	1	40. /ð-/ that	5
17. /-d/ bed	1	41. /-ð/ bathe	8
Velars		Liquids	
18. /k-/ comb	12	42. /l-/ lip	7
19. /-k/ hook	7	43. /-l/ pool	14
20. /g-/ gum	15	44. /r-/ rain	3
21. /-g/ bug	14	45. /-r/ bar	3
22. /-ŋ/ song	13	Clusters	
		46. /sp-/ spin	8
		47. /-ts/ bats	7
		48. /pl-/ plum	14
		49. / tr-/ train	8

A **connected speech sample** was elicited using a wordless book and/or play. Carter's percentage of consonants correct in connected speech was calculated to be 42% and his intelligibility was rated as "severe" (Shriberg & Kwiatkowski, 1982), indicating extremely low intelligibility. In connected speech, Carter frequently deleted velar consonants or replaced them with a front consonant (e.g. d/g). He also substituted /d/ for many sounds and often used glides in place of liquids. He occasionally deleted final consonants and reduced consonant clusters. In connected speech, nine words were unintelligible and could not be included in the calculation. Consonants in the phonetic inventory included: /w, j, h, m, n, p*, b, t, d, k, g*, f*, s, ʃ, tʃ/ and clusters in initial position /fr, br, pr*/ (*indicates only one production in a 100 word sample). The word shape inventory included (C=Consonant, V=vowel): V, CV, VV, VC, CVC, VVC, CVV, CCV, CVVC, CCVV, CVCVC, CCVVC, CVVVC , CVCVV, VVCVV, CVCCVC, CCVVCV, CVCCVV, and CVVCCVC. The most common shape was CVC and the least common was CVCCVV.

Phonological Awareness Screening

The Emergent Literacy Screening from Building Early Literacy and Language Skills was administered to assess skills in language, literacy, and phonological awareness. Carter scored 10/15 for Print Awareness and could identify symbols, identify letters in his name, print random letter strings, and sing most of the alphabet. Carter scored 7/15 for Language Use and could use rhythm patterns, basic concepts, and could relate a past event. Carter's speech was rated as difficult to understand with many grammatical errors. Carter scored 6/15 for Phonological Awareness. He had difficulties with rhyming, blending, and segmenting words. Overall, Carter scored 23/45 and demonstrated emerging literacy skills that were slightly below average for his age.

Summary and Recommendations

Carter Williams, a 5 year, 3 month old boy, was evaluated because of concerns about speech and language skills. Scores on the PLS-4 and PPVT placed overall language skills in the average range. Scores on the HAPP-3 and connected speech sample indicated deficits in phonological skills in the moderate to severe range. Scores on the BELLS Phonological Awareness Screening indicated emergent literacy skills that were slightly below average. Deficits in speech production may make it challenging for Carter to participate in his preschool classroom, engage in age-appropriate activities, develop literacy skills, and express his wants and needs. Prognosis is good because Carter is adaptable across many sounds.

It is recommended that Carter receive speech treatment focused on the following patterns:

1) production of liquid /l/
2) production of s-clusters such as /st-, sn-, or sw-/,
3) production of velars /k, g, ŋ/,
4) production of stridents such as /s, z, f, v, ʃ/.

Amy M. Glaspey, Ph.D., CCC-SLP
Speech-Language Pathologist

Answers to Chapter Review Questions

1. What are the core components of a diagnostic assessment?

A diagnostic assessment should include: child history, standard assessment, dynamic assessment, connected speech sample (with inventory and intelligibility rating), structural-functional examination, phonological awareness screening, and hearing screening.

2. How does a Diagnostic Assessment differ from other forms of assessment?

A Diagnostic Assessment is a comprehensive testing procedure that includes many measures and the purpose is to determine whether a disorder is present and help plan for treatment if necessary. Other assessments are conducted during treatment to determine whether treatment is working and how the child is acquiring skills. The components of a Diagnostic Assessment may be used for these purposes as well.

3. What is the difference between a standard assessment and a dynamic assessment?

A standard assessment is a test that includes procedures that are followed exactly across all children and often generates a standard score that may be based on normative data. A dynamic assessment is individualized based on the child's responses and may be different for each child. Skills are documented and assistance can be given and a normative score is not typically generated.

4. What is the primary benefit of collecting a connected speech sample that may not be assessed on other types of assessments?

A connected speech sample offers greater ecological validity than other measures because it samples speech production in a natural environment.

5. What are three different types of intelligibility measures?

Percentage estimates of glossed conversations, single-word naming tasks, and rating scales.

6. Why is it necessary to conduct a structural-functional examination, hearing screening, and phonological screening when these assessments do not measure speech sound production?

Articulation and phonological disorders may be related to structural/functional deficits, hearing loss, or difficulties with phonological awareness, which can all affect production abilities.

REFERENCES

Abraham, S., Wallace, I., & Gravel, J. (1996). Early otitis media and phonological development at age 2 years. *Laryngoscope*, 106, 727-732.

Bankson, N., & Bernthal, J. (1990). *Bankson-Bernthal Test of Phonology*. Austin, TX: Pro-ed.

Bauman-Waengler, J. (2000). *Articulatory and Phonological Impairments: A Clinical Focus.* Needham Heights, MA: Allyn & Bacon.

Bernhardt, B., & Holdgrafer, G. (2001). Beyond the Basics I: The need for strategic sampling for in-depth phonological analysis. *Language, Speech, and Hearing Services in the Schools,* 32, 18-21.

Brown, R. (1973). *A first language: The early stages.* Cambridge, MA: Harvard University Press.

Carter, E. T., & Buck, M. (1958). Prognostic testing for functional articulation disorders among children in the first grade. *Journal of Speech and Hearing Disorders,* 23, 124-133.

Dodd, B. (2005). *Differential diagnosis and treatment of speech disordered children.* Second edition. London: Whurr.

Fletcher, S. G. (1972). Time-by-count measurement of diadochokinetic syllable rate. *Journal of Speech and Hearing Research,* 15, 763-770.

Flipsen, P., Hammer, J. B., & Yost, K. M. (2005). Measuring severity of involvement in speech delay: Segmental and whole-word measures. *American Journal of Speech-Language Pathology*, 14(4), 298-312.

Fudala, J. (2000). *Arizona Articulation Proficiency Scale—Third Revision,* Los Angelos, CA: Western Psychological Services.

Glaspey, A. M., & Macleod, A. A. N. (2010). A multi-dimensional approach to gradient change in phonological acquisition: A case study of disordered speech development. *Clinical Linguistics and Phonetics, 24,* 283-299.

Glaspey, A. M., & Stoel-Gammon, C. (2007). A Dynamic approach to phonological assessment. *Advances in Speech Language Pathology,* 9, 286-296.

Goldman, R., & Fristoe, M. (2000). *The Goldman-Fristoe Test of Articulation-Second Edition,* Circle Pines, MN: American Guidance Service.

Goldstein, B. (2000). *Cultural and linguistic diversity resource guide for speech-language pathologists.* San Diego: Thomson Delmar Learning.

Gordon-Brannan, M. (1994). *Assessing intelligibility: Children's expressive phonologies.* Topics in Language Disorders, 14(2), 17-25.

Hart Paulson, L., & Moates, L. C. (2010). *LETRS (Language essentials for teachers of reading and spelling) for early childhood educators* (pp. 51-67). Boston, MA: Cambium Learning.

Hodson, B. (2004). *The Hodson assessment of phonological patterns.* Austin, TX: Pro-Ed/Interstate.

Ingram, D. (2002). The measurement of whole-word productions. *Journal of Child Language, 29,* 713-733.

Ingram, D., & Ingram, K. (2001). A whole-word approach to phonological analysis and intervention. *Language, Speech, and Hearing in Schools*, 32, 271-283.

Kent, R., Miolo, G., & Bloedel, S. (1994). The intelligiblity of children's speech: A review of evaluation procedures. *American Journal of Speech-Language Pathology*, 3, 81-95.

Kwiatkowski, J., & Shriberg, L. (1992). Intelligibility assessment in developmental phonological disorders: Accuracy of caregiver gloss. *Journal of Speech and Hearing Research,* 35, 1095-1104.

Morris, S., Wilcox, K., & Schooling, T. (1995). The Preschool Speech Intelligibility Measure. *American Journal of Speech-Language Pathology,* 4(4), 22-28.

Morrison, J. and Shriberg, L. D. (1992). Articulation testing versus conversational speech sampling. *Journal of Speech and Hearing Research,* 35, 259-273.

Nicolosi, L., Harryman, E., & Kresheck, J. (1989). *Terminology of Communication Disorders: Speech-Language-Hearing.* Baltimore, MD: Williams & Wilkins.

Robbins, J., & Klee, T. (1987). Clinical assessment of oropharyngeal motor development in young children. *Journal of Speech and Hearing Disorders,* 52, 271-277.

Secord, W.A., & Donohue, J. S. (2002). *Clinical Assessment of Articulation and Phonology.* Greenville, SC: Super Duper Publications.

Secord, W. A. (1989). The traditional approach to treatment. In N.A. Creaghead, P.W. Newman, & W. A. Secord (Eds.), *Assessment and remediation of articulatory and phonological disorders* (2nd ed., pp. 129-153). Columbus, OH: Merrill.

Shriberg, L., Austin, D., Lewis, B., McSweeny, J., & Wilson, D. (1997). The percentage of consonants correct (PCC) metric: Extensions and reliability data. *Journal of Speech, Language, and Hearing Research,* 40, 708-722.

Shriberg, L., Friel-Patti, S., Flipsen, P., & Brown, R. (2000). Otitis media, fluctuant hearing loss, and speech-language outcomes: A preliminary structural equation model. *Journal of Speech, Language, and Hearing Research*, 43, 100-120.

Shriberg, L. D., & Kwiatkowski, J. (1982). Phonological disorders II: A conceptual framework for management. *Journal of Speech and Hearing Disorders*, 47, 242-256.

Stoel-Gammon, C. (1985). Phonetic inventories, 15-24 months: A longitudinal study. *Journal of Speech and Hearing Research*, 28(4), 505-512.

Stoel-Gammon, C. (1996). Phonological assessment using a hierarchical framework. *Assessment of Communication and Language,* 6, 77-95.

Strand, E., & Skinder, A. (1999). Treatment of Developmental Apraxia of Speech. Chapter in *Clinical Management of Motor Speech Disorders in Children.* Edited by Caruso, A. & Strand, E. New York, NY: Thieme Medical Publishers, Inc.

Van Riper, C., & Emerick, L. (1990). *Speech Correction: An introduction to speech pathology and audiology.* Englewood, NJ: Prentice Hall.

Velleman, S. (1998). *Making phonology functional.* Boston, MA: Butterworth-Heinemann.

Wilcox, K., & Morris, S. (1999). *Children's Speech Intelligibility Measure.* San Antonio, TX: Pearson.

Williams, A. L. (2000). *Speech disorders resource guide for preschool children.* Clifton Park, NY: Singular Publishing Group.

Yorkston, K., & Beukelman, D. (1981). *Assessment of intelligibility of dysarthric speech.* Austin, TX: ProEd.

In: Comprehensive Perspectives …
Editors: Beate Peter and Andrea A. N. MacLeod
ISBN: 978-1-62257-041-6

Chapter 21

EVALUATING THE EVIDENCE OF THERAPY: MANY HANDS MAKE LIGHT WORK - OR AT LEAST LIGHTER WORK

Rebecca J. McCauley

INTRODUCTION

According to recent estimates, children with speech sound disorders (SSDs) account for a large percentage of children with speech and language disorders (Broomfield & Dodd, 2004; Law, Boye, Harris, Harkness & Nye, 2000; McKinnon, McLeod & Reilly, 2007; Shriberg, Tomblin, McSweeny, 1999) and perhaps an even larger percentage of such children who are receiving treatment (ASHA, 2010; Joffe & Pring, 2008; NIDCD, 1994; Zhang & Tomblin, 2000). Most children with SSDs experience challenges that are limited to errored productions of a small number of speech sounds. I would define these as articulation disorders or residual errors (Shriberg, et al. 1999). However, even mild impairments can be associated with significant social impacts (e.g., Hall, 1991; Silverman & Paulus, 1989). In addition, a significant number of children with SSDs (especially those described as exhibiting phonologic disorders) show compromised intelligibility as well as a myriad of associated problems. Some of these are communicative in nature (e.g., oral and written language deficits) and others are broader, more persistent. Nonetheless, all have the potential to imperil affected children's social and vocational futures (e.g., academic failure, psychosocial challenges) (Felsenfeld, Broen, & McGue, 1992; McCormack, McLeod, McAllister, & Harrison, 2009; Shriberg et al., 1999).

Given the prominence of SSDs based on the numbers of affected children, the potential scope of their problems, as well as the long history of interest associated with this disorder in speech-language pathology (Van Riper, 1939), one might expect to find a wealth of powerful treatments that form a widely used basic tool box of validated approaches. This chapter examines this expectation in terms of current research findings, going on to discuss how clinicians can use the information collected by others *and* themselves to secure the best possible results for their individual SSD clients.

Two prominent and complementary strategies for weighing evidence associated with the quality of intervention differ in the scope and nature of evidence they encompass. A **research appraisal of treatments** takes a more global approach that is usually conducted by researchers, depends on the use of research (external) evidence, and focuses on findings aggregated across as many children as possible. In contrast, the **clinical documentation of treatment effects** takes a more local approach that is conducted by individual practitioners, depends on evidence internal to the clinical process, and focuses on findings for an individual child. Within the framework of evidence-based practice (EBP), the individual clinician serving children with SSD takes advantage of the first approach to optimize results obtained in the second (Dollaghan, 2007). Thus, the two approaches are inextricably linked. In this chapter, I survey the results of several recent commentaries on the current state of researched interventions. Then, I discuss several ways in which this kind of external evidence both parallels and informs a clinician's current treatment practices. Finally, I discuss creative strategies that clinicians may use in their practice so that the incorporation of external evidence achieves its potential value.

THE SHARED QUEST: WHAT WORKS?

Both clinicians and researchers share a common question regarding interventions for children with SSD: "What works?" Clinicians ask this question because they want to provide *actual* help to the children they serve, whereas most researchers who undertake intervention research ask it because they want to help a sizeable group of their clinical colleagues in that endeavor. In the scientific realm, answering that question translates into far more specific and answerable (if less appealing) questions of the following sort: "Of those interventions for which research has been conducted, which can be expected to have the desired effects for a particular group of well-described participants when implemented as described?" The terms *efficacy, effectiveness*, and *effects* often figure in the further specifications required (Olswang, 1997) as such questions are asked of specific treatments. Specific and often-cited EBP procedures are usually considered to be the correct methods by which clinicians may answer them (e.g., Johnson, 2006), although there appear to be barriers to this ideal (e.g., Meline & Paradiso, 2003; Zipoli & Kennedy, 2005).

The terms *efficacy* and *effectiveness* can be seen as representing two types of research falling at either end of a continuum of experimental control (e.g., Fey & Finestack, 2009; Robey & Schultz, 1998), as illustrated in Figure 21.1. At one end of the continuum (**efficacy research**), we find highly controlled, "laboratory" studies in which the source of observed effect is credibly identified as the treatment being studied because nuisance variables are eliminated or minimized. At the other end of the continuum (**effectiveness research**), we find more naturalistic studies of treatment. It can be harder to be sure that uncontrolled, extraneous variables weren't active in shaping outcomes in the latter, but there's greater confidence that the treatment can work in conditions approximating those of typical practice. Considered in terms of research validity, efficacy studies favor **internal validity** whereas effectiveness studies favor **external validity**, or generalizability. Both types offer clinicians some hope that the studied treatment is "on to something" that clinicians can implement in their own practice. However, *neither* presents clinicians with a "turn-key" treatment of the type that both researchers and clinicians may crave—one in which the procedure and dosage are empirically driven and outcomes are predictably positive. Because individual responses to interventions vary and even well studied interventions can rarely be implemented exactly as researched, external evidence is always inadequate as the sole support for treatment decisions. Thus, the ultimate in efficacy evidence for a given intervention may lie in clinicians' own assessments of their client's progress.

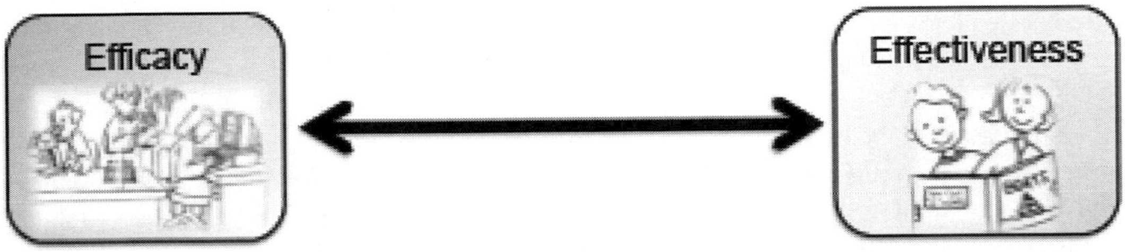

Figure 21.1. The continuum of intervention research evidence.

Treatment effects is the term sometimes used to refer to the array of impacts we hope to have on clients (Olswang, 1997), which vary widely depending on the narrowness of our focus. When we focus more narrowly on speech production, treatment effects can include specific changes in children's *Goldman-Fristoe Test of Articulation* scores or changes in intelligibility ratings on a reading task with the clinician as listener. When we look at the broader impacts on speech sound disorders, treatment effects can include changes in children's level of participation in the classroom, or their attitudes toward speaking. The International Classification of Function (ICF; World Health Organization, 2001) and the ICF-Children and Youth (ICF-CY; WHO, 2007) have helped to formalize how such broader impacts can be conceptualized. In research, the use of this system has resulted in a much richer understanding associated with the impact of SSDs on affected children and their families (e.g., McCormack, McLeod, McAllister, & Harrison, 2009; McLeod & Bleile, 2004; Teverovsky, Bickel & Feldman, 2009). Clinical applications of this system are probably more limited, but may be equally enlightening.

Whereas the complexity of systems like the ICF-CY (WHO, 2007) can be somewhat daunting, it forces us past thinking of the fruits of articulation therapy as a normalized production of /s/ or /r/ toward a consideration of the broader impacts associated with terms like "quality of life." Although a discussion of the considerable body of work generated by this perspective (e.g., Keilmann, Braun, & Napiontek, 2004; McLeod, 2006; Crosbie, Pine, Holm, & Dodd, 2006) is beyond the scope of this chapter, it is yet another way in which asking, "What works?" must be further specified by both researchers and clinicians: "What works for what purpose/to what end?"

Parallels between the concepts of efficacy/effectiveness and effects can be found clinically in the concepts of generalization and progress data, respectively. In terms of treatment progress, clinicians can parallel the efficacy-effectiveness continuum by observing changes in generalization from the child's performance on a treatment target under highly supportive or simplified conditions (e.g., repetition of a standardized test), versus under more realistic, everyday conditions (e.g., generalization probes). In terms of treatment effects, clinicians—like researchers—can collect progress data by tracking a child's progress on measures (effects) representing the child's apparent mastery of a particular production pattern as well as measures reflecting the impact of child-implemented strategies for improving intelligibility.

WHAT CURRENT RESEARCH HAS TO OFFER

As interest in treatment effectiveness has grown to ever-higher levels in the face of external demands, efforts to improve the quality of interventions provided by clinicians have largely focused on how clinicians may best access and synthesize research evidence to help guide their decision-making. In particular, the focus has been on enlisting them to address clinical questions including those related to intervention through the critical appraisal of topics, using methods such as the PICO method (e.g., Gillam & Gillam, 2006; Johnson, 2006). For example, two closely related perspectives on these steps are described in Johnson (2006) and Dollaghan (2007), among numerous others. Despite their differences, both draw on the earliest formulations of EBP, called EBM (M for Medicine) by Sackett and his colleagues who began development of that approach within the context of clinical epidemiology (Sackett, Rosenberg, Gray, Haynes & Richardson, 1996). Essentially, these methods instruct the clinician to construct a question that might be answered by the research literature, seek evidence for it, weigh (appraise) the quality of the evidence, then consider the evidence in light of clinical expertise and client preferences and values--the two other main components of EBP. As final steps, clinicians apply the result of the preceding process and examine the outcomes that follow. As outlined, these several steps, when performed iteratively, are thought to improve clinical practice and therefore intervention effectiveness. Figure 21.2 illustrates this process. The process must be performed iteratively to facilitate the clinician's continued updating as evidence accumulates and as new questions, or variations on old ones, present themselves.

Steeped in the ethos of EBP, clinicians know that **systematic reviews** are considered the pinnacles of scientific evidence that could provide a strong basis for choosing interventions. However, they are also aware that such reviews are about as rare in the literature as Himalayan mountain ranges are in the landscape. As a summary of evidence, the value of systematic reviews is in (a) their rigorous methods (especially their control of bias in how sources of evidence are selected and described); (b) the **transparency of research methods**; and, usually, (c) their greater attention to evidence obtained from more **rigorous research designs** (ones associated with greater control and therefore fewer alternative explanations for findings) (McCauley & Hargrove, 2004). On the other hand, narrative reviews (like this chapter) take their value from their efforts to integrate research evidence when the research base is insufficiently large and of mixed quality, or when the purpose of the review is to guide readers in thinking about that evidence in light of current clinical practices. In this section, I decided to summarize a related pair of systematic reviews (Law, Garrett & Nye, 2004, 2010) and one particularly noteworthy narrative review (Baker & McLeod, 2011) because of their complementary contributions to thinking about what to do in therapy.

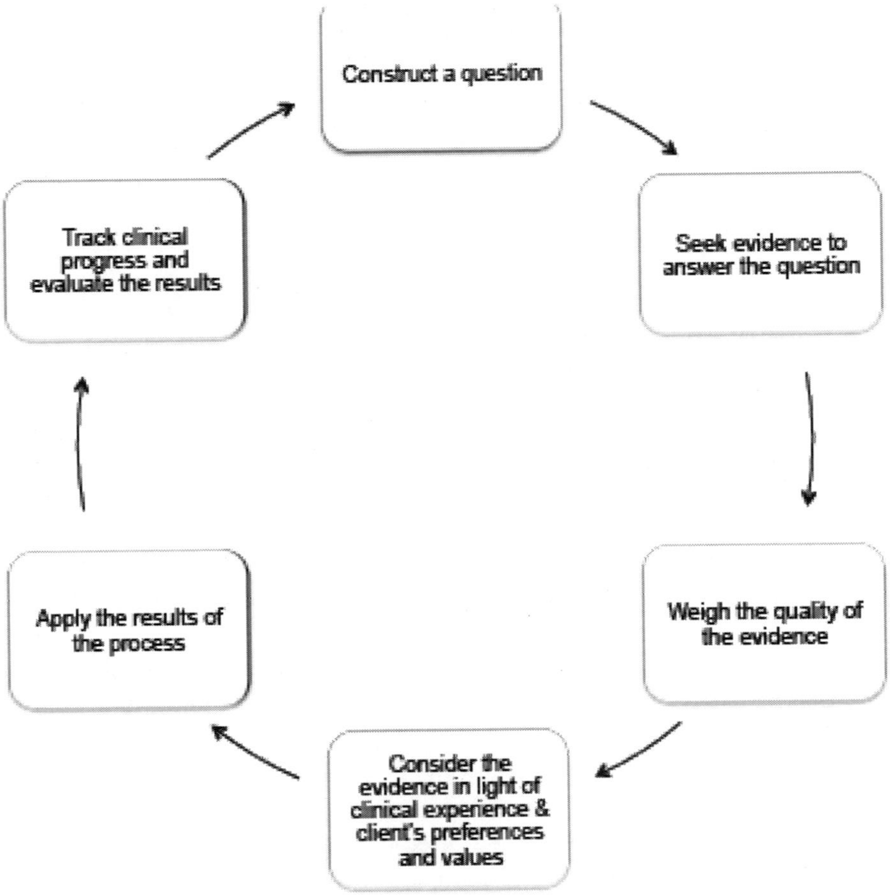

Figure 21.2. The iterative process of evidence-based practice.

In two systematic reviews (Law, Garrett & Nye, 2004, 2010), Law and his colleagues sought to determine the strength of support for speech (*and* language interventions) by using two closely related methods of research syntheses, with a focus on randomized controlled trials (RCTs; i.e., studies in which children were randomly assigned to a treatment or control [delay or no treatment] group). Law and his colleagues used the term "phonological" to refer to interventions and problems that might be more broadly described as those related to "speech sound disorders" and as a means of distinguishing them from those related to expressive or receptive syntax or vocabulary. First, Law et al. conducted a systematic review to identify RCTs that were similar enough in intent and outcome to warrant comparison. Second, they used a meta-analysis to combine data across studies thereby supporting more powerful, reliable statements about the group of studies than could be made in a narrative summary. Although only six studies focusing on *phonological* interventions were identified over a 20-year period, Law and his colleagues' conclusions supported the value of these interventions as a group, especially those phonologic interventions that were administered by SLPs (rather than parents) and those that lasted over 8 weeks. Further, Law et al. found support for efficacy when percentage consonants correct was measured in conversation, but not when the number of target consonants correct was measured in a story-retell.

When Law, Garrett, and Nye updated the 2004 study in 2010, they obtained new findings on language interventions, but added little to their previous findings on interventions for children with SSDs. Specifically, Law et al. (2010) provided continuing support at a bare minimum level, consistent with that from the 2004 study: groups of children with SSDs who received intervention, on average, performed better than those in a control group.

A clinician in the trenches (or a student being initiated into the field) might read this and think, "Well, thank goodness!" or "Did we need a study to tell us this?" However, an SLP-friendly administrator or other policy maker in an era of budget upheavals might breathe a sigh of relief that such information is out there. Still, returning to the idea that all questions about intervention need to be specific, both groups of readers might follow-up with questions about specificity, such as "Which intervention(s) were found to be effective?" and "How old were these children with an SSD and how severe were their problems?" Even the following question could be asked: "Were these efficacy studies or effectiveness studies?" In fact, Johnston (2005) posed questions very similar to these in a Letter to the Editor about the earlier review by Law et al. Responding to that letter, Law et al. (2005) acknowledged these limitations but defended them as necessary, given both the lack of studies for different age groups as well as the lack of study groups looking at any particular intervention or even a type of intervention.

An alternative method for determining what current research on speech sound disorders has to tell us was taken in a narrative review reported by Baker and McLeod (2011). That study focused on interventions for children with phonologic impairments (rather than motor speech or articulation disorders), thus making it an examination of a specific subset of children with SSD, albeit a relatively large and clinically significant one. Baker and McLeod's review shared many of the rigorous methods used in systematic reviews, including a detailed report of methods used first to identify, then to describe relevant intervention studies (e.g., in terms of intervention approach studied, target selection, research design, study duration, and level of evidence). Its primary departure from a strict systematic review was that it "took on all comers," examining not only studies at the highest level of design quality (RCTs), but at all other levels as well. Thus, Baker and McLeod (2011) included case studies, quasi-experimental studies, single-case experimental designs and nonRCTs, in addition to the RCTs, systematic reviews and meta-analyses, designs that are the grist for systematic reviews. Baker and McLeod's goal was to provide a resource falling between the rigor of a review like that of Law et al. (2010) on the one hand, and a more traditional narrative review like that of Gierut (1998) and Tyler (2008) on the other.

Among their results, Baker and McLeod (2011) identified 134 relevant studies during the 30-year time period from 1979 to 2009 that addressed some 46 different intervention approaches. They further noted that 23 of those approaches had been the focus of more than one study and described the levels of evidence associated with these studies using a common classification of research design rigor (American Speech-Language-Hearing Association, 2004; See Table 21.1). Focusing on these 23 approaches, Baker and McLeod found that 74% were associated with levels of evidence falling at Levels IIb (quasi-experimental studies) and III (non-experimental case studies). Further, they noted that the majority of these were studies of efficacy (laboratory condition studies) rather than studies of effectiveness (field condition studies).

Table 21.1. Levels of evidence for studies of treatment efficacy, ranked in terms of quality and credibility from most to least credible (Adapted from Baker &McLeod, 2011a, p. 104; ASHA, 2004)

Level	Description
Ia	Well-designed meta-analysis of > 1 controlled trial
Ib	Well-designed randomized controlled study
IIa	Well-designed controlled study without randomization
IIb	Well-designed quasi-experimental study (Also included at this level in Baker & McLeod were single-case experimental designs such as multiple baselines across participants or behaviors)
III	Well-designed nonexperimental studies (i.e., correlational and case studies)
IV	Expert committee report, consensus conference, clinical experience of respected authorities

Table 21.2. A sample descriptive reference, number of associated research studies and illustrative study for seven SSD interventions identified as having the greatest number of associated studies from the 23 studied interventions included in Baker & McLeod (2011a)

Approach	Number of Studies	Reference describing this approach	Illustrative study: Reference	Illustrative study: Level of Evidence
1 Minimal pairs	42	Baker (2010)	Ruscello, Cartwright, Haynes & Schuster (1993)	Ib
2 Interventions based on complexity	16	Baker & Williams (2010)	Mota, Keske-Soares, Bagetti, Ceron & Melo Filha (2007)	IIb
3 Cycles	8	Prezas & Hodson (2010)	Mota et al. (2007)	IIa
4 Morphosyntax intervention for concomitant phonological and morphosyntax difficulties	6	Tyler & Haskill (2010)	Tyler, Lewis, Haskill & Tolbert (2003)	Ib
5 Core vocabulary	6	Dodd, Holm, Crosbie & McIntosh (2010)	Crosbie, Holm & Dodd (2005)	IIb
6 Traditional articulation therapy	6	Secord (1989)	Pamplona, Ysunza & Espinosa (1999)	Ib
7 Modified cycles	6	Almost & Rosenbaum (1998)	Almost & Rosenbaum (1998)	Ib

For the purposes of this chapter, let's somewhat arbitrarily[1] consider only the top seven of those approaches. These are those approaches scrutinized in 6 or more studies. Even after allowing for the objection that the studies in question used a variety of designs of higher and lower quality; in my view, these seven approaches warrant the attention of practicing

[1] I wanted to choose a relatively small number of approaches to examine, and these were associated with the largest number of studies. The next most-studied approaches (n = 3) had been the subject of only 4 studies each.

clinicians responding to the EBP admonition to look for the "best evidence." They are listed in Table 21.2, along with one or more sources that provide a detailed description of the specific procedures associated with that intervention.

By identifying their review as a "narrative" review, Baker and McLeod were acknowledging that it fell at a level of evidence below what might be considered the best in some ideal sense. However, two aspects of the theory of EBP (Dollaghan, 2007) cause me to champion this review: the first is the idea that empirical evidence must be *relevant* to the clinical question being posed, and the second is that, to be truly relevant, the evidence must interact with another core component in EBP—clinical expertise. Unquestionably, the work by Law et al. (2004; 2010) has paramount relevance for questions of basic efficacy that may be key to defending the value of our professional role for children with SSDs and to alerting researchers to gaping holes in the research literature. However, it seems to have less to say to practicing clinicians who find themselves stretched across those "holes" on a daily basis and who may conclude that all options are equally good because they are equally flawed. In contrast, Baker and McLeod (2011) not only identify a small cohort of interventions that, when compared to many others, are being aggressively studied and are consequently backed by at least some empirical evidence, they also identify weaknesses in the evidence so that clinicians remain suitably alert to their own responsibilities. Thus, their work represents a more clinician-friendly point of entry into EBP.

As a first step, my colleagues and I (McCauley, Williams & McLeod, 2010) have recommended that clinicians consider identifying a well-supported intervention to use, work to become expert at it (in order to maximize the effects they obtain), then expand their expertise to include another well-supported intervention. Based on that idea, the seven interventions listed in Table 21.2 might be entertained as candidates. Thus, they might be considered either for adoption, if the clinician is currently not using any of them, or for re-examination, if the clinician already uses them, but wants to consider revising their implementation or increasing his or her expertise in them based on recent findings.

WHAT CLINICIANS BRING TO THE TABLE

As those choosing, administering, trouble-shooting, and deciding when to end or change interventions, clinicians serve at the front lines of effective treatment and thus provide a critical, last link in the demonstration of treatment effectiveness. This critical role is true regardless of whether the treatment effectiveness concerns the treatment of a specific child, the application of a particular treatment approach across children, or the therapeutic enterprise as a whole. Thus, in a metaphoric sense, what clinicians "bring to the table" of intervention effectiveness is the very "table" itself. The way clinicians practice impacts treatment effectiveness on a daily basis, and the clinicians' tracking of a child's progress during a given treatment serves as a critical, if undervalued, type of efficacy evidence. Both of these aspects of clinicians' contributions to treatment effectiveness will be described below. Figure 21.3 is a schematic of this concept.

Despite a large literature espousing a very large role for research evidence in clinical practice under the auspices of EBP (e.g., Baker & McLeod, 2011; Dollaghan, 2007; Gillam & Gillam, 2006; Johnson, 2006) and an increasing availability of resources intended to facilitate clinician's adoption of that perspective[2], relatively little is known about how clinicians actually practice. Given the large number of children treated for SSDs, the absence of practice information in this area is particularly problematic to the field. A relatively recent pair of research studies (Joffe & Pring, 2008; Lancaster, Keusch, Levin, Pring & Martin, 2010) illustrates the kind of evidence that is beginning to be collected related to SSD treatment and that may benefit from using actual practice patterns as a beginning point.

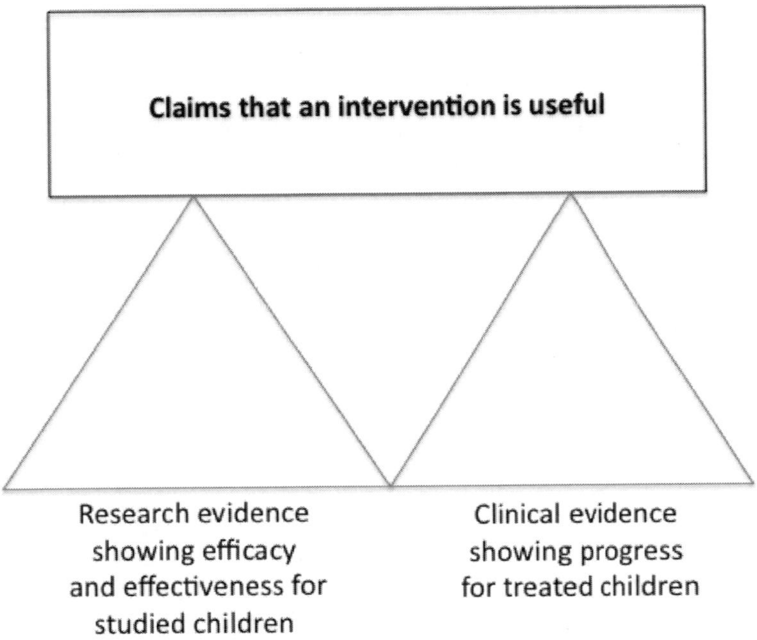

Figure 21.3. Clinical and research evidence as the foundations for demonstrating that a treatment works.

In 2008, Joffe and Pring reported on findings obtained from 98 clinicians in the UK that were surveyed about their work with children with phonological disorders. About 44% of the respondents indicated that more than 40% of their case-load consisted of such children, and all worked with pre-school or primary school children. Choosing from a list of 14 interventions provided by the authors, respondents identified four approaches they used often or always: auditory discrimination, meaningful minimal contrast, phonological awareness and parental involvement. In contrast, they reported rarely using maximal contrast therapy, Cycles, core vocabulary, auditory bombardment and a whole-language approach. The respondents also reported that they often combined interventions, producing what might be termed as an "eclectic approach" to SSD treatment.

In order to examine actual practice patterns, such as the use of an eclectic approach reported in Joffe and Pring (2008), Lancaster, et al. (2010) conducted two small studies, only the first of which will be described here. In that study, Lancaster et al. compared outcomes for 12 preschoolers whom they described as having phonological problems, randomly assigned to

---

[2] Particularly valuable websites for clinicians seeking relevant and pre-appraised research include the American Speech-Language-Hearing Association's Compendium of Systematic Reviews and clinical practice guidelines (http://www.asha.org/members/ebp/compendium) as well as SpeechBITE, a database developed by the University of Sydney and Speech pathology Australia (http://www.speechbite.com).

two experimental groups. The participants' errors were analyzed in terms of speech sounds accuracy; phonological processes were not assessed. The initial-treatment group received an eclectic intervention conducted by clinicians in 8 weekly, 1/2 hour sessions using their typical practice patterns, which reportedly combined listening, phonological awareness, and production tasks similar to those that were most popular in the Joffe and Pring (2008) study. A second, delayed -intervention group was first placed on a waiting list, then treated in the same manner as the initial intervention group after that group had ended treatment. When group performances were examined at 3 points in time, each group showed statistically significant reductions in severity that coincided with the end of the period in which that group received treatment. For reasons not further discussed in that study, the gains were slightly larger in the initial -treatment group compared to the delayed -treatment group.

Although noting the preliminary nature of their study, Lancaster et al. (2010) interpreted their findings as suggesting the potential effectiveness of eclectic approaches, at least as implemented by the practitioners who provided therapy in their study. Those researchers also noted that the intensity of sessions included in their study (1/2 hour per week for 8 weeks) more closely approximated the practice circumstances of most therapists who serve children with SSDs, providing additional support for aspects of clinical practice that may actually prevail in most of the environments in which children with SSDs are served.

Earlier in this section, I introduced these two studies (Joffe & Pring, 2008: Lancaster, et al., 2010) by suggesting that they represent another avenue for pursuing evidence of therapy, one that proceeds from the point of view of what clinicians actually do. Related research endeavors designed to determine how to "scale up" interventions that have been found to be effective at the level of at least some practitioners to a broader range of adopting clinicians has been underway for some time in the area of early literacy practices (e.g., Justice, 2010). However, to my knowledge, this kind of research has yet to be undertaken in the area of speech sound disorders. Both types of research take the demands under which clinicians practice seriously; therefore, both may help promote the best possible interventions for children with SSDs.

One final starting point for thinking about demonstrations and improvements in treatment effectiveness--clinical documentation of treatment effects---resides at the level of the individual clinician-client dyad. Specifically, it consists of the methods clinicians use to examine changes in their client's progress (McCauley, 2001). Even before demands for excellence were framed in terms of EBP, clinicians examined children's progress in treatment to guide their decision-making about advancing from one step of an intervention to the next, moving from one target to others (Bain & Dollaghan, 1991; Glaspey & Stoel-Gammon, 2007; Olswang & Bain, 1985, 1994), or dismissing the child from treatment altogether (e.g., Eger, Chabon, Mient, & Cushman, 1986). Thus, honing skills in the use of standardized norm-referenced and criterion-referenced measures represents yet another way in which clinicians can help insure the best possible outcomes for children with SSDs.

CONNECTIONS

In this chapter, aspects of treatment effectiveness were considered as a means for arguing that the strongest evidence documenting the effectiveness of individual treatments is obtained using data from both clinical practice as well as research. As noted in other chapters in this book, many treatment approaches are specifically designed for certain subgroups of children with SSDs, with the expectation that considering children's specific needs should result in the best treatment outcomes. Chapter 15 describes various ways of classifying children with speech difficulties into more or less discrete subgroups and suggests new and data-driven approaches to disorder subtyping. Chapter 20 shows how insights gained from a comprehensive assessment can flow into the decision making process regarding treatment selection, and Chapter 22 shows how the selected treatment approach is translated into clinical practice as goals and objectives are formulated and treatment sessions are planned. In a relatively new book on interventions for speech sound disorders in children (Williams, McLeod & McCauley, 2010), 23 treatment approaches for children with SSDs are described in a manner intended to emphasize both research evidence and the steps clinicians can take to provide relevant clinical evidence. Being mindful of the mandates of evidence-based practice, including the integration of clinical and research evidence, is a crucial strategy clinicians and their clients can benefit from throughout the clinical decision making process.

Concluding Remarks

In this brief chapter, quite a few beginning points for examining what works in therapy for SSDs were identified as relevant to demonstrating and improving outcomes for children with SSDs: among them, intervention-focused research, clinical practice research, and each clinician's own clinical documentation of treatment effects for individual children with an SSD. Given the ubiquity of calls for external evidence in the speech-language pathology discussions from the last couple of decades, intervention-focused efficacy research has tended to overshadow equally important partners to the EBP enterprise--clinical judgment and client perspectives. Emerging and future efforts to strengthen voices associated with these under-represented perspectives will undoubtedly lead to greater balance as this enterprise proceeds onward.

Chapter Review Questions

1. Compare and contrast differences in perspective and purpose associated with research appraisal of interventions versus clinical documentation of treatment effects.
2. How do studies designed to examine intervention efficacy differ from those
3. designed to examine intervention effectiveness?
4. Name three ways in which the intervention conducted by Lancaster et al. differed from more typically studied interventions?
5. How are clinicians typically advised to demonstrate adherence to the principles of evidence-based practice?
6. How does use of the International Classification of Functions, Disability, and Health: Child and Youth Edition (ICF-CY; WHO, 2007) affect researchers' and clinicians' perspectives on treatment effects?

SUGGESTIONS FOR FURTHER READING

Baker, E., & McLeod, S. (2011a). Evidence based practice for children with speech sound disorders: Part 1 Narrative review. *Language, Speech, and Hearing Research in Schools,* 42, 102-139.

Fey, M.E., & Finestack, L.H. (2009). Research and development in child language intervention: A 5-phase model. In R.G. Schwartz (Ed.), *Handbook of child language disorders* (pp. 513-529). New York, NY: Psychology Press.

Joffe, V., & Pring, T. (2008). Children with phonological problems: A survey of clinical practice. *International Journal of Language and Communication Disorders,* 43, 154–164.

Lancaster, G., Keusch, S., Levin, A., Pring, T., & Martin, S. (2010). Treatment of children with phonological problems: Does an eclectic approach to therapy work? *International Journal of Language and Communication Disorders,* 45(2), 174-181.

McCormack, J., McLeod, S., McAllister, L., & Harrison, L.J. (2009). A systematic review of the association between childhood speech impairment and participation across the lifespan. *International Journal of Speech-Language Pathology,* 11(2), 155-170.

Williams, L., McLeod, S. & McCauley, R. (2010). *Interventions for speech sound disorders in children.* Baltimore, MD: Paul H. Brookes Publishing Company.

SUGGESTIONS FOR STUDENT ACTIVITIES

1. **Clinicians and their access and use of research evidence**. Identify one or more speech-language pathologists who work with children with SSDs. Talk to them about the general, as well as specific methods, they use to "keep up" with research evidence. To gain more information about the specific methods thy use, ask them tell you about (a) a time they believed they were successful in this process and the outcomes associated with its use as well as, and (b) a time when they had a specific question in mind for which they could not find relevant evidence. Finally, use electronic resources identified in this chapter to obtain further information about the question they had posed that had not yielded research evidence in order to determine whether new evidence on the topic is available.
2. **Clinicians and their personal documentation of treatment effects**. Identify a practicing clinician who regularly works with children with SSDs. Without asking the clinician to break confidentiality, have her or him tell you about all the data collected to help make decisions about treatment progress for two clients--one who has a more severe SSD and one whose SSD is more mild or moderate. Consider whether this data provides a full and complete picture of the types of impacts that might be obtained during SSD treatment.

Answers to Chapter Review Questions

1. Compare and contrast differences in perspective and purpose associated with research appraisal of interventions versus clinical documentation of treatment effects.

Both methods seek to examine what helps children with speech sound disorders. Research appraisals of interventions are usually conducted by researchers and focus on external research evidence and findings involving many children. In contrast, clinical documentation of treatment effects are conducted by individual clinicians focusing on data they collect for a single child.

2. How do studies designed to examine intervention efficacy differ from those designed to examine intervention effectiveness?

Whereas efficacy studies are designed to study interventions under ideal or laboratory conditions, effectiveness studies are designed to study interventions under more typical conditions using practitioners, intensity, settings, and stimuli more like those that will be used when an intervention is widely adopted. Because of these differences, efficacy studies allow researchers to make stronger claims about why treatment outcomes were obtained (especially that they were due to treatment) whereas effectiveness studies provide stronger evidence that an intervention is feasible.

3. Name three ways in which the intervention conducted by Lancaster et al. differed from more typically studied interventions?

Unlike most intervention studies, Lancaster et al. had clinicians use the eclectic methods they usually used, intervention was administered less intensively, and the treating clinicians were not experts, but members of the local speech therapy community.

4. How are clinicians typically advised to demonstrate adherence to the principles of evidence-based practice?

They are usually advised to conduct a topic appraisal, a multi-step process in which one prepares a specific clinical question, seeks relevant research to answer the question, appraises the quality and relevance of that research, then considers the results in light of clinical opinion and their clients' values.

5. How does use of the International Classification of Functions, Disability, and Health: Child and Youth Edition (ICF-CY; WHO, 2007) affect researchers' and clinicians' perspectives on treatment effects?

The ICF-CY encourages attention to the broader social effects associated with SSDs, such as how having an SSD affects children's access to learning and social experiences that comprise crucial aspects of their well-being.

References

Almost, D. & Rosenbaum, P. (1998). Effectiveness of speech intervention for phonological disorders: a randomized controlled trial. *Developmental Medicine and Child Neurology,* 40(5), 319-325.

American Speech-Language-Hearing Association (2004). Evidence-based practice in communication disorders: An introduction [Technical report]. Retrieved from *www.asha.org/policy.*

American Speech-Language-Hearing Association. (2010). *Schools Survey report: SLP caseload characteristics trends 1995–2010.* Available from www.asha.org.

Bain, B.A., & Dollaghan, C.A. (1991). Treatment efficacy: The notion of clinically significant change. *Language, Speech, and Hearing Services in Schools,* 22(4), 264-270.

Baker, E. (2010). Minimal pair intervention. In A.L. Williams, S. McLeod, & R. J. McCauley (Eds.), *Interventions for speech sound disorders in children* (pp. 41-72). Baltimore, MD: Paul H. Brookes Publishing, Co.

Baker, E., & McLeod, S. (2011). Evidence based practice for children with speech sound disorders: Part 1 Narrative review. *Language, Speech, and Hearing Research in Schools,* 42, 102-139.

Baker, E. & Williams, A.L. (2010). Minimal pair intervention. In A.L. Williams, S. McLeod, & R. J. McCauley (Eds.), *Interventions for speech sound disorders in children* (pp. 95-116). Baltimore, MD: Paul H. Brookes Publishing, Co.

Broomfield, J., & Dodd, B. (2004). Children with speech and language disability: Caseload characteristics. *International Journal of Language and Communinciation Disorders,* 39(3), 303-324.

Crosbie, S., Holm, A., & Dodd, B. (2005). Intervention for children with severe speech disorder: A comparison of two approaches. *International Journal of Language and Communication Disorders,* 40(4), 467-491.

Crosbie, S., Pine, C., Holm, A., & Dodd, B. (2006). Treating Jarrod: A core vocabulary approach. *Advances in Speech-Language Pathology,* 8(3), 316-321.

Dollaghan, C.A. (2007). *The handbook for evidence-based practice in communication disorders.* Baltimore: Paul H. Brookes Publishing Company.

Dodd, B., Holm, A., Crosbie, S., & McIntosh, B. (2010) Core vocabulary intervention. In A.L. Williams, S. McLeod, & R. J. McCauley (Eds.), *Interventions for speech sound disorders in children* (pp. 117-136). Baltimore, MD: Paul H. Brookes Publishing, Co.

Eger, D.L., Chabon, S.S., Mient, M.G. & Cushman, B.B. (1986). When is enough enough? *ASHA,* 28 (5), 23-25.

Felsenfeld, S., Broen, P. A., & McGue, M. (1992). A 28-year follow-up of adults with a history of moderate phonological disorder: Linguistic and personality results. *Journal of Speech and Hearing Research,* 35, 1114–1125.

Fey, M.E., & Finestack, L.H. (2009). Research and development in child language intervention: A 5-phase model. In R.G. Schwartz (Ed.), *Handbook of child language disorders* (pp. 513-529). New York, NY: Psychology Press.

Gillam, S.L., & Gillam, R.B. (2006). Making evidence-based decisions about language intervention services for children. *Language, Speech, and Hearing Services in Schools,* 37, 304-315.

Glaspey, A., & Stoel-Gammon, C. (2007). A dynamic approach to phonological assessment. *Advances in Speech-Language Pathology,* 9(4), 286-296.

Hall, B.J.C. (1991). Attitudes of fourth and sixth graders toward peers with mild articulation disorders. *Language, Speech, and Hearing Services in Schools,* 22, 334-340.

Joffe, V., & Pring, T. (2008). Children with phonological problems: A survey of clinical practice. *International Journal of Language and Communication Disorders,* 43, 154–164.

Johnson, C.J. (2006). Getting started in evidence-based practice for childhood speech-language disorders, *American Journal of Speech-Language Pathology,* 15, 20-35.

Johnston, J. (2005). Re: Law, Garrett, and Nye (2004a): "The efficacy of treatment for children with developmental speech and language delay/disorder: A meta-analysis" . *Journal of Speech, Language, and Hearing Research, 48*, 1114-1117.

Justice, L. (2010). When craft and science collide: Improve therapeutic practices in schools through evidence-based innovations. *International Journal of Speech-Language Pathology,*

Keilmann, A., Braun, L. & Napiontek, L., (2004). Emotional satisfaction of parents and speech–language therapists with outcome of training intervention in children with speech and language disorders. *Folia Phoniatrica et Logopaedica,* 56, 51–61.

Lancaster, G., Keusch, S., Levin, A., Pring, T., & Martin, S. (2010). Treatment of children with phonological problems: Does an eclectic approach to therapy work? *International Journal of Language and Communication Disorders,* 45(2), 174-181.

Law, J. (2004). The implications of different approaches to evaluating intervention: Evidence from the study of language delay/disorder. *Folia Phoniatrica et Logopaedica,* 56, 199-219.

Law, J., Boye, J., Harris, F., Harkness, A. & Nye, C. (2000). Prevalence and natural history of primary speech and language delay: Findings from a systematic review of the literature. *International Journal of Language and Communication Disorders,* 35(2), 165-188.

Law, J., Garrett, Z. & Nye, C. (2004). The efficacy of treatment for children with developmental speech and language delay/disorder: a meta-analysis. *Journal of Speech, Language, and Hearing Research,* 47, 924-943.

Law, J., Garrett, Z., & Nye, C. (2005). The specificity of a review is the key to its value: A response to Johnston (2005). *Journal of Speech, Language, and Hearing Research,* 48, 1118-1120.

Law, J., Garrett, Z., & Nye, C., (2010). *Speech and language therapy interventions for children with primary speech and language delay or disorder.* The Cochran Library 2010, Issue 5 (Oxford: John Wiley & Sons, Ltd.).

McCauley, R.J. (2001). *Assessment of language disorders in children.* Mahwah, NJ: Lawrence Erlbaum Associates.

McCauley, R.J. & Hargrove, P. (2004). A clinician's introduction to systematic reviews in communication disorders: The course review paper with muscle. *Contemporary Issues in Communication Science and Disorders,* 31, 173-181.

McCauley, R.J., Williams, L., & McLeod, S. (2010). Interventions for children with speech sound disorders: Future directions. In L. Williams, S. McLeod, & R.J. McCauley, (Eds.), *Interventions for speech sound disorders in children* (pp. 601-614). Baltimore, MD: Paul H. Brookes Publishing Co., Inc.

McLeod, S. (2006). The holistic view of a child with unintelligible speech: Insights from the ICF and ICF-CY. *Advances in Speech-Language Pathology,* 8(3), 75-81.

McLeod, S. & Bleile, K. (2004). The ICF: a framework for setting goals for children with speech impairment. *Child Language Teaching and Therapy,* 20(3), 199-219

McCormack, J., McLeod, S., McAllister, L., & Harrison, L.J. (2009). A systematic review of the association between childhood speech impairment and participation across the lifespan. *International Journal of Speech-Language Pathology,* 11(2), 155-170.

McKinnon, D.H., McLeod, S. & Reilly, S. (2007). The prevalence of stuttering, voice, and speech-sound disorders in primary school students in Australia. *Language, speech, and hearing services in schools,* 38(1), 5-15.

Meline, T., & Paradiso, T. (2003). Evidence-based practice in schools: Evaluating research and reducing barriers. *Language, Speech, and Hearing Services in Schools,* 34, 273-283.

Mota, H. B., Keske-Soares, M., Bagetti, T., Ceron, M. I., & Melo Filha, M. G. C. (2007). Análise comparativa da eficiência de três diferentes modelos de terapia fonológica [Comparative analyses of the effectiveness of three different phonological therapy models]. *Pró-Fono Revista de Atualização Cientifica,* 19(1), 67–7.

National Institute on Deafness and Communication Disorders. (1994*). National strategic research plan.* Bethesda, MD: Department of Health and Human Services.

Olswang, C. (1997). Chapter 6. Treatment efficacy research. In C. Frattali, (Ed.), *Measuring treatment outcomes in speech-language pathology* (pp.134-150). New York: Thieme.

Olswang, L., & Bain, B.A. (1985). Monitoring phoneme acquisition for making treatment withdrawal decisions. *Applied Psycholinguistics,* 6(1) , 17-37.

Olswang, L., & Bain, B. (1994). Data collection: Monitoring children's treatment progress. *American Journal of Speech Language Pathology,* 3(3), 55 – 66.

Pamplona, M., Ysunza A., & Espinosa, J. (1999). A comparative trial of two modalities of speech intervention for compensatory articulation in cleft palate children, phonologic approach versus articulatory approach. *International Journal of Pediatric Otorhinolaryngology,* 49(1), 21-26.

Prezas, R.F., & Hodson, B.W. (2010). The Cycles phonological remediation approach. In A.L. Williams, S. McLeod, & R. J. McCauley (Eds.), *Interventions for speech sound disorders in children* (pp. 137-158). Baltimore, MD: Paul H. Brookes Publishing, Co.

Robey, R.R. & Schultz, M.C. (1998). A model for conducting clinical outcome research: An adaptation of the standard protocol for use in aphasiology. *Aphasiology,* 12, 87-810.

Ruscello, D.M., Cartwright, K.R., Haines, K.B. & Schuster, L.I. (1993). The use of different service delivery models for children with phonological disorders. *Journal of Communication Disorders,* 26(3), 193-203.

Sackett, D. L., Richardson, W. S., Rosenberg, W., & Haynes, R. B. (1997). *Evidence-based medicine: How to practice and teach EBM.* New York: Churchill Livingstone.

Secord, W., (1989). Chapter 5: The Traditional approach to treatment. In N. Creaghead, P.W. Newman & W. Secord (Eds.), *Assessment and remediation of articulatory and phonological disorders* (pp. 129-158, 2nd ed.). Columbus, OH: Merrill Publishing Company.

Shriberg, L.D., Tomblin, J.B., & McSweeny, J.L. (1999). Prevalence of speech delay in 6-year-old children and comorbidity with language impairment. *Journal of Speech, Language, and Hearing Research,* 42(6), 1461-1481.

Silverman, F.H., & Paulus, P.G. (1989). Peer reactions to teenagers who substitute /w/ for /r/. *Language Speech & Hearing Services in Schools,* 20(2), 219-221.

Teverovsky, E. G., Bickel, J. O., & Feldman, H. M. (2009). Functional characteristics of children diagnosed with childhood apraxia of speech. *Disability and Rehabilitation: An International, Multidisciplinary Journal,* 31(2), 94-102.

Tyler, A.A. (2008). What works: Evidence-based intervention for children with speech sound disorders. *Seminars in Speech and Language,* 29, 320-330.

Tyler, A.A. & Haskill, A.M. (2010). Morphosyntax intervention. In A.L. Williams, S. McLeod, & R. J. McCauley (Eds.), *Interventions for speech sound disorders in children* (pp. 355-380). Baltimore, MD: Paul H. Brookes Publishing, Co.

Tyler, A. A., Lewis, K. E., Haskill, A., & Tolbert, L. C. (2003). Outcomes of different speech and language goal attack strategies. *Journal of Speech, Language, and Hearing Research, 46,* 1077–1094.

Van Riper, C. (1939). *Speech correction: Principles and methods* Englewood Cliffs, NJ: Prentice-Hall.

Williams, A. L., McLeod, S., & McCauley, R.J. (2010). *Interventions for speech sound disorders in children.* Baltimore, MD: Brookes Publishing.

World Health Organization. (2007). ICF-Y: *International classification of functioning, disability and health: Children and youth version.* Geneva: World Health Organization.

Zhang, X. & Tomblin, J.B. (2000). The association of intervention receipt with speech-language profiles and social-demographic variables. *American Journal of Speech-Language Pathology,* 9, 345-357.

Zipoli, R.P., & Kennedy, M. (2005). Evidence-based practice among speech-language pathologists: Attitudes, utilization, and barriers. *American Journal of Speech-Language Pathology,* 14, 208-220.

In: Comprehensive Perspectives …
Editors: Beate Peter and Andrea A. N. MacLeod
ISBN: 978-1-62257-041-6

Chapter 22

TREATMENT DESIGN AND IMPLEMENTATION

Carol M. Ellis and Barbara Williams Hodson

INTRODUCTION

The history of **speech sound disorders** (SSDs) involves a number of prominent individuals with a variety of beliefs and **treatment** approaches. Although numerous professionals have contributed to this body of knowledge, their beliefs and intervention approaches have not always been compatible. Some speech-language pathologists (SLPs) have shifted from "one-phoneme-at-a-time" programs to a "pattern" perspective, but this shift has been far from universal. Present-day treatment approaches reflect diverse thinking and also demonstrate an abundance of treatment options (e.g., McLeod, 2006; Williams, McLeod, & McCauley, 2010).

The major purposes of this chapter include providing present and future SLPs with basic background information regarding treatment options for children with SSDs, helping them identify major factors to consider when designing a course of treatment, and implementation considerations that support optimal treatment plans. The chapter is divided into five sections: (a) a discussion of major intervention settings, (b) a review of assessment needs/options to consider before treatment begins, (c) a review of current treatment options/approaches, (d) considerations for designing an appropriate treatment, and (e) a discussion of treatment implementation. After reading this chapter, present and future SLPs will have the knowledge to complete more thorough assessments of SSDs, make more informed choices regarding assessment instruments, and understand theories and procedures for a number of treatment options that are currently available. Additionally, students will be better prepared to design and implement an individualized program tailored to optimally meet the needs of their individual clients.

INTERVENTION SETTINGS

SLP services are provided in a variety of settings, including: public schools, private schools, university clinics, hospitals, regular and special preschools (e.g., Head Start), rehabilitation centers, and private providers. Because settings often influence aspects of treatment design and implementation, we begin with a brief overview of some of these settings.

Many children with SSDs receive speech services in the public schools. Federal legislation in the United States (PL 94-142), also called Individuals with Disabilities Act (IDEA), requires local educational agencies (i.e., schools) to provide students who are between the ages of 3 and 21 years with free and appropriate education. The implementation of this law is accomplished through the Individualized Educational Plans (IEPs) that address each student's particular educational needs, including speech and/or language services. Schools are responsible for speech-language services for students both in public and private schools as well as home-schooled children. Services for preschoolers commonly occur in a preschool classroom setting. Sometimes children are transported to a nearby school to receive services; some children receive services in their home. The frequency and duration of treatment depends on many factors such as the severity of the child's needs; sometimes, however, these decisions depend on the physical location of schools, as well as available treatment space, along with numerous other scenarios. Most public school treatment services in the US are provided two times a week in groups for 20-30 minutes.

Federal legislation also provides for children under 3 years of age, who are served through birth-to-three programs. The settings in which services are provided include the child's home, community-based facilities, and birth-to-three centers. The child's family plays an important role in this service delivery model, and the treatment plan is aptly referred to as an Individual Family Service Plan.

University-based, speech-language services commonly occur in speech-language-hearing clinics. Children usually receive services in client treatment rooms that have two-way mirrors and television monitors for observations by clinical supervisors and/or parents. The services are provided by graduate students majoring in speech-language pathology with direct supervision by licensed/certified SLPs.

Hospital speech-language services are provided in a variety of settings. The treatment might occur in the patient's room, in a rehabilitation unit at the hospital, or through home health services. Hospital services are usually more intense than in the schools. For example, they may occur as often as twice a day. Services typically are "ordered" by a physician and carried out by an SLP.

The location of services in other settings (e.g., services from private practice SLPs) depends on the particular situation. For example, SLPs may go to an individual's home to provide speech-language services or they may have their own private office in a separate building. Consequently, speech-language services occur in a variety of settings, and, moreover, treatment frequency and duration vary considerably.

For children who qualify for services in the public schools and birth-to-three programs, service expenses are covered with federal, state, and local funding or by Medicaid in some cases. Some health insurances cover expenses for services provided at hospitals, university clinics, and by SLPs in private practice. Some parents who elect to obtain SLP services in addition to, or instead of, publicly provided services or whose children do not qualify for publicly provided services pay for SLP services out-of-pocket if insurance coverage is not available.

BEFORE TREATMENT BEGINS

Assessment Information Needed. Before any decisions about treatment can be made, primary information needs to be gathered and reviewed. During the diagnostic evaluation, the following basic goals need to be considered: (a) whether there actually is a communication disorder; (b) if so, how severe (e.g., mild, moderate, severe, profound) the disorder/impairment is; (c) possible etiological factors (e.g., hearing loss); (d) prognosis for improvement; and (e) possible direction(s) for intervention. A thorough diagnostic evaluation for a child with highly unintelligible speech includes consideration of: (a) background information, (b) hearing, (c) language, (d) oral mechanism, (e) speech productions, and (f) metaphonological awareness (Hodson, 2010; also see Chapter 20 for further information about the diagnostic process).

The phonological evaluation portion needs to include an assessment of abilities/skills necessary for phonological acquisition (e.g., auditory perceptual, cognitive, phonological, neuromotor), and the results need to be integrated with other evaluation results. In addition, a complete description of a child's productions needs to be obtained through relational and/or independent analyses in cases of children with highly unintelligible speech. These analyses need to provide an in-depth picture of children's speech skills so that appropriate treatment goals can be identified (Stoel-Gammon & Dunn, 1985).

Speech samples may be collected through: (a) continuous speech samples, (b) single word productions (e.g., naming pictures, photos, objects), (c) sentence imitation, and/or (d) oral reading (for school-age children). Samples can be obtained spontaneously, by direct imitation, or by delayed imitation depending on the child's ability level and the examiner's purpose. Shriberg and Kwiatkowski (1980) require that a continuous-speech sample be obtained and analyzed. Stoel-Gammon and Dunn (1985) noted some problems with this requirement, observing that (a) continuous-speech samples are more time-consuming than single-word samples, (b) unintelligible words cannot be analyzed, and (c) the range of phonemes attempted may be narrower. Another factor is that some children are not able (or willing) to provide continuous-speech samples. Nonetheless, continuous speech samples should be recorded and saved whenever possible. They are extremely valuable for comparisons of phonological systems over time even if the initial recordings could not be understood.

Regardless of the methods used to assess phonological systems, an inclusive speech assessment must yield: (a) phonological strengths and weaknesses (e.g., phonetic/phonemic and phonotactic inventories, phonological deviations), (b) a severity rating, (c) intervention targets for treatment, (d) baseline measures for documenting progress, and (e) stimulability information regarding possible targets (Hodson, 2010). This information is needed for the development of appropriate treatment goals and to monitor the effectiveness of treatment. In addition, potential effects of the disorder on the child's social, emotional, and/or educational development needs to be documented for qualification purposes for school services if needed.

Assessment Options. The selection of assessment instruments used to evaluate a child's speech skills is dependent on the severity of the speech difficulty and the investigator's concerns about the child's particular need areas. For example, if the child only has a few phonemes in error, phoneme-oriented "articulation" tools (e.g., Goldman-Fristoe Test of Articulation; Goldman & Fristoe, 2000) are considered appropriate for assessing productions of individual phonemes. These types of errors, however, are scored as totally correct or totally incorrect (i.e., no differentiation for Omissions, Substitutions, and Distortions in the final scores) (Prezas & Hodson, 2010). The information gained from these assessments usually leads to an intervention focus of working on one sound at a time until a pre-specified criterion (e.g., 90%) is reached for each phoneme from isolation to conversation. The typical goal of phoneme-oriented treatment is the correct production of individual phonemes through an **articulation hierarchy** progression (Strattman, 2010).

In addition to phoneme-oriented assessments, SLPs often rely on phoneme acquisition normative data to determine what sounds are acquired by what ages; however, these studies are fraught with inconsistencies (e.g., different methodologies, different sound mastery criteria, differences in scoring of allophonic variations). A specific example of these differences is demonstrated by the Templin (1957) study and the Smit, Hand, Freilinger, Bernthal, and Bird (1990) study. Templin (1957) claimed that /ɹ/ and /s/ are acquired by 4 years of age; Smit et al. (1990), however, reported that these sounds are not acquired until 8 years of age. If traditional speech sound norms are used, it is recommended that they be referred to in a more general categorical manner (e.g., nasals, stops, and glides acquired first). See Chapter 6 for additional details on inconsistent estimates on the age of acquisition of English speech sounds and Chapter 9 for similar inconsistencies in other languages.

If a child has severe/profound speech difficulties, phonologically based assessment instruments (e.g., Hodson Assessment of Phonological Patterns-3rd Edition; Hodson, 2004) can differentiate patterns of errors (e.g., omissions, consonant category deficiencies, substitutions, assimilations). The information obtained from these tests usually leads to an intervention focus of targeting patterns to improve many sounds simultaneously. The goal of a phonologically orientated treatment is to improve speech **intelligibility** as expeditiously as possible rather than perfecting each and every individual phoneme to a criterion. If the disorder appears to be severe, all input and output speech processes (e.g., speech perception, motor programming) need to be considered (e.g., psycholinguistic framework; Stackhouse & Wells, 1997). In addition, if a child continues to have speech intelligibility issues beyond the age of 5;6 (years; months), future literacy skills are likely to be at risk (Bishop & Adams, 1990). Thus, metaphonological awareness skills also need to be evaluated and enhanced.

Once all relevant types of information have been collected, analyses and syntheses lead to a diagnostic conclusion regarding the presence and relative severity of the disorder and, additionally, the nature of the observed deficits. For more information about the diagnostic process see Chapter 20.

Major Treatment Options/Approaches

After a thorough speech evaluation has been completed and the unique needs of an individual child have been identified, the SLP needs to determine what intervention strategies to use and optimal goals for treatment. A major challenge for the SLP at this point is the extensive list of intervention strategies, techniques, and methods for children with an SSD. The task of selecting the optimal approach can be overwhelming. Additionally, this list continues to grow as clinical researchers investigate new techniques and as new clinical applications are developed and refined. Williams, McLeod, and McCauley (2010) provide an extensive description of treatment options, along with information about published evidence of efficacy. Before a decision can be made about which treatment approach is most appropriate, a clinician needs adequate background knowledge associated with the important features of various intervention approaches. A brief theoretical background and description of some current treatment options is presented next. For more information about the history of speech-language pathology, see Chapter 1 of this book. Treatment efficacy evidence is the topic of Chapter 21 in this volume.

Phoneme-Oriented. Several early techniques paved the way for phoneme-oriented approaches. These techniques were described in the 1920s when our profession began to grow at a fast pace due to scientific publications about speech disorders and as universities began to offer courses of study pertaining to the treatment of speech disorders (Paden, 1970). One prominent professional in the early years was May Scripture, who was best known for her 1927 publication, *A Manual of Exercises for the Correction of Speech Disorders,* which was co-authored by Eugene Jackson. Their method, which emphasized placement of the articulators and modification of the airstream, was referred to as "Phonetic Placement." The production of individual speech sounds was demonstrated and described, and visuals such as mirrors or diagrams were used when needed to show placement. The emphasis was on correcting speech errors one sound at a time.

The "Moto-Kinesthetic Method" was another of the early techniques. Sara Stinchfield (who obtained the first Doctor of Philosophy degree in speech "correction" in 1921) gained national recognition for her 1938 book, *Children with Delayed or Defective Speech* (co-authored by Edna Hill Young). Their emphasis was the idea that speech is dynamic, not static (Duchan, 2008b). These investigators believed that speech was a motoric process that involved shaping the exhaled air as it passes through the oral or nasal cavities with an association being made between articulatory movement for a sound and speech output. Although sounds were regarded as dynamic, they were still regarded as single sounds in treatment.

The "Stimulus" approach contributed an "organizational frame" for the development of phoneme-oriented approaches. In 1934, Charles Van Riper published the book, *Speech Correction: Principles and Methods,* which became a "classic" that was followed by eight revised editions. His method, which is often referred to as the "traditional" approach, still serves as the basis for most SLPs today. Van Riper purported that time must be taken for "ear training" prior to the production practice of speech sounds and that each sound must first be clearly produced in isolation before proceeding to higher levels. The five steps of his approach include: (a) sensory-perceptual training, (b) sound elicitation, (c) sound production, (d) transfer, and (e) maintenance. Van Riper's "articulation hierarchy" consists of establishing a targeted phoneme (a) first in isolation; (b) then in syllables, (c) words, (d) phrases, (e) and sentences; and finally, (f) in conversation.

Harris Winitz and Betty Bellerose (1962) (known for their "Discrimination Approach") agreed with Van Riper that teaching a child to discriminate between errors and target sounds before production practice was extremely important. In fact, they believed that the ability to hear the difference between the errors and target sounds was the most critical skill in the whole speech remediation process. Winitz and Bellerose, however, started teaching with word contrasts that were quite dissimilar. They purported that gross contrasts would teach children to discriminate more easily than if the sounds were more alike and that finer contrasts could be worked on later in treatment.

The Sensory-Motor Approach by Eugene McDonald (1964) was another approach that opposed the idea of speech sounds being considered static. He believed that speech consists of a sequence of syllable productions rather than separate phonemes. According to McDonald, the productions of sounds vary as they are coarticulated with other sounds. His treatment involved obtaining a heightened awareness of the speech movement patterns (through bisyllable and trisyllable production practice), practicing sound sequences, and varying the phonetic contexts. This approach incorporates coarticulatory contexts of key words that are placed before and after target phonemes in order to elicit correct productions.

In the 1970s, "Behavior Modification" (adopted from psychology theories) became the major treatment method partially because of the Public Law 94-142 which required IEPs. Objectives that specified observable and measurable behaviors were required for writing IEPs for students. SLPs selected target phonemes based on articulation "norms" (e.g., Templin, 1957) and then followed Van Riper's articulation hierarchy from his stimulus approach. The stimulus-response paradigm was used to change behavior; reinforcement schedules were followed to reinforce correct sound productions; and tangible rewards, such as stickers or food, were used for reinforcement. Charting and tracking speech productions determined whether a child would advance to the next level, and advancement was determined by pre-specified criterion levels. Behavior modification solidified the focus of treating single phonemes within an articulation hierarchy.

A need for increasing efficiency in speech improvement prompted the development of the *Multiple Phonemic Approach* (MPA – McCabe & Bradley; 1975). This phoneme-oriented program, which was extremely behavioristic in nature, involved practicing all phonemes at one time, including those that were already produced correctly.

In summary, phoneme-oriented programs have evolved from many different "pieces". These methods incorporate various early techniques (e.g., phonetic placement, moto-kinesthetic) to help a child produce individual sounds in isolation. They borrowed Van Riper's articulation hierarchy as a framework, and phonemes have usually been selected according to a set of developmental norms (although other selection factors are sometimes considered, such as stimulability and utility). Goals of phoneme-oriented programs include correctly producing individual phonemes in isolation, progressing through more complex levels (e.g., words, phrases) to a criterion, eventually carring over the sounds into conversation. The "one phoneme at a time" treatment approach of the 1920s and 1930s prevailed for an extensive period of time and is still prevalent today. Most SLPs still use phoneme-oriented programs as their only intervention choice for all client cases, including children with extensive sound errors and highly unintelligible speech (personal communications).

Sound Contrasts. The classic "Minimal Pair Approach," which involves contrasting two words that differ by only one phoneme, (i.e., **minimal pairs**: "key" vs. "tea"), has been advocated as an effective treatment method for many years (e.g., Fairbanks, 1960). Some SLPs have used minimal word contrasts in treatment to reduce **phonological processes** (Weiner, 1981). According to Bernthal, Bankson, and Flipsen (2009), minimal contrast therapy is the "signature approach" (p. 304) of linguistic-based treatment. Children learn that different sounds signal different meanings in words. The goal of this approach is to facilitate phonological reorganization and restructuring, thereby reducing homonymy.

Gierut (1989) proposed a phonological treatment approach involving "Maximal Oppositions" rather than minimal pairs. Her study involved one boy, age 4:7, with a repaired cleft palate, who demonstrated word-initial consonant deletion (which is somewhat common in the speech of children with repaired cleft palates [e.g., Magnus et al., 2011]). The treatment utilized one maximal opposition contrast involving the multiple features of voice, place, and manner (e.g., "sad" vs. "mad"). The premise was that a heightened saliency of contrasts would increase the "learnability" that would cause extensive phonemic changes. Fey (1992) has challenged this "interesting twist" (p. 280) to the minimal pairs procedure by pointing out that this approach has limited evidence and that treatment is more limited when implementing "contrived" treatment activities than when using the minimal pairs.

The "Multiple Oppositions Approach," was reported by Williams in 2000. She completed a longitudinal study involving 10 children, ages 4 to 6 years, 5 months, who demonstrated moderate-to-profound phonological impairments. According to Williams, the Multiple Oppositions Approach was efficient in expediting changes in the children's phonological systems and was most appropriate for children with severely impaired speech. This approach is similar to the Minimal Contrast Approach; however, instead of using a single contrastive pair, it involves multiple contrastive pairs of the error with several target sounds (e.g., /t/ vs. /k/, /s/, /st/). The goal of this approach is to help children reorganize their sound systems through practice with several different sound targets. A concern regarding this approach is that for a young child with highly unintelligible speech, the number of simultaneous targets may be overwhelming.

Phonology-Oriented Approaches. A shift toward broader entities occurred partially because of early attempts by practitioners to apply linguistic principles to clinical populations. The distinctive feature method was linguistic-based and consisted of a binary classification system that used features to distinguish phonemes from one another across languages. Phonemes were classified according to the presence or absence of distinctive features: (a) voicing, (b) nasality, (c) front production, (d) back production, (e) continuant, and (f) stridency. Later, distinctive features were used to classify sound changes of a child's speech productions. The next step involved writing phonological rules and specifying underlying representations (as presented in "Sound Pattern of English" [Chomsky & Halle, 1968]). One of the limitations of distinctive feature analyses pertained to the fact that substitutions could be analyzed, but not omissions.

David Stampe's theory of Natural Phonology (1969) was also a major influence in this shift. Stampe purported that children are born with an innate system of phonetically motivated "natural phonological processes" and that these processes occur because of physical properties of speech production. The purpose of these processes was to "maximize the perceptual characteristics of speech and minimize its articulatory difficulties" (Stampe, 1972, p. 9). These natural processes, which applied early in speech, were reduced due to limitation (applying in fewer environments), ordering (an order of application), and suppression (prevented from applying at all). The Natural Phonology theory, which used phonological processes to classify children's speech sound errors in a systematic way, helped SLPs look beyond individual phonemes to patterns of deviations. One of the limitations of natural process analyses (e.g. Shriberg & Kwiatkowski, 1980) was that it was restricted to what was "common" for children around the world (e.g., fronting). Children with highly unintelligible speech often demonstrate uncommon deviations (e.g., backing, initial consonant deletion), which could not be categorized under a natural-process analysis system.

Additionally, following the publication of Ingram's book, *Phonological Disability in Children* in 1976, a rapid growth occurred in phonological-process-based assessments and remediation procedures. Edwards (1994) observed that Ingram's book stimulated this rapid growth in two ways. In general, it played a major role in promoting the clinical usefulness of phonology for clinicians; and, moreover, it promoted the idea of phonological "processes."

The *Cycles Phonological Remediation Approach* (Hodson, 2010, 2011) is an example of a phonological pattern-oriented approach that was designed for children with highly unintelligible speech. Research results reported by Almost and Rosenbaum (1998) provided evidence supporting the effectiveness of the **cycles** approach. The cycles approach focuses on facilitating emergence of phonological patterns and provides opportunities for generalization of these patterns to occur within a child's phonological system. It uses cycles (time periods in which all phonological patterns that need intervention are facilitated sequentially and recycled as needed) to develop intelligible speech patterns in children. Phonemes (e.g, word-final /p/, /t/) are utilized to facilitate development of productions of final consonants, which, in turn, facilitate the emergence of phonological patterns (e.g., final "consonantness"). Potential primary patterns include "syllableness," singleton "consonantness" (if omitted in various positions in words), consonants in clusters/sequences, and also consonant categories (velars, stridents, and liquids). Primary patterns are recycled (repeated) as needed during ensuing cycles until each of the patterns emerges in the child's spontaneous speech. Complexity is then increased gradually as the child demonstrates a generalization of primary target patterns. Secondary target patterns include all other consonant clusters/sequences that are deficient (e.g., medial/final /s/ clusters with /s/ inside the words; three-consonant clusters; palatal sibilants, /ɹ/ in all positions).

Some of the goals of the cycles approach are to increase intelligibility by facilitating a reorganization of the child's phonological system and to help children acquire new phonological patterns. The primary goal of this approach is to increase speech intelligibility more expeditiously. A strength that Stoel-Gammon and Dunn (1985) observed is that the approach has innovative ideas for remediation such as the notion of cycles to stimulate sound classes. An additional strength that Bleile (2004) pointed out was that this approach uses a time criterion for changing treatment targets rather than a percentage correct, which aligns with Ingram's concept that phonological acquisition occurs gradually.

The cycles approach aligns most closely with the "Gestural Phonology Theory" (Browman & Goldstein, 1992). Kent (1997) described this theory as having "articulatory organization" at a phonological representation level. The core representations of this theory include both its movements and its gestures; therefore, both articulation and phonology are "meshed" together. The term "gesture" refers to a class of articulatory movements that takes place during "articulatory events." Gestural scores (or constellations) represent movements on different levels or tiers that specify the movements for an utterance (Kent, 1997). The overlap of gestures in time allows for interaction among articulatory, acoustic, linguistic, psychological, and perceptual aspects.

Whole Language. Hoffman, Norris, and Monjure (1990) conducted a comparison study with 4-year-old twin boys, who apparently had minor speech delays. One child completed minimal pair training involving /s/, /l/, and /ɹ/ clusters, and the other child participated in interactive story-telling tasks. The child's task was to tell a story to a puppet while the clinician provided feedback. Hoffman et al. (1990) reported that the child who received whole language treatment improved more than the other twin. Some questions have arisen regarding how well this method would work for children with severe speech sound disorders and also how much influence the twins had on each other's speech.

Metaphonological Awareness. Gillon (2000) investigated the efficacy of an "integrated" phonological awareness intervention approach for children (ages 5-7 years) with both a spoken language impairment and a reading delay. Sixty-one children with spoken language impairments and 30 children with typically developing speech participated in this study. The results indicated that the children who received phonological awareness instruction improved not only their phonological awareness abilities, but also their reading skills as well as their speech sounds. Gillon recommended that intervention should: (a) occur at the phoneme level, (b) include letter-sound knowledge teaching, (c) incorporate phonemic segmentation skills, (d) use manipulatives, (e) use reflection tasks, (f) be direct and carried out in a small group, and (g) occur after a period of general language instruction.

Phonological awareness approaches have also been used to help children discover characteristics of sounds. The "Metaphon Approach" was designed to teach the awareness and skills necessary to improve a child's metaphonological skills; the child focused on the structures used in a language. The approach centered on the feature differences between sounds; consequently, the child would be able to classify sounds by various characteristics such as "long/short" or "front/back." The goals of this approach are consistent with all phonological approaches: to reorganize the speech sound system and improve a child's speech productions. Evidence of the effectiveness of Metaphon therapy was reported by Dean, Howell, Waters, and Reid (1995) who reported 13 case studies of preschool children with phonological disorders between the ages of 3;7 (years; months) and 4;7. The results indicated that the Metaphon approach reduced phonological processes.

Metaphonological awareness activities (e.g., rhyming, syllable segmentation) are also incorporated in each cycles approach session. Children with highly unintelligible speech have been found to have deficiencies in the area of phonological awareness along with later difficulties in decoding and spelling. Thus, enhancing metaphonological skills along with regular treatment helps children who are particularly at risk to develop these early literacy skills.

Nonlinear/Multilinear Applications. In the 1970s, nonlinear theories began to appear in the linguistics literature. Edwards (2007) stated that these theories focused on the hierarchical relationships between linguistic forms such as segments, syllables, and words that occurred on different tiers or levels. Nonlinear theories typically included stress information and segmental information and were shown as branching tree diagrams. The list of nonlinear (also termed multilinear) phonologies is extensive. One example is *Metrical Phonology* (Liberman, 1975; Liberman & Prince, 1977), which extends a hierarchical-based analysis to characteristics such as stress and syllable boundaries. Another example is *Feature Geometry* (Sagey, 1986), which focuses on the features of phonemes and organizes them into hierarchical relationships with some features dominating others. A workbook by Bernhardt and Stemberger (2000) provides methods for nonlinear analyses and also for intervention.

The Optimality Theory (McCarthy & Prince, 1995) is a constraint-based approach that specifies what a child can or cannot produce. "Output constraints" are limits to the possible alternative pronunciations of a word, and "faithfulness constraints" preserve features and prohibit additions and deletions. These two sets of constraints operate in opposition to each other. The most optimal output is the one that preserves the greatest similarity to the true form while violating the least number of output constraints. It is depicted via a "manual indicator," a pointing finger, and it is selected from a set of alternatives produced by the "generator." This selection is carried out by a mechanism called the "evaluator" that uses language-specific constraints to select an optimal alternative from the set produced by the generator. Variations of language output in different languages and by individual children are accounted for by the relative ranking of constraints that are re-ranked as a child matures (Barlow & Gierut, 1999). In the case of a young child or a child with a speech sound disorder, the evaluator selects a form that violates more faithfulness constraints than output constraints, for example, using a reduced consonant cluster if avoidance of clusters is a highly ranked output constraint for this child. As the child's speech output becomes more adult-like, the "no cluster" output constraint receives a lower ranking, and the form selected by the evaluator may now contain clusters.

Additional Theoretical Applications. More recently, two applications have been introduced and discussed in the current literature by Gierut (2007), and Rvachew and Bernhardt (2010). These applications, "Complexity" and "Dynamic Systems," which were derived from a number of concepts, have been applied to clinical treatments for children with speech sound disorders.

Gierut (2007) identified "Complexity" as a potential generalization tool to shorten the length of treatment. During treatment, a complex cluster (e.g., /stɹ/) is typically selected as the first target, with the goal being to obtain a maximum generalization to other phonemes. This application has evolved through the years from concepts such as "Learnability Theory" (Gold, 1967; a developmental psychology theory involving the acquisition of grammar on the basis of exposure to evidence about different languages) and "least phonological knowledge" (two or more phonemes, that are neither **stimulable** nor early developing, are targeted to effect maximum change.) Gierut (2007) explained that the child's early phonological system is a simpler subset of the adult system that expands over time to become more like adult language. This treatment technique has been challenged by others. Rvachew and Nowak (2001) conducted a randomized-control study to investigate the application of the least phonological knowledge in clinical treatment. These researchers treated four phonemes produced by 48 children with moderate or severe phonological disorders. The children were randomly assigned to a traditional (had the most phonological knowledge) treatment group or a nontraditional (had the least phonological knowledge) treatment group. The results of their research indicated that children who targeted nonstimulable, the least phonological knowledge targets, had poorer treatment outcomes. Rvachew and Nowak concluded that clinicians can be confident that earlier targets, for which a child has greater productive phonological knowledge, will be easier for preschoolers to acquire than unstimulable, later-developing phonemes.

Another clinical application has been presented by Rvachew and Bernhardt (2010). Their "Dynamic Systems" concept borrowed ideas from Fogel and Thelen's (1987) "Dynamic Systems Theory" (a psychological theory involving the complexity of the human organism on many different scales). Rvachew and Bernhardt believe that the development of a given behavior (e.g., speech) arises from system interactions among the same underlying components. The components that create stability may also be involved in shifting the system (and cause temporary instability) so that other stable configurations can occur from the shift. Rvachew and Bernhardt (2010) hypothesized that all new behaviors emerge from dynamic interactions among many aspects which may be internal or external to the individual. For example, a child's phonological development could be a product of various internal complex systems that weave together such as the anatomical units (e.g., muscles), neurological units, (e.g., perception), and various external aspects.

Rvachew and Bernhardt (2010) also challenged the use of "complexity" for treatment goals for children with speech sound disorders. They conducted phonological analyses of pre- and post-treatment performances for six children who received contrasting approaches to target selection. Three children received treatment for simple target phonemes (no new feature contrasts were introduced), and the other three children received treatment for complex targets (targets contained feature contrasts that were not in the children's phonological repertoire). Children who received treatment for simple targets made more progress (i.e., acquisition toward the target sounds, emergence of complex untreated segments, feature contrasts). Children who received treatment for complex targets made little gain in their phonological repertoires. Rvachew and Bernhardt concluded that treatment outcomes will be enhanced if the clinician selects treatment targets that form a foundation for the emergence of later complex phoneme contrasts.

Sidebar 22.1 Target Stimulable Sounds or Non-Stimulable Sounds First?

Traditionally, SLPs have targeted sounds that are "stimulable" (e.g., the client is able to produce the sound with various auditory and visual cues when deciding on intervention goals). It has been reported that an "optimal match" is needed to facilitate a child's progress (Hunt, 1961). After the SLP determines a child's current functioning level, intervention begins one step above that so the child experiences both a challenge and success. Some phonologists (e.g., Gierut), however, argue that treatment should target later-acquired, non-stimulable sounds first (e.g., /str/). The hypothesis is that targeting non-stimulable sounds will lead to a greater generalization of non-targeted sounds. Some investigators have challenged this approach (Rvachew & Nowak, 2001). In addition, the operational definition of stimulability may be part of this issue (Hodson, 2010).

Sidebar 22.2 Oral-Motor Exercises?

Oral-motor exercises have been extremely popular in treatment for children with speech sound disorders over the years, even though theoretical and scientific bases have been questioned. In addition, research evidence is lacking to support their use. Lof and Watson (2008) reported that oral-motor exercises simply do not enhance speech sound development. Nevertheless, many clinicians continue to employ a number of devices (e.g., horns, straws, whistles) to treat children with speech sound disorders.

DESIGNING A COURSE OF TREATMENT

Selecting a Treatment Approach. Kamhi (2006) stated that making treatment decisions is not easy. He concluded, after examining phonological intervention studies, that there are too many treatment methods. The differences in procedures, goal attack strategies, and emphases are extensive. The choices are many; the most difficult part is to select the most appropriate approach that will best fit a particular client's needs and has been shown to be effective.

An illustration of treatment designs includes phoneme-oriented approaches on the one end of a continuum for children with mild impairments and pattern-oriented approaches on the other end of the continuum for children with more severe-to-profound impairments (e.g., children with childhood apraxia of speech). A clinician needs to determine approximately where on the "treatment design continuum" a child's performance falls. Also, treatment techniques may change during intervention. For example, a child may begin with a pattern approach to expedite intelligibility gains and then, later, switch to a phoneme-oriented approach to "clean up" single phoneme errors (e.g., /ɹ/).

Additional Considerations. The severity of a child's speech sound disorder sometimes determines the direction that the intervention will take. In present-day treatment, most SLPs utilize Van Riper's articulation hierarchy with a behavioristic overlay to remediate speech sound disorders regardless of the severity of the disorder. As mentioned earlier, this intervention approach involves establishing a target phoneme, first in isolation, and, ultimately, treatment progresses to the conversational level before progressing on to the next phoneme. The behavioristic overlay from the 1970s remains a strong influence in present-day intervention, including charting and counting correct and incorrect productions. The use of behavioristic rewards (e.g., stickers) also remains prominent in present-day intervention, as well as the use of oral motor devices (e.g., horns, whistles, although their value is controversial). Moreover, early phoneme-oriented methods are still extensively used today for the elicitation and establishment of sounds (e.g., phonetic placement, sensory-motor).

In the case of a child with highly unintelligible speech, some SLPs have expanded their intervention to a pattern-oriented design that focuses on expediting intelligibility gains and phonological reorganization. It is important to match the severity of the speech sound disorder with the approach that will yield the greatest improvement in the shortest amount of time. The specific design implemented may include lexical contrasts, feature contrasts, phonological patterns, hierarchical tiers, etc. Familiarity with the various treatment designs and their goals is essential for determining which approach will provide the most efficacious intervention for a particular child.

Some General Treatment Principles. Although many considerations pertain to a particular setting, there are also general treatment principles to keep in mind no matter what type of approach you decide to use. According to Stoel-Gammon and Dunn (1985), these principles are: (a) develop a plan based on all underlying factors that may relate to the cause of the disorder, (b) remember that each child is an individual, (c) use a comprehensive framework when planning intervention, (d) teach the child to monitor her/his own progress, and (e) measure the child's progress in a systematic way. Perhaps the most critical point to remember is that the treatment plan needs to be comprehensive.

Once an approach has been selected that fits the needs of the child and is feasible with respect to the setting and other factors, goals and objectives are formulated and mapped across a general timeframe. Goals refer to the ultimate targets of treatment, and objectives are the stepwise milestones along the way.

In the public schools, this planning step is accomplished by developing an IEP. In other settings, such as a hospital, the latter usually is called a "speech language treatment plan." Examples of an IEP and a speech-language treatment plan are provided in the sidebars.

A plan is written with a number of considerations in mind: Will treatment be individual or in a group? What dosage is needed? What are the criteria for advancing to another goal or objective? How is generalization achieved? What are the criteria for dismissal from treatment? Often, the particular setting where services are provided has established guidelines for these parameters. Common examples of dosage are 20 minutes twice weekly, 1 hour weekly, or 2 hours weekly.

An effective way to systematically measure the progress of a child with highly unintelligible speech is to collect spontaneous, connected-speech samples to obtain intelligibility percentages at the beginning of treatment and periodically throughout treatment (Ellis & Hodson, 2010). Intelligible speech is the ultimate goal for children with severe speech sound disorders, and collecting connected-speech samples is the most ecologically valid way to document progress for accountability purposes.

In addition, SLPs need to consider a variety of general treatment variables before treatment begins. Stoel-Gammon and Dunn (1985) included: (a) the linguistic content (e.g., syllables for motoric difficulty, establishing sound classes); (b) structure of remediation sessions (e.g., drill, drill play, structured play; Shriberg & Kwiatkowski, 1980); (c) remediation components (e.g., auditory training, self-monitoring, contextual facilitation); (d) the definition of a correct response (e.g., any production of a sound in same category); and criteria for sound mastery if working with a mild disorder (e.g., using new sounds in spontaneous utterances).

Treatment variables for SSD depend on the particular approach used. For example, when an SLP uses the Cycles Approach, there are seven underlying treatment concepts (Hodson, 2010; Hodson & Paden, 1991). These include: (a) Phonological acquisition is a gradual process (Ingram, 1976). Typically developing children do not learn one sound at a time to a particular criterion; (b) Children with "normal" hearing acquire adult speech by listening (Van Riper, 1939); therefore, providing auditory stimulation with slight amplification helps a child "tune in" to targeted speech patterns; (c) Children associate kinesthetic and auditory sensations (Fairbanks, 1954) as they are learning new speech patterns; new accurate kinesthetic images need to be developed through productionpractice; (d) A phonetic environment can facilitate (or inhibit) correct sound productions (Kent, 1982); therefore, production-practice words need to be chosen carefully; (e) Children tend to generalize new speech production skills (McReynolds & Bennett, 1972); targeting optimal patterns facilitates this generalization and increases intelligibility; (f) An optimal "match" facilitates a child's learning (Hunt, 1961); treatment that begins one step above the child's current level results in progress (i.e., children need to be challenged, but have the opportunity to be successful); (g) Children need to be actively involved in treatment.

Treatment in the public schools begins with the IEP. The IEP purpose is to be the vehicle needed for student success in school and, ultimately, for documentation. Multidisciplinary teams (e.g., SLPs, occupational therapists, physical therapists, psychologists, general educators) and parents come together and discuss the needs of each child in a holistic manner. The educators and the parents decide together what skills are needed on the IEP to support a particular student's success in the classroom. The general structure consists of one or more annual goals and a list of stepwise milestones called objectives toward each goal. The individual plan that is developed is good for 1 year and is reviewed at least annually to determine if any changes are needed so that the plan remains appropriate (for an example see 122.3). Full re-evaluations typically are mandated every 3 years.

Sidebar 22.3 Individualized Educational Plan (IEP)

IEPs are developed to ensure that all children receive a free and appropriate education. Services that a child needs in order to be successful in the classroom are listed on the IEP. Some school districts now use special software programs to generate IEPs (A sample IEP follows).

Clarifying Comments

The SLP may be the primary service provider or the only provider for a particular child if no other concerns are identified. A child's goals may be limited to only speech sound production skills or some combination of speech skills, language skills, literacy skills, and/or other issues (e.g., motor). Some controversy has occurred regarding whether certain speech deviations are "educationally relevant" to a student's academic success. For example, SLPs are sometimes challenged to provide evidence that single phoneme errors (e.g., lisps) negatively affect academic areas such as reading or spelling.

The actual treatment design for the implementation of services is defined in the IEP. Traditionally, SLPs have provided speech-language services to all children on their caseloads in groups for 20 minutes twice a week regardless of the severity of the disorder. Traditionally, the amount of speech-language services has remained the same throughout the school year.

Treatment in children's hospitals starts with a Speech-Language Treatment Plan after the evaluation is completed. It may consist of background information, family goals, long-term goals, short-term objectives, an estimate of time for completion of services, and a prognosis for progress. An example of treatment time would be 1 hour once a week. Treatment in most hospitals begins with the physician's "order" for an evaluation and/or a specific amount of treatment. The frequency could be daily or less often, and the specific treatment is defined by the nature of the diagnosis (i.e., traumatic brain injury), the severity, and the specific needs of the patient. Progress is documented for each treatment session for billing purposes. An example of a Hospital Speech-Language Treatment Plan is shown in Sidebar 22.4.

Any School District
Individual Education Program

Student Name Gender: Susie Jones F	Meeting Date 12/11/XXXX	Purpose of Meeting ☐ Initial Eligibility, IEP, Placement ☒ Annual Review of IEP ☐ Three Year Reevaluation ☐ Dismissal from Services Date: ____________ ☐ Parent Request ☐ Other: ____________
Social Security Number 012-345-6789	Age Grade 4 PreK	
Date of Birth 2/14/XXXX	Date Services Begin 12/11/XXXX	Discussed evaluation results/progress/assessment method ☒ Yes ____ (Parent/Guardian initial) Copy of evaluation results received ☐ Yes ____ (Parent initial)
District of Residence Any School District	Annual Review Date 12/10/XXXX	***Transition Planning Needed** ☒ **No** ☐ **Yes (If yes, attach applicable transition pages.)**
Attendance Center Any Head Start	Parent/Guardian Name, Address, Phone Mr. and Mrs. Jones Street Address City, USA Hm: 000-000- 0000 Wk: 000-000-0000	Student is eligible for special education or special education and related services as determined by the IEP team ☒ Yes ☐ No An annual copy of Parent/Guardian Rights was received and reviewed ____________(Date) ________ (Parent/Guardian Initial)
Date of Multidisciplinary Evaluation 10/03/XXXX		
Three Year Reevaluation Due 10/02/XXXX	Parent/Guardian Name, Address, Phone Hm: Wk:	A copy of the IEP was provided to parent/guardian ☒ Yes ______ (Parent/Guardian Initial)

IEP Team Membership	Signature	Date
Parent/Guardian	Mr. and Mrs. Jones	11/11/XXXX
Parent/Guardian		
Student		
Superintendent/Designee	Any Principal	11/11/XXXX
General Classroom Teacher	Any Teacher	11/11/XXXX
Special Education Teacher/Case Manager		
Speech/language Pathologist	Any Therapist	11/11/XXXX
Evaluator		
Title		
Title		
Title		

Child Count Information (District Option to Complete)

Ethnicity: WH **Dismissal Date:** / / **Exit Code:**

Services — **Hrs/Minutes**

A. Hrs/Minutes per week in Special Education		
B. Hrs/Minutes per week in Related Services	40 mins	
C. Transportation ☐yes x no		
D. **A + B = (Total hrs/min. of Special Education/Related Services)**	40 mins	

Placement

☐ 0100 Regular Classroom with Modification
☐ 0110 Resource Room
☐ 0120 Self-Contained Classroom
☐ 0130 Day Program Code: ____________
☐ 0140 24 Hour Program Code: ____________
☐ 0150 Home/Hospital

Placement 3-5

☐ 0305 Home
☐ 0315 Early Childhood Setting
☒ 0325 Part-Time Early Childhood/Part-Time Early Child Special Education Setting
☐ 0335 Early Childhood Special Education Setting
☐ 0345 Separate School
☐ 0355 Residential Facility

Parent/Guardian declines all special education services

Parent/Guardian Signature: ____________________

Present Levels of Performance **Page 2**

Based on evaluation, include academic achievement and functional performance (strengths and weaknesses) in the areas affected by the student's disability, including transition in the IEP to be in effect when the student turns 16; parent concerns; and how the student's disability affects the student's involvement and progress in the general education curriculum. (For a preschool child, how the disability affects his/her participation in appropriate activities.)

Student Name: Susie Jones	IEP Date: 11/11/XXXX

Background Information

Referral Information/Parent Concerns

Strengths

Needs

How disability affects participation in appropriate activities/curriculum

Consideration of Special Factors **Page 3**

Student Name: Susie Jones	**IEP Date: 11/11/XXXX**

Is the student limited English proficient? ☐ Yes ☒ No
If the answer to this question is "yes", please explain the language needs of the student as these needs relate to the student's IEP.

Are there any special communication needs? ☐ Yes ☒ No
If the answer to this question is "yes", what direct instruction will be provided in the student's mode of communication?

Does the student require Braille? ☐ Yes ☒ No
If the answer to this question is "yes", what Braille services will be provided?

Does the student's behavior impede his or her learning or that of others? ☐ Yes ☒ No
If yes, what strategies are required to appropriately address this behavior, including positive behavioral interventions and supports?

<u>Assessment</u> **State and/or District-wide** **(Circle the form(s) of assessment that student will take.)**

1. ☐ Student will be taking the assessment without accommodations.

2. ☐ Student will be taking the assessment with the accommodations identified on Page 6.

3. ☐ Student will be taking an alternate assessment (The alternate assessment is for students working in the alternate achievement standards)
   - ☐ The student meets criteria for significant cognitive disability (cognitive abilities are 2 standard deviations below the mean, goals and objectives focus on alternate content standards, and requires extensive and direct instruction)
   - ☐ Alternate assessments to be administered. ______________________________

4. ☒ Student not required to take district or statewide assessment at this grade level.

Educational Goals and Objectives/Benchmarks **Page 5___**

Student Name: Susie Jones	**Date:** 12/11/XXXX	**Title of personnel responsible to carry out annual goal:** Speech Therapist		
		Procedure Code	Progress Date	Progress Code
Measurable Annual Goal#__1__ Susie will produce the /k/ sound spontaneously in all positions of words on 9 out of 10 trials with auditory and visual cues across 2 sessions.				
Objective/Benchmark (Only required for students who take alternate assessments aligned to alternate achievement standards)				
Objective/Benchmark (Only required for students who take alternate assessments aligned to alternate achievement standards)				
Objective/Benchmark (Only required for students who take alternate assessments aligned to alternate achievement standards)				

Procedure Codes
(Complete at IEP meeting)

1 Teacher-made tests
2 Observations
3 Weekly tests
4 Unit tests
5 Student Conferences
6 Other: ______
7 Work Samples
8 Portfolios
9 Oral Tests
10 Data Response

Progress Codes
P = Progress being made
I = Insufficient Progress to meet goal
X = Not Addressed this Reporting Period
M = Met goal

Reporting Frequency to Parents
☐ Quarterly Reports
X Trimester
☐ Other- describe frequency______

Reporting Method to Parents
☐ Conferences
☐ Report Card
X Copy of Goal Page
☐ Other

See modifications checklist for specific goal modifications.

Educational Goals and Objectives/Benchmarks **Page 5 ___**

Student Name: Susie Jones	**Date:** 12/11/XXXX	**Title of personnel responsible to carry out annual goal:** Speech Therapist		
		Procedure Code	Progress Date	Progress Code
Measurable Annual Goal# __2__ Susie will produce the /g/ sound spontaneously in all positions of words on 9 out of 10 trials with auditory and visual cues across 2 sessions.				
Objective/Benchmark (Only required for students who take alternate assessments aligned to alternate achievement standards)				
Objective/Benchmark (Only required for students who take alternate assessments aligned to alternate achievement standards)				
Objective/Benchmark (Only required for students who take alternate assessments aligned to alternate achievement standards)				

Procedure Codes
(Complete at IEP meeting)

1 Teacher-made tests
2 Observations
3 Weekly tests
4 Unit tests
5 Student Conferences
6 Other: ________________
7 Work Samples
8 Portfolios
9 Oral Tests
10 Data Response

Progress Codes
P = Progress being made
I = Insufficient Progress to meet goal
X = Not Addressed this Reporting Period
M = Met goal

Reporting Frequency to Parents
☐ Quarterly Reports
X Trimester
☐ Other- describe frequency____________

Reporting Method to Parents
☐ Conferences
☐ Report Card
X Copy of Goal Page
☐ Other

See modifications checklist for specific goal modifications.

Educational Goals and Objectives/Benchmarks **Page 5 ___**

Student Name: Susie Jones	**Date:** 12/11/XXXX	**Title of personnel responsible to carry out annual goal:** Speech Therapist		
		Procedure Code	Progress	
			Date	Code
Measurable Annual Goal#__3__ Susie will spontaneously produce the /s/ sound in /s/ blends on 9 out of 10 trials when naming picture cards across two consecutive sessions.				
Objective/Benchmark (Only required for students who take alternate assessments aligned to alternate achievement standards)				
Objective/Benchmark (Only required for students who take alternate assessments aligned to alternate achievement standards)				
Objective/Benchmark (Only required for students who take alternate assessments aligned to alternate achievement standards)				

Procedure Codes
(Complete at IEP meeting)

1 Teacher-made tests
2 Observations
3 Weekly tests
4 Unit tests
5 Student Conferences
6 Other: __________
7 Work Samples
8 Portfolios
9 Oral Tests
10 Data Response

Progress Codes
P = Progress being made
I = Insufficient Progress to meet goal
X = Not Addressed this Reporting Period
M = Met goal

Reporting Frequency to Parents
☐ Quarterly Reports
X Trimester
☐ Other- describe frequency________

Reporting Method to Parents
☐ Conferences
☐ Report Card
X Copy of Goal Page
☐ Other

See modifications checklist for specific goal modifications.

Student Name: Susie Jones	IEP Date: 11/11/XXXX

Modifications and Supplemental Aids/Services or Supports for Student and/or School Personnel Page 6

Describe accommodations/program modifications and frequency of these modifications/program modifications to be used in general and special education, including supplemental aids/services or supports for school personnel, that will be provided to the student.

															Frequency			
All Areas (unless otherwise specified)	English/Language Arts	Mathematics	Science	Social Studies	Health	Fine Arts	PE/Athletics	Reading	Related Services	Goal(s) #	Goal(s) #	Other:	State or district		Daily	Weekly	Monthly	Other: Specify
									x					1. Small group instruction		x		
														2. Guided to unguided instruction				
														3. Taped texts				
														4. Highlighted texts				
														5. Taping lectures				
														6. Note taking assistance				
														7. Extended time for assignment completion				
														8. Shortened assignments				
														9. Assignment notebooks				
														10. Peer tutoring				
														11. Study guides				
									x					12. Repeated review/drill		x		
														13. Preferential seating				
														14. Frequent breaks				
														15. Concrete/positive reinforcers				
														16. Special instructional/adaptive equipment				
														17. Increased verbal response time				
														18. Directions given in a variety of ways (Specify)				
														19. Alternative materials (Specify)				
														20. Adjustments for speech intelligibility/fluency				
														21. Alternative setting				
														22. Oral tests				
														23. Short answer tests				
														24. Extended time for test completion				
														25. Taped tests				
														26. Multiple test sessions				
														27. Other:				
														28. Other:				
														29. Other:				
														Supports For School Personnel				
														30. Consultant service (Specify)				
														31. Specialized material (Specify)				
														32. Other:				

Related Services To Be Provided **Page 7**

Student Name: Susie Jones	**IEP Date: 11/11/XXXX**

	Title of Personnel Responsible	Amount of Services, and Location
☐ A. **Occupational Therapy**		
☐ B. **Physical Therapy**		
☐ C. **Psychological Services**		
☐ D. **Counseling Services**		
☐ E. **Social Work Services**		
☐ F. **Audiological Services**		
☐ G. **Recreation Therapy**		
☐ H. **School Nurse Services**		
X I. **Speech/Language Therapy**	Any Therapist	40 minutes per week at Head Start
☐ J. **Transportation** (Specify when, how often, where, distance, costs, etc.) ☐ Significant physical disability/health condition ☐ Program located other than home school ☐ Student's disability significantly impacts their ability to independently and safely access special education program		
☐ K. **Other**		
☐ L. **Assistive Technology**		
☐ M. **Orientation and Mobility**		
☐ N. **Medical Services** (Diagnostic Services only)		
☐ O. **Interpreting Services**		
☐ P. **Parental Counseling/Training**		

Physical Education

☐ Regular ☒ Not Required ☐ Adaptive Physical Education (Short-Term Objectives attached)

Hearing Aid Maintenance If yes, Title of Personnel Responsible for Monitoring ____________

Monitoring Frequency ____________

☐ Yes ☒ Not Applicable Monitoring Process ____________

Preschool Least Restrictive Environment (Ages 3, 4, and 5) ***Page 8B***

Student Name: Susie Jones	**IEP Date: 11/11/XXXX**

Continuum of Alternative Placements ☐ 0305 Home ☐ 0315 Early Childhood Setting ☒ 0325 Part-Time Early Childhood/Part-Time Early Childhood Special Education Setting ☐ 0335 Early Childhood Special Education Setting ☐ 0345 Separate School ☐ 0355 Residential Facility	**Special Education to be provided: (Specify description of services, amount of services, and location of services)** **Speech/Language Therapy** – Two times per week for 20 minutes for a total of 40 minutes per week in the Speech Therapy room at Head Start **Comments:**

Does child attend a regular education program? Yes ☒ No ☐
(District-run preschool, Head Start, Kindergarten)
If yes, please provide a description:
Susie attends Talking Tots Head Start.

Justification for Placement--An explanation of the extent, if any, to which the child will not participate with non-disabled children in regular classes, and non-academic activities. (Please use accept/reject format for each alternative placement considered.)

Home – Rejected. Susie attends Talking Tots Head Start.

Early Childhood Setting – Rejected. Susie needs to reduce the noise and distractions of the regular classroom in order to concentrate on her individual speech needs.

Part-Time Early Childhood/Part-Time Early Childhood Special Education Setting – Accepted. Susie can interact with her peer models and still receive pullout services to address her individual needs.

☒ The team addressed the potential harmful effects of the special education placement.

Reintegration Plan
Is the student moving from a more to less restrictive environment? ☐ Yes ☒ No
If yes, what strategies are required to appropriately address reintegration?

Extended School Year **Page 9**

Student Name: Susie Jones	IEP Date: 11/11/XXXX

Extended School Year Services: ☐ needed ☒ not needed ☐ to be determined by (Date) ____/____/____

Goal(s) #	*Type of Service	Beginning Date mm/dd/yy	Ending Date mm/dd/yy	Minutes Per Week	Based on **

* Instruction, related services (specify), other (list)

** Regression/Recoupment, Emerging Skills, or Maintenance of Critical Life Skills

Parent/Guardian Consent For Extended School Year Program only

"Consent" means that the parent(s)/guardian(s) have been fully informed of all information relevant to the activity for which consent is sought, in the native language, or other mode of communication; the parent(s)/guardian(s) understand and agree in writing to the carrying out of the activity for which consent is sought, and the consent describes that activity and lists any records which will be released and to whom; and the granting of consent by the parent(s)/guardian(s) is voluntary and may be revoked in writing at any time.

Parent/Guardian Signature ____________ Date ____________

Parent/Guardian Consent Required For Initial Placement Only

"Consent" means that the parent(s)/guardian(s) have been fully informed of all information relevant to the activity for which consent is sought, in the native language, or other mode of communication; the parent(s)/guardian(s) understand and agree in writing to the carrying out of the activity for which consent is sought, and the consent describes that activity and lists any records which will be released and to whom; and the granting of consent by the parent(s)/guardian(s) is voluntary and may be revoked in writing at any time.

Parent/Guardian Signature ____________ Date ____________

Sidebar 22.4 Speech Language Treatment Plan

Treatment plans in specialty hospitals such as children's hospitals contain essentially the same information as an IEP; however, the plan may be much shorter, not as inclusive, and more of a "report" type of organizational form. (A sample SLT Plan follows).

Any Children's Hospital Center
XXXX Any Street
City, State XXXXX
(XXX)-XXX-XXXX

SPEECH LANGUAGE TREATMENT PLAN

Name: Johnnie Smith
Date of Birth: 7/27/20XX
Date Treatment Initiated: 2/10/20XX
Length of Sessions: 60 minutes
Medical Record: 1234567

Date: 12/11/20XX
Age: 4 years
Type: Individual
Frequency: 1 x week
Location: Any Health Center

Background Information History: Therapy was recommended for Johnnie after completing a speech-language evaluation on February 10, 20XX at Any Children's Hospital Center. Johnnie revealed significant difficulties with his speech sound production skills. He produced a /t/ for a /k/ and a /d/ for a /g/. He also omitted the /s/ sound in consonant cluster sequences.

Family Goals: Johnnie's mother wants to understand her child's speech better.

Long-Term Goal: Johnnie will improve his speech production skills to an age-appropriate level.

Short-Term Objectives:

Short-Term Objective #1
Johnnie will demonstrate an accurate production of the velars /k/ and /g/ across word positions at the word level during 80% of opportunities across three consecutive sessions.

Short-Term Objective #2
Johnnie will demonstrate an accurate production of /s/ consonant clusters at the beginning of words during 80% of opportunities across three consecutive sessions.
The prognosis for Johnnie's speech treatment is good with consistent attendance to formal treatment sessions and good follow-through with suggested home practice.
Transition plan/estimated discharge date: It is estimated that Johnnie will require services through 2/20XX.

Any Practioner, MA, CCC-SLP
Certified Speech-Language Pathologist
Any Children's Hospital Center, Pleasant
(XXX) XXX-XXXX

Treatment in university speech-language clinics begins with the collaboration between the clinical supervisor and the student clinician. They meet to discuss the results of the child's performance on evaluations that are given to determine current skill levels. They then decide on the goals together for the academic semester or quarter for that client. Specific targets for each goal are selected and recorded on weekly/monthly summary sheets to keep ongoing documentation of progress towards the goals. Treatment may be on a weekly schedule for an hour or less depending on the client's attention abilities and overall needs. Treatment methods usually depend on the client's individual needs. Re-evaluations typically occur each semester in university clinics because of the need for "progress" reports at the end of semesters.

IMPLEMENTATION

After all the preliminary work of assessment, diagnosis, approach selection, and treatment design is completed, the last step is to actually implement the treatment plan. The lesson plans, materials, and various activities need to be coordinated to support each individual client's needs. Two examples of the implementation of treatment plans are discussed below. The first example will be phoneme-oriented; the second example will be phonological in nature.

Lesson Plan, Materials, and Activities for Client Example #1. Mary is a 6-year-old first grader at an elementary school who has minor speech errors. She was evaluated with the Goldman-Fristoe Test of Articulation. Her only errors were /t/ for /k/ and /d/ for /g/ in all positions of words. These errors were also noted in conversation. A multidisciplinary team met to discuss her speech, and an IEP was developed.

Mary could produce the /k/ and /g/ sounds in all positions of words when given auditory models and visual cues for placement. Because Mary's sounds were stimulable in words, treatment began at the word level of production, and cues were incorporated. A "Phoneme-Oriented Approach" was implemented. Note that many children are not stimulable for sounds that they produce in error. In that case, the child can be taught to produce the sound or possibly "shape" the target sound from another sound in the child's inventory. For more on eliciting target sounds, see resources such as Secord, Boyce, Donahue, Fox, and Shine (2007).

Mary's annual IEP goal stated that "Mary will produce the /k/ and /g/ sounds spontaneously in conversation while conversing with an adult or peer for 2 minutes with 90% accuracy across two different settings." This was the long-term goal or where the SLP wants Mary's productions to be in one year's time. Mary's lesson plan stated that she will play a memory matching game with "k" cards because she was motivated by card games. Selecting activities that the child enjoys is critical for motivating young children to focus on their speech. Mary began working with the /k/ sound in the final position of words rather than the initial position because final /k/ is usually easier. Sidebar 22.5 shows Mary's lesson plan.

Sidebar 22.5 IEP Lesson Plan

> IEP Lesson Plans are usually concise at schools due to time constraints and large caseloads. They may be written differently by each SLP depending on what type of organization works best for that particular person. (A sample IEP Lesson Plan is attached).

Days & Times: Tuesdays @ 11:00AM – 11:30AM	Student(s): Mary Paulson Date: 11/11/20XX

Lesson Plan:
Mary will produce the /k/ sound imitatively in the final position of words while playing a memory matching game with final /k/ picture cards. Auditory models and visual cues will be provided. The criterion is 9 out of 10 correct productions.

Final /k/ words	+	+	-	+	-	+	-	+	+	+	7/10

An articulation hierarchy followed from the word level through the conversational level because Mary had only two speech sounds in error. She simply needed practice producing the sounds correctly at progressively more difficult levels to help her correct productions become more automatic and to help her generalize to spontaneous conversation.

The SLP and Mary played a memory matching game by placing all final "k" cards face down on the table. The cards had matches but were placed randomly on the table. After Mary turned a card over, the SLP modeled the word on the "k" card using auditory and visual cues for Mary to imitate. When she did not produce the word correctly, the SLP incorporated additional prompts and/or cues. If the word was still too difficult, the SLP temporarily pulled that word pair of cards out of the game. This process was repeated when Mary turned over her second card; when a match occurred, Mary could take another turn.

The SLP kept track of correct and incorrect productions in whatever manner was convenient while participating in the activity. School districts usually require consistent data collection or "progress monitoring" throughout treatment sessions so that current "success" levels can be entered on a child's IEP and also so that quarterly progress reports can be sent home to parents to show quarterly progress.

Lesson Plan, Materials, and Activities for Client Example #2. Henry is a 4-year-old boy who came to the speech-language-hearing clinic because his mother was worried about his speech. He was extremely unintelligible in conversation. It was decided that a phonological evaluation would be completed because Henry was extremely difficult to understand. The goal of assessment was to identify his primary error patterns/phonological deviations so the clinician could target those patterns for the most expedient changes in his intelligibility. *The Hodson Assessment of Phonological Patterns-3rd Edition* (Hodson, 2004) yielded a Total Occurrences of Major Phonological Deviations (TOMPD) score of "115" which gave his speech a rating of "Severe."

Following this evaluation, the Potential Target Patterns identified were: (a) /s/ Clusters (combining the targets of Consonant Sequences/Clusters and the Consonant Category Deficiency—Stridents), (b) Velars, and (c) Prevocalic Liquids. The supervisor and the student clinician decided to begin treatment with /s/ clusters because both the Strident Consonant Category deficiency and Consonant Sequence/Cluster omissions were 100% in error. In addition, his /s/ clusters were stimulable and easier than /s/ singletons because the client inserted a stop during productions of words with a singleton /s/ (e.g., *see*—>[sti]). Moreover, enhancing productions of /s/ clusters lead to considerable gains in intelligibility.

Henry's Phonological Remediation Plan began with work on /s/ clusters, which not only improved his productions of consonant clusters in words; it also improved his productions of singleton stridents. His targets were not continued until a pre-determined criterion level was reached, but rather they were cycled because children's sound development is gradual and not linear. A slight amplification was incorporated during his short (approximately 30 seconds) "listening" activity at the beginning and end of each session. Henry had pictures of his production-practice words (on large index cards) that he was able to produce with 100% accuracy (with "assists" as needed) to help him develop new accurate kinesthetic images. He participated in experiential-play motivational activities while practicing his target words. (Specific activities are listed on the remediation plan in Sidebar 22.6.) Future targets were probed for in preparation for his next session. He listened to a rhyme at the end of the session to enhance his phonological awareness skills.

The Role of Caregivers and Home Practice

The role of caregivers in the success of treatment needs to be emphasized. Sessions once or twice a week usually do not provide sufficient practice to expeditiously achieve desired results. Carryover to spontaneous conversation is facilitated by regular home practice. Caregivers can be overwhelmed if extensive practice is requested. They most likely will not complete home practice if a great deal of time is requested. Just a few minutes of speech practice or listening to word lists each day can provide a consistent awareness builder that will help the child develop new accurate auditory and kinesthetic images. Sending practice sheets/cards and listening lists home is highly recommended because daily work enhances progress. Video file 22V1 is an example of a treatment session with a 3-year-old child. The session includes elements from the Cycles treatment approach. Note the variety of activities designed to address the target sound pattern. Also observe the clinician/client interactions and elicitation techniques.

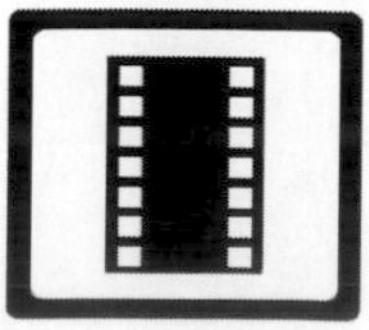

Access Video File 1 (Chapter 22)

22V1 Excerpts from a Cycles treatment session with a 3-year-old child

Sidebar 22.6 Phonological Remediation Plan

Clinics have their own specific forms tailored to their needs; however, they contain essentially the same basic information to document semester progress. Individual supervisors may have a particular lesson plan outline pertaining to that speech-language disability area. (A Phonological Remediation Plan follows).

Remediation Plan for Phonological Intervention

CLIENT: Henry Williams	CLINICIAN: Any
BIRTHDATE: 7/27/20XX	TERM: Fall 20XX
DISORDER: Phonology	SUPERVISOR: Any

Date: *12/11/20XX*Target(s): Pattern: */s/ consonant clusters*-Phoneme: /sp/

1) Review of preceding session's production-practice words.
   Henry just started so he doesn't have previous cards yet.

2) Listening Activity: (Use amplifier with approximately 15 listening list words.)

   Henry will listen to the following /sp/ words while wearing an amplifier: spy, space, spend, spoon, sponge, spot, spell, speed, spill, spin, spa, spear, spook, speak, sport. Henry will say 2 or 3 words from production-practice list into microphone.

3) Production-Practice Activities:

   Selection of 4 or 5 Practice Words: Henry will be presented with the cards: spot, spoon, sponge, spill, and spin. He will choose one card to color.

4) Experiential-play production practice activities:

   Henry will mix up some pudding with a "spoon" & clean up "spills" with a "sponge."
   Henry will "spin" a variety of tops.
   Henry will make "spots" on a paper dog puppet.
   Henry will play a spoon game with target cards under each one.
   Henry will use a flashlight to shine on colored "spots" which have his target cards.

5) Probing for next session:
   /st/ clusters: Supervisor will elicit "stop," "star," and "stamp" to check for /st/ blends.

6) Metaphonological Activity:
   Clinician will read a "Spot" rhyming book.

7) Listening Activity repeated. (Same words listed above.)

(Home program 2-3 minutes per day – Parents read listening list.)

Generalization

Typically, children receive treatment at certain times in a designated facility at various levels of speech complexity, yet the long-term goal is "normalized" speech in all environments and at all times. How do SLPs help children generalize their new speech sounds to conversational speech and carry them over to their daily lives? SLPs can increase the length and complexity of error-free conversations ("Tell me about your last birthday. I'll time you for three minutes and count your good "r" sounds."). SLPs can observe their clients in other contexts, for instance when interacting with a receptionist or in the classroom. The child and his or her classroom teacher can agree on a feedback strategy that is not obtrusive. Parents can be asked to provide feedback to their child at home during certain times. Children can select a personal reminder item, for instance a sticker on the dining table or on the mirror. Children can watch video recordings from a school play to check their own accuracy.

Criteria for Dismissal from Treatment

The child who qualifies for services because of disordered speech will be dismissed from services one day based on one of several possible scenarios. For example, the end goal of treatment, normalized connected speech, has been reached. Note that frequently, children are qualified for services based on a standardized test of articulation or phonology involving the single word level. Children also need to demonstrate carryover into conversational speech. Or, the child has reached his/her potential for improvement. Despite sustained efforts, the child's progress has plateaued. Options include monitoring the child and resuming treatment later. Finally, parents may refuse further services.

Troubleshooting

Despite an SLP's best efforts to plan and prepare for an actual treatment session, unexpected complications often arise. Some challenging situations are listed below, along with some possible solutions.

Q: A 3-year old boy is scheduled for his first treatment session. He keeps jumping up from his chair and is generally extremely uncooperative. How can his attention be directed to the treatment activities?

A: Try a chair and table that fits him, with a block under his feet to keep him stable. Make a session "schedule" using pictures and let the child check off the activities or remove a picture for an activity from a board as he completes them. Stations can be set up around the room for each planned activity. Allow the child to choose the order of some of the activities to provide him with some control and ownership.

Q: A 4-year old boy is terrified of headphones and refuses to wear them for the listening activity list. What can be done to help him overcome his fear?

A: A free-field amplification system can initially be used. Sometimes it helps to incorporate a stuffed animal who wears the headset.

Q: A third-grade girl working on /ɹ/ appears unmotivated to participate in the sessions and to complete her home practice. How can she be motivated?

A: Help her become a stakeholder in her own progress. Show her the IEP and explain the criteria for moving forward through the goals and objectives. Set up a reward schedule at certain milestones along the way. Involve the parents as "cheerleaders" and supporters. Remind them that speech treatment is not unlike soccer practice or piano practice in that the child must practice new skills on a regular basis until they become more automatic.

Q: A first-grader complains to the SLP that his mom corrects his speech "all the time" and that it has become so annoying that he sometimes doesn't feel like talking at all anymore. What can the SLP do to help?

A: Contact the parent and cooperatively set some boundaries. For instance, together, the parent and the child can select a time each day where the parent provides feedback on speech errors but not during any other times so that the conversation then can focus on its content, not its form. The parent needs to be educated about the general progression of treatment and the fact that correcting speech errors in conversational speech is premature when the child is in the early stages of treatment; that type of feedback is best reserved for the generalization phase.

Q: A parent informs the school SLP that the child is now seen by a private SLP for an hour per week in addition to the SLP services at school. How will this affect treatment delivery in both settings?

A: Coordination between the two service providers is imperative and can speed up the child's progress substantially. With the parent's written permission, the two SLPs can communicate and should agree on a treatment plan that is complementary between the two settings. The two SLPs should compare their progress notes periodically and keep each other informed regarding generalization and plans to "exit" the child.

Q: A kindergartner with a severe SSD does not initiate contributions in the classroom and spends most recesses by herself. According to the parent, this child has had so many frustrating experiences with unsuccessful communication attempts that she retreated into a shell. How can she be encouraged to venture out again?

A: The SLP can collaborate with the Social Skills group facilitator in the school and help the child take more social risks. Role-play, video recordings of interactions, and video recorded treatment sessions can help the child gain a better understanding of their own communication needs and successes.

CONNECTIONS

In this chapter, we have provided an overview of treatment design and implementation. In addition, practical information about treatment settings, assessment outcomes, treatment types, and planning actual treatment sessions has been given. (Chapter 20 focuses on assessment and diagnosis in more detail.) Our overview of treatment types links back to the historical and theoretical underpinnings of clinical phonology in Chapter 1. Chapter 21 focuses on published evidence for various treatment approaches and points out, as we have, that SLPs frequently combine elements of different approaches. We have mentioned that the choice of a particular treatment approach may depend on the specific profile and set of needs of a given child. (Additional details about children with SSD are provided in Chapter 15).

Concluding Remarks

A number of SLPs have developed unique approaches and ideas for SSDs. These individuals have added to and expanded our knowledge base regarding how speech sounds are developed, how sounds interact, and how to effect extensive changes in our clients' speech sound systems. The evolution of phonology has added a number of dimensions regarding how we can approach and implement treatment. Some SLPs have changed their treatment mindset from "one sound at a time" to an expanded knowledge level that incorporates important sound classifications, multiple tiers of sound interactions, and/or multidimensional interactions of dynamic language systems at physical, perceptual, and production levels.

The next question is, "Where do we go from here?" It appears that because so many techniques and approaches are available, we need to conduct some "comparative research" (Hodson, 2010, 2011) to enable us to determine which techniques are most effective and efficient for which types of children. For some in-depth consideration of treatment efficacy, see Chapter 21. Another research need is that all of the speech sound intervention techniques seem to produce positive changes in our clients' speech sound production skills. We need to find out why this is so and what components contribute most for which types of clients.

In conclusion, effective treatment is dependent on identifying the specific needs of each individual client, having a strong knowledge base about treatment characteristics that are likely to produce change for that individual, designing an individualized plan, and implementing the intervention plan appropriately. Specifically, SLPs need to remember that although targeting one phoneme at a time may be appropriate for children with mild speech disorders, research-based evidence indicates that phonologically based approaches expedite intelligibility gains for children who have severe/profound speech sound disorders (Hodson, 2010).

Chapter Review Questions

1. What are some of the early landmark approaches for enhancing speech productions? Describe what each approach focused on within treatment.
2. Discuss why behavioristic approaches appeared, and name some of their strengths and limitations.
3. Describe the "cycles approach." Who is this treatment designed for? List some of the goals of this intervention.
4. What are some factors to consider when determining which approach may be most suited to a particular child?
5. Effective treatment is dependent on many factors. Discuss some of those factors.
6. Implementation of a treatment plan involves a variety of factors. Name some.

Suggestions for Further Reading

Hodson, B. (2010). *Evaluating and Enhancing Children's Phonological Systems: Research and Theory to Practice*. Wichita, KS: Phonocomp Publishers.

Hodson, B. (2011). Enhancing phonological patterns of young children with highly unintelligible speech. The ASHA leader. *www.asha.org/Publications/leader/2011/110405/Enhancing-Phonological-Patterns-of-Young-Children-With-Highly-Unintelligible-Speech.htm.*

Secord, W. A., Boyce, S. E., Donohue, J. S., Fox, R. A., & Shine, R. E. (2007). *Eliciting Sounds: Techniques and Strategies for Clinicians*. (2nd ed.). Clifton Park, NJ: Thomson Delmar Learning.

Williams, A., McLeod, S., & McCauley, R. (Eds.) (2010). *Interventions for Speech Sound Disorders in Children. Baltimore*, MD: Paul H. Brookes.

Suggestions for Student Activities

1. Chapter 20 includes a video recording of a child with a speech disorder during conversational speech elicited with a wordless picture book. Alternatively, you can use one of the case examples in Chapter 15 or observe a conversational interaction with a child with disordered speech.

   a. Select two treatment approaches for this child.
   b. Create two IEPs for this child, one for each approach you selected.
   c. Write a basic lesson plan for each approach. Make a list of materials that you would need for a typical session.

2. Record a continuous-speech sample for a child or use one of the sound or video files in Chapters 15 or 20. Write down the words that you can understand. Divide that number by the total number of words in the sample to obtain the percentage of intelligible words for that child.

Answers to Chapter Review Questions

1. What are some of the early landmark approaches that are often used in Phoneme-Oriented Approaches and sometimes in Phonologically Based Approaches? Describe what each approach focused on within their treatment.

   1) Phonetic Placement – Placement of the articulators and modification of the airstream. Moto-Kinesthetic Method – Speech is a motoric process that involves shaping the exhaled air as it passes through the oral and nasal cavities.
   2) Stimulus Approach – Treatment must begin with ear training and sounds must be produced first in isolation, one at a time, before proceeding to higher levels. The

steps include: (a) sensory-perceptual training, (b) sound elicitation, (c) sound production, (d) transfer, and (e) maintenance.

3) Sensory-Motor Method - Speech does not consist of separate phonemes but rather is a sequence of syllable productions. Treatment includes: (a) heightening awareness of speech movement patterns through syllable practice, (b) practicing sound sequences, and (c) varying the phonetic contexts. It incorporates coarticulatory contexts.
4) Discrimination Method – Involves targeting auditory-perceptual ability to hear the difference between the error and target sounds. Treatment starts with discriminating between gross differences in words then, later, finer contrasts.

2. Discuss why behavioristic approaches appeared and name some of their strengths and any limitations.

Behavioristic approaches appeared because of legislation PL 94-142 which involved Individualized Educational Plans that emphasized "accountability" measures. Objectives that specified observable and measureable behaviors were required for writing these educational plans. Strengths include using specific behavioral techniques to change behaviors and the close monitoring of progress; limitations include the use of predetermined specified criterion levels for mastery, which is in contrast to how children actually learn sounds (children learn sounds gradually and not one sound at a time to a specified criterion.). Also, the use of the stimulus-response paradigm was assumed to make positive changes in a child's speech productions.

3. Describe the "cycles approach." Who is this treatment designed for? List some of the goals of this intervention.

The Cycles Phonological Remediation Approach is an example of a pattern-based approach that was designed for children with highly unintelligible speech. The Cycles Approach focuses on facilitating the emergence of phonological patterns and provides opportunities for the generalization of these patterns to occur within a child's phonological system. It uses cycles (time periods in which all phonological patterns that need intervention are facilitated sequentially) to develop intelligible speech patterns in children (Hodson, 2010). Phonemes are utilized to teach deficient target patterns which, in turn, facilitate an emergence of the respective phonological patterns. Potential primary patterns include "syllableness"; singleton consonants (omitted in various positions in words); and omissions of consonants in clusters/sequences, velars, stridents, and liquids. Patterns are recycled (represented) as needed during ensuing cycles, with complexity being increased gradually until each of the patterns begins to emerge in the child's spontaneous speech. Some of the goals of this approach are to increase intelligibility by facilitating reorganization of the child's phonological system and to help children acquire new phonological patterns. This program is an effective approach for increasing speech intelligibility more expediently.

4. What are some factors to consider when determining which approach may be most suited to a particular child?

If a child has only one or two speech errors, a more traditional phoneme-oriented program usually suffices. In the case of a child with highly unintelligible speech, various phonological approaches are more efficient in expediting intelligibility gains and phonological re-organization. It is important to match the severity of the speech sound disorder with the approach that will yield the greatest improvement in the shortest amount of time. The specific design implemented may include lexical contrasts, feature contrasts, phonological patterns, hierarchical tiers, etc. Familiarity with the various treatment designs and their goals is essential for determining which approach is most suited to a particular child. Also remember that treatment could begin with a pattern approach and switch to a phoneme approach if only a couple sound errors remain.

5. Effective treatment is dependent on many factors. Discuss some of those factors.

A variety of factors needs to be considered in order to achieve successful implementation. SLPs need to ask specific questions about implementation for a specific setting. For example, a few questions might be: In what setting will this child receive treatment? Will treatment be individual or in a group? Will this treatment design work in this setting? What is the dosage needed to implement this design? There are also general treatment principles to keep in mind no matter what type of approach you decide to use such as: (a) develop a plan based on all underlying factors that may relate to the cause of the disorder, (b) remember that each child is an individual, (c) use a comprehensive framework when planning intervention, (d) teach child to monitor their own progress (as appropriate), and (e) measure the child's progress in a systematic way.

6. Implementation of a treatment plan involves a variety of factors. Name some.

Implementation involves the actual "action" of a treatment plan. Some things to consider are the appropriateness of the lesson plans, the treatment materials, and the various activities that are used to achieve client goals. All of the details of a treatment session need to be coordinated to effectively lead each client to a successful completion of their goals.

REFERENCES

Almost, D., & Rosenbaum, P. (1998). Effectiveness of speech intervention for phonological disorders: A randomized controlled trial. *Developmental Medicine & Child Neurology,* 40, 319–325.

Barlow, J., & Gierut, J. (1999). Optimality theory in phonological acquisition. *Journal of Speech, Language, and Hearing Research,* 42(6), 1482-1498.

Bernhardt, B., & Stemberger, J. (2000). *Workbook in Nonlinear Phonology for Clinical Applications.* Austin, TX: Pro-Ed.

Bernthal, J. E., Bankson, N. W., & Flipsen, P. (2009). *Articulation and Phonological Disorders: Speech Sound Disorders in Children.* (6th ed.). : Allyn & Bacon.

Bishop, D., & Adams, C. (1990). A prospective study of the relationship between specific language impairment, phonological disorders, and reading retardation. *Journal of Child Psychology and Psychiatry,* 31, 1027-1050.

Bleile, K. M. (2004). *Manual of Articulation and Phonological Disorders: Infancy Through Adulthood* (2nd Edition). Clifton Park, NY: Thomson Delmar Publishing.

Browman, C., & Goldstein, L. (1992). Articulatory phonology: An overview. *Phonetica,* 49, 155-180.

Bowen, C. (2009). *Children's Speech Sound Disorders*. Chichester, West Sussex, PO19 8SQ, UK: John Wiley & Sons.

Chomsky, N., & Halle, M. (1968). *The Sound Pattern of English*. New York: Harper & Row.

Dean, E. C., Howell, J., Waters, D., & Ried, J. (1995). Metaphon: A metalinguistic approach to the treatment of phonological disorder in children. *Clinical Linguistics & Phonetics, 9,* 1-19.

Duchan, J. (2008a). *Sara Stinchfield Hawk (1885-1977).* Retrieved from *http://www.acsu.buffalo.edu/~duchan/history_subpages/stinchfieldhawk.html.*

Duchan, J. (2008b). *Edna Hill Young (1878-19?).* Retrieved from *http://www.acsu.buffalo.edu/~duchan/history_subpages/ednahillyoung.html.*

Edwards, M. L. (1994). Phonological process analysis. In E. Williams and J. Langsam (Eds.). *Children's Phonology Disorders: Pathways and Patterns* (2nd ed., pp. 43-65). Rockville, MD: American Speech-Language-Hearing Association.

Edwards, M. L. (1997). Historical overview of clinical phonology. In B. Hodson and M. Edwards (Eds). *Perspectives in Applied Phonology* (pp. 1-18). Gaithersburg, MD: Aspen.

Edwards, M. L. (2010). Phonological theories. In B. Hodson (2010). *Evaluating and Enhancing Children's Phonological Systems: Research and Theory to Practice* (pp. 145-170). Wichita, KS: PhonoComp.

Ellis, C. M., & Hodson, B. W. (2010, November). *Kindergarteners with disordered phonological systems: Three case studies*. Poster session presented at the American Speech- Language-Hearing Association, Philadelphia, PA.

Fairbanks, G. (1960). *Voice and Articulation Drillbook* (2nd ed.). New York: Harper Brothers.

Fey, M. E. (1992). Phonological assessment and treatment articulation and phonology: An addendum. *Language, Speech, and Hearing Services in Schools,* 23, 277-282.

Fogel, A., & Thelen, E. (1987). Development of early expressive and communicative action: Reinterpreting the evidence from a dynamic systems perspective. *Developmental Psychology,* 23, 747-761.

Gierut, J. A. (1989). Maximal opposition approach to phonological treatment. *Journal of Speech and Hearing Disorders, 54*, 9-19.

Gierut, J. A. (2007). Phonological complexity and language learnability. *American Journal of Speech-Language Pathology*, 16, 6-17.

Gillon, G. (2000). The efficacy of phonological awareness intervention for children with spoken language impairment. *Language, Speech, and Hearing Services in Schools,* 31, 126-141.

Gold, E. M. (1967). Language identification in the limit. *Information and Control,* 10, 447-474.

Goldman, R., & Fristoe, M. (2000). *Goldman-Fristoe Test of Articulation-2.* Circle Pines, MN: American Guidance Service.

Hodson, B. (1997). Disordered phonologies: What have we learned about assessment and treatment? In B. Hodson and M. Edwards (Eds). (1997). *Perspectives in Applied Phonology* (pp. 197-224), Gaithersburg, MD: Aspen.

Hodson, B. W. (2004). *Hodson Assessment of Phonological Patterns-Third Edition.* Austin, TX: Pro-Ed.

Hodson, B. (2010). *Evaluating and Enhancing Children's Phonological Systems: Research and Theory to Practice.* Wichita, KS: PhonoComp Publishing.

Hodson, B. (2011). Enhancing phonological patterns of young children with highly unintelligible speech. The *ASHA Leader.* *www.asha.org/Publications/leader/2011/110405/Enhancing-110405.htm.*

Hodson, B. W., & Paden, E. P. (1991). *Targeting Intelligible Speech: A Phonological Approach to Remediation* (2nd Edition). Austin, TX: Pro-Ed.

Hoffman, P. R., Norris, J. A. & Monjure, J. (1990). Comparison of process targeting and whole language treatments for phonologically delayed preschool children. *Language, Speech, and Hearing Services in Schools* 21, 102-109.

Hunt, J. (1961). *Intelligence and Experience.* New York: Ronald Press.

Ingram, D. (1976). *Phonological Disability in Children.* London: Cole & Whurr.

Jacobson, R., Fant, G., & Halle, M. (1952). *Preliminaries to Speech Analysis: The Distinctive Features and their Correlates* (Tech. Rep. No. 13, MIT Acoustics Laboratory) Cambridge, MA: MIT Press.

Kamhi, A. G. (2006). Treatment decisions for children with speech-sound disorders. *Language, Speech, and Hearing Services in Schools*, 37, 271-279.

Kent, R. D. (1982). Contextual facilitation of correct sound production. *Language, Speech, and Hearing Services in Schools,* 13, 66-76.

Kent, R. D. (1997). Gestural phonology: Basic concepts and applications in speech-language pathology. In M. Ball & R. Kent (Eds.), *The New Phonologies: Developments in Clinical Linguistics*. San Diego: Singular.

Liberman, M. (1975). *The Intonational System of English.* Doctoral dissertation, Massachusetts Institute of Technology, Cambridge, MA.

Liberman, M., & Prince, A. (1977). On stress and linguistic rhythm. *Linguistic Inquiry,* 8, 249-336.

Lof, G., & Watson, M. (2008). A nationwide survey of nonspeech oral motor exercise use: Implications for evidence-based practice. *Language, Speech, and Hearing Services in Schools,* 39, 392-407.

Magnus, L., Hodson, B., & Schommer-Aikins, M. (2011). Relationships of speech-related and nonspeech variables to listener ratings of speech of children with lip and palatal anomalies. *Canadian Journal of Speech-Language Pathology and Audiology.* 35, 32-39.

McCabe, R. B., & Bradley, D. P. (1975). Systematic multiple phonemic approach to articulation therapy. *Acta Symbolica*, 6(1), 2-18.

McCarthy, J. J., & Prince, A. S. (1995). Faithfulness and reduplicative identity. In J. N. Beckman, L. W. Dickey, & S. Urbaczyk (Eds.), *University of Massachusetts Occasional Papers,* 18 (pp. 249-384). Amherst, MA: Graduate Linguistic Student Association, University of Massachusetts.

McDonald, E. T. (1964). *Articulation testing and treatment: A sensory motor approach.* Pittsburgh, PA: Stanwix House.

McLeod, S. (Ed.) (2006). Intervention for a child with unintelligible speech. *Advances in Speech-Language Pathology,* 8.

McReynolds, L.V., & Bennett, S. (1972). Distinctive feature generalization in articulation training. *Journal of Speech and Hearing Disorders,* 37, 462-470.

Paden, E. (1970). *A History of the American Speech and Hearing Association 1925-1958.* Rockville, MD: American Speech and Hearing Association.

Prezas, R., & Hodson, B. (2010). Phonological cycles remediation approach. In L. Williams, S. McLeod & R. McCauley (Eds.) *Interventions for Speech Sound Disorders in Children* (pp. 137-157). Baltimore: Brookes.

Rvachew, S., & Bernhardt, B. M. (2010). Clinical implications of dynamic systems theory for phonological development. *American Journal of Speech-Language Pathology*, 19, 34-50.

Rvachew, R. H., & Nowak, M. (2001). The effect of target selection strategy on phonological learning. *Journal of Speech, Language, and Hearing Research, 44,* 610-623.

Sagey, E. (1986). *The representation of features and relations in non-linear phonology.* Unpublished doctoral dissertation, Massachusetts Institute of Technology, Cambridge, MA.

Secord, W. A., Boyce, S. E., Donohue, J. S., Fox, R. A., & Shine, R. E. (2007). *Eliciting Sounds: Techniques and Strategies for Clinicians*. (2nd ed.). Clifton Park, NJ: Thomson Delmar Learning.

Scripture, M. K., & Jackson, E. (1927). *A Manual of Exercises for the Correction of Speech Disorders*. Philadelphia, PA: F. A. Davis.

Shriberg, L., & Kwiatkowski, J. (1980). *Natural Process Analysis*. New York: John Wiley.

Smit, A., Hand, L., Freilinger, J., Bernthal, J., & Bird, A. (1990). The Iowa articulation norms project and its Nebraska replication. *Journal of Speech and Hearing Disorders*, 55, 779-798.

Stackhouse, J., & Wells, B. (1997). *Children's speech and literacy difficulties.* London: Whurr.

Stampe, D. (1969). The acquisition of phonetic representation. In R. T. Binnick, A. Davison, G. M. Green, & J. L. Morgan (Eds.). *Papers from the fifth regional meeting of the Chicago Linguistic Society* (pp. 443-454). Chicago, IL: Chicago Linguistic Society.

Stampe, D. (1972). *A dissertation on natural phonology*. Doctoral dissertation, University of Chicago, IL.

Stinchfield, S. M., & Young, E. H. (1938). *Children with Delayed or Defective Speech.* Stanford, CA: Stanford University Press.

Stoel-Gammon, C., & Dunn, C. (1985). *Normal and Disordered Phonology in Children.* Baltimore, MD: University Park Press.

Strattman, K. (2010). Overview of intervention approaches, methods & targets. In B. Hodson . *Evaluating and Enhancing Children's Phonological Systems: Research and Theory to Practice*. Wichita, KS: PhonoComp Publishing, pp. 65-84.

Templin, M. (1957). *Certain language skills in children.* Minneapolis, MN: University of Minnesota Press.

Van Riper, C. (1934). *Speech Correction: Principles and Methods.* Englewood Cliffs, NJ: Prentice-Hall.

Van Riper, C. (1939). *Speech Correction: Principles and Methods* (2nd ed.). Englewood Cliffs, NJ: Prentice-Hall.

Weiner, F. (1981). Treatment of phonological disability using the method of meaningful minimal contrast: Two case studies. *Journal of Speech and Hearing Disorders*, 46, 93-103.

Williams, A. L. (2000). Multiple oppositions: Case studies of variables in phonological intervention. *American Journal of Speech-Language Pathology,* 9, 289-299.

Williams, A. L. (2005). A model and structure for phonological intervention. In A. G. Kamhi and K. E. Pollock (Eds.), *Phonological Disorders in Children: Clinical Decision Making in Assessment and Intervention* (pp. 189-199), Baltimore, MD: Paul H. Brookes.

Williams, A., McLeod, S., & McCauley, R. (Eds.) (2010). *Interventions for Speech Sound Disorders in Children.* Baltimore, MD: Paul H. Brookes.

Winitz, H., & Bellerose, B. (1962). Sound discrimination as a function of pretraining conditions. *Journal of Speech and Hearing Research,* 5, 340-348.

APPENDICES

In: Comprehensive Perspectives …
Editors: Beate Peter and Andrea A. N. MacLeod
ISBN: 978-1-62257-041-6

Appendix 1

REPRESENTING SPEECH SOUNDS WITH WRITTEN SYMBOLS: INTRODUCING THE IPA AND THE EXTENDED IPA

Martin J. Ball

Children who receive treatment for a speech-sound disorder are not, by definition, using the normal phonology of their target language variety. Therefore, if we wish to record their speech in writing, we cannot use the normal orthography of the language concerned (even if, unlike in English, there is good phoneme-grapheme correspondence). Carol Stoel-Gammon noted the importance of this in her paper on transcribing the speech of young children (Stoel-Gammon, 2001). Reduction of disordered speech to writing is usually a necessity, even in cases where instrumental analyses are used, as usually it is necessary to annotate with written symbols the graphic results of instrumental investigations.

Further, the work of Carol Stoel-Gammon and her colleagues and other researchers in the field of speech sound disorders in children has clearly demonstrated that these clients often use speech sounds from outwith the phonological system of their target variety, and sometimes sounds that are not attested in natural language (i.e. any known language). It became clear early, therefore, in speech language pathology that phonetic transcription was a necessary part of the analysis and recording of disordered speech, and that the International Phonetic Alphabet (IPA; see IPA 1999) was the only internationally recognized symbol system.

That the full IPA, rather than just those symbols needed to transcribe the non-disordered target language, is needed in the speech clinic has been shown in a number of studies in the literature. For example, a review by Ball and Müller (2007) showed that the full range of non-pulmonic egressive sounds had been recorded from clients whose target language was English. Thus, pulmonic ingressive sounds had been noted (e.g. in the case of a dysfluent speaker); ejectives (in the speech of children with speech sound disorders); implosives (in children with cochlear implants); and clicks (among other instances in cases of children with velopharyngeal inadequacy, but also in cases of speech sound disorder).

For speech sound disordered clients with English as their target language, there are also many examples of the use of non-English, but pulmonic egressive sounds. Indeed, virtually every consonant and vowel type included on the IPA chart has been recorded with this client group. This variety includes consonants at non-English places of articulation (such as retroflex, uvular, and pharyngeal), non-English combinations of place and manner (such as bilabial and velar fricatives, palatal plosives, and labiodental approximants); and non-English manners of articulation (such as lateral fricatives and trills – though an alveolar trill may be normal in Scottish English). A review of such consonant usage is available in Ball, Müller, Rutter and Klopfenstein (2009).

Also found are non-English vowels. These include front rounded vowels, back unrounded vowels, and a range of non-English diphthongs. These are reviewed in Ball, Müller, Klopfenstein and Rutter (2010), a tutorial that also illustrates the need to be able to use the range of IPA diacritics in recording disordered speech. Carol Stoel-Gammon was in the forefront of the growth of interest in vowel disorders, and her study on vowel disorders in children (Stoel-Gammon and Herrington 1990) showed the importance of detailed phonetic transcription. Of course, phonetic transcription is not restricted to the segmental level of speech. The IPA provides means of transcribing some prosodic features: for example, stress, length and tone (although it does not mandate any particular intonation transcription system). Examples of the transcription of disordered suprasegmentals are given in Rutter, Klopfenstein, Ball and Müller (2010), where ways to denote other aspects such as tempo, loudness, and voice quality are also described.

The IPA chart has been subject to continuous revision and expansion since the alphabet was first drawn up in the late nineteenth century. Included here is the most recent revision of 2005, which saw the addition of a symbol for a labiodental flap; while this has yet to be reported in disordered speech, it would be surprising if it does not turn up sooner or later!

As stated earlier, children with speech sound disorders sometimes use sounds that are not only beyond their native phonological system but are unattested in natural language. Transcribing these sounds was previously difficult, as the IPA was devised to provide symbols for natural language only. For a long time, as noted in the Phonetic Representation of Disordered Speech Group (PRDS, 1983), clinical phoneticians and speech-language clinicians had to rely on their own ad hoc symbols to capture these atypical sounds. In 1983, the PRDS Group published a report that contained suggestions on how to transcribe a wide range of atypical speech sounds (1983). Later, in 1989, the IPA Congress at Kiel adapted this report with some changes and additions (see IPA, 1989). This became the Extensions to the IPA for the transcription of disordered speech (Duckworth, Allen, Hardcastle and Ball, 1990). This "extIPA" system has been under the control of the International Clinical Phonetics and Linguistics Association ever since, and the most recent 2008 update of the extIPA chart is included here. The extIPA chart contains atypical manners of articulation (such as percussives and simultaneous median and lateral fricatives); atypical places of articulation (such as dentolabial, labioalveolar and velopharyngeal); and atypical oro-nasal resonance types (such as nasal fricatives, and velopharyngeal friction). There are a number of diacritics that allow the marking of phonetic characteristics such as lack of aspiration, alveolar place of articulation, and lip spreading, that are not found on the IPA chart. There are also diacritics to mark connected speech phenomena such as pausing, tempo, loudness, and the timing of voicing. The other main innovation of the extIPA system is granting the transcriber the ability to denote how certain (or uncertain) they are about a particular symbol. The system allows the transcriber to note anything from an indeterminate sound, through "probably a consonant," "probably a voiceless plosive," up to "probably [t]," and so forth. Naturally, the use of this indeterminacy system will make inter- and intra-transcriber reliability measures more complex. As research on child speech disorders progresses, we are beginning to see more examples of extreme variability in the realization of target sounds (see, for example, Müller, Ball and Rutter, 2006). This variability goes beyond substitutions at the phonemic level, and to record it accurately we need to be able to use the full resources of the International Phonetic Alphabet, and sometimes too the Extensions to the IPA for the transcription of atypical speech. This Appendix contains the most recent versions of both those charts.

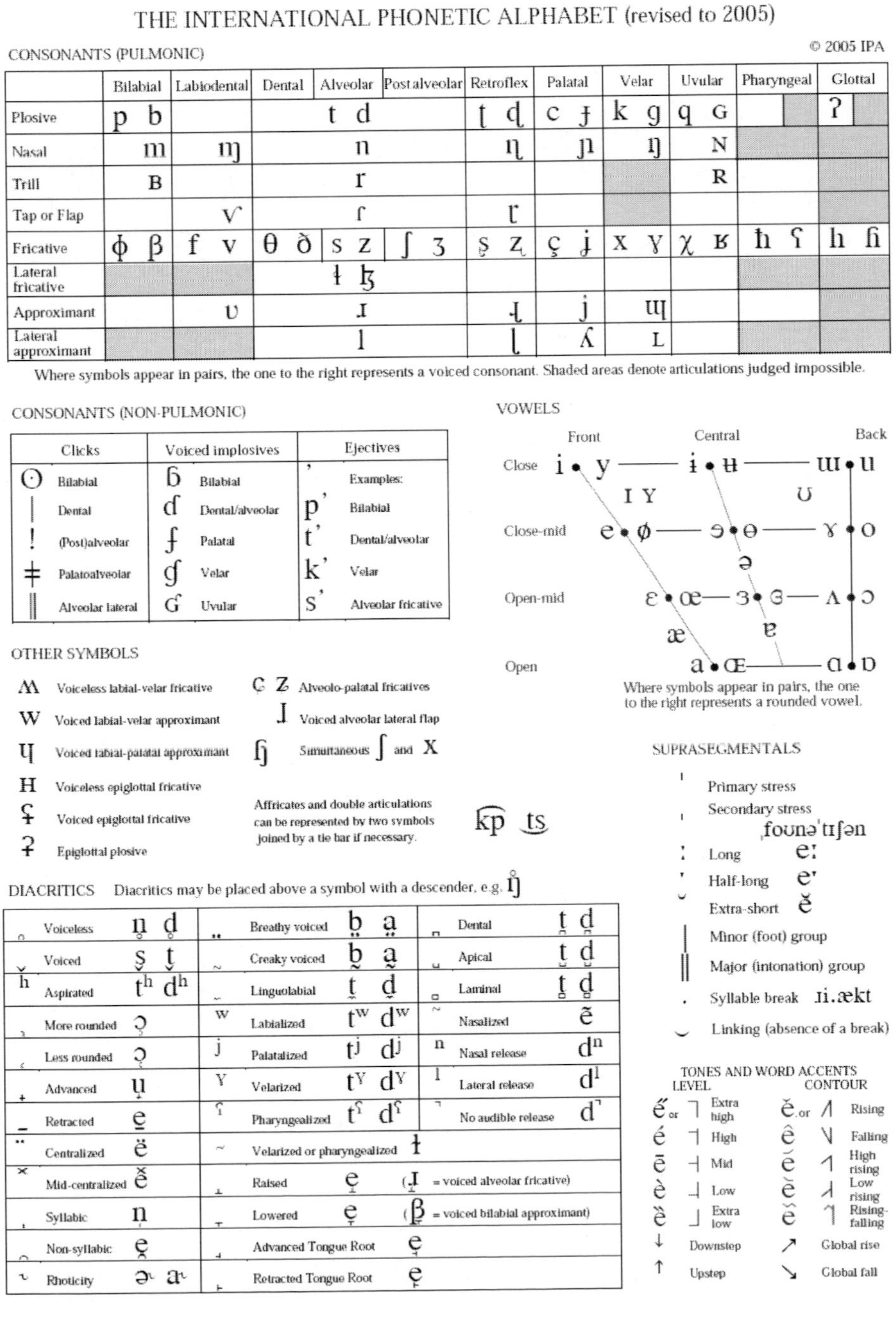

The IPA Chart. Reproduced by permission of the International Phonetic Association.

extIPA SYMBOLS FOR DISORDERED SPEECH

(Revised to 2008)

CONSONANTS (other than on the IPA Chart)

	bilabial	labiodental	dentolabial	labioalv.	linguolabial	interdental	bidental	alveolar	velar	velophar.
Plosive		p̪ b̪	p͆ b͆	p͇ b͇	t̼ d̼	t̪͆ d̪͆				
Nasal			m͆	m͇	n̼	n̪͆				
Trill					r̼	r̪͆				
Fricative median			f͆ v͆	f͇ v͇	θ̼ ð̼	θ̪͆ ð̪͆	h̪͆ ħ̪͆			ʩ
Fricative lateral+median								ʪ ʫ		
Fricative nareal	m͊							n͊	ŋ͊	
Percussive	ʬ						ʭ			
Approximant lateral					l̼	l̪͆				

Where symbols appear in pairs, the one to the right represents a voiced consonant. Shaded areas denote articulations judged impossible.

DIACRITICS

͍	labial spreading	s͍	͈	strong articulation	f͈	͋	denasal	m͋
͆	dentolabial	v͆	͉	weak articulation	v͉	͊	nasal escape	v͊
̪͆	interdental/bidental	n̪͆	\	reiterated articulation	p\p\p	͌	velopharyngeal friction	s͌
͇	alveolar	t͇	͎	whistled articulation	s͎	↓	ingressive airflow	p↓
̼	linguolabial	d̼	͢	sliding articulation	θ͢s	↑	egressive airflow	!↑

CONNECTED SPEECH

(.)	short pause
(..)	medium pause
(...)	long pause
f	loud speech [{*f* laʊd *f*}]
ff	louder speech [{*ff* laʊdɚ *ff*}]
p	quiet speech [{*p* kwaɪət *p*}]
pp	quieter speech [{*pp* kwaɪətɚ *pp*}]
allegro	fast speech [{*allegro* fɑst *allegro*}]
lento	slow speech [{*lento* sloʊ *lento*}]
crescendo, ralentando, etc. may also be used	

VOICING

ˬ	pre-voicing	ˬz
ˬ	post-voicing	zˬ
₍̥₎	partial devoicing	₍z̥₎
₍̥	initial partial devoicing	₍z̥
̥₎	final partial devoicing	z̥₎
₍̬₎	partial voicing	₍s̬₎
₍̬	initial partial voicing	₍s̬
̬₎	final partial voicing	s̬₎
˭	unaspirated	p˭
ʰ	pre-aspiration	ʰp

OTHERS

(◌), (C̄), (V̄)	indeterminate sound, consonant, vowel	ʞ	velodorsal articulation
(P̄l.vls), (N̄)	indeterminate voiceless plosive, nasal, etc	¡	sublaminal lower alveolar percussive click
( )	silent articulation (ʃ), (m)	!¡	alveolar and sublaminal clicks (cluck-click)
(( ))	extraneous noise, e.g. ((2 sylls))	*	sound with no available symbol

The extIPA Chart. Reproduced by permission of the International Clinical Phonetics and Linguistics Association.

REFERENCES

Ball, M. J. and Müller, N. (2007). Non-pulmonic egressive speech sounds in disordered speech: a brief review. *Clinical Linguistics and Phonetics, 21,* 869-874.

Ball, M. J., Müller, N., Rutter, B. and Klopfenstein, M. (2009). My client's using non-English sounds! A tutorial in advanced phonetic transcription. Part 1: Consonants. Contemporary Issues in Communication Sciences and Disorders, 36, 133-141.

Ball, M. J., Müller, N., Klopfenstein, M. and Rutter, B. (2010). My client's using non-English sounds! A tutorial in advanced phonetic transcription. Part 2: Vowels and Diacritics. Contemporary Issues in Communication Sciences and Disorders, 37, 103-110.

Duckworth, M., Allen, G., Hardcastle, W. and Ball, M. J. (1990). Extensions to the International Phonetic Alphabet for the transcription of atypical speech. *Clinical Linguistics and Phonetics, 4,* 273-280.

IPA (1989). Report on the 1989 Kiel Convention. Journal of the International Phonetic Association, 19, 67-80.

IPA (1999). Handbook of the International Phonetic Association. Cambridge: Cambridge University Press.

Müller, N., Ball, M. J. and Rutter, B. (2006). A Profiling Approach to Intelligibility Problems. Advances in Speech-Language Pathology, 8, 176-189.

Rutter, B., Klopfenstein, M., Ball, M. J., and Müller, N. (2010). My client's using non-English sounds! A tutorial in advanced phonetic transcription. Part 3: Prosody and Unattested Sounds. Contemporary Issues in Communication Sciences and Disorders, 37, 111-122.

PRDS Group (1983). The Phonetic Representation of Disordered Speech. London: The King's Fund.

Stoel-Gammon, C. (2001). Transcribing the speech of young children. *Topics in Language Disorders, 21,* 12-21.

Stoel-Gammon, C. and Herrington, P. (1990). Vowel systems of normally developing and phonologically disordered children. *Clinical Linguistics and Phonetics, 4,* 145-160.

In: Comprehensive Perspectives …
Editors: Beate Peter and Andrea A. N. MacLeod

ISBN: 978-1-62257-041-6

Appendix 2

A GENERAL GUIDE TO PHONOLOGICAL PATTERNS

Kristina Findlay and Andrea A. N. MacLeod

An **error pattern** is a way to group together errors that occur in a child's speech based on similar elements at the segmental, syllable, or word level. Error patterns are also called "**phonological patterns**" or "**phonological processes**." When identifying error patterns, it is important to remember to keep a global view of the child's productions and thus using only one method of describing an error could limit the ability to gain a comprehensive understanding of the child's abilities. Keeping a global view entails three elements. First, we must consider that multiple processes may act of the same segment, and need to be identified as such. For example, cluster reduction, prevocalic voicing, and velar fronting are all present in the production of "clown" /klaʊn/ as [daʊn]. Second, we should elicit multiple opportunities to identify the error pattern accurately. For example, "cat" produced as [tæt] could be assimilation or velar fronting. If subsequent utterances show "take" /teɪk/ produced as [keɪk] we might infer that the error pattern is assimiliation; conversely, if key /ki/ is produced as /ti/, then we would infer that the error pattern is more likely velar fronting. Third, the occurrence of an error pattern, within the analysis, can be related to the age of child. Certain errors, regardless of the child's age, are atypical and may be associated with severe forms of speech sound disorders.

The description of error patterns varies across studies since they differ in theoretical orientation. In this appendix, we have attempted to provide commonly reported phonological patterns seen in typically developing children and in children whose speech development is delayed or disordered. However, you may encounter other patterns reported in research or used in your clinical setting, or different terms to refer to the error patterns we have named here. When faced with different terms to describe the same errors, we suggest focusing on what errors the child is producing and consistently using one term to refer to these patterns. For example, deleting final consonants could be described as either "word final consonant deletion" or "omission of word final consonants." We suggest that you choose one of these terms, and stick to it when writing your evaluation report and in planning treatment goals.

Table A2.1. Summary of different patterns organised by broad category, type of phonological pattern, a definition, and examples from published data

Phonological Pattern	Definition	Examples
Broad Category: Assimilation		
Assimilation of place, manner or voicing [1, 4, 7, 9, 12, 14, 15, 16, 29, 31]	One consonant is replaced by another that is the same or similar to another consonant within the word	Labial Assimilation: "bake" /beɪk/ produced as [beɪb] Alveolar assimilation: "take" /teɪk/ produced as [teɪt] Voicing assimilation: "goat" /goʊt/ produced as [koʊt] Manner assimilation: "candy" /kændi/ produced as [næni]
Context-sensitive voicing [3, 15, 17] (could also be categorized within Substitution Errors)	A consonant's voicing is influenced by the surrounding context. Most commonly seen patterns are prevocalic voicing (anticipating the voicing from the vowel) and postvocalic devoicing (anticipating the end of voicing after the word)	"penny" /pɛni/ is produced at [bɛni] "tag" /tæg/ produced as /tæk/
Reduplication [7, 15, 17]	The repetition of a single syllable of the target word. This pattern could be total (repetition of same syllable) or partial (vowels differed, consonants the same or consonants differed, vowels the same).	"basket" /bæskɪt/ produced [bæbæ] "pudding" /pʊdɪŋ/ produced as [pʊpʊ]
Broad Category: Substitution		
Affrication[15, 23, 30]	A consonant is produced as an affricate.	"fit" /fɪt/ is produced as [tʃɪt] "shoe" /ʃu/ produced as [tʃu]
Backing [11, 15, 17]	A consonant is produced further back in the oral cavity.	"do" /du/ is produced as [gu]
Deaffrication [1, 4, 15]	An affricate is realized as a fricative or as an stop If a stop is produced, this could also be called stopping.	"chip" /tʃɪp/ is produced as [ʃɪp] "pitch" /pɪtʃ/ is produced as [pɪt]
Deaspiration[27, 30]	The loss of aspiration of a stop consonant resulting in an unaspirated consonant (may overlap with "prevocalic voicing").	"paw" /pɑ/ is produced as [bɑ]
Denasalisation [13, 15]	A nasalized consonant is substituted by another non-nasal consonant while maintaining same place of articulation	"nose" /noʊz/ is produced as [doʊz]
Depalatization (palatal fronting)1, [15, 17, 19]	A palatal consonant is realized as a consonant produced further forward in the oral cavity	"fish" /fɪʃ/ is produced as [fɪs] "match" /mætʃ/ is produced as [mæts] "shoe" /ʃu/ is produced as [su]
Velar fronting [1, 2, 3, 4, 6, 7, 8, 11, 13, 15, 16, 17, 20, 21, 28, 30, 32, 34]	A velar consonant is realized as a consonant produced further forward in the oral cavity (typically an alveolar)	"car" /kɑɹ/ is produced as [tɑɹ]

Phonological Pattern	Definition	Examples
Broad Category: Substitution		
Gliding (liquid simplification; liquid deviation)[1, 2, 3,6, 7, 11, 13, 15, 16, 17, 21, 25, 27, 29, 30, 32, 33]	A liquid consonant (e.g., /l, ɹ/) is replaced by a glide (e.g., /w, j/)	"rabbit" /ɹæbɪt/ is produced as [wæbɪt] "look" /lʊk/ is produced as [wʊk] or [jʊk]
Glottal replacement [11, 17]	The substitution of a glottal stop for a consonant target	"hat" /hæt/ is produced as [hæʔ]
Stopping [1, 2, 3, 4, 6, 7, 8, 10, 11, 16, 17, 18, 21, 28, 29, 30, 32, 33]	A fricative or affricate consonant is realized as a stop. In the case of the affricate, this could also be called deaffrication.	"sun" /sʌn/ is produced as [tʌn] "juice" /ʤus/ is produced as [dus]
Vowelization (vocalization) [2, 3, 16, 18, 33]	A consonant, typically a liquid, is replaced by a vowel	"door" /dɔɹ/ is produced as [dɔʊ]
Vowel errors [18]	A vowel target is realized as another vowel; this can be affected by dialectic variation	"dog" /dɑg/ is produced at [dʊg]
Broad Category: Syllables		
Epenthesis (addition) [7, 12, 13, 22, 26]	A segment that was not present in the matching target syllable was produced; often seen in clusters where a vowel is inserted in a cluster to simplify the syllable structure	"blue" /blu/ is produced as [bəlu]
Cluster reduction [1, 2, 3, 6, 7, 8, 11, 13, 16, 17, 18, 19, 23, 27, 28, 30, 32, 33, 34]	The deletion of one or more members of a cluster; most frequently, the stop consonant is retained	"plane" /pleɪn/ is produced as [peɪn] or [leɪn]
Deletion (omission)_ [1,2, 3, 7, 8, 10, 11, 13, 15, 16, 18, 19, 21, 24, 33]	A target consonant (or vowel) in any position is deleted during production	"bus" /bʌs/ is produced as [bʌ]
Metathesis [7, 17, 15]	The reversal of letters in a word	"basket" /bæskət/ is produced as [bæksət]
Migration [15]	A target consonant is moved to another position in the word during production	"stick" /stɪk/ is produced as [tɪks]
Cluster reduction[22]	Omission of a cluster member (typically, the stop element is retained)	"stop" /stɑp/ is produced as [tɑp] "hand" /hænd/ is produced as [hæn] "glass" /glæs/ is produced as [læs]
Phonemic similarity effect [22]	Vowels interact with vowel, consonants with consonants	"clear blue sky" /klɪɹ blu skaɪ/ is produced as [glɪɹ plu skaɪ]
Syllable deletion (reduction)[1, 3, 7, 10, 11, 13,15]	Also called "weak syllable deletion", it is the deletion of the unstressed syllable	"giraf" /dʒɹæf/ is produced as [ræf]

In Table A2.1, we have grouped error patterns into three broad categories based on those proposed by Stoel-Gammon and Dunn (1985). The first broad category is *assimilation patterns*, which describe error patterns that lead to changes in place, manner or voicing in the context of a neighboring phoneme. This group of patterns includes labial, velar, or nasal assimilation; prevocalic voicing; or final devoicing. The second broad category is *substitution patterns*, which describe error patterns that lead to changes in place, manner, or voicing of the target consonants. This group of patterns includes gliding, vowelization, stopping, depalatization, and velar fronting. The third broad category is *syllable structure patterns,* which describe changes to the syllable structure of the target word. This group of patterns includes syllable deletion, cluster reduction, consonant deletion, and phoneme addition (epenthesis).

REFERENCES

[1] Bernthal, J. E., Bankson, N. W., & Flipsen, P. (2009). Articulation and Phonological Disorders: Speech Sound Disorders in Children, 6th Ed. Boston, MA: Pearson.

[2] Bland-Stewart, L. M. (2003). Phonetic inventories and phonological patterns of African American two-year-olds. *Communication Disorders Quarterly*, *24*(3), 109-120.

[3] Crary, Michael A., Landess, Susan and Towne, Roger(1984) 'Phonological error patterns in developmental verbal dyspraxia', Journal of Clinical and Experimental Neuropsychology, 6: 2, 157 — 170

[4] Dinnsen, Daniel A, Gierut, Judith A., Morrisette, Michele L., Green, Christopher R. (2011). On the interaction of deaffrication and consonant harmony*. J. Child Lang. 38 (2011), 380–403.

[5] Dodd, B. (1985). Procedures for classification of sub-groups of speech disorder. In B. Dodd (ed.), Differential Diagnosis and Treatment of Children with Speech Disorder (London: Whurr), p. 49

[6] Dodd, B., Holm, A. Zhu Hua & Crosbie, S. (2003). Phonological development: a normative study of British English-speaking children. *Clinical Linguistics & Phonetics*, 17(8): 617-643.

[7] Dunn, C., & Davis, B. (1983). Phonological process occurrece in phonologically disordered children. Applied Psycholinguistics, 4: 187-207.

[8] Dyson, A. T., & Paden, E. P. (1983). Some phonological acquisition strategies used by two-year-olds. *Communication Disorders Quarterly*, *7*(1), 6-18.

[9] Edwards, M.L. (1983). Issues in phonological assessment. Seminars in Speech and Language, 4:351-374.

[10] Fey, M. E. (1992). Clinical Forum: Phonological Assessment and Treatment Articulation and Phonology: Inextricable Constructs in Speech Pathology. Language, Speech and Hearing Services in Schools, 23, 225-232.

[11] Gildersleeve-Neumann, C. E., Kester, E. S., Davis, B. L., & Peña, E. D. (2008). English speech sound development in preschool-aged children from bilingual english-spanish environments. *Language, Speech, and Hearing Services in Schools*, *39*(3), 314-28.

[12] Girbau, D., Schwartz. R.G. (2008). Phonological working memory in Spanish-English bilingual children with and without specific language impairment. Journal of Communication Disorders. 41 124–145

[13] Goldstein, B.A. & Iglesias, A. (1996). Phonological pattersn in normally developing Spanish-speaking 3- and 4-yearls-olds of Puerto Rican descent. Language, Speech and Hearing Services in Schools, 27:82-90.

[14] Goldstein, B.A. & Swasey Washington, P. (2001). An initial investigation of phonological patterns in typically developing 4-year-old Spanish-English bilingual children. Language, Speech and Hearing Services in Schools, 32:153-164.

[15] Gordon-Brannan, M.E. & Weiss, C.E. (2007). *Clinical management of articulatory and phonologic disorders* (3rd Ed). Baltimore, MD: Lippincott, Williams & Wilkins.

[16] Haelsig, P. C., & Madison, C. L. (1986). A study of phonological processes exhibited by 3-, 4-, and 5-year-old children. *Language, Speech, and Hearing Services in Schools*, *17*(2), 107-114.

[17] Hodson, B. & Paden, E. (1981). Phonological processes which characterize unintelligible and intellible speech in early childhood. Journal of Speech and Hearing Disorders, 46, 369-373.

[18] James, D. G. H. (2001). Use of phonological processes in Australian children ages 2 to 7; 11 years. *International Journal of Speech-Language Pathology*, *3*(2), 109-127.

[19] James, D. G., van Doorn, J., McLeod, S., & Esterman, A. (2008). Patterns of consonant deletion in typically developing children aged 3 to 7 years. *International Journal of Speech-Language Pathology*, *10*(3), 179-192.

[20] Lowe, R. J., Knutson, P. J., & Monson, M. A. (1985). Incidence of fronting in preschool children. *Language, Speech, and Hearing Services in Schools*, *16*(2), 119-123.

[21] McIntosh, B., & Dodd, B. J. (2008). Two-Year-Olds' phonological acquisition: Normative data. *International Journal of Speech-Language Pathology*, *10*(6), 460-469.

[22] Meyer, Antje S. (1992). Investigation of phonological encoding through speech error analyses: Achievements, limitations, and alternatives. Cognition. 42:181-211.

[23] Peter, B. (2010). Complex disorder traits in a three-year-old boy with a severe speech-sound disorder. In: S. Chabon & E. Cohn (Eds), *Communication disorders: A case-based approach*, pp. 156-163. Delaware: Pearson.

[24] Prather, E. M., Hedrick, D. L., & Kern, C. A. (1975). Articulation development in children aged two to four years. *Journal of Speech and Hearing Disorders*, *40*(2), 179-191.

[25] Preisser, D. A., Hodson, B. W., & Paden, E. P. (1988). Developmental phonology: 18-29 months. *Journal of Speech and Hearing Disorders*, *53*(2), 125-130.

[26] Preston, J & Edwards M. (2010). Phonological Awareness and Types of Sounds Errors in Prechoolers with Speech Sound Disorders. Journal of Speech, Language and Hearing Research. 53: 44-60.

[27] Ray, J. (2002). Treating Phonological Disorders in a Multilingual Child: A Case Study. American Journal of Speech-Language Pathology. 11:305-315.

[28] Roberts, J. E., Burchinal, M., & Footo, M. M. (1990). Phonological process decline from 2 1/2 to 8 years. *Journal of Communication Disorders*, *23*(3), 205-217.

[29] Roulstone, S., Loader, S., Northstone, K., & Beveridge, M. (2002). The speech and language of children aged 25 months: Descriptive data from the avon longitudinal study of parents and children. *Early Child Development and Care*, *172*(3), 259-268.

[30] So, L & Dodd, B. (2007). Phonological Awareness Abilities of Cantonese-speaking Children with Phonological Disorder. *Asia Pacific Journal of Speech Language and Hearing*, 10, 189-204

[31] Stoel-Gammon, C., & Dunn, C. (1985). *Normal and disordered phonology in children*. Austin, TX: Pro-Ed.

[32] Thoonen, G., Maassen, B., Gabreëls, F., & Schreuder, R. (1994). Feature Analysis of Singleton Consonant Errors in Developmental Verbal Dyspraxia (DVD). *Journal of Speech Hearing Research. 37:1424-1440*

[33] Watson, M. M., & Scukanec, G. P. (1997). Profiling the phonological abilities of 2-year-olds: A longitudinal investigation. *Child Language Teaching & Therapy*, *13*(1), 3-14.

[34] Wells, B., Peppé, S. and Goulandris, N. (2004) *Intonation development from five to thirteen.* Journal of Child Language, 31 (4). pp. 749-778.

In: Comprehensive Perspectives …
Editors: Beate Peter and Andrea A. N. MacLeod
ISBN: 978-1-62257-041-6

Appendix 3

Statistical Properties of Standardized Tests: How to Interpret a Child's Test Score

Beate Peter

Standardized Tests in Clinical Practice

Speech-language pathologists (SLPs) routinely use standardized tests to evaluate children's communicative abilities, for instance in the areas of speech production, language comprehension, verbal expression, and fluency. Here, we focus on standardized tests of articulation and phonology. Typically, a test protocol sheet has spaces to enter test points such as number of incorrectly produced speech sounds across word positions or number of observed phonological processes ("raw scores"), along with various types of standardized scores. The standardized information helps SLPs make decisions about diagnosis and treatment by comparing the results from testing one child against a distribution of scores from a norming sample, also referred to as reference or standardization sample. Norming samples are created by giving the same test to a large number of children, divided into age cohorts and, in some cases, even further into subgroups of same-aged boys and girls. These cohorts are created because children's articulation and phonological abilities change with increasing age and these trajectories may differ in girls and boys. Consequently, the score from one tested child can be compared to the performance of other children of the same age and sex.

Frequently, standardized tests are part of a comprehensive assessment. To interpret the results and to explain them to a child's parents, SLPs need to answer questions such as these: What is the interpretation of a standard score of 6 when the mean is 10? Or of a standard score of 83 when the mean is 100? How low can a child's score be and still be considered "within normal limits"? What is the cutoff score to qualify for treatment? To address these questions, it is useful to understand some major concepts behind test construction.

Constructing a Hypothetical Standardized Test of Articulation

Raw Scores

Let's say we want to publish a new articulation test and obtain reference data by giving the test to approximately 4,000 children of various ages, including representative proportions of children with and without communication disorders including speech and language disorders. These will be the children against whom an SLP will compare a child who is being tested with our test in the future. We begin by evaluating the scores from 400 children age 4;0 (years;months) to 4;6. Because we know that boys and girls may develop their speech sound abilities at slightly different rates, we make sure our sample includes 200 girls and 200 boys and calculate raw scores separately for these two subgroups, starting with the girls. Let's further assume that the highest possible raw score in our hypothetical test is 50 and the lowest, 0. Most of the 200 girls in the young 4-year-old cohort obtain scores between 30 and 40 but a few girls score close to the full 50 points and a few get scores around 20 points. If we line up their scores like dots along the test score scale, we would get a few scattered low points and a few scattered high points and lots of scores crowded in the middle, as shown in Figure A3.1.

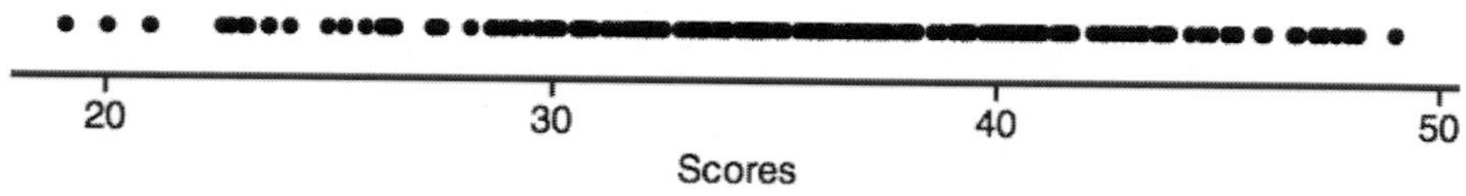

Figure A3.1. Dot plot of hypothetical test scores.

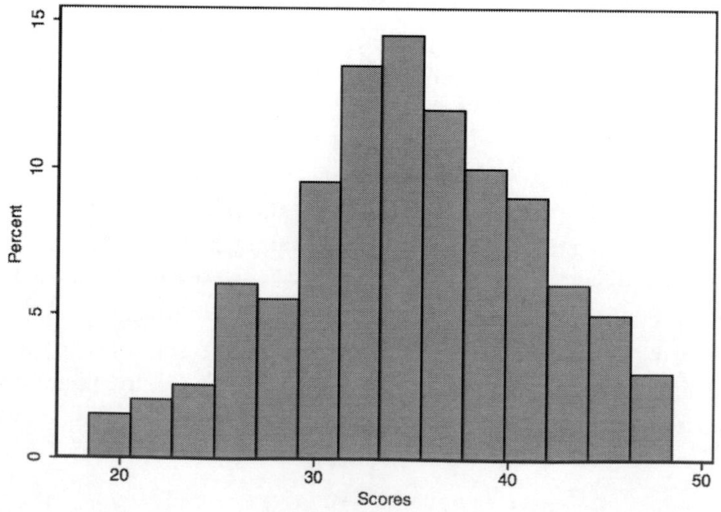

Figure A3.2. Histogram of test scores consolidated into 14 bins.

Next, we divide the point scale into equal score intervals called bins and observe how many girls in the sample obtained scores that fell into each bin. The number of girls within each bin is converted into a proportion or percentage. Figure A3.2 shows a bar graph of these percentages as a function of the test score bins. In this case, 14 bins were generated. A bar graph of score frequencies as a function of score ranges is called a histogram. Note that in this hypothetical example, the histogram is not completely symmetrical, in part because many of the 4-year-olds in the sample already have a well-developed speech system and approached the maximum point score, whereas a few trailed behind in their speech development.

DESCRIPTIVE STATISTICS

Next, we calculate some descriptive statistics to help us understand how the raw scores were distributed. The mean score *m* achieved by our hypothetical subgroup of young 4-year-old girls is found by adding up all scores *x*, then dividing that sum by the number *n* of girls in the subgroup following equation (1). The mean score in our hypothetical example turns out to be approximately 35.

$$m = \frac{\sum_{i=1}^{n} x}{n} \tag{1}$$

If we want to know how variable the scores were, we calculate the variance of the scores, which is a first measure of variability in a dataset. The variance *s* is the average of the squared differences from the mean, based on equation (2) and its simplified form in equation (3). The squaring is done because some scores are lower than the mean and some, higher, and if we simply summed the differences between the actual scores and the mean, they would add up to close to zero. By squaring the differences, we have a measure of divergence from the mean that is always positive. We subtract 1 from *n* to avoid underestimating the variance in very small samples.

$$s^2 = \frac{\sum_{i=1}^{n}(x_i - m)^2}{n-1} \tag{2}$$

$$s^2 = \frac{1}{n-1}\sum_{i=1}^{n}(x_i - m)^2 \tag{3}$$

Here are a few examples. If a child obtained a score of only 20, then her squared difference is $(20\text{-}35)^2 = 225$. Another child with a test score of 34 has a squared difference of $(34\text{-}35)^2 = 1$. Children with high scores contribute to the variance as well, so that a child with the full score of 50 contributes a squared difference of 225, just like the child with the score of 20, and a child with a test score of 36 contributes the same squared difference of 1 as the child with a test score of 34. All squared differences in the data are summed and divided by the number of children minus 1, as shown in equations (2) and (3), in this case 199, and the result is the variance. The variance is small when the datapoints are scattered closely about the mean, and it is large when the distribution is scattered widely about the mean or contains outliers far above or below the mean. In our hypothetical example, the variance is approximately 39.7. Another way of stating this is that the sum of squared differences, on average, was 39.7.

To obtain a measure of variability that is converted back to the same scale as the raw test scores, the square root of the variance is calculated, and that measure is called standard deviation, denoted by the letter s, following equation (4). In research papers, you will also see the abbreviation SD.

$$s = \sqrt{\frac{1}{n-1}\sum_{i=1}^{n}(x_i - m)^2} \quad (4)$$

It turns out that the standard deviation s in our hypothetical dataset is 6.3. Thus, child A with a test score of 29 places approximately 1 standard deviation below the mean and child B with a test score of 22 places approximately 2 standard deviations below the mean. The term z score was created to express a raw score in units of standard deviations that were derived from a reference sample. For child C with a point score of 32, the z score is calculated as follows (5):

$$z = \frac{32-35}{6.3} = -\frac{3}{6.3} = -.48 \quad (5)$$

In normal distributions of data, as a general rule, approximately 68% of the data fall into the range of scores between 1 standard deviation below and above the mean, 34% below the mean and 34% above. If we widen the range to 2 standard deviations below and above the mean, approximately 95% of the data are captured, leaving just 5% unaccounted for, 2.5 % at each tail of the distribution. The interval between 3 standard deviations below and above the mean captures approximately 99% of the data. These properties allow us to estimate a percentile score for each child. Child C obtained a test score equal to the mean score (z = 0), and this score falls at the 50th percentile, which is another way of saying that 50% of the children in the set had a lower test score than Child C. Back to Child A with a test score of 29 and a z score of -1. This score fell at the 16th percentile (remember that one standard deviation below the mean accounts for 34% of the data, so: 50 – 34 = 16). Child B with a test score of 22 and a z score of -2 obtained a percentile score of 2.5, because only 2.5 % of all scores in the low tail of the distribution fall below 2 standard deviations below the mean.

Speech and language tests vary in how they report normed scores. Some, in the tradition of IQ tests, scale the z score to a distribution with $m = 100$ and $s = 15$; other scales are 50 (8) or 10 (3) for m (s). In these three types of scales, a z score of -1 would be equivalent to a standard score of 85, 42, and 7, respectively. Some tests report a T score, which is a linear transformation of the z score that is obtained by multiplying the z score by 10 and adding 50.

The result is a scale with a range of mostly positive numbers. Some educators and clinicians prefer this type of scale because it allows them to describe a child's tested abilities without using negative numbers.

As mentioned, the distribution of scores in a reference sample for measures of speech ability may not always be symmetrical. As a result, you may see in published tests that a standard score of 100 (or 10 or 50, depending on the scale), which typically represents the mean score, is not necessarily equivalent to a percentile ranking of 50. To describe the distribution of scores in our hypothetical example more fully, we could calculate skewness, a measure of asymmetry in a distribution. Negative skewness is present when the left tail of the distribution is longer than the right tail, and the reverse is true for positive skewness. Our hypothetical sample had a skewness value of -.13, which implies a slightly longer left tail, compared to the right, consistent with visual inspection of Figure A3.2. To describe how flat or peaked the distribution is, we could calculate kurtosis. A flat and broad distribution line is called platykurtic and a narrow distribution with a high peak is called leptokurtic. Our hypothetical sample yielded a kurtosis score of 2.61, which is slightly lower than the expected value of 3 for a normal distribution and indicates a slightly flatter distribution.

To finish the norming process for our hypothetical test, we would have to calculate descriptive statistics for the young 4-year-old boys and collect similar samples for the boys and girls all other age groups we want to include, then create data distributions for each subgroup. The final product would be a standardized test where the raw score of any child can be converted to a standard score and a percentile by comparing the child to the reference cohort of the same age and sex.

With data collected from all age ranges to be included in the reference sample, we are now ready to create a chart for age equivalents. Separately for boys and girls, we create subgroups of children of similar ages, for instance age 4;3 plus/minus 3 months (which fits our hypothetical subgroup of 200 girls), 4;9 plus/minus 3 months, and so on.

Within each age group, we obtain the median score, which is simply defined as that score that was exceeded by half the children. In our subgroup, the median score was 34.8. If a younger or older girl obtains a test score of 34.8, then age 4;3 plus/minus 3 months would be the age equivalent. Bear in mind, however, that a wide range of scores is within normal limits for each age group, and that tying the age equivalence to just the median score of that subsample is not a meaningful way of comparing a child's test performance to the performance of other children.

For standard scores and percentiles, confidence intervals can be calculated as a measure of the reliability of the obtained test score. It indicates how many times the true value would be found within a specified range if the rest were to be repeated many times. A 90% confidence interval of 87 to 94 means that if the test were to be repeated 100 times, 90 times the true value would be found in the interval between 87 and 94.

If we wanted to increase the confidence level to 95%, this usually requires a broader interval of scores.

THE QUALITY OF A STANDARDIZED TEST

Test manuals typically describe how the test was constructed, and before selecting it as an assessment tool, SLPs should inform themselves. For instance, it is important to know the nature of the sample against which an individual is being compared when interpreting a standard test score. Some reference samples are population-based and include representative proportions of individuals with high, average, and low ability, whereas others deliberately exclude individuals with disabilities. If a child with a speech sound disorder is compared to a reference sample that excluded children with speech sound disorders, the tested child may obtain a lower standard score than when compared to a reference sample that included children with speech sound disorders. Additional aspects of the reference sample include its size, male:female ratio, ethnicity, geographic distribution, and socioeconomic diversity.

Various aspects of the test's validity and reliability attest to the test's overall quality. Different types of validity address questions about ***what*** the test presumes to measure, whereas the different types of reliability address ***how*** the test performs its purpose. Concurrent validity is a measure of how well the test correlates with other tests that were designed to assess similar or different but related skills when these tests were given to the same individuals at about the same time. For example, different tests of articulation measuring the accuracy of consonants may correlate highly with each other but not as highly with tests of phonological processes because these two types of tests are designed to measure different aspects of speech production. Predictive validity captures the correlations between the test and others that are given to the same individuals later in time. For instance, a test of phonological processing administered to preschoolers might have predictive validity for tests of reading or spelling ability given to the same children after they enter school. Construct validity describes how well the test measures what its authors intended to measure. For instance, a test of phonological processing ability should address the underlying and theorized concept of phonological processing ability as established and validated by several other measures.

A reliable test produces consistent results. High inter-rater reliability results in similar scores when the test is administered to the same individuals by different clinicians. High test-retest reliability results in similar scores when the test is re-administered to the same individual. If the test items are divided into two randomly assigned groups and administered separately, the scores from both halves are highly correlated if the test has high internal consistency.

FROM STANDARDIZED TEST SCORES TO CLINICAL DECISIONS

Back to the crucial questions about how to interpret a child's score (What is the interpretation of a certain standard score? How low can a child's score be and still be considered within normal limits? What is the cutoff score to qualify a child for treatment?). The savvy SLP knows where a given standard score falls in terms of standard deviations; for instance, a standard score of 7 when the population mean is 10 is equivalent to 1 standard deviation below the mean. Similarly, a standard score of 115 when the mean is 100 is equivalent to 1 standard deviation above the mean. An important caveat, as previously mentioned: In some articulation tests, standard scores and percentile rankings are not based on a normal (symmetrical) distribution of scores, so that a 50th percentile does not necessarily equate a standard score at the population mean.

When is a standard score considered to be within normal limits? In part, the answer depends on whose definition of normal limits is used. Most agree that scores within one standard deviation of the mean are safely considered within normal limits. To qualify a child for intervention, however, federal, state, and local guidelines vary. Some clinicians are required to show that the child's score was below -1.5 *s* (approximately equivalent to the 7th percentile), or even -2 *s* (2nd percentile).

A standard score from a well-designed and carefully normed articulation or phonology test is certainly a meaningful measure of a child's speech ability. It should, however, be supplemented with other relevant information and integrated with clinical judgment as diagnostic and treatment-related decisions are made.

KEY TERMS

Acceleration: A phonological unit (segmental or suprasegmental) is acquired faster than what typically occurs in monolingual development.

Accent modification: A program through which non-native speakers learn to change pronunciation and improve speech intelligibility minimizing pronunciation and prosodic differences between the native language and the target language.

Accent: See **stress**.

Accentedness: The extent to which a non-native speaker's individual's speech pattern differs from that of the target language community.

Accuracy measures: Measures that compare whether a child's production is correct in comparison to a target, and for example, may include accuracy of consonants, vowels, or syllable shapes. Also may be considered a relational analysis.

Acoustic phonetics: A subfield of phonetics that sets out to explore acoustic (mechanical wave) features of speech sounds. Acoustic phonetics investigates, among other features, waveforms, duration measures, fundamental frequency of sounds, frequency spectrums, etc., and the relationship of these properties to other sub-fields of phonetics.

Adult language learner: An individual who learns a new target language after childhood.

Afferent: Directional term of information flow, toward the brain.

Age of arrival: The age at which a speaker first arrives in the environment where the target language is spoken.

Age-effect approach: An approach used to understand how differences in age of second language exposure impacts proficiency in one's first and second languages.

Algorithm: A set of explicit calculations to solve a mathematical problem.

Apraxia: A condition interfering with the planning, programming, and/or execution of intended movements. This results in the loss of the ability to produce learned purposeful movements, (or in the case of children difficulty learning these movements) despite having the desire and the physical ability to perform the movements. See also **Childhood Apraxia of Speech**.

Articulation: The motoric process of producing speech sounds.

Auditory-articulatory feedback loop: Auditory and articulatory input that a child receives when vocalizing; as a baby vocalizes, he is able to both hear and feel the result of the movement, allowing him to associate a specific movement pattern with a specific acoustic signal.

Aural–oral communication: Aural-Oral Communication emphasizes the use of speech capitalizing on residual hearing. The use of visual processing of the speaker's lip movements, lipreading, is also often encouraged. Signing is not used in this approach.

Bifid: Forked or divided into two parts.

Binary oppositions: Contrasts created by the presence vs. absence of a feature, for instance sounds produced in the front of the mouth, as opposed to sounds produced further back in the mouth.

Canonical babble: Consonant-vowel (CV or VC) syllables that resemble speech syllables in that they are characterized by rapid formant transitions and full vowels.

Canonical syllables: Syllables that contain a minimum of one consonant and a vowel and are produced with adult-like timing; often represented with "CV" notation where C stands for any consonant sound and V stands for any vowel sound.

Categorical perception: Perception of speech sounds that differ acoustically, yet are classified as part of the same phonemic category.

Category assimilation: The mechanism by which a new target language phoneme is assimilated into a similar, existing native language phoneme.

Category dissimilation: The mechanism by which a distinct phonetic category is created for a new target language phoneme.

Caudal: Directional term with respect to location, toward the tail of the organism.

Central nervous system: Brain and spinal cord; essentially those parts of the nervous system that are physically encased in bone. Technically also includes the retina of the eye.

Central nervous system: Part of our nervous system that includes the brain and spinal cord.

Child-directed speech: Adults addressing children frequently alter their speaking style in terms of grammar, word choice, and prosody. Child-directed speech is slower and higher-pitched, compared to speech addressed to adults, and it has wider pitch ranges. Also referred to as Motherese.

Childhood Apraxia of Speech (CAS): A childhood neurological speech sound disorder in which planning of motor goals for each sound and/or programming sequential speech production movements are impaired. Inconsistent errors on consonants and vowels in repeated productions of syllables or words are one major feature proposed among the literature to be characteristic to CAS. Other features that have gained some consensus among researchers include lengthened disrupted coarticulatory transitions between sounds and syllables, and inappropriate prosody, while there is no validated set of symptoms which differentiates CAS from other types of childhood speech sound disorders (American-Speech-Language-Hearing-Association, 2007).

Click: Popping sound created as negative air pressure is equalized.

Closant: Sound produced with closure along the articulatory tract, resulting in a sound that resembles a consonant.

Cluttering: A fluency disorder characterized by rapid speaking rate and erratic rhythm giving rise to reduced speech intelligibility. The breakdown in fluency also involves jerky spurts that are usually associated with faulty phrasing patterns.

Coarticulation: Producing a speech sound that shows articulatory features of the preceding or subsequent sound(s).

Code-switching: A linguistic act of changing the language spoken within or between utterances and is motivated by contextual factors such as the interlocutor, the context, or the topic.

Communicative intent: A desire to communicate one's needs, wants, or ideas to another person.

Comorbidity: The co-occurrence of two or more disorders in the same individual. In the more traditional definition of the term, the co-occurring disorders could be unrelated or related. In the newer definition, disorders are said to be comorbid if they are causally related.

Comprehensibility: A listener's perception of how difficult it is to understand a speaker.

Congenital deafness: Deafness refers to the complete loss of hearing ability in one or two ears. In congenital deafness, the hearing loss is present at birth. It can include genetic hereditary hearing loss or hearing loss due to other factors present either prenatally or at the time of birth. Congenital deafness contrasts with acquired deafness, which occurs after birth.

Connected speech sample: A sample of speech that the child has spoken consecutively which may be analyzed for the presence of specific syllables, consonants, vowels, or other phonological patterns.

Criterion based score: Indicates the presence or absence of a certain ability defined by cut-off score, for instance the presence or absence of an expressive vocabulary of at least 50 words at age 18 months.

Critical period hypothesis (CPH): The CPH maintains that changes in neuroplasticity during puberty make it much more difficult for individuals beyond that age to attain complete mastery of a new language.

Critical period: The period beyond which a defined goal cannot be achieved, for instance becoming a proficient speaker of a first or second language.

Cry: Reflexive expression of distress with a characteristic respiratory pattern; more intense and loud than fuss or whimper.

Deceleration: A phonological unit (segmental or suprasegmental) is acquired slower than what typically occurs in monolingual development.

Decode: The process of sounding out an unfamiliar word or a nonword is referred to as decoding.

Deep orthography: A writing system where the letter/sound associations are complex, such that a given grapheme can stand for more than one phoneme and/or a given phoneme can be represented by more than one grapheme. Also referred to as opaque orthography.

Dendrogram: A tree-like graphical representation of datapoints, frequently used to show the output from cluster analysis.

Denotation: The literal, core meaning of a word. This is in contrast to the term "connotation" that refers to the associated emotional undertones. For example, the terms "delayed" and "retarded" have the same denotional content but the negative connotations associated with "retarded" have caused researchers to replace that term with "delayed" when referring to areas of child development.

Diadochokinetic (DDK) tasks: Rapid repetition of monosyllables (/papapapa …,/, /tatatata …/, /kakakaka …/ and multisyllables (e.g., /patapata …/ and /patakapataka/) to assess motor speech function in repetitive and alternating movements.

Diadochokinetic rate: The rate at which consonant-vowel sequences can be produced, for instance /papapa …/ or /patakapataka …/

Differential diagnosis: The process of selecting the most likely diagnostic label from a set of possible labels after considering the evidence collected during an assessment.

Digraph: A sequence of two letters that represents a single sound.

Dual System Hypothesis: The hypothesis that the language systems of bilinguals are separate from a young age.

Dynamic assessment: A test that is individualized during administration to each child's needs and responses. It assesses whether a specific set of skills are present and may include instruction or cueing to produce these skills.

Dysarthria: A motor speech disorder resulting from damage to the central or peripheral nervous system that decreases a person's ability to accurately produce speech. This results in disordered speech due to paralyzed, weak, or uncoordinated musculature.

Dyslexia: A disorder that interferes with the acquisition of written language at the word level, characterized by deficits in accurate and/or fluent word recognition, decoding, and spelling in the presence of generally normal oral language skills.

Ecological validity: The extent to which a procedure (assessment or treatment) relates to the experiences in real life.

Efferent: Directional term of information flow, away from the brain.

Egressive: Direction of airflow from the lungs outward, during exhalation.

Elision: A phonotactic phenomenon of French that describes the process whereby a vowel in a clitic is deleted when the clitic appears before vowel initial words.

Enchainement: A phonotactic phenomenon of French that describes the process whereby word final consonants that are pronounced become the onset for the following word if it begins with a vowel.

Error patterns: This term refers to systematic error patterns that a child produces. These patterns may be common in typical development at certain ages, or may be particular to certain child. Also referred to as **phonological patterns** or **phonological processes**.

Etiology: Generally, the study of causation; in medicine, the cause of a disease or disorder.

Expression: In genetics, the process of synthesizing protein products from DNA and, by extension, the observable results in the organism. SSD expression can vary by severity and also in terms of speech characteristics. The same genetic disruption sometimes causes variable expression among carriers of the risk variant.

F1–F2 range: Perceived vowel qualities are dependent on the relative values of the formants, which show acoustic resonances characteristics of the vocal tract shapes associated with the production of specific vowels. The first formant, or F1, corresponds to vowel openness (vowel height), and the second formant, or F2, corresponds to vowel frontness. Thus, the F1-F2 range indicates how wide the tongue, jaw, and lips move during vowel productions.

Factor analysis: A statistical tool designed to identify those variables in a multivariate dataset that are closely correlated with each other.

Familial: Disorders that appear to run in families are called familial disorders. This descriptor does not directly imply genetic and/or environmental causes.

First words period: Early stage of language development spanning the period from the child's acquisition of the first word through an expressive vocabulary of approximately 50 words.

Fluency: A listener's perception of how smooth and free-flowing a speaker's speech is.

Focus: Use of prosody to highlight informational content.

Foot: A metrical unit that consists one or more syllables. A trochaic foot consists of a strong syllable followed by a weak syllable (e.g., "baker"); an iambic foot consists of a weak syllable followed by a strong syllable (e.g., "guitar"). Feet can combine to form a lexical word ("macaroni" consists of two trochaic feet).

Full vowel: A vowel with a perceptual quality of a postured articulatory configuration, with deliberate positioning of the mouth and tongue in a speech-like way, yielding a vowel quality distinct from that corresponding to an at rest position of the tract.

Fundamental frequency (F_0): The frequency at which the vocal folds vibrate. It is perceived as vocal pitch.

Fuss: Reflexive expression of distress, but less intense and loud than crying (may also seem more volitional than cry in some instances).

Genetic association: In genetic studies, chromosomal markers can be tested for genetic association to a trait, e.g., presence of a disorder or a score on a test task. Certain variants of these markers may be found more frequently in individuals with the disorder, compared to individuals without it, or more frequently in individuals with low test scores, compared to individuals with average test scores. If this is the case, the marker is said to be associated with the trait.

Genetic linkage: Regions of DNA located closely near each other on the same chromosome tend to be inherited together and, hence, are in genetic linkage with each other. If a certain genetic marker variant is usually inherited with a certain disorder, one can suspect that the genetic region causing the disorder is located near the genetic marker.

Gibberish: Babbled productions that resemble conversational speech in terms of intonational and durational aspects but do not include meaningful words. This type of utterance is often also referred to as jargon. No examples of Gibberish are presented in the chapter.

Glottal stop sequence: Phonation interrupted by at least one glottal stop, producing the perception of distinct syllables.

Goo: Sounds formed by primitive tongue closure somewhere in the back of the oral cavity, usually occurring during phonation and often accompanied by either quasivowels or full vowels. The timing of the primitive articulation in gooing does not resemble that of canonical babbling. Gooing can be considered a special case of particularly primitive marginal babbling.

Grapheme: A unit of written language; a letter unit.

Gray matter: Brain tissue consisting primarily of the cell bodies of neurons.

Growl: Vocalization with either low fundamental frequency (often with glottal fry) or with fundamental frequency in the speaker's habitual range accompanied by substantial vocal harshness.

Harmony: Phonological process resulting in all consonants or vowels in a word being produced with similar articulatory features (e.g., all consonants in a word produced with a labial place of articulation; *book* produced as [bʊp]).

Hearing aid: A hearing aid is a small electroacoustic device designed to amplify and modulate sound for the wearer, and it consists of three basic components: a microphone, amplifier, and speaker. It typically fits in or behind the wearer's ear. Two main types of electronics are analog and digital. Analogue hearing aids convert sound waves into electrical waves, which are amplified. Digital aids convert sound waves into numerical codes using mathematical calculations before amplifying them.

Hearing screening: A sample of hearing ability that typically includes an assessment of pure-tones at 500, 1000, 2000, and 4000 Hz at 20dB.

Hearing thresholds: A hearing threshold is the lowest sound level for a person to detect a sound at a given frequency.

Heterogeneous: When a disorder is caused by different genetic mechanisms in different families, the disorder is heterogeneous. An example is autism spectrum disorder.

Hierarchical agglomerative clustering: Statistical procedure to generate clusters of data that are maximally similar within clusters and maximally different between clusters. The most similar datapoints are merged into clusters, the most similar clusters are merged into the next tier of clusters, and so forth, until all clusters are linked to a single cluster node. The result is a tree-like structure of clusters called a dendrogram.

History: Information gathered regarding a child including developmental, educational, medical, and other personal information that will help the clinician interpret test results and prepare for treatment if needed.

Homophonous: An adjective referring to words that have different meanings but are produced with the same phonetic form; they may or may not be spelled the same (e.g., *wait/weight*).

Hypernasal: Hypernasal speech is a resonance disorder that occurs when sound enters the nasal cavity inappropriately during speech, for instance during vowels.

Hypoglossal Nerve: Twelfth cranial nerve that innervates the tongue and controls tongue movements for speech, feeding and swallowing.

Hyponasal: The opposite of hypernasal resonance. Air that normally would be emitted through the nose during a nasal consonant is emitted through the mouth.

Iamb: An unstressed syllable followed by a stressed syllable, together forming a **foot** (see keyword definition). An example is the word "guitar."

Idiopathic: A disorder that arises from unknown causes.

Implicational hierarchy: The presence of one feature necessarily implies the presence of another. For instance, if a language has plural forms, it automatically also will have singular forms. In terms of child phonology, if a child can produce a fricative, then it is very likely that he or she can produce a stop, stops being easier to produce and generally earlier acquired.

Incidence: The rate of occurrence of a disease (how often does it occur within a given time period, e.g., per year, in a given place?). This is in contrast to prevalence rates, which refer to the overall proportion of affected individuals in a population at a given place and point in time.

Independent analysis: An analysis of a child's speech (consonants, vowels, syllable structure, tones etc.) without reference to an adult target.

Indexical: Prosodic characteristics that are specific to an individual speaker or a group of speakers.

Individual bilingualism: A focus of research on understanding how bilingual people learn and use their language.

Ingressive: Direction of airflow inward into the lungs, during inhalation.

Intelligibility: The degree to which a speaker's utterance (or utterances) can be understood by a listener. Measures include percentage estimates of glossed conversations, scores based on naming tasks, and rating scales.

Inter-word variability: Variable production of a specific sound when it occurs in different words (e.g., /s/ produced as [s] in the word *house* but as [t] in the word *sun*).

Interaction: A phonological unit (segmental or suprasegmental) influences a unit in the other language.

Interlocutor: Another word for "speaker."

Intonation: Pattern of pitch changes across words, phrases, or sentences.

Intra-word variability: Variable production of a single word (e.g., the word *sun* produced as [sʊn], [tʊn], and [dʊn]).

***K* means clustering**: Grouping of items using multiple variables, where one selects the number of groups ("*k*") one wishes to generate. The *k* means algorithm generates groups with high within-group similarities and maximal between-group differences.

Kinesthesia: The perception of the position and movement of one's own muscles and joints.

Knowledge of Performance: Specific feedback regarding the way a sound was produced.

Knowledge of Results: General feedback regarding whether a production was correct or incorrect.

Language impairment: Difficulty comprehending and/or formulating language in the presence of otherwise typical development.

Language rights: Human and civil rights that give individuals and communities the freedom to communicate in their chosen language across a variety of contexts.

Language-specific tendency: A pattern of usage or acquisition that is characteristics of a specific language only.

Laryngeal: Related to the larynx, or vocal folds.

Laugh: A reflexive expression of positivity, which, like cry, has a characteristic respiratory pattern but with distinct contours.

Laws of irreversible solidarity: Regularities observed by Roman Jakobson about the relationship between less frequently used speech sounds mandating the presence of more basic sounds in sound inventories cross-linguistically that also pre-determine a universal order in the acquisition of speech sounds. See also "**implicational hierarchy**."

Lexical selection: A child's preference for words based on their phonological properties.

Liaison: A phonotactic phenomenon of French that describes the process whereby word final consonants that appear in the orthography but are not pronounced become the onset of the following word if the word begins with a vowel.

Linkage analysis: A group of statistical procedures to determine genetic regions that are inherited along with a disorder or an observable characteristic.

Liter: A metric unit of volume, approximately equivalent to 1.06 quarts.

Loi de position: A phonotactic phenomenon of French that describes the preference for the appearance of lax vowels in closed syllables and tense vowels in open syllables.

Mand-model: A demonstration of how to request something.

Marginal babble: Resembles canonical babble except that it does not include rapid formant transitions from consonant-like element to full vowel. A marginal babble can also consist of a supraglottal consonant-like element paired with a quasivowel.

Marked: In linguistics, marked forms are the more exceptional (or complex) forms whereas the **unmarked** forms are more basic. See also **markedness**.

Markedness (in phonology): Explanatory principle in phonology for proposing a binary feature system for speech sounds where the less basic feature (e.g., [+voiced]) is characterized by the addition of certain phonetic characteristics to the more basic feature (e.g., [-voiced]).

Mental age: An index of intelligence, and is expressed as the equivalent average age of normally developing children at which a particular child is performing intellectually. The mental age of the child is tested with intelligence tests.

Meter: A metric unit of length, approximately equivalent to 1.09 yards.

Microcephaly: A substantially smaller head circumference, given the age and sex of a child.

Mild to moderate hearing loss: Hearing impairment is ranked according to the severity as measured in decibels. In mild hearing loss, the smallest sounds that children can hear with their better ear are between 26 and 40 dB HL. In moderate hearing loss, children's hearing thresholds are between 41 and 55 dB HL (Clark, 1981).

Millimeter: A metric unit of length defined as one thousandth of a meter, approximately equivalent to the thickness of a small coin. Ten millimeters (mm) equal one centimeter (cm). One inch equals 2.54 cm.

Mitosis: Cell division by cleaving a mother cell into two identical daughter cells.

Monolingual comparison approach: An approach used to understand how bilinguals differ from monolingual speakers of each of their languages.

Mora: Unit of syllable weight.

Morphology: The study of form. In anatomy, the study of form and structure of organs or organisms.

Motherese: See **child-directed speech.**

Motor Speech Disorders: A collection of communication disorders involving the retrieval and activation of motor plans for speech, or the execution of movements for speech production

Multifactorial inheritance: A phenotype that is the result of a combination of many genes at different loci and/or factors from the environment; the combination of genes and other factors all have a small added effect to form the characterics in the phenotype.

Nasendoscopy/nasopharyngoscopy: A minimally invasive endoscopic procedure that allows visual observation and analysis of the velopharyngeal mechanism or larynx during speech through the use of a scope that is inserted through the nose until it reaches the nasopharynx; can be used to evaluate velopharyngeal function, phonation, or swallowing.

Native language (NL): The first language acquired and spoken by an individual in early childhood.

Neural plasticity: Neural plasticity refers to the ability of the brain and nervous system to change the structure, function, and organization of neurons in response to new situations or to changes in the environment.

Normative score: A score that can be used to compare one individual's actual score to the scores in a given reference group such as children of the same age and sex. Examples are standard scores and percentile rankings.

Nosology: Classification of diseases into groups or subtypes.

Ontogeny: The study of the origin of a characteristic within an individual.

Opaque orthography: See **deep orthography**.

Oral proficiency: A speaker's oral command of a language as evidenced by pronunciation skills, comprehensibility and fluency.

Penetrance: The proportion of risk genotype carriers who show evidence of the associated trait.

Percent Consonants Correct (PCC): Although there are different ways to calculate PCC, essentially this measure is calculated by dividing the number of correctly produced consonants (i.e., consonant that match the adult target and are in the right place in the word) by the number of consonants in the adult target.

Percent Phoneme Correct (PPC): Although there are different ways to calculate PPC, essentially this measure is calculated by dividing the number of correctly produced consonants and vowels by the number of consonants and vowels in the adult target.

Percent Vowel Correct (PVC): Although there are different ways to calculate PVC, essentially this measure is calculated by dividing the number of correctly produced vowels (i.e., vowels that match the adult target and are in the right place in the word) by the number of vowels in the adult target.

Peripheral nervous system: All components of the nervous system that lie outside bony encasement. Two subdivisions are the somatic peripheral nervous system and the autonomic ("visceral") peripheral nervous system.

Pharyngeal arch apparatus: Arched bulges that form by the fourth week of embryonic development; precursors for structures of the head and neck.

Pharyngeal flap: A surgical procedure where tissue from the posterior pharyngeal wall is sewn into the velum to assist with closing the velopharyngeal port.

Pharyngoplasty: A surgical procedure of the pharynx that is designed to correct velopharyngeal dysfunction.

Phonemic awareness: Well-specified mental representation of speech sounds. This involves understanding that words are composed of individual units of speech sounds; understanding the unique features of each sound; understanding the order of speech sounds in a syllable or word; and understanding the concept of rhymes and similar word onsets when comparing two or more words. Also referred to as **phonological awareness.**

Phonemic inventory: A phonemic inventory refers to a list of phonemes that a child can produce that is in the correct place in the target and that matches the target word. Also referred to as **phonological inventory**.

Phonetic inventory: An independent analysis where the clinician creates a list of phonemes from a connected speech sample that the child can produce, even if the phoneme is not in the correct place in the target word.

Phonological awareness: See **phonemic awareness**.

Phonological inventory: See **phonemic inventory**.

Phonological pattern: See **error patterns** or **phonological process**.

Phonological process: A speech sound error that follows systematic patterns, e.g., fricatives are replaced by stops. Also referred to as **error patterns** or **phonological patterns**.

Phonological representation: Information stored in an individual's mental lexicon regarding the sound structure of a word.

Phonology: The systematic study of the speech sounds, phonotactics, and prosody of a language.

Phonotactic inventory: A list of syllable shapes that a child can produce, even if the shape does not match the target word.

Phrase-final lengthening: Prolongation of the final syllable in a phrase or utterance.

Phylogeny: The study of the origin of a characteristic within a species as a whole.

Prelingual deafness: Prelingual deafness refers to the complete loss of hearing ability due to an impairment which is congenital or otherwise acquired before the individual has acquired speech and language. This condition renders disadvantages over postlingual deafness because the child is unable to access spoken language models from the outset.

Profound hearing loss: Profound hearing loss refers to the condition in which the person is unable to hear sounds below 91dB HL (Clark, 1981).

Proprioception: Perception of the position of one's own body parts in space.

Prosodic word: A unit of language that consists of at least one foot and may or may not coincide with lexical words. "Doesn't" is an example of a prosodic word that merges two lexical words.

Protophone: Any of the pre-speech vocalizations (not including vegetative sounds or fixed signals such as laugh or cry).

Protoword: A relatively stable sound pattern used by a child in a consistent meaningful context that does not have an identifiable adult target form; often used by children during the transition from babble to meaningful speech.

Quantitative trait: A trait that can vary within a range of values, for instance body height.

Quasivowel: Vowel sound produced with normal phonation and a neutral (unpostured) vocal tract configuration. Quasivowels are typically quiet and short, but are not always so. They differ from full vowels in that full vowels are produced with deliberate posturing of the articulatory tract.

Raspberry: Trills or vibrants formed most often with the lips or the tongue and lips, and occasionally by the tongue body against the toothless alveolar ridge.

Reduplicated babble: Type of canonical babbling where syllables are perceived to be repeated, e.g., [bababababa …], although they are not required to be phonetically identical.

Reduplication: Phonological process involving the exact or partial repetition of a syllable (e.g. [baba] for "bottle").

Relational analysis: An analysis of a child's speech (consonants, vowels, syllable structure, tones etc.) with reference to the adult target.

Relational inventory: See **phonemic inventory**.

Residual hearing: Residual hearing refers to the degree of hearing sensitivity a person has left after a loss of hearing.

Rhotics: A class of speech sounds defined as "r-like," including the consonant /ɹ/ and r-colored vowels such as in the words "b<u>ir</u>d" and "teach<u>er</u>."

Rhythm of speech: Overall pattern of timing and prominence effects in utterances.

Rime: The vowel and final consonant segments of a syllable, i.e. all syllabic segments except the consonantal onset.

Root node: A bundle of phonetic features that characterize a single speech sound. Manner features are considered to be "attached" to the Root.

Rostral: Directional term with respect to location, toward the head of the organism.

Segment: A consonant or vowel.

Segmental: Relating to segments, which are units of speech sounds (synonymous with phonemes).

Sensitive period model: A model of second language learning that broadens the age range during which native-like proficiency of a target language can be achieved.

Sensitive period: The period during which a person continues to be able to learn a new ability.

Sequence (in anatomical or physiological development of an organism)**:** The occurrence of a pattern of multiple anomalies within an individual that arise from a single known or presumed prior anomaly or mechanical factor; where one anomaly leads to the development of the other anomalies as in Pierre Robin sequence.

Sequential bilingual: A person who can speak and understand two languages, but one of these languages was learned after the other.

Sexual dimorphism: Differences in form or appearance between males and females of the same species.

Shallow orthography: A writing system where the letter/sound associations are unambiguous, such that a given grapheme represents just one sound and a given phoneme can be written by just one grapheme. Also referred to as **transparent orthography**.

Shared-separate approach: An approach to understand the extent to which bilingual's two languages overlap.

Sibilant consonants: A class of speech sounds produced by forcing an air stream through a narrow constriction, resulting in a sound with aperiodic acoustic energy (e.g., /s, f/) and a hissing quality.

Sight word: A word whose spelling does not follow standard spelling rules and is recognized visually by the word shape. An example is the "sight" part of the term "sight word."

Simultaneous bilingual: A person who can speak and understand two languages that were acquired very early in childhood.

Societal bilingualism: A focus of research on understanding how societies preserve languages, manage language interactions, and plan language policies.

Speech adaptability: A child's ability to respond to cues and changes in linguistic environment to produce phonemes or patterns that were previously produced in error.

Speech Learning Model (SLM): A model proposed by Flege (1995) to explain the presence of foreign accents in second language learners.

Squeal: Vocalization produced at a high pitch level, above the habitual range of the vocalizer.

Standard assessment: A test that includes all necessary materials, an established protocol for elicitation, scoring, and analysis. The test manual typically includes reference information so that a tested child's performance can be compared to same-age peers. Also referred to as **standardized test.**

Standardized test: See **standard assessment**.

Stimulability testing: A procedure to determine whether a child is able to produce a target sound under simplified conditions after it was produced incorrectly during standardized assessment.

Stress: Use of pitch, duration, and/or intensity to add prominence. Changes in pitch which serve to make a syllable more prominent are called accent, stress, or pitch **accent**.

Structural-functional examination: An evaluation conducted to determine whether any structural or functional abnormalities are present when viewing a child's face, oral cavity, and articulators.

Successive Single-Word Utterance (SSWU): Sequence of individual words that are produced without syntactic, semantic, or prosodic coherence, in which each word represents a single utterance

Suprasegmental: Aspects of speech that exceed the level of individual segments. This includes rhythm, stress, intonation, pitch.

Syllable structure: The elements of syllables include onsets and rimes, which, in turn, consist of a nucleus (usually a vowel, but optionally a syllabic consonant) and sometimes a consonantal ending (coda). In English, syllables are composed of an optional onset (zero to three consonants), a vowel nucleus, and an optional ending (zero to four consonants).

Syllable: One or more segments can be grouped into syllables, whereby a vocalic nucleus is required and consonantal onsets and offsets can vary in number.

Synapse: The point of contact between two neurons. The two neurons don't actually physically touch each other; a tiny space called synaptic cleft separates the two neurons.

Syndrome: A disorder characterized by a variety of characteristics co-occurring in the same individual; pattern of multiple anomalies or malformations that regularly occur together, are pathogenically related, and have a common known or suspected cause. An example is 22q11.2 deletion syndrome, also known as velo-cardio-facial syndrome, which affects the formation of the velum, the heart, and facial structures.

Target language (TL): Any new language to be acquired by an adult learner, regardless of how many languages the learner already speaks.

Taxonomy: Systematic classification of items, often arranged into a hierarchical structure.

Teratogen: An external chemical or physical agent, such as cigarette smoke, drugs, viruses, or radiation, that can interfere with normal embryological development and result in congenital malformations.

Timing (in prosody): Durations of syllables and pauses in an utterance.

Transfer: A phonological unit (segmental or suprasegmental) that only exists in one language is used in the other language.

Transparent orthography: See **shallow orthography**.

Trochee: A stressed syllable followed by an unstressed syllable, together forming a foot (see keyword). An example is the word "picture."

Unitary System Hypothesis: The hypothesis that the language systems of bilinguals are shared at a young age and become gradually differentiated.

Universal trends: Tendencies in speech and language that are detectable across several (many) languages.

Unmarked: See **marked.**

Untrained Probes: Target syllables, words, phrases that have not been practiced during treatment.

Vagus Nerve: Tenth cranial nerve that innervates the larynx and various organs within the torso.

Variegated babble: Type of canonical babbling where successive syllables are perceived to differ substantially from each other, e.g., [mana] or [mami].

Vegetative sounds: Unintentional sounds resulting from non-speech behaviors, e.g., sneezes, coughs, hiccups, and grunts.

Velopharyngeal: Area that includes the velum and pharyngeal areas of the oral cavity that are active in the valving between the oral and nasal cavities.

Videofluoroscopy: Visualizing structures and their movements using a contrast material and X-ray video technology.

Videonasoendoscopy: Visualizing the structures of the upper respiratory tract using a fiberoptic tool by inserting into the nasal cavity.

Vocal motor schemes: Sound production patterns observed frequently in the babble of an individual child that often carry over into meaningful speech.

Vocant: Vowel-like sound produced by infants (the term is meant to encompass both quasivowels and full vowels). Vocants contrast with closants (another term for consonant-like elements), which are produced with narrowing of the articulatory tract and resemble consonants.

Whisper: Speech or pre-speech utterance that is produced without full voicing.

White matter: Brain tissue consisting primarily of oligodendrocytes wrapping the axons of neurons.

Word template: Whole word articulatory pattern (including segmental, phonotactic, and prosodic information) that a child may use for the production of multiple words.

Word: A true word has a stable semantic referent together with a (relatively) stable phonetic form that in some way

Yell: Vocalizations produced at high amplitude, above the habitual amplitude range of the vocalizer.

INDEX

#

A

D

E

I

J

K

L

O

P

Q

R

S

T

U

V

W

X

Y